Efficient Oculofacial Surgery

Jeremiah P. Tao
Editor

Efficient Oculofacial Surgery

Springer

Editor
Jeremiah P. Tao
Division of Oculofacial Plastic and
Orbital Surgery
Department of Ophthalmology
University of California, Irvine
Irvine, CA, USA

Chief Video Editor
Jenny N. Wang

Chief Illustrator
Michael M. Han

Associate Editors
Teresa H. Chen
Seanna R. Grob

International Associate Editors
Maria A. Belen Camacho
Roberto M. Limongi

ISBN 978-3-031-63177-1   ISBN 978-3-031-63178-8 (eBook)
https://doi.org/10.1007/978-3-031-63178-8

This Springer imprint is published by the registered company Springer Nature Switzerland AG
The registered company address is: Gewerbestrasse 11, 6330 Cham, Switzerland

Foreword

> Look to the essence of a thing, whether it be a point of doctrine, of practice, or of interpretation.
>
> —Marcus Aurelius

Many process descriptions are overly complicated and have limited practical ramifications. This is typical for many of today's textbooks and the medical literature describing surgeries. A plethora of operating advancements requires special instrumentation or new technologies that are often not pragmatic for the typical surgeon in practice. Importantly, many of these options add complexity or cost without meaningfully improving quality.

With the trust and responsibility of his or her patients, there are many things the oculofacial surgeon needs to consider whether in the office or operating room setting. These include subtleties in diagnosis and assessment. Next are the requirements of safety and efficacy in the operating room where an awareness of common and unusual complications is also key.

With an ever-increasing demand for oculofacial plastic surgery, high-quality and cost-effective interventions are also a must. It is for this situation that Dr. Jeremiah Tao has compiled and edited this book. Each chapter describes the essence of surgical procedures that require no sophisticated instrumentation nor costly device to treat the most encountered orbit, eyelid, or lacrimal problems.

This book is a needed and very valuable contribution to the field of oculofacial plastic surgery. A group of excellent and experienced oculofacial plastic surgeons contributed to the book and have included valuable details of surgical approaches with text, illustrations, and very helpful videos, which also show subtleties of the surgical procedures in a graphic manner.

I highly recommend this book conceived and produced by my good friend and colleague who has accompanied me on surgical missions to Africa and collaborated with publications, Dr. Tao.

Clinton D. (Sonny) McCord MD
Past President, American Society of Ophthalmic Plastic
and Reconstructive Surgery
Hailey, Idaho, USA

Preface

Oculofacial plastic surgery has seen tremendous advances in recent decades. Innovations in lasers, implants, endoscopes, pharmacotherapies, and neuroimaging have enriched the field. Many of these developments, while interesting and useful in some scenarios, have increased complexity and cost. Especially in underdeveloped regions but even in the first world, special devices, pharmacotherapies, or equipment are not readily available. Importantly, many do not meaningfully improve outcomes while others de-emphasize surgical fundamentals. For instance, reliance on stereotactic navigation may be rearing a new generation of surgeons with less ability to identify directly visualized intraoperative landmarks and hence who cannot perform certain surgeries without this special equipment.

Minimally complex, safe, and effective interventions are a must for any cost-effective practice or healthcare system. High-quality surgery is the essence of the oculofacial plastic surgery discipline.

This textbook is dedicated to minimal complexity, safe, and proven effective, "scalpel and suture" surgery for periorbital conditions. The chapters offer a systematic approach to wide-ranging congenital, acquired, reconstructive, and aesthetic disorders of the orbit, eyelids, lacrimal system, and midface. The authors provide a comprehensive discussion, pearls, and step-by-step description of techniques.

Expert oculofacial surgeons contributed to this book which includes photographs, diagrams, and video, for multi-format skills and knowledge transfer. In the spirit of efficiency, videos have been edited to be short and to demonstrate key steps. The included interventions do not require costly or otherwise inaccessible equipment, instrumentation, or pharmaceuticals. For instance, autologous grafts are focused in lieu of implants or special devices that add cost and complexity.

Lastly, oculofacial surgeons suffer a disparate risk for musculoskeletal injuries due to intraoperative positioning and the delicate and often microscopic nature of the surgeries. Their patients are also exposed to unique special risks, such as surgical fire due to electrosurgical devices used near oxygen supplementation. This textbook will highlight ergonomics and other safety measures in oculofacial surgery.

The efficiency theme aims to advance the quality and safety of oculofacial plastic surgery. The hope is that this textbook will inspire and help surgeons at any level of training and across diverse disciplines.

Jeremiah P. Tao
Professor, Department of Ophthalmology
University of California, Irvine
Irvine, CA, USA

Contents

Set Up and Ergonomics in Oculofacial Surgery

1

Johsias A. Maru, Jeremiah P. Tao, and Seanna R. Grob

Abstract

Efficient and safe oculofacial surgery starts with operating room set up. This includes proper patient positioning and draping. Equipment and supplies should be organized. Attention to ergonomics improves the quality of surgery and forestalls musculoskeletal injury. Oculofacial plastic surgeons are at particular risk for developing work-related neck or back disorders due to repetitive motions, static loading, or sustained exertions. Moreover, injudicious use of loupes or headlights can further lead to strain or injury. This chapter describes operating room set up and ergonomics that maximize efficiency and safety of oculofacial surgeries and mitigate risk of injury to surgeons.

Keywords

Oculofacial surgery set up · Draping · Operating room lighting · Ergonomics · Posture · Loupes · Headlights

J. A. Maru
University of California, San Francisco, San Francisco, USA

J. P. Tao (✉) · S. R. Grob
Division of Oculofacial Plastic and Orbital Surgery, University of California, Irvine, Irvine, CA, USA
e-mail: jeremiat@hs.uci.edu

Section I: Set Up in Oculofacial Surgery

Introduction

Efficient oculofacial surgery starts with proper patient positioning and draping. An organized approach with instrumentation and surgical supplies also improves safety, maintains sterility, minimizes waste, and saves time.

Operating Room Set Up

Pre-operative Tray Set Up

A typical pre-operative tray consists of local and topical anesthesia, needles, syringes, alcohol swabs, marking pen, and a ruler or caliper (sometimes a forceps if a skin pinch test is planned), among other items for specific surgeries (Fig. 1.1). Antiseptic skin prep supplies are often included (e.g., betadine and gauze) on this or a separate tray. Local anesthesia syringes should be a marked and labeled clearly.

The most common surgical skin prep for oculofacial plastic surgery is povidone iodine. For ocular or eyelid prep, 5% povidone iodine is recommended to avoid ocular surface toxicity. 10% povidone iodine is acceptable for the non-periocular face, but care must be taken to avoid significant exposure to the eyes. Alcohol, hydrogen peroxide, or chlorhexidine are generally

J. Tao (ed.), *Efficient Oculofacial Surgery*, https://doi.org/10.1007/978-3-031-63178-8_1

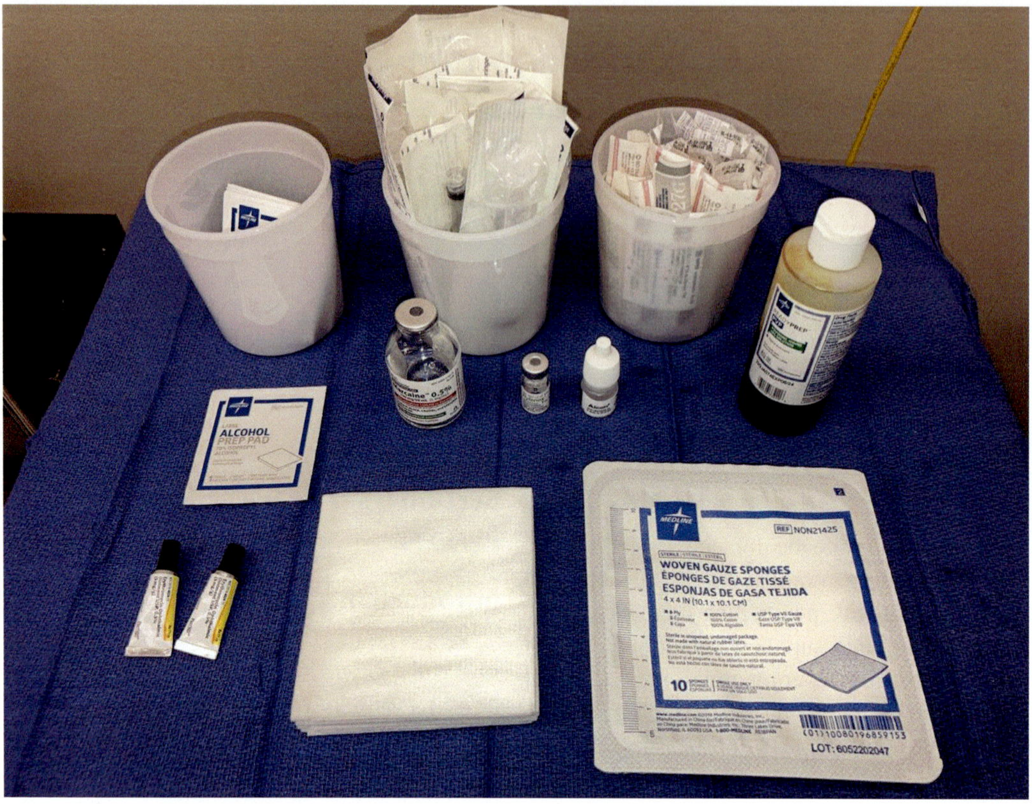

Fig. 1.1 Example of pre-operative table set Up

avoided for oculofacial surgery due to corneal toxicity. Baby shampoo or hypochlorous acid may be acceptable alternatives if patients have allergies to povidone iodine.

Mayo Stand or Surgical Table Set Up

Instruments, gauze, cotton tip applicators, scalpels, corneal protectors, wound dressings, and sutures should be organized on a Mayo stand or a back table (Figs. 1.2 and 1.3). Special instrumentation, implants, or devices should be available here prior to the incision (Fig. 1.4). Sutures that are likely needed for the case should be placed on the table. Each surgeon's preferences should be recorded and surgical trays should be updated to exclude unnecessary supplies or instruments [1–3].

Patient Positioning

The oculofacial surgery patient should be in a comfortable supine position that allows for wide access to the face and for proper surgeon ergonomics. An eye gurney or height adjustable operating room table/bed is preferred. The operating chair should wheel freely and have a kickstand to easily adjust height. A chair with lumbar support is ideal, but a rolling backless stool is acceptable. A donut pillow or other cushion should be placed under the head. For orbital surgery or facial bone surgery, and other cases under general anesthesia, more stable head immobilization is necessary to forestall movement. In addition, cases with longer duration require a cushioned headrest to prevent decubitus ulcer formation. A fluidized

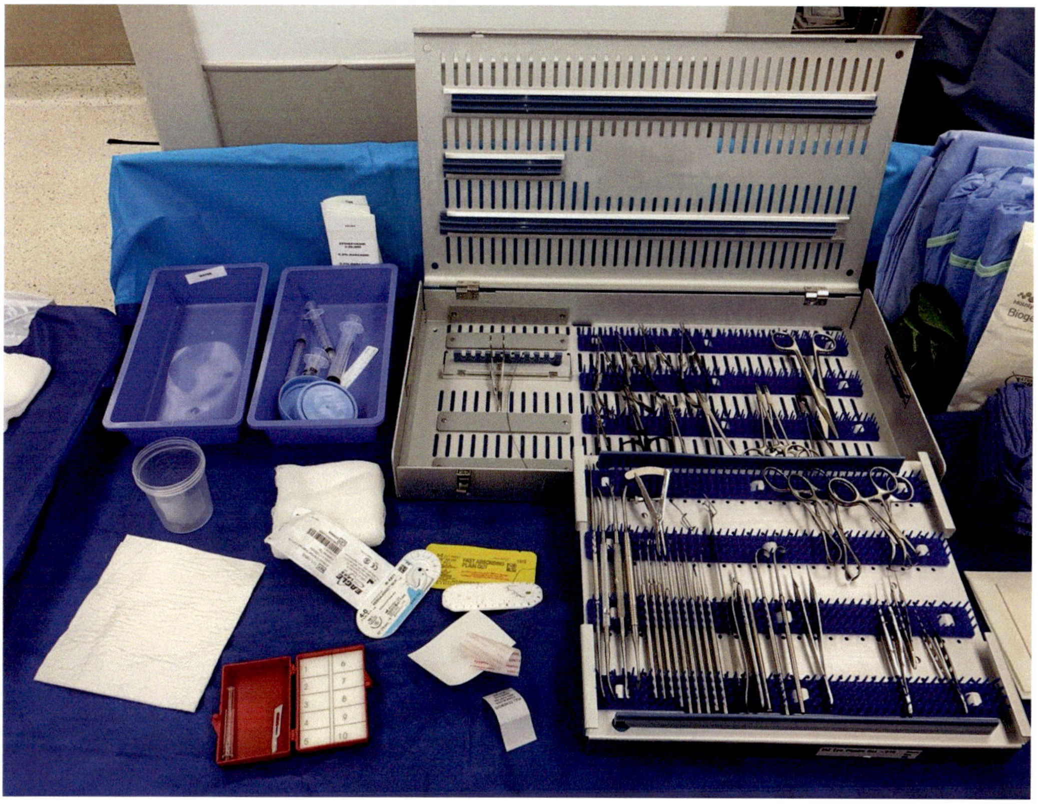

Fig. 1.2 Instrument tray set up

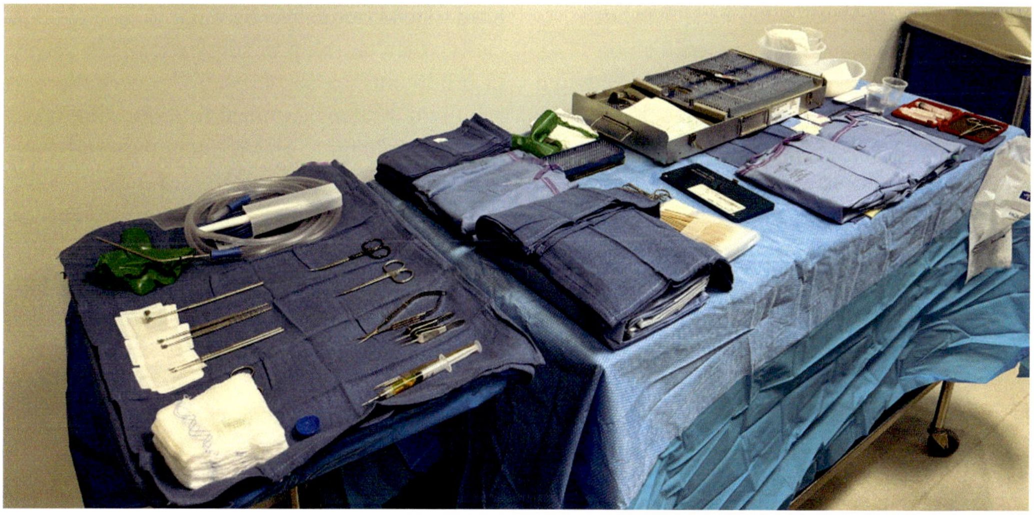

Fig. 1.3 Surgical table set up

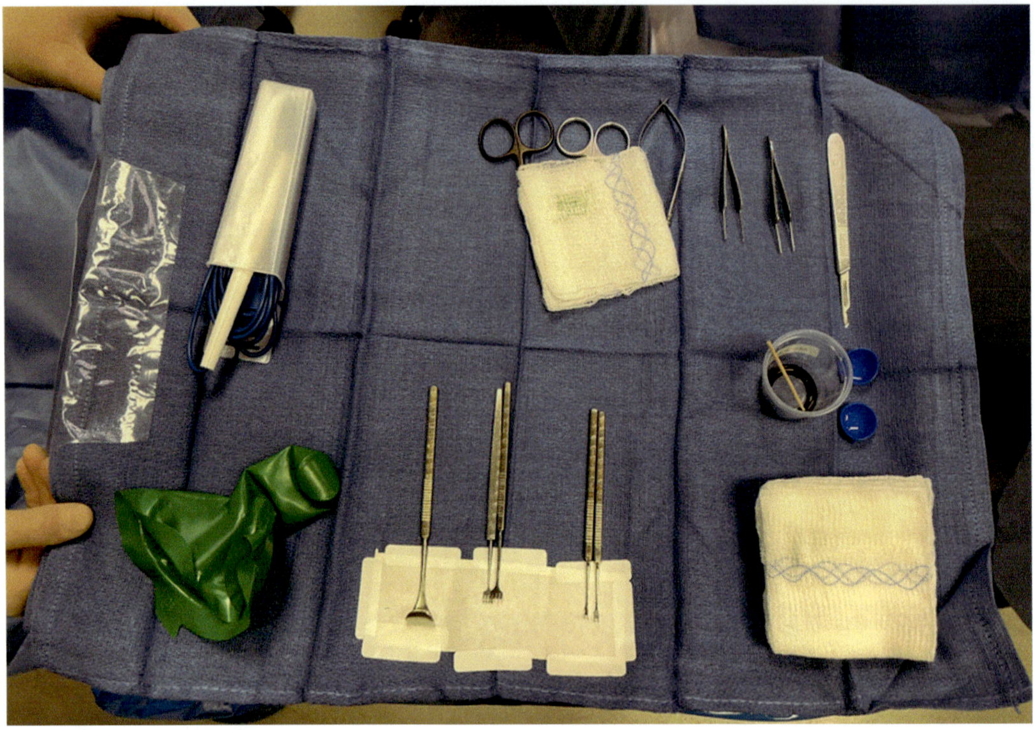

Fig. 1.4 Mayo stand set up

positioner (Z-Flo™ Fluidized Positioner, Mölnlycke® Health Care, Peachtree Corners, GA) obviates focal scalp and head pressure risks while providing some head immobilization.

There are special instances where standing or sitting to one side of the patient achieves better access, but in general, the primary surgeon is seated or standing at the head of the table. The surgical field (the patient's face) should be at the level of the surgeon's forearms parallel to the ground. The assistant surgeon(s) are seated to either side of the patient's head. The scrub technician is usually on the side opposite to the anesthetist, away from the head at the level of the patient's torso or abdomen.

Surgical Field Lighting

The oculofacial surgical field should be well illuminated. A dual overhead ceiling mounted operating room light system with multidirectional arms is ideal. Modern operating lamps include shadowless technology, however a second light is useful for instances for older lamps and when the beam from the first arm is blocked, i.e., behind an assistant surgeon's head. Head mounted lighting is useful especially when working in surgical cavities such as in orbitotomy or nasolacrimal surgery. Portable headlight systems are ideal to reduce inefficiencies of unplugging and re-plugging cords, e.g., from the fiberoptic lightbox or power source and when there are co- or assistant surgeons and frequent positional changes. The ideal headlight system should also be lightweight and comfortable. (The authors use the Ronin® X6 headlight, Ronin Surgical, Los Angeles, CA, but there exist other systems with these attributes). Importantly, the authors recommend using surgical headlights only when overhead surgical illumination is inadequate, since neck and back strain are risks from craning to the spotlight position.

Patient Draping

Draping is important to maintain sterility. The drape should be comfortable for the patient especially when she/he is awake. Good surgical drape technique allows good exposure of the surgical field and is secure to ensure sterility, and prevent fluid or blood egress from the surgical field.

The authors use two surgical towels and a half sheet placed under the patient's head. The top towel is wrapped to form a turban and secured with a towel clip to keep the patient's hair out of the surgical field. The wrapped head is then placed on the donut pillow or head immobilizer. An additional towel is then placed under the patient's chin.

If oxygen supplementation via nasal cannula is required, a 45 cm × 30 cm 3 M 1000 Steri-drape™ is placed over the patient's nose and cheeks creating a midface seal and covering the nasal cannula. A vent opening is cut over the mouth using scissors; the plastic drape at the inferior edge of the cut is placed flatter against the inferior face while the superior edge is tented (Fig. 1.5). This midfacial seal drape reduces fire risks by blocking oxygen egress from the nasal cannula oxygen to the surgical field (please see fire safety chapter) [4].

Next, the authors place a U-drape over the patient's body with the U opening under the patient's chin (Fig. 1.5). The authors recommend securing the U drape at the top of the patients head with a towel clip instead of exposing the adhesive that may adhere to and inadvertently dislodge an endotracheal tube or laryngeal mask if the drape is tugged during the case or when it is removed at the end of the case.

Conclusion

Good operating room set up considers safety and efficiency. Beyond the particulars described here, good communication between the surgeon and operating room staff and assistants is paramount.

Section II: Ergonomics in Oculoplastic Surgery

Introduction

The Human Factors and Ergonomics Society (HFES), defines ergonomics as a body of knowledge about human abilities, limitations, and characteristics that are relevant to design. Ergonomic design is that application of this knowledge to the design of tools, machines, systems, tasks, jobs, and environments for

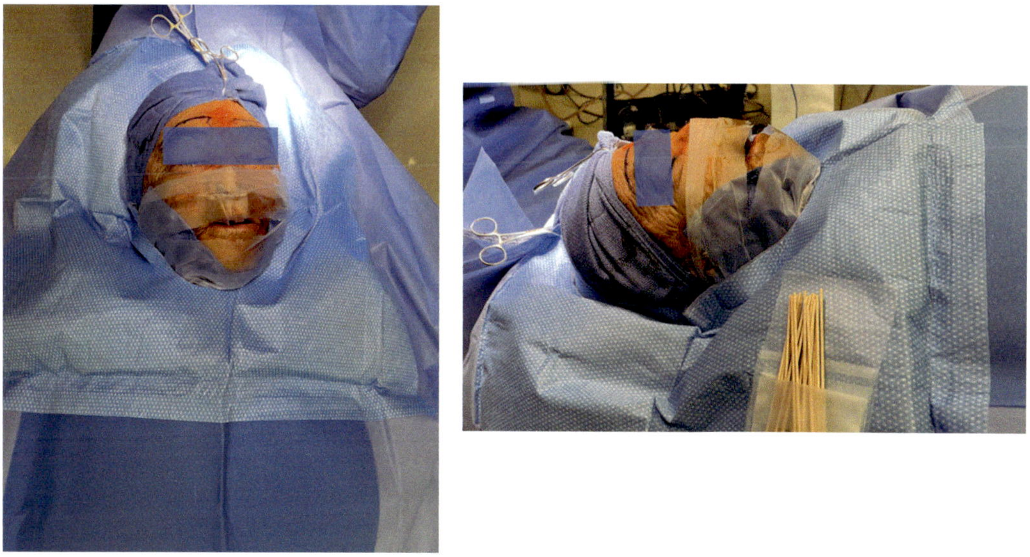

Fig. 1.5 Patient draping during monitored sedation and nasal cannula oxygen supplementation

safe, comfortable, and effective human use [5]. The goal of ergonomics is to optimize performance and minimize the risk of user injury. Proper ergonomic practices correlate to efficiency. In addition to safe and effective patient results, another goal is minimized risk of sustaining a work-related musculoskeletal disorder (WRMSKD) for the surgeon.

In a 2005 survey of practicing ophthalmologists in the United States, 51.8% reported job-related neck, upper body, or lower back pain, and 15% confirmed limitations in their work [6]. Furthermore, among oculofacial plastic surgeons, approximately 70% self-reported pain with operating [7]. Despite the pervasiveness of injuries due to poor ergonomic configuration, the impact is often either unknown or grossly understated among surgeons [8]. In this chapter, the authors describe risk factors and recommendations surrounding a surgical WRMSKD.

Risk Factors

Surgeons are at high risk of developing a WRMSKD [9]. Predisposing factors include repetitive motions, static loading, sustained exertions, and awkward postures.

Performing the same or similar motions repeatedly can result in trauma to the joints and surrounding tissues. Without sufficient time for rest and recovery, repetition can lead to injury [10]. Particularly in oculofacial plastic surgery, where fine movements are required, focal strain is placed on select muscles and joints. Patient volume has been directly correlated with probability of physical pain. Among practicing ophthalmologists, seeing more than 100 patients per week, performing $\geq$4 surgeries, and $\geq$6 lasers per week have been associated with increased neck, upper extremities, or lower back symptoms [6].

Static loading, which occurs when a muscle holds part of the body in a single position for a long period of time, can also increase one's risk of incurring a WRMSKD [10–12]. This lack of movement reduces circulation and causes muscle tension, which can contribute to or aggravate already existing WRMSKDs. Sustained exertions are a type of static loading where force is applied continuously for long periods of time. These typically occur with prolonged visual focus, often in postures dictated by limited adjustability of a surgical instrument or limited visibility, such as when operating in the orbit.

Lastly, for each joint in the body, there is a specific range of motion. Exceeding this range repeatedly and for prolonged periods of time poses high risk of WRMSKDs [10, 12]. Postures that force joints into positions where they are more likely to sustain an injury are termed awkward postures. According to one study, the most common awkward postures are extreme forward head tilt and overstretched neck, trunk inclination and rotation towards one side, the raising of one or both shoulders, increased curvature of the thoracic vertebral column, and incorrect positioning of the lower limbs with thigh-leg angle of less than 90° [13]. In oculofacial plastic surgery, awkward postures are frequent, especially in orbital surgery and attention to minimizing or eliminating them prevents injury.

Ergonomics During Oculofacial Surgery

Operating in a Seated Position

Oculofacial plastic surgery is frequently in a seated position. Improper positioning can precipitate excess strain. Prolonged sitting time has been identified as a significant risk factor for the development of lower back pain [14]. Several variables determine the posture of a seated person, including the design of the chair, sitting habits, and the task performed.

The height and inclination of the seat of the chair, the backrest, and other types of support affect posture. A good chair should wheel easily and permit quick adjustments in position and posture. Ideally, the operating stool should also have a backrest.

The ergonomically ideal seated posture is called the balanced or neutral posture (Fig. 1.6) [15]. It is a reference point recommended to be maintained within the limits imposed by practice conditions. This posture is comfortable and causes minimal muscular contractions or tensions. This position is stable across all body segments and joints. This position is also symmetrical – the defining element for postural balance. The notion of neutral derives from the fact that each joint of the body has a neutral zone to which the movements are natural. Recurrent exceeding of the neutral zone can generate joint and muscle strain.

The balanced posture features can be summarized as follows:

- a straight back and respect for body symmetry; avoiding rounding the back into "C" shape.
- forward inclination of the head up to 20–25° from the trunk.
- forward inclination of the trunk of a maximum of 20°; a greater forward inclination, or tilting to a side or trunk rotation are undesirable.
- the arms placed along the body, forearms parallel to the ground, with wrists flexed/extended<15°.
- the thighs should be slightly angled downwards, flexed from the spine between 90 and 105°.
- the angle between the thighs and shins should be 90–130°.
- the shins oriented perpendicular to the floor.
- the feet on the floor-oriented forwards in the same plane with the shins; when the feet are symmetrically positioned below the operator hands, the posture is balanced.

Microscopes

Strain associated with improper seating configuration can be further aggravated using microscopes (Fig. 1.7). A survey of plastic surgeons found that microscope usage while seated significantly exacerbated neck and back pain during surgery [16]. An increased prevalence of cervical symptoms is associated with jobs that require neck flexion in excess of 15 degrees [17, 18].

Similarly, studies by Lakhiani et al. and Fisher et al. elaborated on cervical spine biomechanics and the increased risk of injury for microsurgeons, highlighting the common occurrence of flexion of the lower cervical spine into a sustained forward head posture (FHP) [19, 20]. Oculofacial surgeons are a risk of sustained FHP, especially in the setting of orbital surgery and use of loupes. If left unopposed over long periods of time, FHP results in increased compressive load on surrounding tissues, which can adversely affect various soft tissue components, bony structures, and neural elements [21].

Nicholas and Marx et al. have recommendations to minimize overexertion of the back, hip, and neck during seated procedures [22]:

I. To minimize stress on the lumbar spine and hips, the physician's feet should be positioned flat on the floor with the back against the backrest of the chair. The bed should be positioned to allow the wheels of the surgeon's chair to slide under; this will help reduce the degree of forward flexion at the hips required.
II. Keeping the neck in a neutral position also is critical; adjusting the oculars or using loupes with appropriate focal distance that allow a neutral surgeon neck position.
III. A soft elbow rest can reduce strain on the shoulder and elbow. It is also important to be mindful of the wrist position, as the wrist should be kept in a neutral position without extension or flexion. The physician should always reposition themselves or the patient to realign themselves when addressing the alternate eye or assuming a new position to avoid torquing the back or acquiring an abnormal posture.

An eye gurney is ideal since it allows for the surgeon in a seated position to slide his/her legs under the patient's headrest to reduce forward flexion. The surgeon should keep their neck in as close to a neutral position as possible, minimizing sustained neck flexion. Regular checks on posture to ensure the most neutral posture possible, as described above, is recommended. Asking a colleague to photograph or video postures during surgery can highlight ergonomic flaws.

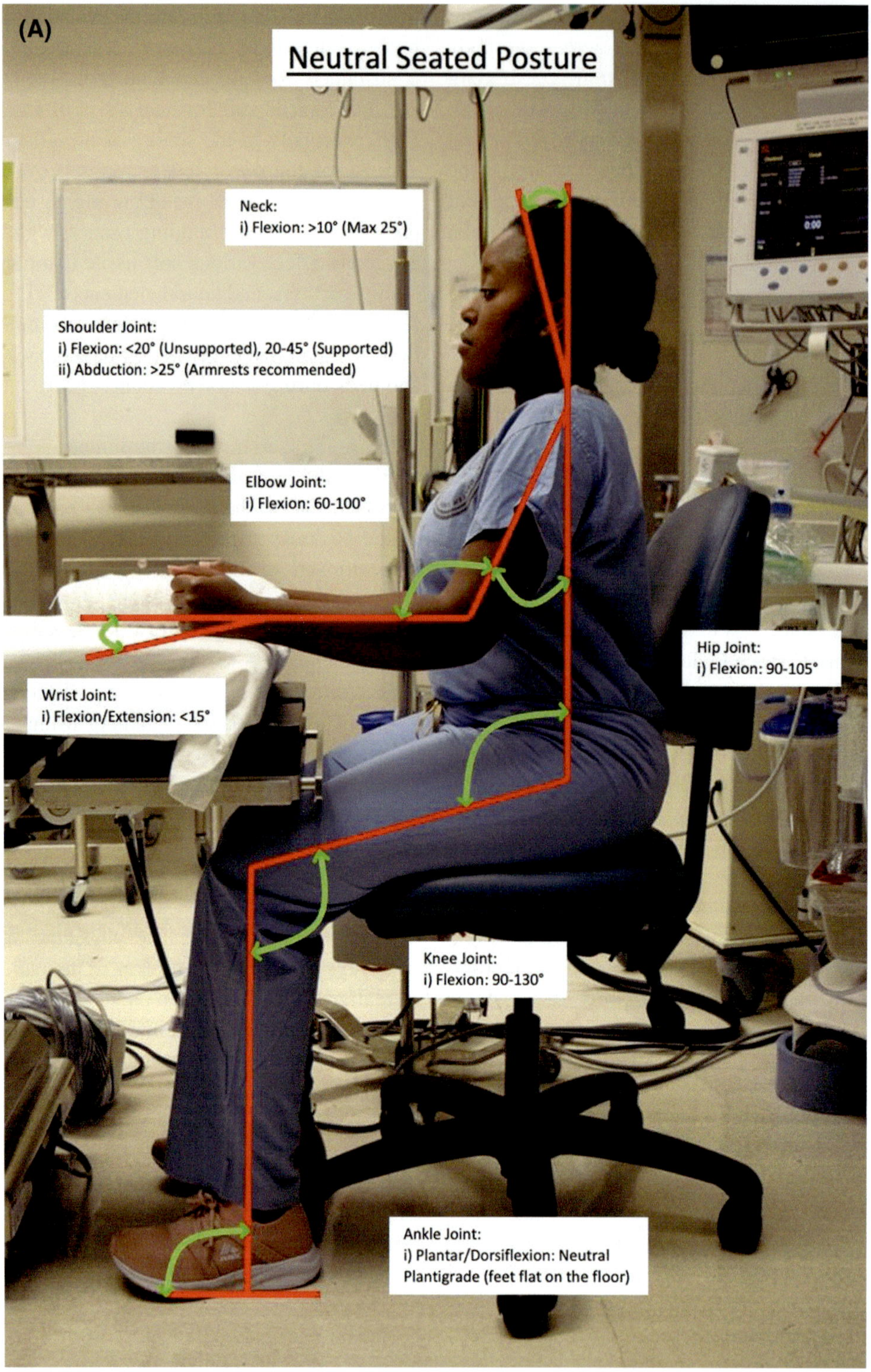

Fig. 1.6 Diagram of neutral seated (**A**) and standing (**B**) posture with key joint angles highlighted

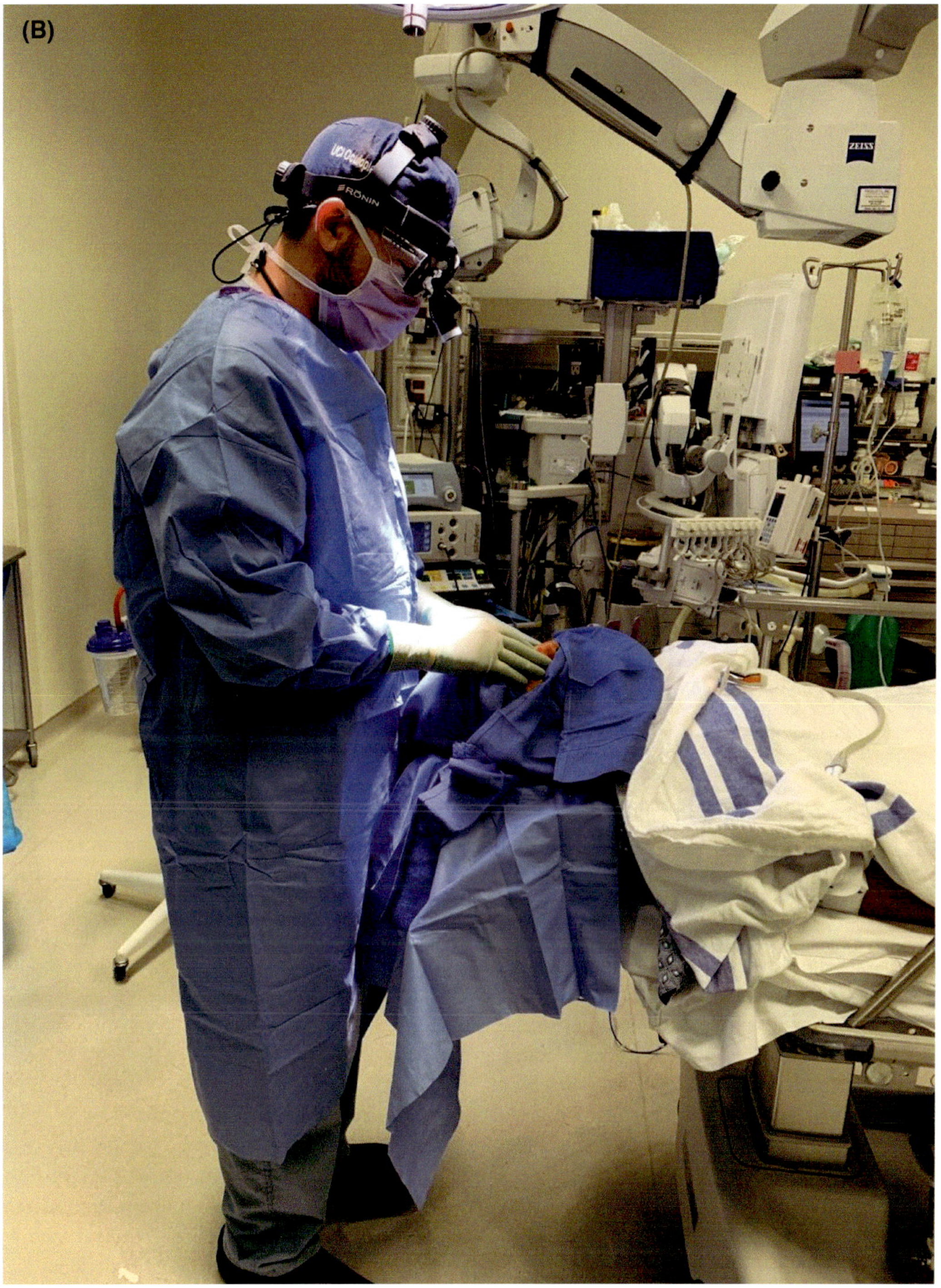

Fig. 1.6 (continued)

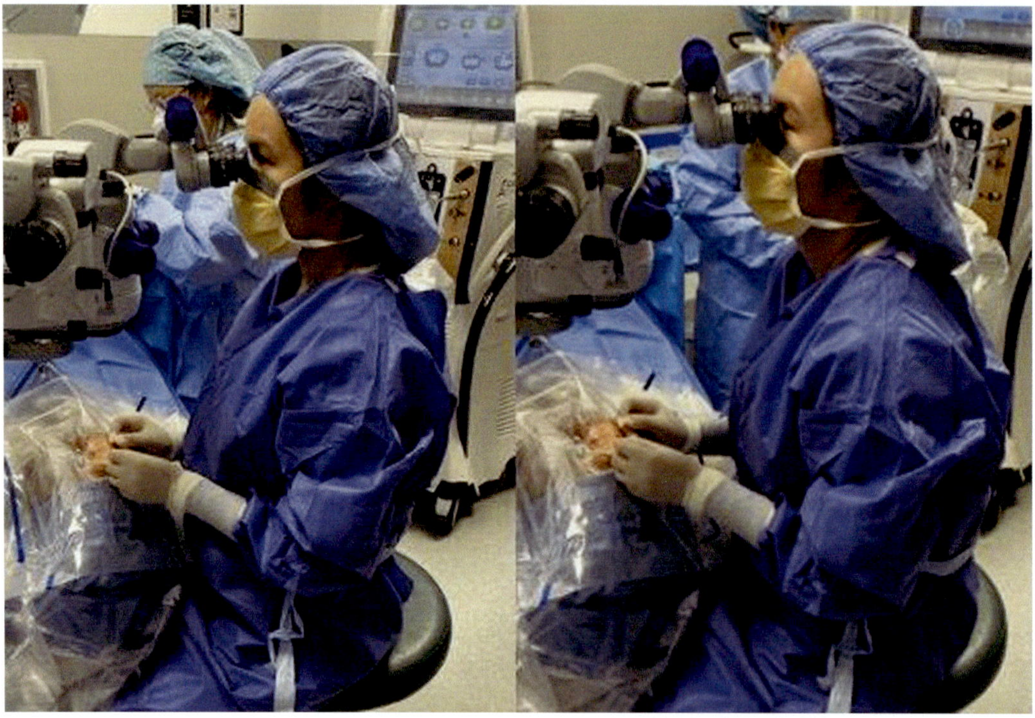

Fig. 1.7 Ergonomics at the operating microscope. The figure on the left demonstrates proper neck positioning at the microscope with the neck in a neutral position. The figure on the right demonstrates poor positioning at the microscope where the neck is hyperextended owing to poor posture

Operating While Standing

The following are three common ergonomic errors made while operating in a standing position (Fig. 1.8):

1. Forward head position: Surgeons often unconsciously drift their heads forward, lengthening the moment arm of the head on the neck and increasing the effective weight of the head by 10 pounds for every inch that the head moves forward. This leads to accelerated degenerative changes in the midcervical spine.
2. Sustained and improper shoulder elevation and internal rotation: This causes fatigue to the deltoid and trapezius muscles. This error is most observed when the operating table is too high compared to the surgeon's height. Akin to operating while seated, the forearms should be parallel to the ground.
3. Pelvic girdle asymmetry: An example of this is placing most of one's weight on one foot, which causes asymmetrical loading, and back and leg pain. This error is most observed when a surgeon is reaching across the patient to the contralateral side, or when a surgeon is twisting their body to align their visual field with the longitudinal axis of the patient's body.

Ergonomics of Headgear

Loupes and headlamps are important factors for neck strain in oculofacial surgery [19]. Studies on the effects of loupe magnification have shown an increased mean cervical load by 40% at all postures and across all cervical levels [23, 24]. This poses a significant threat to cervical health; furthermore, more than 80% of surgeons who routinely use loupe magnification report symptoms of neck strain. While loupes may be useful for some microsurgical tasks,

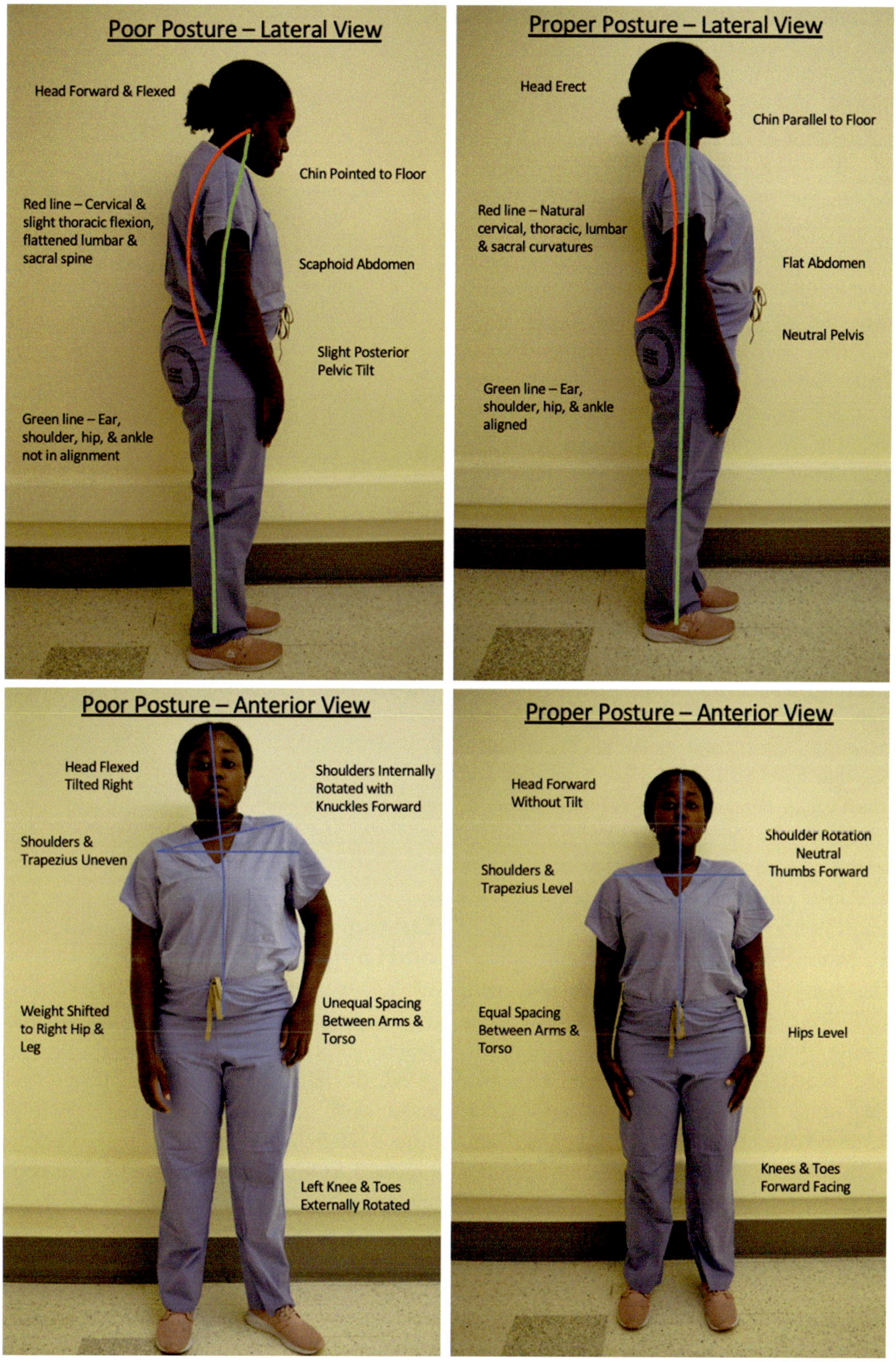

Fig. 1.8 Contrasting poor and proper standing posture from both the lateral and anterior perspectives. Common features of each are highlighted

many oculofacial surgeries can be performed without magnification.

When it is incumbent to use loupes, diligence in finding a proper fitting device may help to minimize prolonged neck hyperflexion. Frame weight, declination angle, and working distance of the lens are pertinent factors. Another factor is the necessary level of magnification. The least sufficient magnification should be sought since increasing levels of magnification significantly increase the weight of the device. Fortunately, carbon fiber and stainless-steel frame designs may alleviate lens weight. Front-mounted loupes pose a significant disadvantage compared to through-the-lens mounted loupes in terms of cervical strain; due to the forward-shifting effect of front mounting on one's center of gravity, neck extensors work harder to hold the added weight during flexed posture thereby increasing cervical muscle strain. Although the working distance and declination angle of the lens do not directly influence axial load or cervical strain, they significantly contribute to the overall line of sight of the surgeon and thus play a role in maintaining appropriate posture. Specifically, loupes that have an improper working distance for the task at hand and/or a declination angle less than 25° predispose surgeons to strain-evoking postures [25] (Fig. 1.9). Lastly, a narrower field of view induced by loupes may predispose to sharps injuries to assistants whose hands may not be within the surgeon's view.

The use of headlamps is common, with nearly 70% of oculofacial plastic surgeons endorsing intraoperative use [7]. Akin to loupes, headlights often force the surgeon's cervical spine into non neutral positions. Sahni et al. demonstrated that spinal surgeons who frequently used both headlamps and loupes reported an increased frequency and severity of neck symptoms due to strain [25]. The added weight yields concomitant increases in cervical loads at all angles, which may precipitate degeneration. Additionally, any discrepancy between the focal lengths of one's loupes and headlamp may provide greater opportunity for the surgeon to assume and maintain threatening postures [26]. To avoid protracted exposure to harmful postures, surgeons must be diligent in their selection and judicious in the use of headlamps.

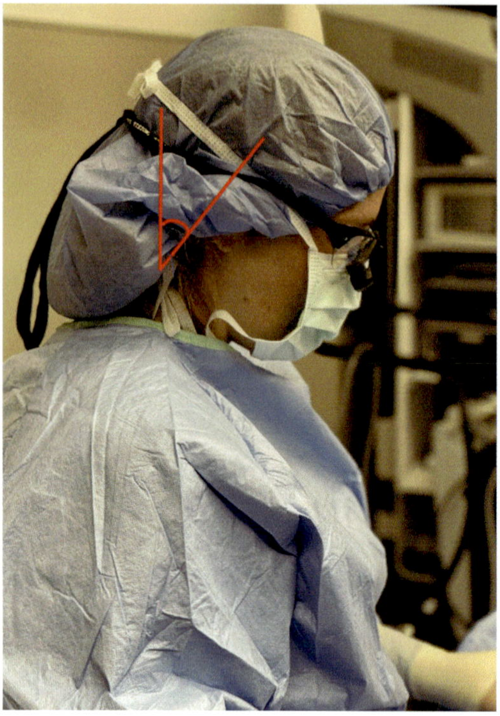

Fig. 1.9 Head position with use of loupes demonstrating forward flexion of the neck

Strategies to Improve Ergonomics and Longevity

Proper ergonomic positioning in oculofacial plastic surgery is not widely taught or emphasized. It is imperative to implement harm-reducing strategies and techniques early in one's career. Surgical postural habits form quickly and are hard to break, especially once one is years into practice.

Besides intraoperative posturing, other strategies exist to mitigate excess strain. These include targeted stretching microbreaks (TSMBs) and strength training.

TSMBs are intraoperative breaks with the intention of initiating targeted stretching exercises—particularly exercises that focus on concentric and eccentric contractions with slow lifting velocity (e.g., front shoulder raises, lateral shoulder raises, dumbbell flies, and shoulder shrugs)—of muscle groups prone to surgical strain. According to the US Occupational Safety and Health Administration (OSHA), participating in five-minute breaks or "micro-pauses" for each hour of a prolonged session is recommended as a method to provide time for muscles and tendons to recover [27]. TSMBs have been found to improve surgeon post-procedure pain scores in the neck, lower back, shoulders, upper back, wrists/hands, knees, and ankles for both laparoscopic and open procedures [28, 29]. Moreover, surgeons perceived improvements in physical performance and mental focus. Surgeons consistently endorsed a desire to continue incorporating TSMBs in their practice [30].

A 2019 study found promising results with a novel WRMSKD prevention program aimed at reducing the prevalence of WRMSKD among surgeons [8]. The program was developed with physical therapists who had expertise in WRMSKDs and consisted of 2 phases: 1) the awareness and application of ergonomic principles, according to the needs of the subjects, to decrease the stress on the musculoskeletal system and 2) an early standardized, easy-to-remember self-treatment of the most affected areas, which is also easily reproducible. At 3 months from the beginning of the study, a significant improvement in the quality of life was observed, measured as General Health (GH) item in the SF-36 questionnaire. The benefit of the program became more evident after 6 months, with a decreased lower back pain (LBP) prevalence and a significant reduction of analgesic consumption (30.9 vs. 15.5%; $P=0.03$). The improvement of the GH was also confirmed after 6 months. Even if only lower back WRMSKD was significantly improved by the program, a positive trend was reported for almost all the considered bodily areas [8].

Physical fitness and exercise are other ways to obviate cervicospinal and lower back strain. Both targeted and general fitness prevent and ameliorate neck injuries by improving posture and reducing reported symptoms [31]. Furthermore, FHP can be corrected by stretching foreshortened trapezius, sternocleidomastoid, and levator scapulae muscles and by strengthening the deep cervical flexors [32]. While alterations in posture may translate to an overall improvement in spinal health over time, both targeted and general fitness should also be emphasized for symptomatic management. Regular exercise directly reduces WRMSKD symptoms in surgeons, with studies supporting the performance of exercise of>5 h/week and/or>3 days/week [10]. Targeted exercises that focus on concentric and eccentric contractions with slow lifting velocity (e.g., front shoulder raises, lateral shoulder raises, dumbbell flies, and shoulder shrugs) have also been shown to reduce neck and shoulder pain [33].

Technological advancements in loupe and microscope technology may also ameliorate WRMSKD of the neck and upper extremities in surgeons. Deflection prismatic lenses, for example, are equipped with a built-in declination angle that permits the viewing field to reside at a fixed angle 5° below a true horizontal line of sight. These lenses clinically reduce neck and shoulder pain by minimizing the degree of neck flexion required to visualize the viewing field [34]. Similarly, the development of stereoscopic video displays may serve to eliminate the duration of forward head posturing during microsurgery using a three-dimensional (3-D) video screen and lightweight lenses are recent developments. In a recent study by Yu et al. examining the postural changes in microsurgical trainees on traditional stereoscopic microscopes versus 3-D video display, the authors observed that neck angles were a mean 9° to 13° more neutral, and that the time trainees spent in neck extension was significantly higher (30 vs. 17%) [35]. An additional merit of stereoscopic 3-D video microscopy is that of enhanced team engagement in the operation, as the display makes the microscopic field visible to all in the operating room.

Conclusion

Oculofacial plastic surgeons are at high risk for WRMKDs due to the physical and repetitive nature of the work. To mitigate these disorders, proper operating ergonomics should be adopted as early as possible in a surgeon's career. In addition to general posture and body positioning during surgery, thoughtfulness about using loupe magnification or headlight illumination are keys to improving career longevity as an oculofacial surgeon. While loupes may be useful in certain micro surgeries, developing a dependence upon them for all oculofacial procedures should be avoided. Small breaks and targeted stretches, as well as good physical fitness, may mitigate strain.

References

1. Fu T, Msallak H, Namavarian A, Chiodo A, Wlmasri W, Hubbard B, Xu J, Pegoraro R, Higgins K, Enepekides D, Monteiro E, Eskander A. Surgical tray optimization: a quality improvement initiative that reduces operating room costs. J Med Syst. 2021;45(8):78.
2. Lonner J, Goh G, Sommer K Niggeman G, Levicoff E, Vernace J, Good R. Minimizing surgical instrument burden increases operating room efficiency and reduces perioperative costs in total join arthroplasty. J Arthropl. 2021;36(6):1857–63.
3. Whitmer H, Dhiman A, Jones A, Laffan A, Adelman D, Turaga K. Systematic review of operative team familiarity on metrics of efficiency, patient outcomes, cost and team satisfaction. Ann Surg. 2022. https://doi.org/10.1097/SLA.0000000000005531.
4. Tao J, Hirabayashi K, Kim B, Zhu F, Joseph J, Nunery W. The efficacy of midfacial seal drape in reducing oculofacial surgical field fire risk. Ophthal Plast Reconstr Surg. 2013;29(2):109–12.
5. Hfes.org. What is Human Factors and Ergonomics | HFES 2022. https://www.hfes.org/About-HFES/What-is-Human-Factors-and-Ergonomics. Accessed 7 April 2022.
6. Dhimitri KC, McGwin G Jr, McNeal SF, et al. Symptoms of musculoskeletal disorders in ophthalmologists. Am J Ophthalmol. 2005;139(1):179–81. https://doi.org/10.1016/j.ajo.2004.06.091.
7. Sivak-Callcott JA, Diaz SR, Ducatman AM, Rosen CL, Nimbarte AD, Sedgeman JA. A survey study of occupational pain and injury in ophthalmic plastic surgeons. Ophthalmic Plast Reconstr Surg. 2011;27(1):28–32. https://doi.org/10.1097/IOP.0b013e3181e99cc8.
8. Giagio S, Volpe G, Pillastrini P, Gasparre G, Frizziero A, Squizzato F. A preventive program for work-related musculoskeletal disorders among surgeons: outcomes of a randomized controlled clinical trial. Ann Surg. 2019;270(6):969–75. https://doi.org/10.1097/SLA.0000000000003199.
9. da Costa BR, Vieira ER. Risk factors for work-related musculoskeletal disorders: a systematic review of recent longitudinal studies. Am J Ind Med. 2010;53(3):285–323. https://doi.org/10.1002/ajim.20750.
10. Kitzmann AS, Fethke NB, Baratz KH, Zimmerman MB, Hackbarth DJ, Gehrs KM. A survey study of musculoskeletal disorders among eye care physicians compared with family medicine physicians. Ophthalmology. 2012;119(2):213–20. https://doi.org/10.1016/j.ophtha.2011.06.034.
11. Chatterjee A, Ryan WG, Rosen ES. Back pain in ophthalmologists. Eye. 1994;8(Pt 4):473–4. https://doi.org/10.1038/eye.1994.112.
12. Bernard BP (ed). Musculoskeletal disorders and workplace factors. A critical review of epidemiologic evidence for work-related musculoskeletal disorders of the neck, upper extremity, and low back. Cincinnati: DHHS (NIOSH) Publication Number 97-141; 1997. www.cdc.gov/niosh/docs/97-141/default.html. Accessed 27 Dec 2019.
13. Kanteshwari K, Sridhar R, Mishra AK, Shirahatti R, Maru R, Bhusari P. Correlation of awareness and practice of working postures with prevalence of musculoskeletal disorders among dental professionals. Gen Dent. 2011;59(6):476–85.
14. Baradaran Mahdavi S, Riahi R, Vahdatpour B, Kelishadi R. Association between sedentary behavior and low back pain; a systematic review and meta-analysis. Health Promot Perspect. 2021;11(4):393–410. https://doi.org/10.34172/hpp.2021.50.
15. Pîrvu C, Pătraşcu I, Pîrvu D, Ionescu C. The dentist's operating posture—ergonomic aspects. J Med Life. 2014;7(2):177–82.
16. Capone AC, Parikh PM, Gatti ME, Davidson BJ, Davison SP. Occupational injury in plastic surgeons. Plast Reconstr Surg. 2010;125(5):1555–61.
17. Cagnie B, Danneels L, Van Tiggelen D, De Loose V, Cambier D. Individual and work related risk factors for neck pain among office workers: a cross sectional study. Eur Spine J. 2007;16(5):679–86. https://doi.org/10.1007/s00586-006-0269-7.
18. Hansraj KK. Assessment of stresses in the cervical spine caused by posture and position of the head. Surg Technol Int. 2014;25:277–9.
19. Lakhiani C, Fisher SM, Janhofer DE, Song DH. Ergonomics in microsurgery. J Surg Oncol. 2018;118(5):840–4. https://doi.org/10.1002/jso.25197.
20. Fisher SM, Teven CM, Song DH. Ergonomics in the operating room: the cervicospinal health of today's

surgeons. Plast Reconstr Surg. 2018;142(5):1380–7. https://doi.org/10.1097/PRS.0000000000004923.
21. Moustafa IM, Diab AA. The effect of adding forward head posture corrective exercises in the management of lumbosacral radiculopathy: a randomized controlled study. J Manipulative Physiol Ther. 2015;38(3):167–78. https://doi.org/10.1016/j.jmpt.2014.11.009.
22. Nichols M, Marx J. Ergonomics for the retinal physician. Retinalphysician.com. https://www.retinalphysician.com/issues/2019/may-2019/ergonomics-for-the-retinal-physician. Accessed 6 April 2022.
23. Nimbarte AD, Sivak-Callcott JA, Zreiqat M, Chapman M. Neck postures and cervical spine loading among microsurgeons operating with loupes and headlamp. IIE Trans Occup Ergon Hum Factors. 2013;1(4):215–23.
24. Nimbarte AD, Zreiqat M, Chapman M, Sivak-Callcott JA. Physical risk factors for neck pain among oculoplastic surgeons. In: Proceedings of IIE annual conference expo; Orlando, FL; 2012
25. Sahni D, James K, Hipp J, et al. Is there an increased incidence of cervical degenerative disease in surgeons who use loupes and a headlight? J Spine 2015;04(5):256. https://doi.org/10.4172/2165-7939.1000256
26. Rohrich RJ. Why I hate the headlight and other ways to protect your cervical spine. Plast Reconstr Surg. 2001;107(4):1037–8.
27. OSHA. Extended unusual work shifts. https://www.osha.gov/emergency-preparedness/guides/extended-unusual-work-shiftshours.html
28. Park AE, Zahiri HR, Hallbeck MS, et al. Intraoperative "Micro breaks" with targeted stretching enhance surgeon physical function and mental focus: a multicenter cohort study. Ann Surg. 2017;265(2):340–6. https://doi.org/10.1097/SLA.0000000000001665.
29. Hallbeck MS, Lowndes BR, Bingener J, et al. The impact of intraoperative microbreaks with exercises on surgeons: a multi-center cohort study. Appl Ergon. 2017;60:334–41. https://doi.org/10.1016/j.apergo.2016.12.006.
30. Abdelall ES, Lowndes BR, Abdelrahman AM, Hawthorne HJ, Hallbeck MS. Mini breaks, many benefits: development and pilot testing of an intraoperative microbreak stretch web-application for surgeons. Proc Human Factors Ergonom Soc Annu Meeting. 2018;62(1):1042–6. https://doi.org/10.1177/1541931218621240.
31. Ruivo RM, Carita AI, Pezarat-Correia P. The effects of training and detraining after an 8 month resistance and stretching training program on forward head and protracted shoulder postures in adolescents: randomised controlled study. Man Ther. 2016;21:76–82.
32. Lynch SS, Thigpen CA, Mihalik JP, Prentice WE, Padua D. The effects of an exercise intervention on forward head and rounded shoulder postures in elite swimmers. Br J Sports Med. 2010;44:376–81.
33. Zebis MK, Andersen LL, Pedersen MT, et al. Implementation of neck/shoulder exercises for pain relief among industrial workers: a randomized controlled trial. BMC Musculoskelet Disord. 2011;12:205.
34. Lindegård A, Nordander C, Jacobsson H, Arvidsson I. Opting to wear prismatic spectacles was associated with reduced neck pain in dental personnel: a longitudinal cohort study. BMC Musculoskelet Disord. 2016;17:347.
35. Yu D, Green C, Kasten SJ, Sackllah ME, Armstrong TJ. Effect of alternative video displays on postures, perceived effort, and performance during microsurgery skill tasks. Appl Ergon. 2016;53:281–9.

Sutures and Wound Closure Fundamentals

2

Mark A. Prendes, Peter J. Timoney, and Lalita Gupta

Abstract

Wound closure is fundamental to oculofacial surgery. The face is highly visible and minimizing conspicuous scarring with proper suture selection and good placement technique are keys. There exist many suture materials and needle options as well as suturing styles to consider for oculofacial surgeries. These particulars should be individualized to the type of surgery being performed and other specifics about the patient including age. In this chapter, the authors describe the fundamentals of sutures and wound closure in oculofacial surgery.

Keywords

Wound closure · Sutures · Needles · Interrupted suture · Mattress suture

Supplementary Information The online version contains supplementary material available at https://doi.org/10.1007/978-3-031-63178-8_2.

M. A. Prendes
Department of Ophthalmology and Visual Sciences, Case Western Reserve University, Cleveland, OH, USA

P. J. Timoney (✉) · L. Gupta
Department of Ophthalmology, University of Kentucky, Lexington, KY, USA
e-mail: pjtimo2@uky.edu

Introduction

In oculofacial surgery, wound closure affects functional and cosmetic outcomes. Suture is generally favored over staples or adhesives on the face. Other variables include suture needle type and size, suture material, and how the sutures are placed. Patient age and other particulars such as past reaction to suture types are important variables to consider. In the pediatric population, absorbable sutures are generally preferred since removal of nonabsorbable sutures may require sedation or general anesthesia.

Good wound closure is with the wound tightly apposed but without excessive tension. Overly tight sutures may strangulate incorporated tissue. For thicker skin away from the eyelids, deep sutures are often useful to approximate the wound together so that superficial sutures can hold skin edges with minimal tension. Optimal suture placement involves gentle tissue handling. Eversion of wound edges forestalls a depressed scar with the closure of thicker non-eyelid skin.

Sutures

Needles

The anatomy of a suture needle include its point, body, and the swaged end (Fig. 2.1). The

J. Tao (ed.), *Efficient Oculofacial Surgery*, https://doi.org/10.1007/978-3-031-63178-8_2

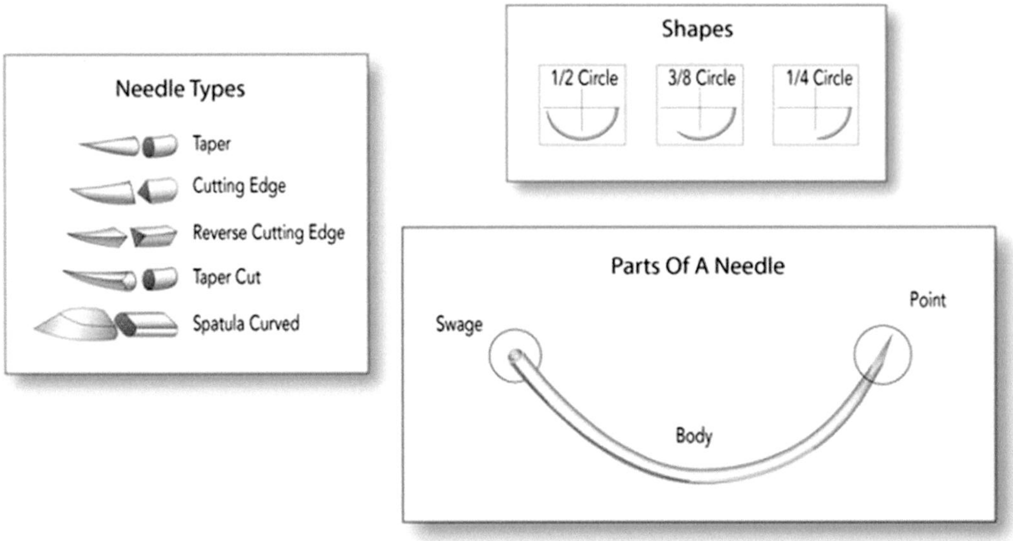

Fig. 2.1 Needle types and anatomy of a suture needle

needle is grasped with a needle holder three-fourths of the way from the point, to allow for optimal control of the needle while minimizing damage to the needle itself. The commonly used needle holders are the spring handle Castroviejo or ring handle Webster for 4–0 or greater size suture. Needles can be various sizes. The curve or shape of a needle may be a 3/8 circle, 1/2 circle, or 1/4 circle. The 3/8 circle is versatile. The 1/2 circle is used for tight spaces, such as within a dacryocystorhinostomy wound to secure mucosal flaps or within a lateral canthotomy wound to anchor the lateral lower eyelid tarsus to periosteum.

The suture needles vary in ease of passage and the degree of tissue trauma [1]. The cutting needle has sharp edges along the curvature of the needle. It can be reverse cutting or conventional cutting. While a conventional cutting needle has a sharp edge on the inner curvature, the reverse cutting needle has the sharp edge on the outer curvature. With the cutting edge is on the inner curvature, the needle tends to be pulled up when being passed through a tissue. A conventional cutting needle cuts superiorly enlarging the needle tract when passed. Reverse cutting needles are commonly used in oculofacial surgery as they are less traumatic to the tissue. Spatulated needles are shaped such that the sides of the needle cut but the top and bottom of the needle do not. They are used for lamellar passes such as through the tarsus or sclera. Tapered have a round body that tapers to a sharp point and are preferred textures that are easy to penetrate such as vessels or nerves; they are less commonly used in oculofacial surgery.

Caliber and Material

Sutures come in a variety of sizes and materials and with variable characteristics [2]. In oculofacial surgery, 3-0–8-0 caliber suture are common. Suture materials vary in whether they are natural or synthetic (including metallic), absorbable or nonabsorbable, and monofilament or multifilament (Table 2.1). Catgut or gut suture comes from the wall of sheep or goat intestines. Gut sutures are degraded by enzymatic action. Chromic gut is gut treated with chromic oxide solution to slow the breakdown and increase the strength retention time. Synthetic absorbable sutures such as polyglactin are less reactive and are degraded by hydrolysis. Nonabsorbable sutures retain their tensile strength for years. They are mostly inert and less inflammatory than absorbable sutures except

Table 2.1 Suture materials

	Absorbable (strength retention time) versus nonabsorbable	Natural versus synthetic versus metal	Monofilament versus multifilament
Nylon	Nonabsorbable	Synthetic	Monofilament
Polypropylene (Prolene®)	Nonabsorbable	Synthetic	Monofilament
Silk	Nonabsorbable	Natural	Multifilament
Polyester (Mersilene®)	Nonabsorbable	Synthetic	Multifilament
Steel	Nonabsorbable	Metal	Mono or Multifilament
Catgut	Absorbable • Fast absorbing (3–5 days) • Plain (7–10 days) • Chromic (10–14 days)	Natural	Monofilament
Monocryl	Absorbable (1–2 weeks)	Synthetic	Monofilament
Polyglactin (Vicryl®)	Absorbable (2–4 weeks)	Synthetic	Multifilament
Polydiaxonone (PDS)	Absorbable (4–6 weeks)	Synthetic	Monofilament

for silk. Nonabsorbable skin sutures are usually removed in 1 week. Made of a single strand, monofilament sutures allow for easy passage and are less reactive. Multifilament sutures are made of braided strands. This allows for effective knots that hold better but spaces between braids theoretically more likely potentiate infection.

Wound Closure

The quality of wound closure affects the outcome of surgery [3]. A well-constructed wound begins with its design. Skin incisions should be placed within skin tension lines if possible (Fig. 2.2, video 2-1) These lines are perpendicular to underlying skeletal muscle striations and corresponding to wrinkles or other skin creases. Incisions that traverse these creases tend to be more conspicuous.

The sides of a wound edge should generally be perpendicular to the skin plane. During wound closure, the tissue must be handled delicately. Toothed forceps allow less crush injury and better grasp of the tissue. To minimize vascular compromise, skin hooks can be used to gently grasp skin edges especially when manipulating a skin flap.

Superficial sutures are placed in the skin in an interrupted or running fashion. Placement must avoid inadvertent traction on the eyelid. Simple interrupted sutures are useful in complex lacerations in which the first sutures are placed in the midpoint of the wound and subsequent sutures between the first sutures and the end of the wound and continuing in a wound dividing fashion. Temporary sutures may be useful to align the wound and reduce tension. Simple interrupted sutures are also effective in creating eversion of the wound edges which compensates for contraction of the wound reducing

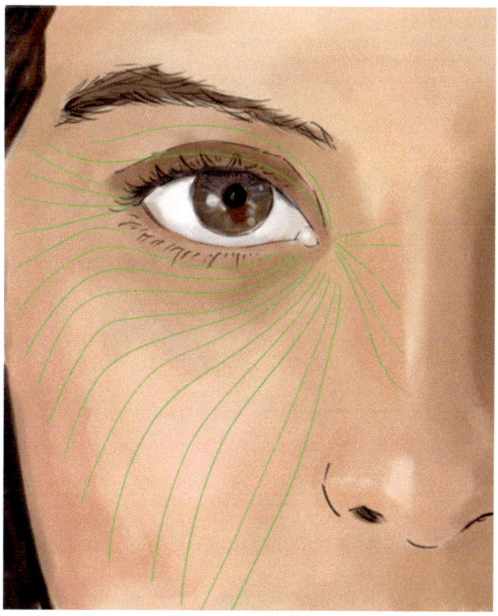

Fig. 2.2 Periorbital relaxed skin tension lines (*illustration by* Michael Han, MD)

the risk of a depressed scar. Running sutures help distribute tension evenly along the wound. They can be placed and removed more quickly than interrupted sutures. A running subcuticular suture can forestall suture tracks or scars. Exteriorized at the wound ends, the suture is passed in an S-shape through the subcutaneous tissue. Upper blepharoplasty incisions may be closed in a subcuticular manner, but more commonly they are closed with running sutures with minimal and inverting skin bites to encourage crease formation (Fig. 2.3). In general, subcuticular sutures elsewhere on the face may potentiated a depressed scar due to the lack of wound eversion.

Wider and deeper suture passes across a wound that incorporate more deep tissue especially at the lateral aspects of the base of the wound achieve better wound eversion. Wider passes, however, may leave the skin edge less apposed. A vertical mattress suture obviates these issues (Fig. 2.4). The suture is first passed far to far for a deep pass to incorporate deep tissue for eversion effects. Then, in the opposite direction but directly above and parallel to the first pass, the suture is passed near to near for a

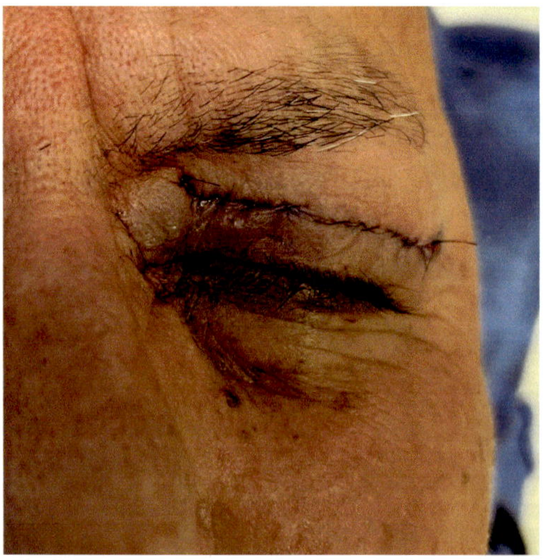

Fig. 2.3 Blepharoplasty wound closure with small inverting bites to encourage wound inversion and crease formation

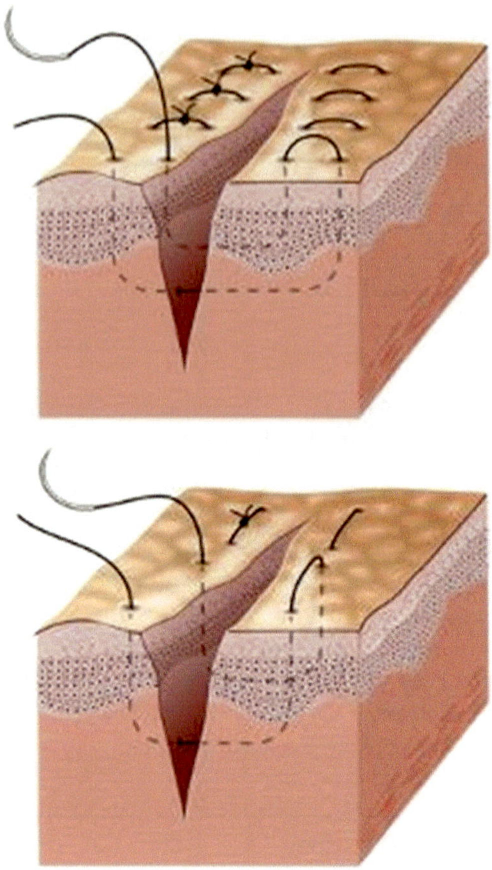

Fig. 2.4 Vertical mattress sutures (top) and horizontal mattress sutures (bottom)

superficial pass to precisely appose the skin. A running vertical mattress captures additionally allows for broader distribution of suture tension (Fig. 2.5). Horizontal mattress sutures distribute tension along a longer length of wound. Two passes are made next to each other in opposite directions and then tied. Horizontal mattress sutures also achieve good wound eversion (Fig. 2.3).

To close subcutaneous or deeper tissue, deep sutures are placed in a buried fashion with absorbable sutures, commonly polyglactin. This helps stabilize the wound and relieve skin tension. Closing dead space also prevents formation of a hematoma. Tension also may be relieved during wound closure by placing

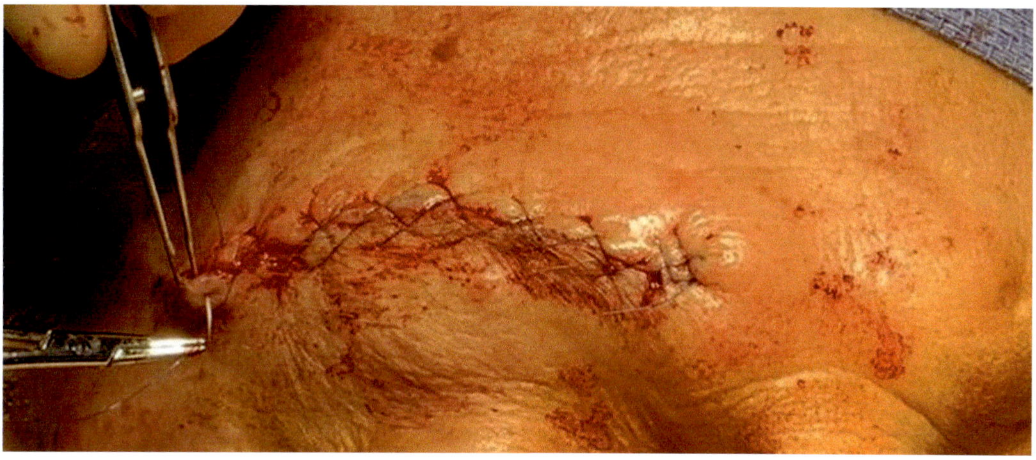

Fig. 2.5 Direct brow lift closure with a running vertical mattress suture. Note incorporation of increased tissue both across the wound and deep evert the wound to forestall a depressed scar

temporary sutures or traction sutures. Too much tension on a wound closure, potentiates a depressed or widened scar that may be disfiguring. Undermining the skin from underlying tissues may also help relieve tension. Redundant, or "dog ear deformity" tissue at the end of a wound may be excised in a triangle, by first extending the incision.

While sutures are generally preferred for facial skin closure, skin staples have occasional roles in oculofacial surgery and offer high efficiency in wound closure. In particular, post trichial incisions for forehead lift or temporal artery biopsy may be closed with staples since the wound is well hidden in the hair bearing scalp. Nevertheless, staples should be placed with the wound edge meticulously approximated and elevated to encourage staple bites that are even, precisely approximate the wound edge, and are everted to depressed scar formation (Video 2.2).

Conclusion

Wound closure is very important in oculofacial surgery. Suture selection and technique contribute to good functional and aesthetic outcomes.

References

1. Nerad JA. The art of surgical technique. In: Nerad JA, editor. Techniques in ophthalmic plastic surgery. 2nd ed. Philadelphia: Elsevier; 2021. p. 1–28.
2. Lever J, Nesi FA, Levine MR. Basic wound repair: surgical techniques, flaps, and grafts. In: Levine MR, Allen RC, editors. Manual of oculoplastic surgery. Cham: Springer International Publishing; 2018. p. 31–8.
3. Golan S, Zoumalan CI, Nesi FA, Lelli GJ. Basic principles of ophthalmic plastic surgery. In: Servat JJ, Black EH, Nesi FA, Gladstone GJ, Calvano CJ, editors. Smith and Nesi's ophthalmic plastic and reconstructive surgery. Cham: Springer International Publishing; 2021. p. 65–85.

3 Fire Safety in Oculofacial Surgery

Michael M. Han, Christopher R. Dermarkarian, and Jeremiah P. Tao

Abstract

Operating room fires are a critical danger in oculofacial surgery owing to the proximity of oxygen, ignition sources, and fuels. The best practices to reduce the risk of a surgical fire include minimizing oxygen in the surgical field, strategic draping, coordinating the use of electrocautery and laser devices, and managing fuel sources such as antiseptics and draping. In the event of a fire, turning off oxygen sources is a key first step. Next steps are extinguishing the fire and removing fuels from the surgical field. Operating room fires are preventable and safety measures described in this chapter can forestall serious injuries.

Keywords

Operating room fires · Fire safety · Oxygen · Ignition · Fuel · Fire response

Introduction

Operating room fires are termed "never events" since they are preventable and can cause serious harm [1]. Oculofacial surgery poses high risk for fires owing to the close proximity of oxygen supplementation devices near ignition sources. In a 2018 survey of 258 members of the American Society of Ophthalmic Plastic and Reconstructive Surgery (ASOPRS), 32.2% of surgeons had experienced at least one operating room fire in their careers [2]. It is estimated that approximately 600 operating room fires occur annually in the United States, although the number may be higher since many go unreported [3]. Surgical fires can cause serious harm and even death.

The three necessary elements for a fire are oxygen, heat, and fuel (Fig. 3.1). Surgery of or around the face places heat sources in proximity with supplemental oxygen devices. Fuel is abundant in the operating room, and includes surgical drapes, cleansing solutions, and even the patient's own tissues. In this chapter, we aim to provide an overview of operating room fire prevention and management strategies.

Minimizing Oxygen in the Surgical Field

The use of supplemental oxygen in the operating room is common, especially when patients are sedated [3]. In oculofacial surgery, oxygen administered via nasal cannula or mask naturally and easily egresses to the surgical site. Oxygen saturation can cause ignition of materials or

M. M. Han · C. R. Dermarkarian · J. P. Tao (✉)
Division of Oculofacial Plastic and Orbital Surgery, University of California, Irvine, Irvine, CA, USA
e-mail: jeremiat@hs.uci.edu

J. Tao (ed.), *Efficient Oculofacial Surgery*, https://doi.org/10.1007/978-3-031-63178-8_3

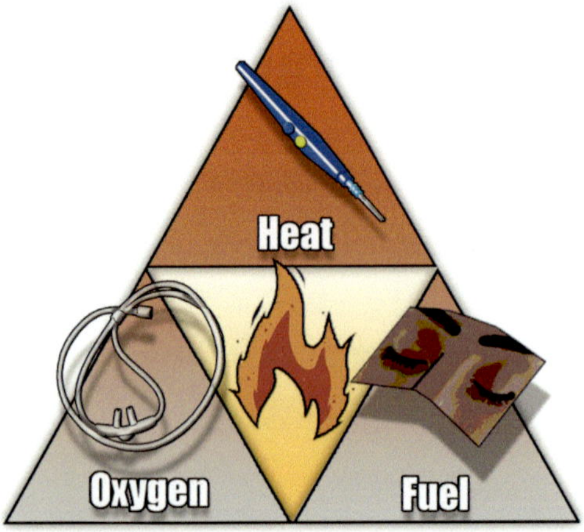

Fig. 3.1 The fire triangle

tissues that are otherwise not flammable in room air. High levels of oxygen not only potentiates ignition times, but also causes faster fire propagation [4]. The risk of fire is likely higher in monitored anesthesia care (MAC), as the supplemental oxygen is not delivered in a closed systems as it is with an endotracheal tube [5].

Woven cotton operating room towels are highly permeable to oxygen and frequently lead to oxygen contamination of the surgical field when used as barriers. Conversely, while plastic occlusive drapes provide a good barrier against oxygen contamination, they may contribute to pooling of higher concentrations of oxygen just outside the surgical field. Sudden combustion is possible if ignition sources reach these oxygen saturated materials. Strategies to mitigate fire aim to avoid oxygen saturation of combustible materials and the patient's tissues in the surgical field.

The American Society of Anesthesiologists recommends stopping supplemental oxygen for at least one full minute prior to the use of electrocautery, laser, or other potential devices that could serve as an ignition source. This approach is fraught with user error and requires additional coordination between anesthetist and surgeon. Moreover, bleeding may be abrupt and trigger prompt use of electrocautery. Importantly, stopping supplemental oxygen may not be desirable when blood oxygenation is already suboptimal. Patients with cardiopulmonary disease are at risk with this strategy that deprives oxygen. Also, healthy patients may need supplemental oxygen due to decreased frequency or depth of respiration effects of sedatives. The authors recommend trialing patients off oxygen supplementation whenever feasible. If patients breathe normally on room air and there is no blood oxygen desaturation, leaving the oxygen off for the majority of the case is sensible.

Draping to shunt oxygen away from the surgical field is another strategy. In experiments, a plastic drape with an adhesive (3M 1000 drape state, USA) was able to maintain oculofacial surgical field oxygen saturation under the threshold for combustion risk [6]. As such, the authors routinely use a midfacial seal drape in MAC cases (Fig. 3.2). The midface must be dry to achieve a tight seal. In addition, the authors cut a horizontal slit over the mouth region to create a vent that shunts oxygen inferiorly and avoids oxygen pooling under the drape. While some oxygen may pool in crevices formed by

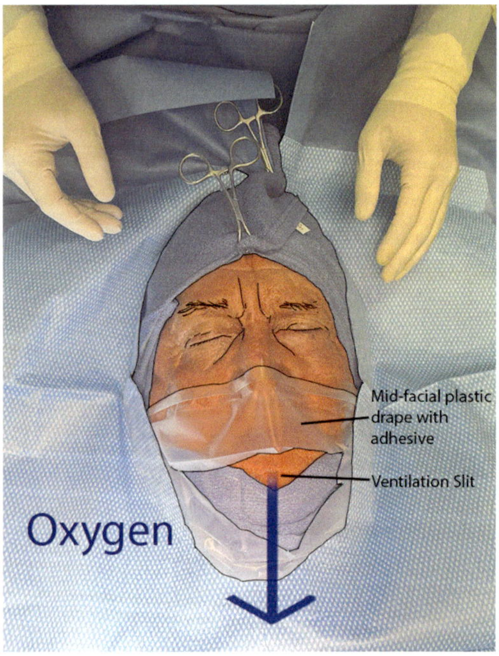

Fig. 3.2 **Mid-facial draping to reduce oxygen contamination**. An example of a mid-facial drape with an adherent seal superiorly and a ventilation slit in the inferior oral region to shunt oxygen away from the surgical field [6]

the non-adherent aspect of the drape, this system obeys fire safety principles so long as no ignition sources reach these areas.

Other strategies to keep oxygen away from the surgical field and ignition sources might include utilizing vacuum suctioning to scavenge oxygen. Of note, nitrous oxide is another oxidizing anesthetic agent sometimes used in oculofacial surgery; the same fire safety principles apply [7].

Managing Ignition Sources

The most common ignition source for an oculofacial operating room fire is cautery, with monopolar and thermal cautery contributing to the vast majority of reported cases of fire [5]. Using the lowest power needed for the procedure is advised. It is also recommended to keep cautery instruments within their holders when not in use due to the risk of inadvertent activation while in the operating field. As aforementioned, cessation of supplemental oxygen for a period prior to the use of electrocautery can reduce the chance of combustion even if the ignition source reaches potential fuels [7].

Carbon dioxide laser is another important ignition source often employed in eyelid or facial surgery [8]. Especially for broader facial resurfacing applications, wet towels should be strategically placed around the surgical area to prevent the ignition of surgical drapes. Endotracheal tubes should also be selected on the basis of laser resistance [7]. Another recommendation is filling the cuffs of endotracheal tubes with saline tinted with dye such as methylene blue rather than air to more readily expose a puncture.

Managing Fuels

Common sources of fuel include tracheal tubes, sponges, drapes, gauze, alcohol containing preparatory solutions, hair, ointments, and packaging materials among others [7]. Interestingly, regulations for the fire resistance of gowns and personal protective equipment exists, but as of 2021 there are no similar regulations for the fire resistance of surgical drapes [3]. Sponges and gauze are less likely to ignite if wet, so moistening these items before using them near an ignition source can be considered.

The pre-procedural antiseptic is important to consider in the context of fire prevention. Alcohol-based antiseptics are particularly high-risk [9]. Commonly used antiseptics for skin preparation include povidone-iodine and chlorhexidine gluconate. The risk of ignition with these solutions is greatly reduced by allowing for sufficient time for drying, usually with a wait time of at least 2–3 min and up to 5 min. In addition, pooling of antiseptic solutions should be minimized as much as possible; sponge applicators are notorious for contributing to this as they often contain more preparatory solution than is necessary.

Another fire hazard is make-up and beauty products such as eyelash extensions, adhesives for which can be composed of a flammable cyanoacrylate that can ignite with thermocautery [10]. These should be addressed on pre-operative evaluation especially for small same-day office-based procedures.

Other Features of Fire Safety

All operating room staff should have fire safety education. In addition, other steps include fire drills, a dedicated fire response protocol, and equipment for fire management readily available in the operating room. Fire risk should be assessed during surgical time-outs.

Responding to a Fire

In the event a surgical fire occurs, each operating room team member should have a dedicated role. Early signs can include a flash, unusual sounds, odors, smoke, or heat. Oxygen (or nitrous oxide) should be shut off immediately. The patient's airway should be checked and managed. The surgeon should stop any oxidation sources in the operating field and help remove all drapes and flammable material from the patient. The fire should be extinguished with saline or by smothering the flames. Subsequently, the patient should be evaluated for burns and inhalation injury.

If the fire cannot be controlled with the above methods, a carbon dioxide extinguisher should be utilized. If the flames persist, fire alarms should be activated and the patient should be evacuated. Operating room doors should be closed and the supply of medical gas to the room should be stopped. The fire should be reported to local regulatory agencies and to the hospital as an adverse event. As such, the event should be reviewed to identify practices that can be improved upon to reduce the risk of fires and improve fire response.

Conclusion

The consequences of operating room fires are borne by both the patient and the surgery team. For the patient, these events can be fatal, especially if ignition of oxygen sources lead to endotracheal burns. In less extreme examples, fires can lead to unpredictable results in post-procedural outcomes and patient cosmesis. Fires can physically injure the surgeon or staff as well. From a medicolegal risk perspective, since a surgical fire is considered a never event, it may be tantamount to negligence. The risk and consequences of an oculofacial surgical fire can be greatly diminished, if not averted, with thoughtful best practices.

References

1. Lembitz A, Clarke TJ. Clarifying "never events and introducing "always events." Patient Saf Surg. 2009;3(1):26. Available from https://www.ncbi.nlm.nih.gov/pmc/articles/PMC2814808/.
2. Maamari RN, Custer PL. Operating room fires in oculoplastic surgery. Ophthal Plast Reconstr Surg. 2018;34(2):114–22. Available from https://pubmed.ncbi.nlm.nih.gov/28263248/.
3. Culp WC, Muse KW. Preventing operating room fires: impact of surgical drapes on oxygen contamination of the operative field. J Patient Saf. 2021;17(8):e1846–50. Available from https://journals.lww.com/journalpatientsafety/Fulltext/2021/12000/Preventing_Operating_Room_Fires__Impact_of.161.aspx.
4. Culp WC, Kimbrough BA, Luna S. Flammability of surgical drapes and materials in varying concentrations of oxygen. Anesthesiology. 2013;119(4):770–6. Available from http://www.apsf.org/resources_video.php.
5. Connor MA, Menke AM, Vrcek I, Shore JW. Operating room fires in periocular surgery. Int Ophthalmol. 2018;38(3):1085–93. Available from https://pubmed.ncbi.nlm.nih.gov/28528356/.
6. Tao J, Hirabayashi K, Kim B, Zhu F, Joseph J, Nunery W. The efficacy of a midfacial seal drape in reducing oculofacial surgical field fire risk. Ophthal Plast Reconstr Surg. 2013;29(2):109–12.
7. Apfelbaum JL, Caplan RA, Barker SJ, Connis RT, Cowles C, Ehrenwerth J, et al. Practice advisory for the prevention and management of operating room fires an updated report by the american society of anesthesiologists task force on operating room fires. Anesthesiology. 2013;118(2):271–90. Available from http://pubs.asahq.org/anesthesiology/article-pdf/118/2/271/491312/20130200_0-00013.pdf.
8. Mak S, Ophth F, Cuhk MPH. Carbon dioxide laser safety issues in blepharoplasty and eyelid surgery. 16(1):6–10.
9. Ebecca R, Ooher T, Uy G, Addern JM, Ohn J, et al. Surgical fires and alcohol-based skin preparations. ANZ J Surg. 2004;74(5):382–5. Available from https://doi.org/10.1111/j.1445-1433.2004.02997.x.
10. Michaels JPS, MacDonald P. Ignition of eyelash extensions during routine minor eyelid surgery. Ophthal Plast Reconstr Surg. 2014;30(3). Available from https://journals.lww.com/op-rs/Fulltext/2014/05000/Ignition_of_Eyelash_Extensions_During_Routine.25.aspx.

Anesthetic and Systemic Considerations for Oculofacial Surgery

4

Robert Victor, Ashley Broussard, and Kyle Paredes

Abstract

Anesthetic plans for oculofacial surgery usually include topical local anesthetics and/or nerve blocks, or regional anesthesia (RA). They may also involve monitored anesthetic care (MAC) or full general anesthesia (GA). RA uses local anesthesia (LA) within peribulbar, retrobulbar, and sub-Tenon's nerve blocks to achieve pain control and akinesia of specific orbital structures. Retrobulbar, peribulbar, and sub-Tenon's nerve blocks allow for anesthesia of the cornea, uvea, and conjunctiva alongside providing akinesia of extraocular muscles. MAC involves sedative, anxiolytic, and analgesic medication alongside continual monitoring to maintain moderate to deep sedation. GA, in which a patient is maintained within an unarousable state, may be necessary in the context of more invasive procedures or with certain patient conditions. This chapter details safe and effective anesthesia protocols for oculofacial surgery.

Keywords

Oculofacial anesthesia · Topical local anesthetics · Facial nerve blocks · Regional anesthesia (RA) · Monitored anesthesia care (MAC) · General anesthesia (GA)

Introduction

This chapter will review anesthetic strategies and considerations for procedures within the oculofacial plastic and orbital surgery subspecialty. Topics span anesthetic approaches and plans for varying oculofacial procedures, perioperative management, patient positioning, strategies specific to oculoplastic anesthesia, and safety concerns.

Innervation of Orbit and Periorbital Structures

An understanding of the general sensory and motor innervation of the orbit and periorbital structures is necessary to control regional pain and provide akinesia of structures, if needed. Specific nerve blocks that target varying structures will be expanded upon within the chapter section discussing regional anesthesia.

R. Victor · A. Broussard · K. Paredes (✉)
University of California, Irvine, Irvine, CA, USA
e-mail: paredesk@hs.uci.edu

J. Tao (ed.), *Efficient Oculofacial Surgery*, https://doi.org/10.1007/978-3-031-63178-8_4

The Orbit [1]

Sensory innervation of the orbit and globe is mostly provided by the ophthalmic nerve—the first branch of the trigeminal nerve or cranial nerve (CN) V1. The frontal and nasociliary branches of the ophthalmic nerve pass through the muscular cone while some of the floor of the orbit is supplied by the infraorbital branch of the maxillary nerve (the second branch of the trigeminal nerve). The frontal nerve courses inferior to the orbital roof and branches into the supraorbital nerve, which innervates the forehead, and the supratrochlear nerve, which innervates the medial canthus. The nasociliary nerve provides sensory innervation to the eye alongside the nasal and sinus mucosa. The nasociliary nerve terminates as the infratrochlear nerve, which provides sensory innervation to the skin of the medial canthus and lateral nose, conjunctiva, and caruncle.

The trochlear nerve (CN IV) provides motor innervation to the superior oblique muscles and the abducens nerve (CN VI) provides motor innervation to the lateral rectus muscle. The oculomotor nerve (CN III) innervates all other extraocular muscles: superior rectus, inferior rectus, medial rectus, and inferior oblique muscles. CN III also controls the levator palpebrae superioris, which raises the upper eyelid. All except CN IV pass through the muscular cone and can be targeted by a regional block accordingly.

Periorbital Structures

The maxillary division of the trigeminal nerve (CN V2) innervates the lower eyelid, mainly via the infraorbital nerve. The infraorbital nerve passes through the foramen rotundum and along the floor of the orbit within the infraorbital groove and canal to emerge out of the infraorbital foramen below the infraorbital rim. The infraorbital nerve supplies sensation to the lower eyelid, cheek, upper gingiva, and teeth. The zygomaticotemporal and zygomaticofacial nerves also arise from CN V2 and supply cutaneous sensation over the lateral orbital rim and malar region, respectively.

The lower face is innervated by branches of the mandibular nerve (CN V3). The nerve passes through the foramen ovale and branches into the lingual nerve, inferior alveolar nerve, and auriculotemporal nerve. These branches provide overlapping sensory input to the lower jaw, lip, and chin. Redundant innervation makes the use of mandibular nerve blocks less effective for eyelid surgery.

The facial nerve (CN VII) provides motor innervation to the orbicularis muscle and the other muscles of facial expression. The facial nerve exits the skull at the stylomastoid foramen, deep to the tragus of the ear, and enters the parotid gland to divide into five peripheral branches: the temporal, zygomatic, buccal, mandibular, and cervical branches.

- The temporal branch supplies the orbicularis, procerus, corrugator, and frontalis muscles.
- The zygomatic branch innervates the orbicularis of the lower lid.
- The lower branches (buccal, mandibular, and cervical) innervate the facial muscles inferior to the orbit, extending to the platysma of the neck.

Approaches to Oculofacial Anesthesia

Anesthetic approaches for oculoplastic surgery involve topical local anesthetics and/or regional anesthesia (RA). The anesthetic plan may also include monitored anesthetic care or general anesthesia (GA) may be necessary depending on the medical history of the patient, procedure type, patient preference, and surgeon preference.

Topical Anesthesia

Overview

Topical anesthesia is a relatively simple and fast option to achieve superficial anesthesia of the orbit. Local anesthetic (LA) gel or eye drops are placed on the cornea and conjunctiva shortly before surgery. LAs inhibit voltage-gated sodium channels in the neuronal cell membrane to increase action potential thresholds and effectively decrease muscle contraction and pain perception without altering the level of consciousness. Commonly used topical agents include eye drop solutions of proparacaine hydrochloride 0.5% or tetracaine hydrochloride 0.5% alongside lidocaine hydrochloride 3.5% gel [2].

Indications

Adjuvants to RA nerve blocks to decrease the pain involved with needle injection, especially when pursuing a peribulbar or Sub-Tenon's approach, in children, or in needle-phobic patients [3].

- Minimize the stinging of antiseptic agents.
- Reduce the discomfort of corneal protectors [3].
- Patients on anticoagulation therapy (do not cause intraocular bleeding) [2–4].

Benefits and Drawbacks

If used for standalone anesthesia, topical anesthetics do not alter vision and avoid the need for LA to be injected near the eye, effectively eliminating needle-stick injury. Topical anesthetics cause less wound distortion than injectable LAs, do not increase IOP, and have been shown to be safer than the retrobulbar and peribulbar blocks used for RA [2, 5, 6]. However, topical agents do not provide akinesia of the eye and provide insufficient standalone anesthesia for oculoplastic procedures [2, 4, 5].

Technique

Topical anesthetic agents for the skin should be applied preoperatively 30–60 min before the desired time of peak effect [3]. For the ocular surface, the onset of effects is quicker. A few drops (1–2) are applied to the eye to produce conjunctival anesthesia within minutes. Cotton swabs soaked in the solution can be placed in the inferior fornix for 5 min to enhance the anesthetic effect [3]. The cotton-swab method can also be utilized to inject LA into the posterior lamella of the lower lid [7]. When used to reduce injection pain during RA nerve block, topical anesthetic ointment should be applied to the needle entry sites.

Regional Anesthesia

Overview

RA employs targeted nerve blocks with LA to achieve pain control of facial and orbital structures and akinesia of the extraocular muscles [2]. Nerve blocks have been suggested to aid in hemostasis and enhance patient cooperation [8]. Lidocaine, mepivacaine, bupivacaine, and ropivacaine are the most used agents used for RA [2]. Shorter acting LAs are preferred to avoid prolonged postoperative orbicularis weakness and lagophthalmos. Lidocaine and mepivacaine have a duration of 1–3 h after infiltration whereas bupivacaine can last more than 6–8 h.

Lidocaine hydrochloride [2]	• Onset of action: 2–3 min • Duration: 1–3 h depending on the strength of the preparation, with the duration of action extended when mixed with epinephrine • Maximum safe dose: 4.5 mg/kg and with epinephrine 7 mg/kg. One milliliter of 1% lidocaine contains 10 mg of lidocaine
Bupivacaine hydrochloride	• Onset of action: 10 min • Duration: 6–8 h • ~~Maximum safe dose: 2–2.5 mg/kg without epinephrine and 2.5–3 mg/kg with epinephrine~~

Hyaluronidase is sometimes used to enhance the spread of LA through connective tissue, optimizing the rate of anesthesia onset and surface area covered [2]. Epinephrine can be mixed with LA to achieve local vasoconstriction and hemostasis, thereby augmenting analgesia and limiting systemic spread [2]. An epinephrine concentration of 10 μg/mL (1:100,000) in LA provides adequate vasoconstriction for eyelid surgery, and hemostasis is usually observed within 1 min [3]. The anesthetist should be alerted if epinephrine is used because its systemic absorption can lead to cardiopulmonary complications.

Tranexamic acid (TXA) may be given along with local anesthetics to decrease postoperative edema and ecchymosis. TXA is a synthetic antifibrinolytic, which binds to plasminogen and prohibits its binding to fibrin and subsequent conversion to plasmin. The textbook editor (JT) uses the admixture of 1% lidocaine with 1:100,000 epinephrine, 0.5% bupivacaine, and TXA 100 mg/1 mL in equal parts for most oculofacial surgeries.

Injection site pain can be reduced with topical anesthetics for facial nerve blocks, but topical agents cannot control pain for nerve blocks that target deeper structures, such as in the retrobulbar block. Additional strategies to manage injection site pain include adding sodium bicarbonate 7.5% to RA agents to increase the overall injectate pH, premedicating with a sedative or opioid of short duration of action, and injecting slowly and incrementally [9]. If premedication is used for sedation, supplemental oxygen (O_2) should be given during the block to reduce risk of hypoxemia.

Multiple techniques exist for RA nerve block in oculoplastic surgery, but the most common are the retrobulbar, peribulbar, and Sub-Tenon's approaches [10]. These techniques can be supplemented with varying blocks of structures innervated by facial nerve branches and will be discussed below.

Indications

- Regional pain control in conjunction with MAC or GA
- Akinesia of extraocular muscles
- Postoperative pain control.

Benefits and Drawbacks

Advantages of RA include the ability to perform a procedure without GA, thus allowing faster recovery times in the post-anesthesia care unit (PACU) and a reduced need for systemic opioids and other analgesics for pain control [11]. Further, avoiding GA reduces complications associated with volatile anesthetic agents and with airway manipulation.

Drawbacks to RA involve risks of injection site pain, needlestick injury, wound distortion, conjunctival chemosis, and damage to the globe, tear drainage system, and superficial structures [3, 11, 12]. Blindness may occur in the event of retrobulbar hemorrhage, optic nerve damage, or ocular perforation. Inadvertent intravascular injection may lead to systemic toxicity and cardiopulmonary arrest, whereas optic nerve sheath injection may lead to anesthesia of the brainstem [1, 2, 11, 12]. Additional risks include myotoxicity with high concentrations of LA and allergic reactions.

Retrobulbar block has the highest incidence of adverse events, spanning globe perforation, respiratory arrest, severe vision loss due to retrobulbar hemorrhage, and optic nerve compression from LA infiltration [10, 12]. Complications occur less frequently with the peribulbar approach, although conjunctival chemosis secondary to the accumulation of LA within the orbit may occur [12].

General Technique

Patients must be requested to look straight ahead to protect the ophthalmic artery and optic nerve from damage caused by the injection needle [3]. The non-injecting hand should be anchored to the forehead or cheek for better stability. The injection should be ceased if the globe moves in the direction of the needle, if a sneezing reflex occurs, or if restriction of advancement is noted.

Gentle negative aspiration of the syringe should be performed after initial needle entry to rule out intravascular injection. LA should be administered slowly and in an advancing fashion that causes the tissue ahead of the needle to balloon [3].

Targeted Blocks

Retrobulbar block [1]	
Overview	The retrobulbar block targets the retrobulbar space, located behind the globe, to provide anesthesia and akinesia through infiltration of the intraconal space. LA is injected within the muscular cone and, accordingly, targets nerves that run through this space. Anesthesia of the cornea, uvea, and conjunctiva are provided through block of the ophthalmic nerve while akinesia is achieved in all extraocular muscles except for the superior oblique muscle
Goal effect	• Anesthesia of the cornea, uvea, and conjunctiva • Akinesia of all extraocular muscles other than the superior oblique
Technique	Identify the space lateral of the junction of middle and lateral thirds of the inferior orbital rim [3]. After the inferior orbital rim is palpated, the globe should be displaced superiorly to expand the space between the orbital floor and the globe. A 23–25 gauge needle of length 1.5 inches is inserted superior to the inferior orbital rim, bevel-up, and advanced upward and inward until the space behind the globe is entered [3]. The needle is advanced along the orbital floor until the first "pop" is felt when it is passed through the orbital septum and met with resistance. Following this signal, the needle is redirected approximately 45° medially and superiorly and advanced through a second "pop" that demonstrates passage through the muscular cone and entry into the target intraconal space. The needle should not advance more than 24 mm from the skin in total The syringe should be drawn back to confirm that the needle has not entered a vessel, at which point approximately 3–5 ml of LA should be injected into this space. Anterior displacement of the globe, drooping of the upper lid, and dilation of the pupil are expected during injection and signify that the injectate is entering the intraconal space. The needle is then withdrawn, and pressure is applied to the globe with gauze for 5–10 min to tamponade any potential retrobulbar hemorrhage

Peribulbar block [1]	
Overview	In a peribulbar block, LA is delivered to the extraconal space via two injections. One injection occurs inferotemporal and the other between the caruncle and the medial canthus. Enough LA can be deposited into the extraconal space such that it diffuses into the intraconal space because there are no discrete barriers that separate the two. The needle tip is farther away from the globe and retrobulbar structures than with a retrobulbar block, so a peribulbar approach may reduce the risk of injury at the cost of a slightly lower success rates of appropriate analgesia and akinesia
Goal effect	• Anesthesia of the cornea, uvea, and conjunctiva • Akinesia of all extraocular muscles other than the superior oblique
Technique	A peribulbar block can be achieved by combined inferotemporal and medial injections. To begin, the lower fornix should be exposed by pulling down on the lower lid and the needle should be inserted through the fornix below the lateral limbus. The needle should be directed slightly downwards and passed inferiorly and laterally. Total needle depth should not exceed 24 mm **Inferotemporal** The inferotemporal injection is divided into three injections, totaling 4–5 ml LA injectate in total. Inject 1 ml immediately posterior to the orbicularis oculi, another 1 ml anterior to the equator, and 2 ml after the needle is advanced past the globe **Medial** The medial injection of 3–4 ml LA is given between the caruncle and medial canthus. To ensure proper needle placement, the needle should be passed inferiorly and medially away from the globe for roughly 24 mm prior to injecting. Injecting through the caruncle can cause bleeding

Sub-Tenon's block [1]	
Overview	A sub-Tenon block is achieved by injecting LA into the space between the sclera and the overlying sub-Tenon capsule (episcleral space) via needle or cannula. If the conjunctiva is lifted off the sclera posterior to this fusion, the sub-Tenon capsule is also elevated, allowing injection of LA between the scleral and exposed episcleral space. Sub-Tenon's block does not require a sharp needle, and thus has been suggested to have a lower risk profile than retrobulbar and peribulbar approaches while maintaining similar anesthesia and akinesia

Sub-Tenon's block [1]	
Goal effect	• Anesthesia of the cornea, uvea, and conjunctiva • Akinesia of all extraocular muscles other than the superior oblique
Technique	To begin, topical LA drops are often instilled to improve patient comfort. Cauterizing the incision space may also assist with reducing subconjunctival hemorrhage. An eyelid speculum, or the finger of an assistant, should be used to keep the eyelids apart. The patient is asked to look upwards and outwards to expose the inferonasal quadrant and the conjunctiva. The Tenon's capsule is gripped with a non-toothed forceps 5–10 mm away from the limbus and the sclera is exposed via a small incision made with blunt-tipped scissors. A sub-Tenon cannula should be inserted along the curvature of the globe and 3–5 ml of LA agent is carefully injected

Retrobulbar Versus Peribulbar Versus Sub-Tenon's Blocks

Different block types ultimately correspond to the same final location of LA within the muscular cone, and it is important to evaluate the success of the block by assessing for globe or extraocular muscle motion [13].

The major benefit of the retrobulbar block is that it provides rapid akinesia to the extraocular muscles, has a longer duration of effect, and is associated with less chemosis than the peribulbar block due to lower injection volumes. However, retrobulbar block has increased risks compared to peribulbar and Sub-Tenon's techniques. These risks span injury to the globe, optic nerve, or extraocular muscles alongside retrobulbar hemorrhage and brainstem anesthesia. Accordingly, it is not the suggested approach for patients with coagulopathies or myopia, which generally involves an axial length greater than 25 mm.

Because the retrobulbar cone is not sealed by an intermuscular membrane, a large-volume peribulbar (extraconal) nerve block can theoretically provide as effective anesthesia and akinesia as a targeted small-volume retrobulbar nerve block. Compared to a retrobulbar block, a peribulbar block allows for decreased insertion depth, a shorter needle, and a more gradual needle trajectory that all decrease the likelihood of adverse events [14, 15]. As such, a peribulbar block should always be used in anticoagulated or myopic patients. While a peribulbar approach is safer, the major drawback is that it has a slower onset than the retrobulbar approach (approximately 5 min) and may require multiple injections. It also runs a higher risk of conjunctival chemosis secondary to the higher volume of injectate [14, 17].

A sub-Tenon's block is generally administered as a supplement when a retrobulbar or peribulbar block does not provide adequate anesthesia and akinesia. As a standalone block, the sub-Tenon's block provides excellent anesthesia and akinesia without requiring a sharp needle and is less likely to cause systemic complications than retrobulbar or peribulbar blocks. Sub-Tenon's block has been suggested to be efficacious in vitreoretinal, strabismus, and trabeculectomy procedures. A Sub-Tenon's block is unsuitable for procedures that require intact conjunctiva (such as in glaucoma procedures) or akinesia and in patients with prior scleral buckling, local infection, or highly myopic eyes.

Overview of periorbital nerve blocks	
Upper and lower eyelid blocks	The eyelid blocks involve infiltration of LA directly into the eyelids to achieve akinesia of the orbicularis oculi. An upper eyelid block is completed at 1 cm above the medial canthus whereas the lower eyelid block is performed 0.5 cm below the medial canthus
Supraorbital block	A supraorbital block provides anesthesia to the upper eyelid, brow, forehead, and anterior scalp. A large area is anesthetized with a smaller volume of LA. The block is administered at the supraorbital foramen, roughly 2 cm from the midline of the face. The needle is inserted inferolateral and 0.5 cm below the supraorbital foramen. Care should be taken to avoid penetration of the foramen

Overview of periorbital nerve blocks	
Supratrochlear block	The supratrochlear nerve block is often used in conjunction with the supraorbital block to maximize forehead anesthesia. Block location is at the supraorbital margin, approximately 3 mm medial to a vertical line from the medial canthus. A needle is placed at this site and advanced
Nasociliary block	The nasociliary block allows for anesthesia of mucosal surfaces of the sphenoid, ethmoid, frontal sinuses and the anterior septum, lateral nasal cavity, ala, and apex of the nose. The anesthetic can be aimed toward the anterior and posterior ethmoidal foramina to deliver additional anesthetic to the infratrochlear nerve. Epinephrine should not be used to reduce the risk of retinal artery spasm
Infratrochlear block	The infratrochlear block provides anesthesia to the inferior portion of the medial canthus, the lateral nose, medial conjunctiva, and caruncle and is often used during nasal surgery or skin laceration repairs. Infiltration occurs at the superomedial orbit below the trochlea
Anterior ethmoid block	The anterior ethmoid block allows for anesthesia of the anterior nasal septum, the lateral nasal cavity wall, and the tip of the nose. The anterior ethmoidal foramen is at a halfway point between the posterior palpebral fold and the eyebrow, found medially at a depth of 1.5 cm
Infraorbital block	The infraorbital nerve provides sensory innervation to the lower eyelid, lateral nose, upper lip, and maxillary teeth. Accordingly, this block is useful for lower eyelid and maxillofacial procedures. The maxillary branch of CN V2 courses within the infraorbital groove before emerging 1 cm below the inferior orbital rim at the infraorbital foramen The block is performed through either an intraoral or extraoral approach. The intraoral approach is accomplished by inserting a needle into the mucosa superiorly, parallel to the upper second bicuspid, and advancing it toward the foramen. Careful palpation is necessary to prevent injection into the foramen. The extraoral approach approaches the foramen subcutaneously and is considered more straightforward
Zygomaticofacial, zygomaticotemporal block	The zygomaticofacial branch innervates the skin overlying the zygomatic bone and can be targeted by injecting laterally at the inferolateral orbital rim The zygomaticotemporal branch provides sensory innervation to the temporal skin alongside secretomotor innervation to the lacrimal nerve. A zygomaticotemporal block should begin at the concave surface of the posterolateral orbital rim and advance inferiorly to the level of the lateral canthus

Monitored Anesthesia Care

Overview

MAC involves the administration of sedative, anxiolytic, and analgesic medications alongside the continual monitoring and support of patient vitals by a qualified anesthesia provider. Patients under MAC show a purposeful response under repeated stimulation and are not intubated, as opposed to patients under GA who are unarousable and have ventilation support measures in place. While MAC is not defined by depth of sedation, MAC is indicated when deeper levels of analgesia and sedation beyond moderate sedation may occur [19]. Compared to GA, MAC allows for faster operating room (OR) turnover time and less postoperative nausea and vomiting: both of which are preferable for oculofacial procedures that adhere to a day procedure schedule. MAC must be supplemented with regional anesthesia to allow the patient to properly tolerate the procedure, however, and some cases may involve surgical areas that cannot be reliably anesthetized with LA. In these cases, GA is required.

Sedation is a continuum ranging from minimal anxiolysis to moderate and deep sedation. The depth of sedation during MAC should be assessed regularly by assessing patient responsiveness to stimulus and with Bispectral index (BIS) [14]. Patients may respond variably to sedative agents and thus an anesthetist intending to produce a given level of sedation should be able to rescue the patient if the level of sedation becomes deeper than initially intended. For example, providers individuals intending to administer deep sedation should be able to manage and rescue patients who exhibit airway distress or cardiovascular instability [15].

Drugs selected for use in MAC ideally have a fast onset and short duration of action [16]. These most commonly include benzodiazepines, propofol, opioids, dexmedetomidine, and ketamine [14]. Benzodiazepines (most commonly midazolam) are anxiolytic, amnesic, and sedative but do not provide analgesia, may cause respiratory depression, and are contraindicated in patients with angle-closure glaucoma or reported memory loss. Propofol allows for rapid induction and emergence but may cause pain on injection, respiratory and cardiac depression, and vasodilation. Opioids, most commonly the short-acting fentanyl, allow for sedation and analgesia but may cause respiratory depression and perioperative nausea and vomiting. Dexmedetomidine allows for sedation, anxiolysis, and analgesia with an effect that mimics natural sleep, but may cause hypotension and require a loading dose with continuous drip to maintain proper depth of sedation. Lastly, ketamine produces a dissociative amnesic state with significant analgesia alongside having minimal effect on blood pressure and heart rate but may increase secretions that interfere with the airway and may also cause nystagmus. During MAC, the potential for conversion to GA is always possible and may be required in circumstances such as respiratory distress, hypoventilation, hypoxia, or aspiration [17].

Indications

MAC is most appropriate for surgical procedures that are short in duration and when the procedure can be reliably performed with pain control via LA and moderate to deep sedation. As such, many oculofacial procedures can be performed under MAC.

Benefits and Drawbacks

The main benefit of MAC is fewer side effects than full GA. Drawbacks of MAC include patient awareness during the procedure and lack of total postoperative amnesia. Patients undergoing a procedure with MAC must be able to tolerate a degree of awareness throughout surgery and should be counseled accordingly beforehand. Additional concerns include respiratory complications from aspiration and complications related to patient movement, such as damage to the orbit from sharp surgical tools near the eye [14].

General Anesthesia

Overview

GA is necessary when intraoperative pain cannot be mitigated with LA alone, such as in the repair of ocular trauma and enucleation, orbital surgery, and exenteration procedures. Certain contexts and patient conditions also indicate GA as the preferred approach, such as contexts where psychological awareness during surgery would not be tolerated or when the airway must be secured with intubation. A stable state of sedation must be maintained during GA to optimize patient safety and comfort. The patient should follow fasting guidelines, and an attempt should be made to maintain a day-case surgery by using drugs that are rapidly metabolized and eliminated [9]. These agents include propofol, fentanyl or remifentanil, NSAIDs, and short- or intermediate-acting muscle relaxants.

Airway management is crucial in all procedures under GA. In the context of oculoplastic surgery, the relationship between GA agents, intubation, and intraocular pressure (IOP) requires additional consideration. These concerns will be elaborated upon below.

Indications

Patient conditions warranting GA include [9]:

- Conditions
  - Moderate or severe trauma
  - Severe anxiety or claustrophobia
  - Localized infection
  - Uncontrolled tremors
- Patient history
  - Severe language or communication barriers
  - Abnormalities of airway (e.g. hypognathia)
  - Allergy to LA solutions
  - Prior complication with RA
  - Pediatric patients
- Prolonged or invasive procedures
- Patient or surgeon request

Benefits and Drawbacks

Benefits of GA involve the ability to provide unconscious sedation throughout procedures that involve intraoperative pain that cannot be controlled sufficiently with LA and would be inappropriate for patients to endure in a semiconscious state.

Drawbacks of GA include greater associated risks and more rigid perioperative restrictions. Volatile agents used in GA are associated with increased risk of complications that span transient confusion, nausea, vomiting, respiratory depression, urinary retention, emergence delirium, and hypotension alongside the rare risk of malignant hyperthermia.

Airway Management

Airway management is key to patient safety in GA and can be achieved via endotracheal intubation (ETI) or with a supraglottic airway device (SGA), which includes the laryngeal mask airway (LMA) [9, 18]. The choice between standard ETI and SGA for an oculoplastic procedure is mostly based on patient factors that may compromise the airway or impose aspiration risk, such as GERD or obesity.

- ETI offers a more secure airway than SGA and should be used if the patient has an elevated risk of aspiration secondary to a history of gastric reflux disease, obesity, hiatal hernia, or gastroparesis from diabetes mellitus (DM). A secure airway device is of heightened relevance during oculofacial procedures because it can be difficult to adjust a dislodged device with limited access to the patient's head [22]. However, ETI may inadvertently increase IOP due to increased risk of straining and coughing during extubation [18]. This can be managed with pretreatment of fentanyl, remifentanil, or dexmedetomidine before extubation [24]. ETI also requires that a nondepolarizing neuromuscular blocking agent be administered and titrated.

- SGA may offer a reduced risk of coughing during extubation due to smoother removal [18]. SGA use also produces a smaller increase in IOP than ETI. However, an SGA can accidentally become displaced due to inadvertent surgeon contact and should be reevaluated regularly.

Intraocular pressure (IOP)

GA is associated with significant changes in IOP throughout the perioperative period.

Decreases in IOP occur during induction and with volatile agents. Propofol, thiopental, and etomidate can decrease IOP by approximately 30%. This drop in IOP is exacerbated by use of volatile anesthetics to maintain anesthesia after induction [19, 20].

Increases in IOP occur with succinylcholine and ketamine use and during valsalva. Depolarizing neuromuscular blocking agents like succinylcholine cause a transient increase in IOP. If nondepolarizing neuromuscular blockade is pursued, neostigmine and glycopyrrolate reversal agents will also increase IOP [21]. Vomiting increases IOP by approximately 30–40 mm Hg, so postoperative prophylaxis of nausea and vomiting should be given [22]. Antiemetics are given prophylactically to reduce this risk, commonly ondansetron or dexamethasone. External pressure applied to the eye by the surgeon will increase IOP, although this is not specific to GA [22–25].

Anesthetic Strategy by Surgical Approach

RA with or without MAC [26, 27]	GA
• Eyelid surgery • Blepharoplasty • Entropion and ectropion repair • Ptosis surgery • Chalazion operations • Operations on the upper lacrimal apparatus	• **Bony orbital procedures** • **Enucleation** • **Evisceration** • **Exenteration** • **Dacryocystorhinostomy and other lower lacrimal surgery** • **Rhytidectomy (forehead, face, or midface)** • **Traumatic eye injury**

Preoperative Considerations

Oculofacial surgical procedures are generally low risk and thus the impact of chronic medical conditions often have less of an impact than they may be within other surgical settings. A review of pertinent medical history and medication regimens should always occur to optimize safety.

Preanesthetic exam assessment	
Surgical requirements	• **Communication and cooperation** – Does the patient understand the instructions? – Will the patient communicate discomfort to the surgical team? • **Positioning** – Can the patient lie flat comfortably during eye surgery with no movement?
Focused history	• **Screen for common comorbidities** – DM, HTN, obesity, COPD • **Screen for contraindications to surgery** – Recent myocardial infarction (within 30 days) – Recent percutaneous coronary intervention (within 14 days without stenting or within 30 days with stenting) – New onset of clinically significant arrhythmia(s) – Decompensated heart failure – New onset severe pulmonary condition or exacerbation of a severe chronic condition – New onset neurologic condition – Malignant hypertension with evidence of acute end-organ damage – Recent episode of diabetic ketoacidosis or hyperosmolar hyperglycemic nonketotic syndrome
Focused physical	• Standard airway assessment • Assessment for abnormalities or conditions that interfere with the ability to lie supine comfortably when topical or regional anesthesia is planned
Medication screening	• Anticoagulants • Beta-adrenoreceptor antagonists • Muscarinic agonists • Phenylephrine • Alpha-2 adrenergic agonists • Atropine • Pilocarpine • NSAIDs • Glucagon-like peptide-1 receptor agonists • Ecothiopate

Preanesthetic exam assessment	
Fasting screening	• 6 h of fasting from non-clear liquids and food prior to elective procedures requiring anesthesia or sedation • 8 h of fasting following a large or fatty meal • Patients may drink clear liquids (e.g., water, juices without pulp, coffee or tea without milk, carbohydrate drinks) until two hours before elective procedures requiring anesthesia or sedation but should consume no liquids within two hours of surgery

Diabetes Mellitus

Diabetes mellitus (DM) is frequently encountered as a comorbidity in the ophthalmic surgical population and thus is of relevance. Patients with DM should be preferentially scheduled for morning procedures to better avoid disturbance to their daily routine and insulin regimen [28]. Sequelae of poor glycemic control in DM include obesity and cheiroarthropathy, and these factors pose a challenge to securing the airway with LMA or ETI in GA or in maintaining a patent airway during MAC sedation [29]. Fasting blood glucose should be monitored preoperatively and kept below 180 mg/dL (10 mmol/L) using subcutaneous rapid-acting insulin or continuous infusion of regular insulin therapy if necessary [30]. Poor intraoperative glycemic control may impair cerebrovascular reactivity, exacerbate neurologic insults, and increase the risk for adverse cardiovascular events while under anesthesia [29].

Anticoagulants

Patients actively taking anticoagulant agents are at increased thrombotic and hemorrhagic risk [3]. Patients with high thromboembolic risk who undergo procedures associated with higher levels of blood loss, such as orbital and lacrimal surgery, should stop antiplatelet agents, direct oral anticoagulants, and warfarin prior to the procedure with permission from the patient's cardiologist. Low-risk patients can cease all anticoagulant agents [31]. Thrombotic risk is assessed on a patient-specific basis. The following are instructions according to specific agents.

- Aspirin—reduce to 81 mg/day (1 baby aspirin/day) if higher dose and need to continue, stop 5–7 days for normal platelet count and secondary prevention, stop 7–10 days if primary prevention or thrombocytopenia, restart day 1–2 after surgery unless you have active bleeding.
- Aggrenox® (dipyridamole)—stop 3 days before your surgery, restart day 1–2 after surgery unless you have active bleeding.
- Brilinta® (ticagrelor)—stop 5 days before surgery, restart day 2 after surgery.
- Coumadin® (warfarin)—INR 1.5–3, then stop 5 days before surgery; INR 3–4.5, then stop 6 days before surgery; INR more than 4.5, Vitamin K and delay surgery.
- Effient® (prasugrel)—stop 5 days before surgery, restart day 2 after surgery.
- Eliquis® (apixaban)—Creatinine clearance (CrCl) more than 50, stop 2 days before surgery restart day 3 after surgery; CrCl less than 50, stop 3–4 days before surgery, restart day 4–6 after surgery.
- Plavix® (clopidogrel)—stop 5 days before surgery, restart day 2 after surgery.
- Pradaxa® (dabigatran)—CrCl more than 50, stop 2 days before surgery, restart day 3 after surgery; CrCl less than 50, stop 3 4 days before surgery, restart day 4–6 after surgery.
- Savaysa® (edoxaban)—CrCl more than 50, stop 2 days before surgery, restart day 3 after surgery; CrCl less than 50, stop 3–4 days before surgery, restart day 4–6 after surgery.
- Ticlid® (ticlopidine)—stop 5 days before surgery, restart day 2 after surgery.
- Xarelto® (rivaroxaban)—CrCl more than 50, stop 2 days before surgery, restart day 3 after surgery; CrCl less than 50, stop 3–4 days before surgery, restart day 4–6 after surgery.
- Other nonsteroidal anti-inflammatory drugs—most (ibuprofen, naprosyn) stop 1–3 days before surgery; long-acting (Meloxicam®/Piroxicam®/Nabumetone®)

stop 10 days before surgery, restart postop day 2 after surgery as needed.
- Avoid substances that thin the blood, for example turmeric, ginger, garlic, gingko biloba, etc. for 14 days.

Other Medications

Ecothiopate, an acetylcholinesterase inhibitor historically used in the treatment of glaucoma, can result in prolonged paralysis when succinylcholine is administered due to irreversible inhibition of pseudocholinesterase [21]. Additional medications that should be screened for include beta blockers, muscarinic agonists, phenylephrine, alpha-2 blockers, atropine, pilocarpine, and NSAIDs. Glucagon-like peptide-1 receptor agonists (GLP-1 RA) delay gastric emptying. The American Society of Anesthesiologists (ASA) recommends that patients taking glucagon-like peptide-1 receptor agonists (GLP-1 RAs) withhold the medication before surgery. If taken daily, GLP-1 RAs should be stopped on the day of surgery. If taken weekly, GLP-1 RAs should be stopped a week before surgery.

Patient Positioning

Supine position in a flatbed is standard for most oculoplastic procedures because it allows for the best surgical and anesthetic access while preserving patient comfort [32].

- The anesthetist should be stationed to the side of the patient with the IV cannula and pulse oximeter probe placed on that side for access.
- The patient should be positioned beneath the operating microscope with the headrest lying flat and the face pointing upward.
- The head should be taped in a steady position above the level of the heart to avoid increased venous pressure in the eye. Substantial neck flexion or extension should be avoided.
- The nasal oxygen cannula should be secured to avoid displacement.
- The non-operative eye should be protected, especially in the case of patients undergoing GA.
- The arms should be secured at the sides to avoid unexpected movements of the extremities.
- The body should be secured with safety straps to reduce fall risk.
- The lumbar spine should be supported with pillows placed beneath the knees.

Non-standard positioning may be required when a medical condition prevents normal positioning. Common examples include orthopnea, chronic obstructive pulmonary disease, spinal deformity, and obesity. Strategies for patient positioning when supination is contraindicated include upright seating with the head reclined, Trendelenburg, and repositioning of the surgeon or microscope. GA may be advantageous in these cases.

Additional Strategies

A sneezing reflex may occur during RA block of the orbit. It has been suggested that this reflex occurs more often with a peribulbar block than with a retrobulbar block [33]. Unexpected and sudden head movements associated with sneezing during RA injection may cause injury to the globe, ocular vasculature, or optic nerve [16]. If sneezing occurs, time should be given for the sneezing to completely abate before proceeding with a block.

A small dose of fentanyl, dexmedetomidine, or antihistamines have been found to suppress the sneeze reflex during peribulbar and retrobulbar block [16].

Post-anesthesia Recovery

All patients should undergo postoperative care in a recovery area that is equipped to detect respiratory or cardiovascular compromise. Most oculoplastic procedures adhere to a day procedure schedule, and patients who are breathing spontaneously, alert, speaking, responding appropriately to commands, and hemodynamically stable can be prioritized for discharge [26]. The timeline of recovery is as follows:

1. **Early recovery**
   a. Operative room or the post-anesthesia care unit (PACU).
   b. Patient recovers protective reflexes and motor function.
2. **Intermediate recovery**
   a. After discharge from the PACU but before discharge home.
   b. Patient recovers coordination and physiologic function.
3. **Late recovery**
   a. After discharge from the hospital or the ambulatory surgery facility.
   b. The patient recovers completely from surgery and is ready for routine daily activities.

Patients should have an escort to transport them to their home. Patients should be instructed to avoid driving and operating machinery until vision has been restored to baseline, sedative effects have dissipated, and the eye patch has been removed. This occurs the day after surgery at minimum. Alcohol consumption should also be delayed similarly [26].

Safety Concerns

Fire Risk

OR fire is a major safety concern in oculoplastic procedures due to the close proximity of oxygen gas, cautery equipment, and patient draping within a relatively small operative field [34]. These elements form a fire triad: enriched oxygen, a source of ignition, and a fuel source [35]. All members of the surgical team—anesthesiologist, surgeon, and nursing staff—are involved in management of these factors and thus the management of fire risk is a shared responsibility.

Careful control of O_2 is essential. An impermeable barrier should be established between the patient's nares and the surgical field by securing drapes to the face. Compressed medical air should be continually flushed under the draping at 10 L/min during the procedure to reduce O_2 and CO_2 buildup [34, 36]. Vacuum suctioning can be used to further vent the surgical field. If supplemental O_2 is required, an air and O_2 blender should be used to deliver the lowest O_2 concentration needed—ideally less than 30% [34]. Adequate O_2 saturation should be ensured by pulse oximetry.

Closed-loop communication is crucial when O_2 concentrations above 30% are expected to be used. The surgeon should alert the anesthesiologist when an ignition source (e.g. cautery) is to be used and to turn the "oxygen off". The anesthesiologist then should reduce the O_2. Once O_2 concentration has dropped below 30% the anesthetist should inform the surgeon that the "oxygen is off" and the heat source is safe to use.

Fuel sources for OR fire include alcohol-based prep solutions, draping, tubing, and organic matter. Care should be taken to separate these from ignition sources, which include electrosurgery units (ESUs), lasers, and fiberoptic lights.

Table 1 OR fire triad components

Fire risk	*Agent*	*Risks and management*
Oxidizers	**Oxygen:**	• O_2 is the oxidizer in 95% of OR fires [35]. • The lowest concentration should be used.
	Nitrous oxide:	• Has the same oxidizing potential as O_2. • Should be avoided when possible.

Fire risk	*Agent*	*Risks and management*
Fuels	**Alcohol-based prep solutions** *Alcohol-based surgical prep solutions contain 70–75% isopropyl alcohol and are excellent fuels*	• Allow to dry for at least 3 min before use of an ignition source. • The prep solution should be completely dry before draping. • Alcohol-based fires have a nearly invisible flame. • Povidone-iodine solutions and chlorhexidine soaps are not flammable.
	Draping *Surgical drapes, towels, sponges, and gauzes manufactured from cotton, paper, or plastics are flammable.*	• Oxygen can be trapped within cotton towels or drapes. • Configure drapes to minimize O_2 accumulation. • Suction or flush the field with medical air to minimize O_2 buildup. • Moisten sponges and towels if used near an ignition source. • Have sterile water or saline available for fire suppression. • Keep excess drapes and towels in an area far removed from ignition sources.
	Tubing *Endotracheal tubes and laryngeal masks made from either silicone or polyvinyl chloride*	• Use an ETT that is laser- and fire-resistant. • Tubing should have a dual cuff. • Both tube cuffs should be filled with saline that is colored with methylene blue.
	Organic matter *Hair*	• Remove ignitable organic material before use of an ignition source.
Ignition sources	**Electrosurgery unit (ESU)** *Bovie*	• Greatest risk: Holding the Bovie tip above the tissue or touching the tip to a hemostat. • Use of a bipolar ESU lowers the risk of spark or arcing [35].
	Surgical lasers	• High-power lasers can ignite dry materials. • Check to ensure laser fibers are not broken or cracked.
	Fiberoptic lights	• Fiberoptic lights can create high temperatures when focused. • Direct burn injury or melting surgical drapes.

Fire Management

Early warning signs of OR fire include a smell of smoke, a popping sound, or a flash of light [36]. If fire is suspected, the procedure should be halted when it is safe and the source should be investigated. If a fire is confirmed all efforts should be directed toward controlling and extinguishing it.

If the fire is on the patient:

- Stop the flow of airway gases.
- Pour water or saline on hot spots.
- Remove drapes and burning material.
- Extinguish small fires by patting them with wet towels or sponges.
- Use a fire extinguisher if the first attempt to control the fire fails.
- Assess for smoldering elements and flames that may be hidden underneath the drapes.

If the fire is in the airway:

- Immediately remove the ETT and stop the flow of airway gases.
- Pour water or saline into the airway to extinguish residual burning materials.
- Resume ventilation after the fire is extinguished—ideally without O_2 or nitrous oxide.
- Search the upper airway via laryngoscopy for melted plastic and any soft tissue swelling that could lead to airway compromise.
- Assess the lower conducting airways via bronchoscopy for injury or inflammation due to inhalation of smoke or superheated gas.

Begin the RACE fire protocol if a fire persists despite the above efforts:

1. **Rescue**—Remove the patient from burning source.
2. **Alarm**—Activate the fire alarm system.
3. **Confine**—Close OR doors after evacuation. Turn off medical gas supply lines.
4. **Extinguish**—Use a fire extinguisher as you retreat from the area.

After rescuing the patient, assess the airway and the posterior and anterior body surfaces for burn injuries [36]. A dry, sterile dressing should be applied to injured areas. The patient and all OR personnel should be screened for smoke inhalation. Inhalation injury may not initially be symptomatic but can quickly progress toward severe respiratory distress. Other severe injuries include full thickness burns that encompass 10% or more of the total body surface and any burns involving the eyes, ears, face, hands, feet, or perineum. Severe burn injuries warrant transfer of care to a burn center.

Conclusion

An understanding of different anesthetic approaches to oculofacial surgery is important when evaluating the appropriate strategy for a specific patient or procedure. Strategies covered in this chapter include topical anesthetics, RA blocks, MAC, and full general anesthesia. Variables to consider include desired depth of sedation, surgical requirements, and patient or provider preference.

References

1. Nerad J. Clinical anatomy. 2nd ed. In: Techniques in ophthalmic plastic surgery; 2021.
2. Mahan M, Flor R, Purt B. Local and regional anesthesia in ophthalmology and ocular trauma; 2022.
3. Lodhi O, Tripathy K. Anesthesia for eye surgery. StatPearls Publishing; 2022.
4. Nanji KC, Roberto SA, Morley MG, Bayes J. Preventing adverse events in cataract surgery: recommendations from a Massachusetts expert panel. Anesth Analg. 2018;126(5):1537–47. https://doi.org/10.1213/ANE.0000000000002529.
5. Zhao LQ, Zhu H, Zhao PQ, Wu QR, Hu YQ. Topical anesthesia versus regional anesthesia for cataract surgery: a meta-analysis of randomized controlled trials. Ophthalmology. 2012;119(4):659–67. https://doi.org/10.1016/j.ophtha.2011.09.056.
6. Lee RM, Thompson JR, Eke T. Severe adverse events associated with local anaesthesia in cataract surgery: 1 year national survey of practice and complications in the UK. Br J Ophthalmol. 2016;100(6):772–6. https://doi.org/10.1136/bjophthalmol-2015-307060.
7. Moody BR, Holds JB. Anesthesia for office-based oculoplastic surgery. Dermatol Surg. 2005;31(7 Pt 1): 766–9. https://doi.org/10.1097/00042728-200507000-00007.
8. Ing EB, Philteos J, Sholohov G, et al. Local anesthesia and anxiolytic techniques for oculoplastic surgery. Clin Ophthalmol. 2019;13:153–60. https://doi.org/10.2147/OPTH.S188790.
9. Imtiaz WR, Chaudry IA. Anaesthesia for oculoplastic surgical procedures. Oxford Specialist Handbooks in Anaesthesia; 2012.
10. Duker JS, Belmont JB, Benson WE, et al. Inadvertent globe perforation during retrobulbar and peribulbar anesthesia. Patient characteristics, surgical management, and visual outcome. Ophthalmology. 1991;98(4):519–26. https://doi.org/10.1016/s0161-6420(91)32262-0
11. Folino TB, Mahboobi SK. Regional anesthetic blocks; 2022.
12. Kumar CM. Orbital regional anesthesia: complications and their prevention. Indian J Ophthalmol. 2006;54(2):77–84. https://doi.org/10.4103/0301-4738.25826.
13. Ripart J, Lefrant JY, de La Coussaye JE, Prat-Pradal D, Vivien B, Eledjam JJ. Peribulbar versus retrobulbar anesthesia for ophthalmic surgery: an anatomical comparison of extraconal and intraconal injections. Anesthesiology. 2001;94(1):56–62. https://doi.org/10.1097/00000542-200101000-00013.

14. Das S, Ghosh S. Monitored anesthesia care: an overview. J Anaesthesiol Clin Pharmacol. 2015;31(1):27–9. https://doi.org/10.4103/0970-9185.150525
15. Continuum of depth of sedation: definition of general anesthesia and levels of sedation/analgesia; 2018.
16. Hakim KY, Alsaeid MA. Comparative study between the efficacy of fentanyl, antihistamines, and dexmedetomidine in suppressing photic sneeze reflex during peribulbar block. Anesth Essays Res. 2019;13(1):40–43. https://doi.org/10.4103/aer.AER_174_18
17. Kim S, Chang BA, Rahman A, et al. Analysis of urgent/emergent conversions from monitored anesthesia care to general anesthesia with airway instrumentation. BMC Anesthesiol. 2021;21(1):183. https://doi.org/10.1186/s12871-021-01403-9
18. Lamb K, James MF, Janicki PK. The laryngeal mask airway for intraocular surgery: effects on intraocular pressure and stress responses. Br J Anaesth. 1992;69(2):143–7. https://doi.org/10.1093/bja/69.2.143.
19. Mirakhur RK, Shepherd WF, Darrah WC. Propofol or thiopentone: effects on intraocular pressure associated with induction of anaesthesia and tracheal intubation (facilitated with suxamethonium). Br J Anaesth. 1987;59(4):431–6. https://doi.org/10.1093/bja/59.4.431.
20. Self WG, Ellis PP. The effect of general anesthetic agents on intraocular pressure. Surv Ophthalmol. 1977;21(6):494–500. https://doi.org/10.1016/s0039-6257(77)90001-7
21. Greenstein SH, Abramson DH, Pitts WR. Systemic atropine and glaucoma. Bull N Y Acad Med. 1984;60(10):961–8.
22. Hsu YP, Chu KC, Bai CH, Huang CJ, Chen C, Hsu CW. Safety and efficacy of clonidine on postoperative vomiting and pain in pediatric ophthalmic surgery: a systematic review and meta-analysis. Paediatr Anaesth. 2019;29(10):1011–23. https://doi.org/10.1111/pan.13712
23. Sheen MJ, Chang FL, Ho ST. Anesthetic premedication: new horizons of an old practice. Acta Anaesthesiol Taiwan. 2014;52(3):134–42. https://doi.org/10.1016/j.aat.2014.08.001.
24. Gan TJ, Diemunsch P, Habib AS, et al. Consensus guidelines for the management of postoperative nausea and vomiting. Anesth Analg. 2014;118(1):85–113. https://doi.org/10.1213/ANE.0000000000000002.
25. Sinclair DR, Chung F, Mezei G. Can postoperative nausea and vomiting be predicted? Anesthesiology. 1999;91(1):109–18. https://doi.org/10.1097/00000542-199907000-00018.
26. Gasanova I, Joshi G. Opthalmic anaesthesia: postoperative management. Oxford Specialist Handbooks in Anaesthesia; 2012.
27. Abdeldayem OT, Amer GF, Abdulla MG. Postoperative analgesic efficacy of Sub-Tenon's block with levobupivacaine in retinal surgery under general anesthesia. Anesth Essays Res. 2019;13(3):437–40. https://doi.org/10.4103/aer.AER_116_19.
28. Kumar C, Dodds C, Gayer S. Preoperative assessment and preparation. In: Ophthalmic anaesthesia. Oxford University Press; 2012.
29. Sreedharan R, Abdelmalak B. Diabetes mellitus: preoperative concerns and evaluation. Anesthesiol Clin. 2018;36(4):581–97. https://doi.org/10.1016/j.anclin.2018.07.007.
30. Duggan E, Chen Y. Glycemic management in the operating room: screening, monitoring, oral hypoglycemics, and insulin therapy. Curr Diab Rep. 2019;19(11):134. https://doi.org/10.1007/s11892-019-1277-4.
31. Kim C, Pfeiffer ML, Chang JR, Burnstine MA. Perioperative considerations for antithrombotic therapy in oculofacial surgery: a review of current evidence and practice guidelines. Ophthalmic Plast Reconstr Surg. 2022;38(3):226–33. https://doi.org/10.1097/IOP.0000000000002058.
32. Eke T, Palte H. Opthalmic anesthesia: patient positioning for eye surgery. Oxford Specialist Handbooks in Anaesthesia; 2012.
33. Ahn ES, Mills DM, Meyer DR, Stasior GO. Sneezing reflex associated with intravenous sedation and periocular anesthetic injection. Am J Ophthalmol. 2008;146(1):31–5. https://doi.org/10.1016/j.ajo.2008.02.013.
34. Day AT, Rivera E, Farlow JL, Gourin CG, Nussenbaum B. Surgical fires in otolaryngology: a systematic and narrative review. Otolaryngol Head Neck Surg. 2018;158(4):598–16. https://doi.org/10.1177/0194599817746926.
35. Mehta SP, Bhananker SM, Posner KL, Domino KB. Operating room fires: a closed claims analysis. Anesthesiology. 2013;118(5):1133–9. https://doi.org/10.1097/ALN.0b013e31828afa7b.
36. Apfelbaum JL, Caplan RA, Barker SJ, et al. Practice advisory for the prevention and management of operating room fires: an updated report by the American society of anesthesiologists task force on operating room fires. Anesthesiology. 2013;118(2):271–90. https://doi.org/10.1097/ALN.0b013e31827773d2.

5 Pain Management in Oculofacial Surgery

Charlotte L. Marous and Edward J. Wladis

Abstract

The management of discomfort after oculofacial surgery is critical. Postoperative pain may be inadequately treated in approximately half of all surgical procedures, with 10% of these patients going on to suffer from long-term postoperative discomfort (Carroll et al. in J Reconstr Microsurg 29:213–222, 2013 [1]). Historically, opioid analgesics were used to manage postoperative pain following orbital and periorbital surgery, although the side effect profile of these medications poses serious concerns, including risks of nausea, emesis, sedation, pruritus, urinary retention, delirium, respiratory depression, and long-term dependence (Benyamin et al. in Pain Physician 11:S105–S120, 2008 [2]). Coupled with tighter prescriber legislation, enhanced awareness of these issues has resulted in a shift towards employing alternatives to narcotic analgesics in perioperative patients (Xie et al. in JAMA Ophthalmol 139:157–162, 2021 [3]). This chapter characterizes the armamentarium of agents and optimal administration practices to enhance the oculofacial surgical experience.

Keywords

Analgesia · Postoperative pain · Orbit · Eyelid · Lacrimal · Orbitotomy

Understanding Pain

Types of Pain

Pain is categorized into nociceptive, neuropathic, and psychogenic subtypes.

Nociceptive pain results from tissue irritation and injury, culminating in release of prostaglandins and activation of local nociceptors that transmit impulses via peripheral nerves and the spinal cord to the brain. Traditional opioids and antinociceptive agents, including non-steroidal anti-inflammatory drugs (NSAIDs), reduce afferent input from both intact and traumatized tissue [4].

Neuropathic pain occurs secondary to nerve injury or malfunction in either the peripheral or central nervous system. Acute activation of nociceptor fibers may turn into irreversible modifications of the peripheral and/or central nociceptive

C. L. Marous · E. J. Wladis (✉)
Ophthalmic Plastic Surgery, Lions Eye Institute, Department of Ophthalmology, Albany Medical College, 1220 New Scotland Road, Suite 302, Slingerlands, NY, USA
e-mail: wladise@amc.edu

J. Tao (ed.), *Efficient Oculofacial Surgery*, https://doi.org/10.1007/978-3-031-63178-8_5

system, resulting in neuropathic pain [4]. Pain may persist for months to years well beyond apparent structural healing of any damaged tissue and is poorly responsive to conventional opioids and NSAIDs [5]. Anticonvulsant agents such as gabapentin and pregabalin are efficacious in reducing conversion of acute pain into chronic pain by reducing the hyperexcitability of neurons induced by tissue damage [4].

Psychogenic pain refers to psychological factors contributing to the patient's presentation of the pain problem.

Postsurgical Pain

Pain specifically induced by surgery is complex and involves physiologic and psychologic factors. Postoperative pain may delay recovery, increase complications, prolong hospital stays, augment post-discharge caregiver requirements, and reduce patient well-being [6].

Postsurgical pain is grouped into acute and chronic variants. Acute pain is precipitated by surgical trauma and may be of nociceptive or neuropathic origin. Its onset is experienced immediately after surgery (up to 7 days), whereas pain lasting more than 3 months after surgery is considered chronic. Both acute and chronic pain can arise from cutaneous, deep somatic, visceral, and neuropathic structures.

Perioperative Timing of Analgesic Administration

Timely administration of analgesia may avert the development of postoperative discomfort inherent to invasive surgery.

Prophylactic agents as adjuncts to intraoperative and postoperative medications should be considered. Randomized trials have documented benefit in using acetaminophen, ketorolac, and pregabalin 30 minutes to 1 hour preoperatively to reduce pain preceding eyelid surgery (including blepharoplasty, ptosis repair, eyelid retraction, wedge resections, post-Mohs reconstructions), lacrimal surgery (dacryocystorhinostomy), and orbital surgery [7–11]. Both oral and intravenous routes can be administered. Timely pre-emptive administration of these non-narcotic alternatives can result in dramatic reduction of self-reported pain and the need for postoperative opioid and antiemetic medication [8]. This approach safely improves the patient experience, while also inherently optimizing surgical outcomes by reducing wound manipulation associated with increased discomfort.

Intraoperative analgesia can be achieved with local topical or infiltrative anesthetic agents administered by the surgeon, or in concert with monitored anesthesia care by an anesthesiologist. Local infiltrative lidocaine or bupivacaine provides excellent anesthesia and can be administered topically as a viscous solution, subcutaneously, or regionally as a retrobulbar or peribulbar nerve block. Lidocaine acts quickly within 2–5 minutes of injection, and lasts approximately 2 hour, or 3 hour if combined with epinephrine [12]. Bupivacaine has a slower onset of action at around 5–10 minutes, but lasts much longer (4–8 hour post injection), making it an excellent adjunct for post-operative pain control [12]. The addition of epinephrine to local anesthetic increases duration of action of the medication via its vasoconstrictive properties that prevent quick dissemination. Adding hyaluronidase or sodium bicarbonate can reduce pain associated with injection by buffering the solution while maintaining solubility of the anesthetic [13]. Tranexamic acid may be added to the local admixture to reduce postoperative edema and ecchymosis.

Postoperative pain following oculofacial procedures is well controlled with over-the-counter oral NSAIDs, and in rare cases prescribed oral opioids as outlined in Sect. 5.2.

Patient Selection

Patient specific comorbidities should be considered when tailoring treatment plans. Analgesic

Table 5.1 List of agents with documented efficacy in managing pain after oculofacial surgical procedures

Agent	Types of surgery with documented efficacy	Adverse effects, complications
Acetaminophen-hydrocodone, oxycodone, acetaminophen-oxycodone, tramadol, hydromorphone, and acetaminophen-tradamol	Enucleation with orbital implant, orbitotomy with bone flap decompression, orbital fracture repair	Respiratory depression, death, high risk addiction and dependence. Should be avoided unless severe, unrelenting pain
Pregabalin, Gabapentin	Eyelid surgery (blepharoplasty, canthoplasty, ptosis repair, eyelid retraction repair, pentagonal wedge resection, and MOHS reconstruction), dacryocystorhinostomy	Somnolence, dizziness, ataxia, confusion, dysarthria, blurred vision, diplopia
Acetaminophen	Orbital surgery, eyelid surgery, MOHs surgery	Should not be used in patients with hepatic disease
Ibuprofen	Eyelid surgery	Should be avoided in patients with severe renal disease, gastrointestinal ulcers
Ketorolac	Orbital surgery, ptosis repair, dacryocystorhinostomy	Should be avoided in patients with severe renal disease, gastrointestinal ulcers
Memantine	Dacryocystorhinostomy	Confusion, insomnia, gastrointestinal side effects
Local anesthesia	Enucleation, evisceration, secondary orbital implant placement, dacryocystorhinostomy	Not applicable
Ice	Eyelid, lacrimal, and orbital surgery	Should not be used in full thickness skin grafts
Manuka honey	Blepharoplasty	Not recorded
Saireito	Blepharoplasty	Not recorded

medications have well known side effects, especially in patients with baseline renal, hepatic, gastrointestinal, and respiratory dysfunction (Table 5.1). Elderly patients are not optimal candidates for opioids agents as they can result in excessive sedation, respiratory depression, and reduced coordination leading to falls.

The nature of oculofacial surgery performed should also be used to guide medication choice. Primary versus revisional surgery, operative time, and nature of procedure are important considerations. Eyelid surgery is typically shorter in length, involves more superficial tissue that responds well to short term, oral NSAID analgesics, and less frequently requires opioid prescription [3]. In contrast, patients undergoing orbital surgery, specifically orbital floor fracture repair, enucleation with orbital implant, and orbitotomy with bone flap for decompression, have been shown to require higher amounts of prescribed analgesics including opioids [3]. This may be due to higher risk for structural nerve injury, longer operative time, use of heat-producing tool instrumentation for hemostasis and bone work creating more broad tissue injury and inflammation. Lastly, revisional procedures may involve additional manipulation of scar tissue that may be more sensitive than virgin tissues, necessitating higher pain control demands [6].

Awareness of Opioid Epidemic

Opioid abuse was declared a public health emergency in the United States in 2017 and recently accounted for more deaths in the United States than motor vehicle accidents [14–16]. While prescription opioids, especially in the postoperative patient cohort, may represent well-intended efforts to address pain, they may also contribute to inappropriate use and dependency.

In opioid-naïve patients, surgical procedures are associated with an increased risk of chronic, persistent opioid use in the post-operative period and 67–92% of patients report having unused opioids after surgery [17]. Excessive prescription and unused narcotics are a recognized hazard for later abuse or improper use, with one study identifying that patients who filled an opioid prescription after surgery were more likely to use them persistently during the 90–180-day postoperative period [17]. Furthermore, an estimated 63% of patients in a review of oculofacial plastic surgery did not dispose of unused opioid medication in accordance with FDA-recommended guidelines including pharmacy take-back, trash disposal by mixing with cat litter/coffee grounds, or flushing down the toilet [18]. Instead, these patients stored them in their homes, which is a known risk to future abuse. In a study of intravenous heroin users, 60% grew up in households or visited family member's homes where opioids had been prescribed, and among those households, one third reported initiating with an opioid scavenged from a family members home [19]. Recognizing and understanding the threatening implications of opioid dispensing and disposal after oculofacial plastic surgery may aid in efforts to alleviate the public health crisis.

Opioid prescriptions represent approximately 16.5% of all prescriptions written by American Society of Ophthalmic Plastic and Reconstructive Surgery members between 2013–2016, which is lower than the 36.5% average among other surgical subspecialties [20]. Opioid needs understandably vary according to subtype of surgery, and requirements for these agents may be minimal after oculofacial plastic surgery compared to other specialties. Higher requirement for postoperative opioid pain control may still be needed following orbit procedures such as fracture repair and enucleation compared to eyelid or lacrimal surgery, and should be factored into conservative prescribing patterns of controlled substances [3, 18]. Younger age may be associated with higher opioid needs, although the literature is conflicting [18]. Ultimately, a shift towards alternatives to opioids in these types of procedures yields encouraging results and should be considered in the appropriate clinical setting for pain control.

Potential Agents

Opioids

Opioids act in the central nervous system to block the transfer of pain signals from the spinal cord to the brain [5]. The most commonly prescribed opioids by oculofacial surgeons for postoperative pain include, in reducing sequential order: acetaminophen-hydrocodone, oxycodone, acetaminophen-oxycodone, tramadol, hydromorphone, and acetaminophen-tramadol.3 These medications may be administered intravenously or orally, and should be reserved for conservative use in orbital surgeries that are more likely to result in considerable discomfort, such as orbitotomies with bone flap decompression, enucleations with implant placement, and orbital fracture repair. When opioid alternatives are insufficient at controlling pain postoperatively, outpatient dosing of narcotics for orbital surgery may range from 10 tablets of hydrocodone/acetaminophen 5/325 mg, or 5 tablets for patients undergoing eyelid or lacrimal surgery [18]. Refills are not typically indicated.

Pregabalin and Gabapentin

Pregabalin and its predecessor gabapentin are anticonvulsants that have emerged as a treatment for neuropathic pain. They work by inhibiting calcium channels, resulting in reduced calcium entry into the nerve terminals, decreased substance P, noradrenaline, calcitonin gene related-peptide, and glutamate release into the spinal cord [21]. This reduction in postsynaptic excitability is believed to inhibit pain transmission and central sensitization [6]. Unlike gabapentin, pregabalin has greater bioavailability due to amino acid substitution that enables improved absorption via the small intestines [6]. As such, pregabalin is the preferred drug choice. US Food and Drug Administration has approved pregabalin for use in treating epilepsy, postherpetic neuralgia, diabetic neuropathy, and fibromyalgia [7]. Its use in reducing postoperative pain and chronic neuropathic pain is increasingly well documented in dental surgery, spine surgery, podiatric surgery, laparoscopic abdominal surgery, and more recently oculoplastic surgery [6, 7, 11].

Pre-emptive pregabalin 30 minutes to 1 hour prior to incision time, ranging from 50 to 300 mg orally, can help reduce need for postoperative pain medication, notably the need narcotic analgesics, and lower pain scores [7, 11]. This algorithm has shown success in eyelid procedures including blepharoplasty, canthoplasty, ptosis repair, eyelid retraction repair, pentagonal wedge resection, and Mohs reconstruction, as well as in lacrimal surgery when performing dacryocystorhinostomy [7, 11]. Following these one-time doses, side effects are less likely. However, drug reactions following long time use l may include dizziness, somnolence, blurred vision, diplopia, confusion, ataxia, and dysarthria [16]. Pregabalin is contraindicated in patients with a history of angioedema, depression, renal failure, and heart failure [16].

Acetaminophen

Acetaminophen blocks pain impulses to the brain itself by inhibiting the cyclooxygenase pathway in the central nervous system, but not in peripheral tissues [5]. Pre-operative and intraoperative intravenous infusion of acetaminophen using standard 1 g dosing in orbital surgery is associated with reduced pain scores, lower opioid requirements, and less need for postoperative antiemetic agents [8]. Acetaminophen should be used with caution in patients with a history of hepatic dysfunction.

Ibuprofen

Ibuprofen exerts its anti-inflammatory and analgesic effects by blocking the cyclooxygenase pathway, thereby reducing production of prostaglandin. Ibuprofen 400 mg has been found as effective as acetaminophen/codeine 600/60 mg for pain relief following cosmetic facial surgery, including eyelid surgery [22]. Furthermore, pure ibuprofen is better tolerated with fewer side effects compared to combined acetaminophen with codeine, making it an excellent choice for postoperative pain[22]. Ibuprofen should be used sparingly in patients with renal insufficiency, peptic ulcer disease, and gastritis.

Ketorolac

Ketorolac is another NSAID that works by reducing pain via inhibition of cyclooxygenase, which is required to produce prostaglandins [23]. Intravenous(IV) forms of the medication act as potent non-narcotics with rapid onset of action and an efficacy similar to opioid medication [10]. IV ketorolac analgesia peaks 75–150 minutes following administration, and has a short half-life of 5–6 hour, accounting for its marked reduction in immediate postoperative pain[24]. Historically surgeons have been hesitant to use ketorolac due to concerns of hemorrhagic complications, however studies in oculofacial surgery suggest these limitations are unfounded both in terms of bleeding-related complications and grading scores of ecchymosis [10, 25, 26]. Implementing a standard weight-based dosing of intravenous ketorolac (15 or 30 mg) in patients immediately before undergoing orbital, lacrimal (specifically external dacryocystorhinostomy), and eyelid ptosis repair surgery can reduce pain scores immediately after surgery as well as on subsequent postoperative days, and reduce the likelihood of needing opioid analgesics [9, 10, 24]. While these benefits are encouraging, ketorolac should not be used in patients with a history of allergy to the medication or with renal impairment.

Memantine

Memantine is an antagonist of N-methyl-D-aspartate receptor that reduces neuronal excitability within the dorsal horn of the spinal cord [6]. It is generally used to treat Alzheimer's disease but more recently is showing promise in treating neuropathic pain. Oral administration ranging from 50 to 200 mg in patients undergoing dacryocystorhinostomy is associated with lower pain scores and lower consumption of opioids in the first 48 h postoperatively [6, 27]. Although the medication is generally well tolerated, patients should be made aware of potential side effects including confusion, insomnia, and gastrointestinal changes [16].

Other Agents

Ice pack application following surgery, or any tissue injury, has been used for years due to its well-known ability to ease pain [28]. Cold reduces the transmission rate of impulses along nerve fiber, especially at temperatures 27 °C or lower, thus nerve conduction fails, and the sensation of pain is reduced [29]. Additionally, cool temperatures reduce muscle spasm and edema after tissue injury, compounding its analgesic effect. Ice pack application to the surgical site has been shown to significantly reduce subjective pain scales up to postoperative day five, and represents a safe, easy, and low cost means to improve patient comfort [29]. Ice should be avoided in full thickness skin grafts to prevent tissue ischemia and rejection.

Manuka honey applied topically following eyelid surgery has shown preliminary evidence in reduced long-term postoperative pain following blepharoplasty [30]. Oral saireito following blepharoplasty has also shown benefit in faster resolution of discomfort [31]. Cannabis has not yet been shown to result in significant reduction in postoperative pain following oculofacial plastic surgery. The literature does not support the use of other homeopathic agents such as Arnica montana for oculofacial surgeries in the context of pain or recovery.

Role of Local Anesthesia

Local anesthetics intercept pain signals ascending the nerve by binding to sodium-channels and preventing nerve depolarization. Lidocaine and bupivacaine have multifaceted involvement in nociceptive transmission as they interact with muscarinic agonists, glycine inhibitors, release of endogenous opioids, and reduce production of excitatory amino acids, neurokinins, and thromboxane A2 [6]. Thus, benefits are analgesic, anti-hyperalgesic, and anti-inflammatory in nature. Self-administration of local anesthetic agents after enucleation, evisceration, and secondary orbital implant surgery have shown benefit in pain scores and patient comfort. 18-guage catheter placement through the skin towards the orbital apex, 23-guage needle injection inferotemporal within the orbit, and an on-Q pump placed intraconal delivering bupivacaine in patients following surgery showed lower pain scores and significant reduction in narcotic analgesic needs [32–35]. No side effects or infections have been reported following these methods. Paranasal injection of bupivacaine in dacryocystorhinostomy patients has also been shown to alleviate post-operative discomfort and reduced need for opioids [36]. Intravenous lidocaine has documented benefits in mitigating post-surgical pain but has not been trialed specifically in the oculofacial surgery literature [6].

Cost Considerations

Financial burden of analgesic medication and associated healthcare costs is an important consideration and has yet to be formally outlined with respect to the above narcotic-alternatives in oculofacial surgery. Although specific financial implications remain uncertain and can vary substantially case by case, improving patient experience by optimizing pain control may result in faster discharge, reduced need for postoperative care, and reduced need for long term narcotic and antiemetic medication.

Conclusions

Appropriate management of postoperative pain is key to successful oculofacial surgery. While opioid analgesics are available and appropriate in select cases, a wide variety of non-narcotic analgesics are available. Understanding the various options, their indications, risks, and side effects may improve the quality of the oculofacial surgical experience for patients.

References

1. Carroll I, Hah J, Mackey S, Ottestad E, Kong JT, Lahidji S, Tawfik V, Younger J, Curtin C. Perioperative interventions to reduce chronic postsurgical pain. J Reconstr Microsurg. 2013;29(4):213–22. https://doi.org/10.1055/s-0032-1329921. PMID: 23463498; PMCID: PMC4852210.
2. Benyamin R, Trescot AM, Datta S, Buenaventura R, Adlaka R, Sehgal N, Glaser SE, Vallejo R. Opioid complications and side effects. Pain Physician. 2008;11(2 Suppl):S105–20. PMID: 18443635.
3. Xie Y, Joseph AW, Rudy SF, Elner VM, Demirci H, Kim DS, Nelson CC, Joseph SS. Change in postoperative opioid prescribing patterns for oculoplastic and orbital procedures associated with state opioid legislation. JAMA Ophthalmol. 2021;139(2):157–62. https://doi.org/10.1001/jamaophthalmol.2020.5446.
4. Dahl JB, Mathiesen O, Møiniche S. Protective premedication': an option with gabapentin and related drugs? A review of gabapentin and pregabalin in in the treatment of post-operative pain. Acta Anaesthesiol Scand. 2004;48(9):1130–6. https://doi.org/10.1111/j.1399-6576.2004.00484.x. PMID: 15352959.
5. Gupta A, Kaur K, Sharma S, Goyal S, Arora S, Murthy RS. Clinical aspects of acute post-operative pain management & its assessment. J Adv Pharm Technol Res. 2010;1(2):97–108. PMID: 22247838; PMCID: PMC3255434.
6. Rai A, Meng H, Weinrib A, Englesakis M, Kumbhare D, Grosman-Rimon L, Katz J, Clarke H. A review of adjunctive CNS medications used for the treatment of post-surgical pain. CNS Drugs. 2017;31(7):605–15. https://doi.org/10.1007/s40263-017-0440-1. PMID: 28577135.
7. Wei LA, Davies BW, Hink EM, Durairaj VD. Perioperative pregabalin for attenuation of postoperative pain after eyelid surgery. Ophthalmic Plast Reconstr Surg. 2015;31(2):132–5. https://doi.org/10.1097/IOP.0000000000000219. PMID: 25000214.
8. Wladis EJ, Kattato DF, De A. Intravenous acetaminophen in orbital surgery. Ophthalmic Plast Reconstr Surg. 2016;32(3):211–3. https://doi.org/10.1097/IOP.0000000000000470. PMID: 25902387.
9. Wladis EJ, Dennett KV, Chen VH, De A. Preoperative intravenous ketorolac safely reduces postoperative pain in levator advancement surgery. Ophthalmic Plast Reconstr Surg. 2019;35(4):357–9. https://doi.org/10.1097/IOP.0000000000001265. PMID: 30407996.
10. Wladis EJ, Lee KW, De A. Intravenous ketorolac reduces pain score and opioid requirement in orbital surgery. Ophthalmic Plast Reconstr Surg. 2020;36(2):132–4. https://doi.org/10.1097/IOP.0000000000001484. PMID: 31743284.
11. Alimian M, Imani F, Hassani V, Rahimzadeh P, Sharifian M, Safari S. Effects of single-dose pregabalin on postoperative pain in dacryocystorhinostomy surgery. Anesth Pain Med. 2012;2(2):72–6. https://doi.org/10.5812/aapm.4301. PMID: 24223341; PMCID: PMC3821116.
12. NIH US National Library of Medicine. Bupivacaine versus lidocaine local anesthesia. Updated 2015. https://clinicaltrials.gov/ct2/show/NCT01751347. Accessed 1 Jan 2022.
13. Rüschen H, Aravinth K, Bunce C, Bokre D. Use of hyaluronidase as an adjunct to local anaesthetic eye blocks to reduce intraoperative pain in adults. Cochrane Database Syst Rev. 2018;3(3):CD010368. https://doi.org/10.1002/14651858.CD010368.pub2. PMID: 29498413; PMCID: PMC6494176.
14. Patel S, Sternberg P Jr. Association between opioid prescribing patterns and abuse in ophthalmology. JAMA Ophthalmol. 2017;135(11):1216–20. https://doi.org/10.1001/jamaophthalmol.2017.4055. PMID: 28983558; PMCID: PMC5710378.
15. Coppens M, Versichelen L, Mortier E. Treatment of postoperative pain after ophthalmic surgery. Bull Soc Belge Ophtalmol. 2002;285:27–32. PMID: 12442340.
16. Wladis EJ, Rothschild MI, Rubinstein TJ. Management of postoperative pain in ophthalmic plastic surgery: a major review. Orbit. 2021;40(4):269–73. https://doi.org/10.1080/01676830.2020.1793373. PMID: 32669009.
17. Olds C, Spataro E, Li K, Kandathil C, Most SP. Assessment of persistent and prolonged postoperative opioid use among patients undergoing plastic and reconstructive surgery. JAMA Facial Plast Surg. 2019;21(4):286–91. https://doi.org/10.1001/jamafacial.2018.2035. PMID: 30844024; PMCID: PMC6583832.
18. Vu PQ, Yu JJ, Charlson ES, Grob SR, Kshirsagar RS, Tao JP. Opioid use after orbital, eyelid, or lacrimal surgery. Ophthalmic Plast Reconstr Surg. 2021;37(3S):S62–5. https://doi.org/10.1097/IOP.0000000000001813. PMID: 32852374.
19. Lankenau SE, Teti M, Silva K, Jackson Bloom J, Harocopos A, Treese M. Initiation into prescription opioid misuse amongst young injection drug users. Int J Drug Policy. 2012;23(1):37–44. https://doi.org/10.1016/j.drugpo.2011.05.014. Epub 2011 Jun 20. PMID: 21689917; PMCID: PMC3196821.
20. Charlson ES, Feng PW, Bui A, Grob S, Tao JP. Opioid prescribing patterns among American society of ophthalmic plastic and reconstructive surgery members in the medicare part D database.

Ophthalmic Plast Reconstr Surg. 2019;35(4):360–4. https://doi.org/10.1097/IOP.0000000000001266. PMID: 30439721.
21. Kumar N, Laferriere A, Yu JS, Leavitt A, Coderre TJ. Evidence that pregabalin reduces neuropathic pain by inhibiting the spinal release of glutamate. J Neurochem. 2010;113(2):552–61. https://doi.org/10.1111/j.1471-4159.2010.06625.x. PMID: 20132471; PMCID: PMC4492734.
22. Chen T, Adamson PA. Comparison of ibuprofen and acetaminophen with codeine following cosmetic facial surgery. J Otolaryngol Head Neck Surg. 2009;38(5):580–6 PMID: 19769830.
23. Cashman JN. The mechanisms of action of NSAIDs in analgesia. Drugs. 1996;52(Suppl 5):13–23. https://doi.org/10.2165/00003495-199600525-00004. PMID: 8922554.
24. Agarwal A, Patidar N, Gabba HS, Sood D, Piush P. Pain score assessment using single-dose IV ketorolac only, after external dacryocystorhinostomy: a randomized double/triple-blind placebo-controlled trial. Ophthalmic Plast Reconstr Surg. 2021;37(2):173–5. https://doi.org/10.1097/IOP.0000000000001730. PMID: 32467522.
25. Gobble RM, Hoang HLT, Kachniarz B, Orgill DP. Ketorolac does not increase perioperative bleeding: a meta-analysis of randomized controlled trials. Plast Reconstr Surg. 2014;133(3):741–55. https://doi.org/10.1097/01.prs.0000438459.60474.b5. PMID: 24572864.
26. Chang M, Gould A, Gur Z, Buhbut O, Hosalkar H, Liu CY, Korn BS, Kikkawa DO. Does intraoperative ketorolac increase bleeding in oculoplastic surgery? Ophthalmic Plast Reconstr Surg. 2020;36(4):355–8. https://doi.org/10.1097/IOP.0000000000001549. PMID: 31809483.
27. Rahimzadeh P, Imani F, Nikoubakht N, Koleini Z, Faiz SHR, Sayarifard A. A comparative study on the efficacy of oral memantine and placebo for acute postoperative pain in patients undergoing dacryocystorhinostomy (DCR). Anesth Pain Med. 2017;7(3):e45297. https://doi.org/10.5812/aapm.45297. PMID: 28856113; PMCID: PMC5561447.
28. Ernst E, Fialka V. Ice freezes pain? A review of the clinical effectiveness of analgesic cold therapy. J Pain Symptom Manage. 1994;9(1):56–9. https://doi.org/10.1016/0885-3924(94)90150-3. PMID: 8169463.
29. Akan M, Misirlioğlu A, Yildirim S, Cakir B, Taylan G, Aköz T. Ice application to minimize pain in the split-thickness skin graft donor site. Aesthetic Plast Surg. 2003;27(4):305–7. https://doi.org/10.1007/s00266-003-3014-1. PMID: 15058555.
30. Malhotra R, Ziahosseini K, Poitelea C, Litwin A, Sagili S. Effect of Manuka honey on eyelid wound healing: a randomized controlled trial. Ophthalmic Plast Reconstr Surg. 2017;33(4):268–72. https://doi.org/10.1097/IOP.0000000000000743. PMID: 27429228.
31. Morimoto N, Kakudo N, Mitsui T, Kuro A, Ueda Y, Hihara M, Tanaka Y, Ozaki Y, Suzuki K, Kusumoto K. The effectiveness of Saireito, a traditional Japanese herbal medicine, in reducing postoperative edema after acquired ptosis surgery: a prospective controlled trial. Evid Based Complement Alternat Med. 2018;2018:4742305. https://doi.org/10.1155/2018/4742305. PMID: 30050587; PMCID: PMC6040292.
32. Ing E, Al-Anezi F, Abuhaleeqa K. Postoperative analgesia with a transcutaneous parabulbar butterfly catheter. Can J Ophthalmol. 2008;43(5):604–5. https://doi.org/10.3129/i08-095. PMID: 18982046.
33. Samimi DB, Erb MH, Perry AC, Burnstine MA, Dresner SC. On-Q pump for pain control after orbital implant surgery. Ophthalmic Plast Reconstr Surg. 2014;30(5):396–9. https://doi.org/10.1097/IOP.0000000000000127. PMID: 24777268.
34. Fezza JP, Klippenstein KA, Wesley RE. Use of an orbital epidural catheter to control pain after orbital implant surgery. Arch Ophthalmol. 1999;117(6):784–8. https://doi.org/10.1001/archopht.117.6.784. PMID: 10369590.
35. Merbs SL, Grant MP, Iliff NT. Simple outpatient postoperative analgesia using an orbital catheter after enucleation. Arch Ophthalmol. 2004;122(3):349–52. https://doi.org/10.1001/archopht.122.3.349. PMID: 15006848.
36. Scawn RL, Allen MJ, Rose GE, Verity DH. Randomised, masked study of local anaesthesia administered prior to external dacryocystorhinostomy under general anaesthesia. Eye (Lond). 2019;33(3):374–379. https://doi.org/10.1038/s41433-018-0201-5. Epub 2018 Sep 18. PMID: 30228368; PMCID: PMC6460689.

Autologous Grafts in Oculofacial Surgery

6

Suzana Matayoshi and Ivana Cardoso Pereira

Abstract

Grafts and flaps are essential in oculofacial plastic surgery. Autologous grafts have the advantage of tissue compatibility and lower probability for rejection. Common surgeries in which grafts are used are eyelid reconstruction, frontalis suspension ptosis surgery, and anophthalmic socket rehabilitation. This chapter details harvesting techniques, donor site care, and complications for common autologous tissue grafts in oculofacial surgery.

Keywords

Graft · Eyelid reconstruction · Anophthalmic socket · Frontalis suspension · Skin graft · Mucous membrane graft · Hard palate graft · Fascia graft

Supplementary Information The online version contains supplementary material available at https://doi.org/10.1007/978-3-031-63178-8_6.

S. Matayoshi (✉) · I. C. Pereira
University of São Paulo, São Paulo, Brazil
e-mail: suzana.matayoshi@gmail.com

Introduction

Tissue replacement is core to oculofacial surgery. In eyelid reconstructions, it is vital to consider the tissue replacements for the anterior and posterior lamellae. Frontalis suspension surgery for eyelid ptosis is frequently performed with autologous fascia. Anophthalmic socket surgeries commonly require grafts to increase volume as well as increase the socket and forniceal surface area. This chapter describes technique and indications for common autologous grafts in oculofacial surgery.

Part 1—Eyelid Surgery

Anterior Lamella

The anterior eyelid lamella is composed of skin and orbicularis oculi muscle. Isolated anterior lamellar defects may need not only skin coverage but also orbicularis muscle reconstruction (transposition flap or cheek rotation flap).

Skin Graft

Skin grafts are commonly used to repair simple anterior lamellar defects with a healthy orbicularis base or for use in combination with vascularized posterior lamellar replacements for bilamellar defects [1].

J. Tao (ed.), *Efficient Oculofacial Surgery*, https://doi.org/10.1007/978-3-031-63178-8_6

FULL-THICKNESS SKIN GRAFT. Composed of epidermis and dermis, including adnexal structures, such as hair follicles and sweat glands, full thickness skin grafts are commonly used for eyelid reconstruction. Attention should be given to skin color, texture, and thickness, in relation to the recipient site to provide an excellent cosmetic result. Wound contraction is minimal and dermal adnexal structures are left intact. Recipient sites must be able to provide a rich vascular supply for capillary ingrowth and fibroblasts for graft adherence.

Donor site considerations

Skin is always best replaced with skin and donor site selection is relevant (Fig. 6.1). In general, eyelid skin is the best to replace eyelid defects. Commonly, grafts taken from redundant upper eyelid skin repair lower eyelid defects very well. Grafts of thinner skin, however, should be oversized by at least 100% to prevent contraction and possible ectropion. Preauricular skin provides a good source of a thicker skin with a degree of sun exposure and can be used to repair nasal defects. This donor site heals excellently with an inconspicuous scar; however, care should be taken not to harvest hair-bearing skin from this site. Conchal bowl grafts provide an option where a sebaceous texture is needed, as with the nasal tip on some patients. Skin from the nasolabial fold also may be used to close small nasal tip defects. Prospective donor skin should be carefully examined for malignancies, to avoid transfer to a recipient site. Clavicular skin may be used for larger defects. Harvest wounds need to be placed carefully and closed meticulously to avoid a visible scar.

Aesthetically, skin tissues from the ipsilateral or contralateral eyelid, preauricular, retroauricular, inner brachial and supraclavicular areas that provide similar color, thickness, and texture are considered ideal donor sites for the periocular region. There is minimal donor site morbidity and usually there exists sufficient skin for eyelid reconstruction [2].

PARTIAL THICKNESS SKIN GRAFTS: Composed of the epidermis and a portion of the dermis, partial (a.k.a. split) thickness skin grafts vary from 0.25 to 0.75 mm in thickness and are categorized as thin (0.0125–0.275 mm), medium (0.275–0.4 mm), or thick (0.40–0.75 mm). A manual Blair skin-graft knife or dermatome are tools to harvest split thickness skin (Fig. 6.2).

These grafts may be placed over almost any recipient bed, including those with only mild vascularization. They may be meshed to increase their surface area and to facilitate drainage of blood and exudate from beneath the graft [3]. Their semi-transparent nature allows visualization

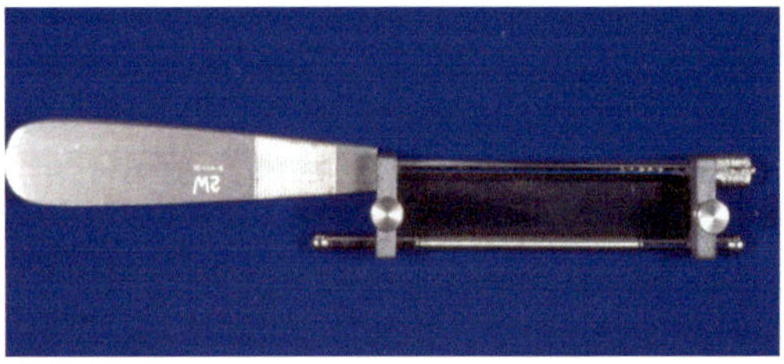

Fig. 6.2 Blair skin-graft knife

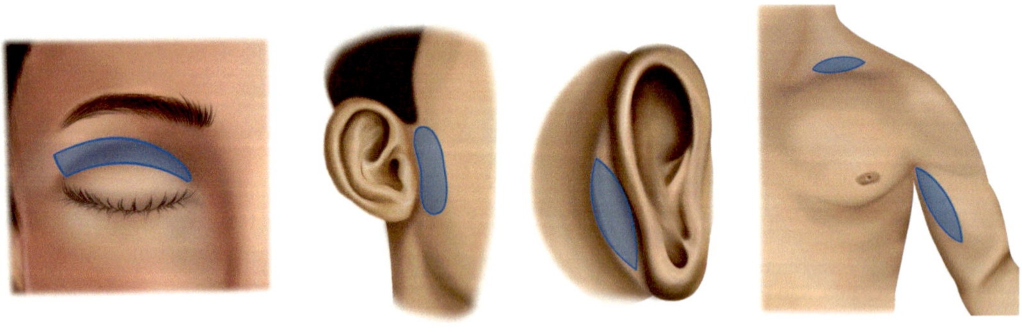

Fig. 6.1 Common skin donor sites

of the wound bed of an excised aggressive tumor to monitor for recurrence. This very thinness often contributes to a greater tendency to contract and a less cosmetically acceptable result. In addition, the donor site is usually left to heal by second intention and may be associated with a scar.

Donor site selection

Selection of the donor site is based on cosmesis, size of the graft, accessibility of the site for postoperative care, and patient activity. Common sites include the anterior, medial, and lateral thighs, the inner and outer aspects of the upper arm, and the inner aspect of the forearm.

The disadvantages are relatively high rates of graft contraction and hypertrophy. Hypertrophic scarring is the most common complication and can be treated with massage, steroid ointment, steroid injection, 5 fluorouracil injection, or silicone gel application.

Posterior Lamella

The posterior eyelid lamella is composed of conjunctiva and tarsus, so the replacement must provide a smooth, mucosal surface to avoid corneal and conjunctival friction damage and maintain supporting structure.

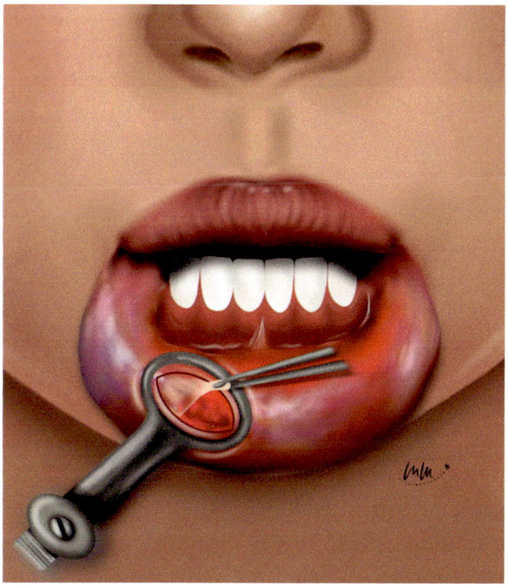

Fig. 6.3 Lower lip mucosa exposed—donor site

Mucous membrane harvesting

Oral mucosa can replace both the bulbar and tarsal conjunctiva [4, 5]. If used for bulbar conjunctival replacement, however, full thickness oral mucosa grafts can appear excessively red or thick. Amucotome can help achieve a sufficiently thin graft that is a better match to transparent bulbar. It can be harvested from the inner surface of the lower lip (most used), the upper lip, and the cheek region (Fig. 6.3). The harvest site should not be apparent externally nor too deep in the labial fornices.

After local asepsis with povidone-iodine or chlorhexidine, the mucosa is infiltrated with local anesthetic. Large chalazion forceps can aid vasoconstriction and facilitate exposure of the labial mucosa for removal. The incision is made with a 15-blade scalpel and dissects the submucosal tissue with a scalpel and delicate scissors. Cautery should be minimal because it can cause pain and impair healing. Although these oral wounds can be left to heal by second intention, suturing the defect may offer better postoperative comfort and faster healing. 5-0 or 6-0 polyglactin or chromic sutures are used. Care in the jugal region to avoid injury to the Stensen's duct, located at upper 1st–2nd molar level. Oral rinses with saltwater or antiseptic mouthwash are encouraged in the first seven postoperative days.

The labial mucosa can thus be used to repair deficiency of the tarsal and bulbar conjunctiva and anterior surface of anophthalmic sockets. Video 6.1 shows trichiasis correction using lower lip mucosa. In addition, in dry eye situations, the mucosa containing the lacrimal gland can be transplanted into the inferior or superior fornix, allowing for improved hydration of the ocular surface.

Complications in the donor area are rare but generally related to the friction of the suture thread on the tongue, accumulation of food debris on the thread, and delay in oral healing (Fig. 6.4). In the recipient area, as in any graft,

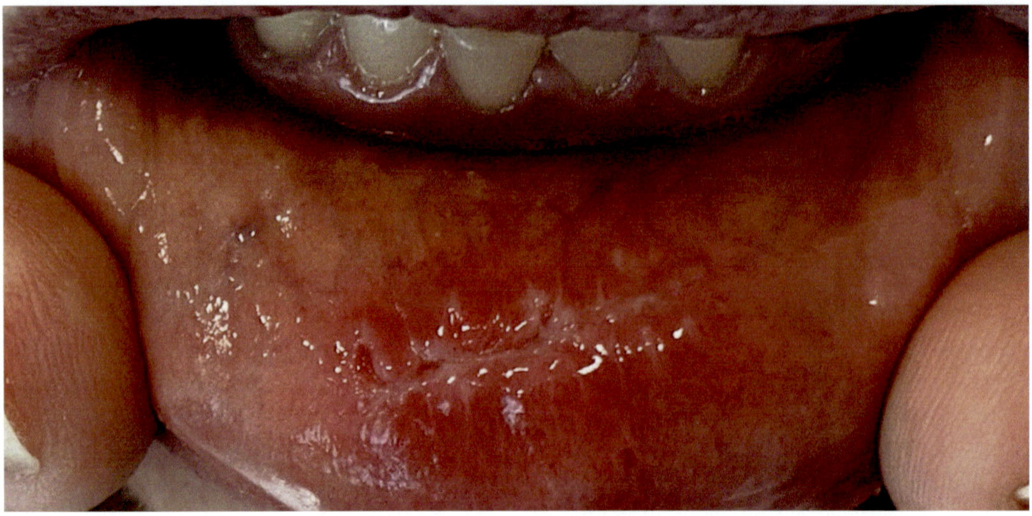

Fig. 6.4 Donor area healing process at 14th post-operative day

there may be a retraction, necrosis, and non-integration of the same in the transplant area. When located on the bulbar conjunctiva, yellow-white spots can be seen in some cases, corresponding to the salivary glands.

Ear Cartilage

Although the tarsus is not cartilage, ear cartilage is a suitable replacement because it is rigid and offers good eyelid support for reconstructions or retraction repair. Cartilage can be harvested from the concha, scapha, or antihelix [6]. The upper antihelix may be preferable since it is flatter, and offers the ability to harvest grafts of slightly larger dimensions (Fig. 6.5). The auricular cartilage is covered by the perichondrium, which epithelializes with mucosa when exposed posteriorly and sewn into the eyelid.

Subcutaneous infiltrative anesthesia distends the area, making it easier to dissect the cartilage, which lies just under the skin. Generally, rectangular or elliptical grafts are harvested with a scalpel. The skin on either side of the cartilage is dissected free. Often the graft may have an undesirable convex surface. Partial-thickness incisions on the convex face can help eliminate this curvature. Bleeding is usually minimal, but a postoperative hematoma may form, so a gentle pressure patch may be useful. Interrupted or running 5-0 nylon sutures approximate the edges of the skin and are removed within 7–10 days. Healing is excellent, usually with

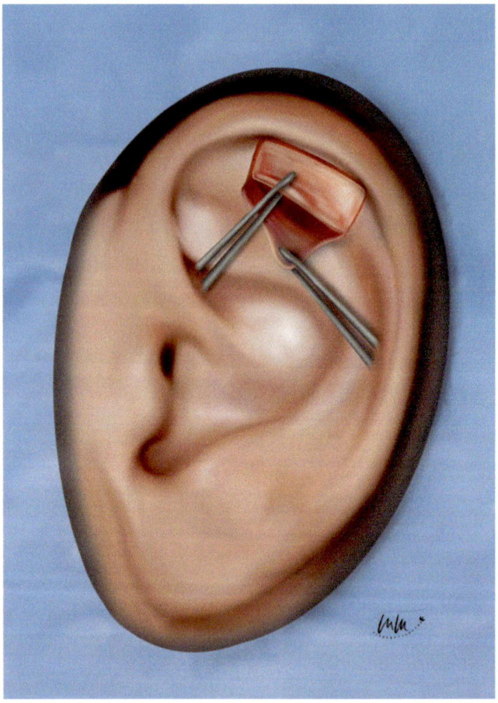

Fig. 6.5 Ear cartilage donor site—scapha portion

an imperceptible external appearance, with only a slight difference in the thickness of the donor region.

At the recipient site, cartilage grafts may cause some deformity in the contour of the eyelid or the graft may be apparent, projecting through the skin. When this occurs, minor interventions to resect and flatten the cartilage may be necessary.

Hard Palate

The hard palate is an excellent graft that transfers mucosa and support to the posterior lamella [7]. The surgical access is more complicated than other grafts owing to the small surgical space of the mouth. A sweetheart retractor is useful. The endotracheal tube, if the patient is under general anesthesia, needs to positioned away from access to the roof of the mouth. There exist significantly vascularized areas that should be avoided: the region of the incisive foramen (anterior midline) and palatine foramen (laterally at the height of the molars), keeping the incision in the paramedian area (Fig. 6.6).

In general, the height of the graft should be double the desired lower eyelid elevation in lower eyelid retraction repair. After local anesthesia is administered the palate incision is created with a 15 or 11 scalpel. The lamellar graft can be dissected from the bed with a spatulate blade (crescent blade). Hemostasis must be performed sparingly. Fibrin glue or other hemostatic agents such as methylcellulose sponges can be placed in the harvest wound to minimize bleeding and facilitate healing. The insertion of pre-shaped palate plates can provide comfort to this wound. Oral saltwater or antiseptic mouthwash rinses are advised for the first postoperative week (Fig. 6.7). Complications are usually bleeding, which can be intense if the arterial arcades are injured. Ischemia with a nonhealing wound or fistula formation with the maxillary sinus are also possible [8].

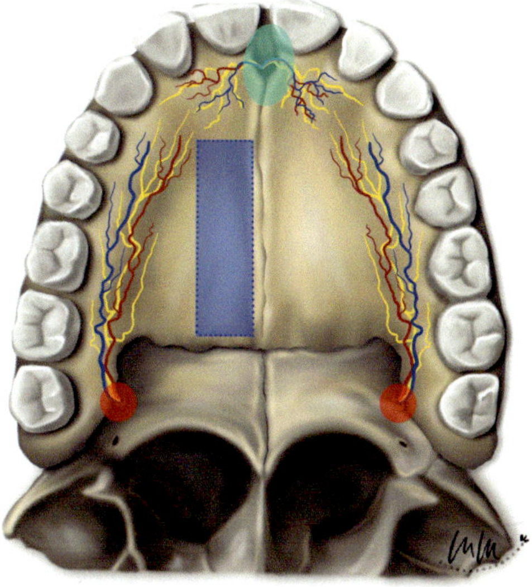

Fig. 6.6 Anatomy of hard palate: the incisive foramen in green, the palatine foramen in red. In blue, the safest area to obtain the palate graft

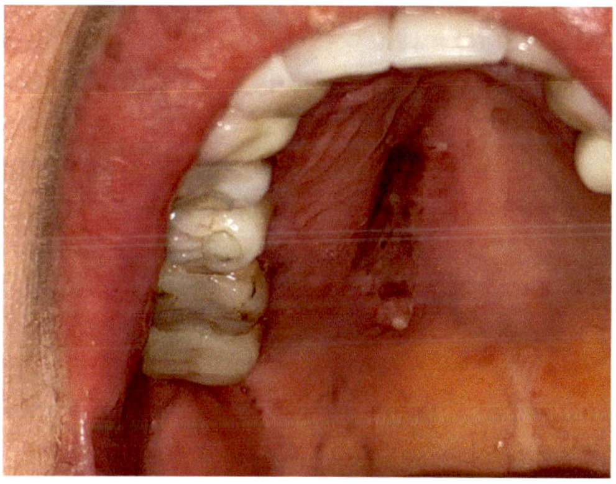

Fig. 6.7 Hard palate cicatrization after three days

Dermis

Autologous dermis is an excellent choice to lengthen the eyelid retractors especially in patients with hollowed lower eyelids or other malar soft tissue atrophy [9]. Dermis or dermis-fat is easily harvested, and large quantities are available. Postoperative recovery is less painful than other grafts, such as auricular cartilage and hard palate. A non-hair bearing area on the lower abdominal region is ideal (Fig. 6.8).

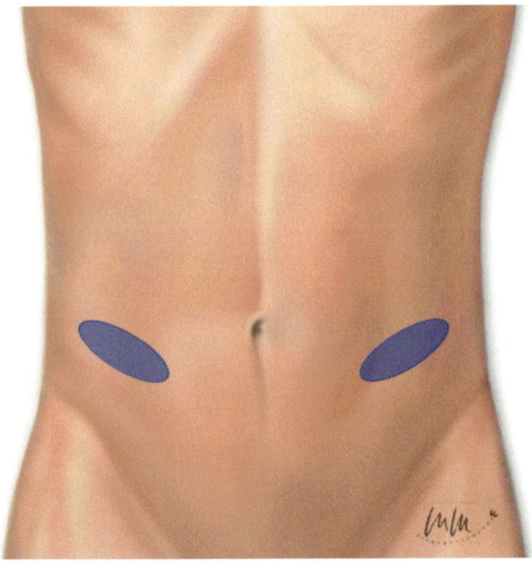

Fig. 6.8 Lower abdominal dermis donor area marked

Alternatively, an ellipse may be taken at the umbilical area or prior abdominal scar sites (if any) to avoid creating an abdominal scar.

After infiltration of local anesthetic, the epidermis is removed with a scalpel or drill. If a thicker dermal component is desired, a diamond burr is useful. Next, cuts are deepened and a 20–25 mm long graft is harvested. Generally, the width is 2 times the desired improvement in lower eyelid height. Bleeding from the donor site is minimal. Closure can be performed with 3-0 or 4-0 polyglactin sutures to the deep tissues and chromic or nylon sutures to the skin (video 2). An additional layer of tissue glue (Dermabond®) can be useful to forestall wound dehiscence.

The main complication is the incomplete removal of the epidermis that can irritate the ocular surface, owing to residual hair follicles or keratinized tissue. As with any wound, risks of granulomas, dehiscence, and infections in the donor and recipient areas are possible.

Part 2—Ptosis Surgery Grafts

Fascia Lata

Fascia lata is a material that is abundant and safe to harvest. It has multiple uses as a graft material. One of the most common uses is as a frontalis sling in brow suspension ptosis surgery in patients over 3 years of age [10]. Patients younger than 3 usually have insufficient leg length for an appropriately long graft.

The fascia lata is collected using a fasciatome or a fascia lata stripper through a 3–4 cm linear skin incision in the lateral aspect of the thigh superior to the knee joint over the ileotibial tract. A strip of tissue 1–2 cm wide and 11–15 cm in length is excised (Fig. 6.9, video 6.3). The wound is closed in one or two subcutaneous layers with 4.0 polygalactin and interrupted nylon sutures to the skin. An additional layer of tissue glue (Dermabond®) can be useful to prevent wound dehiscence.

Very few complications related to harvesting fascia lata have been reported. Postoperative hematoma and muscle herniations are possible. Serious issues such as weakness of hip flexion, numbness, pain, hemorrhage, superficial phlebitis, and wound infection are uncommon. The wound can lead to a conspicuous scar, especially when wearing shorts or a skirt.

Temporalis fascia

Fascia taken from the temporalis muscle may have the following advantages: (1) ease of harvest under local anesthesia, usually in the same operative field, (2) hidden scar, and (3) minimal postoperative morbidity [11, 12]. A vertical incision approximately 7 cm in length is made over the temporalis muscle within the hairline (Fig. 6.10).

The incision is beveled parallel to the hair follicles to minimize damage and subsequent development of localized alopecia. After the scalp has been incised, a loose areolar layer beneath is encountered which contains the superficial temporal artery. This has been designated the superficial temporal fascia (or temporoparietal fascia). After this layer, the deep temporalis fascia is identified covering the temporalis muscle (Fig. 6.11). This layer consists of multiple condensations of fibrous tissue that assume a fan configuration coursing obliquely in an anterior and inferior direction and converging in the area of the zygomatic arch. The temporalis muscle usually measures 7–9 cm vertically

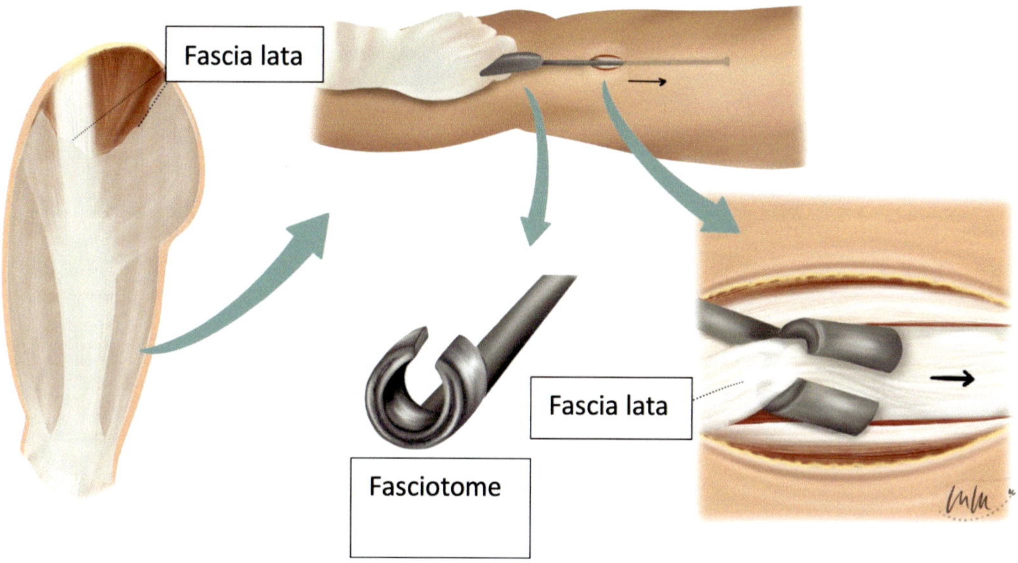

Fig. 6.9 Fascia lata harvesting procedure

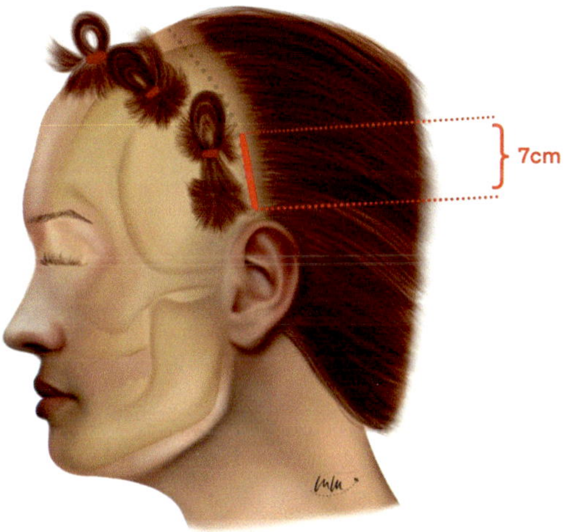

Fig. 6.10 Skin incision to harvest temporalis fascia

and 8–11 cm horizontally. Although individual variation is significant, a sheet of fascia approximately 4 × 6 cm can be obtained from each temporalis muscle.

When obtaining the deep temporal fascia, two structures deserve attention: the superficial temporal artery and its branches, and the posterior branch of the temporal trunk of the facial nerve.

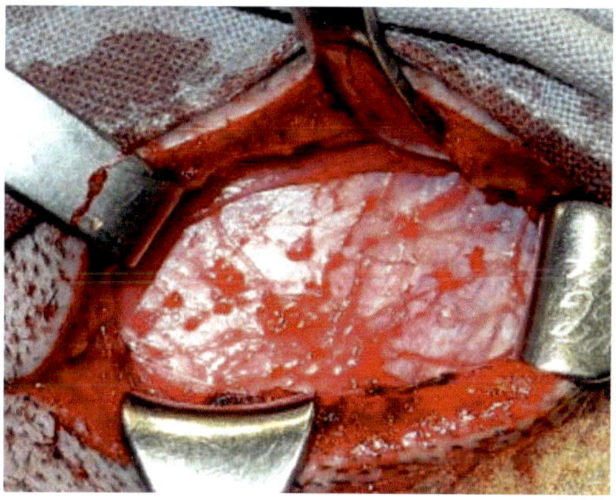

Fig. 6.11 Image of deep temporalis fascia

Perioperative hemostasis of bleeding vessels is important to prevent hematoma formation.

Part 3 Anophthalmic Socket

Enophthalmos and loss of volume from the anophthalmic orbit occur over time in many patients. Dermis-fat and isolated fat grafts can correct and improve this type of deformity.

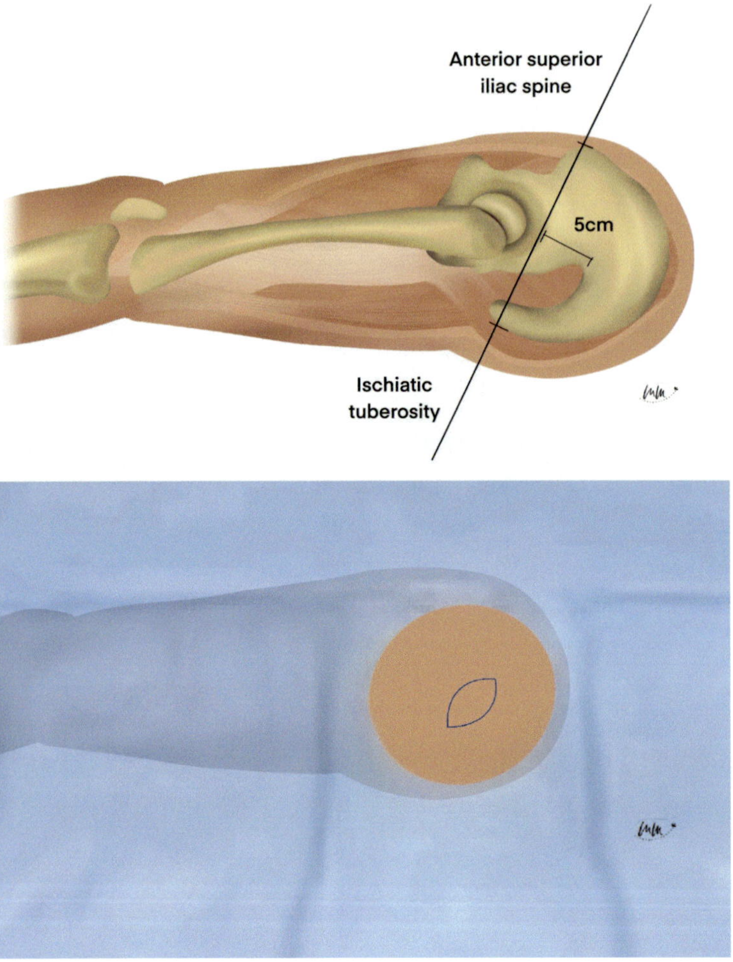

Fig. 6.12 Dermis-fat graft donor site

Dermis-Fat Graft

As described in 1978 by Smith and Petrelli, dermis-fat graft has been essential especially when alloplastic implants are unavailable or undesirable. Indications are in post-enucleation/evisceration, post- extrusion, or alloplastic implant rejection [13].

The graft harvesting sites are the buttocks and abdomen, where there is enough adipose tissue to harvest a graft. In the abdomen, it is customary to remove from the umbilical or lumbar region. If there exists any prior abdominal scar, harvest may be taken from these areas to avoid introducing a new scar. If taken from the buttock region, areas covered by underwear or swimwear may be ideal. The buttock incision should not be too low and be on an area compressed while seated (Fig. 6.12).

The skin is marked, in general, as a circle of 20 mm in diameter, complemented by two lateral triangles to facilitate closure. The incision can be made with a 15-blade scalpel, proceeding with the removal of the epidermis. Next, the incision is deepened to obtain a specimen of about 20–25 mm in height, including the dermis and fat. Hemostasis is performed. Closure is in layers with 3-0 or 4-0 polyglactin sutures to the deep tissues and 5-0 chromic or nylon to the skin (Video 6.3). An additional layer of tissue glue (Dermabond®) can be useful to forestall wound dehiscence.

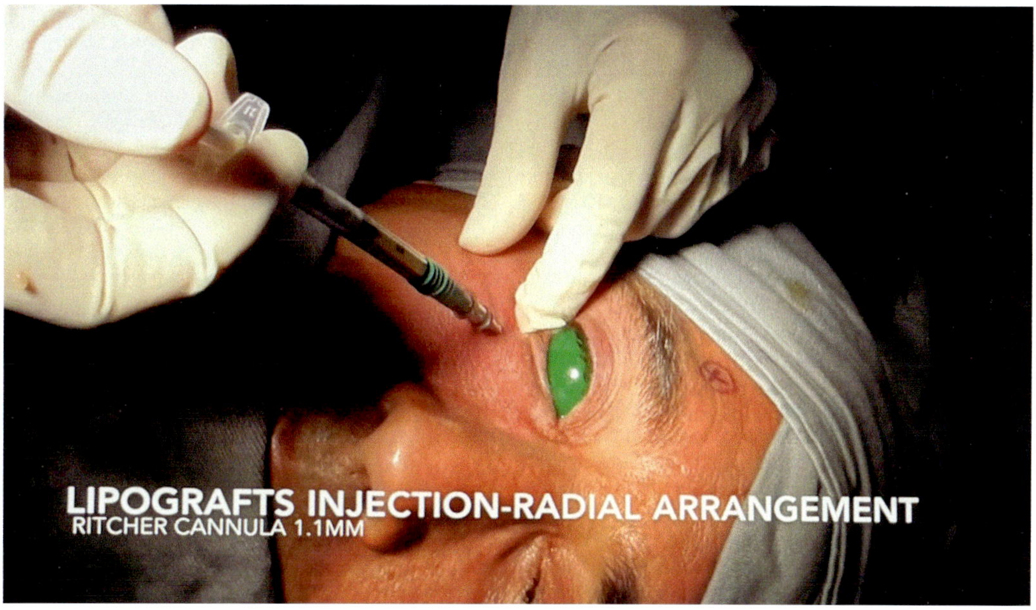

Fig. 6.13 Lipofilling using a 1.1 cannula to volumize enophthalmic orbit. Photo courtesy of Dr. Maria AG Nascimento

The graft is transferred to the recipient anophthalmic socket. The conjunctiva is sewn to the perimeter of the dermis component. Mucosa migrates over the face of the graft over the ensuing weeks to months. These grafts may undergo partial resorption over time. In rare instances the graft may not survive as well. Conversely, especially in children, the hypertrophy of the grafted fat may occur with weight gain. In these cases, the fat lobules are thinned, resected, and reduced.

Fat can be aspirated from the inner thighs or abdomen, centrifuged, and injected into various places of the face, including the anophthalmic orbit, with volumization and improvement of enophthalmos (Fig. 6.13) [14]. Reabsorption is a concern with injected fat, which can occur between 30 and 50%, and repeat fat transfer may be indicated.

Conclusions

There exists a wide range of grafts for various procedures in oculofacial surgery. Autologous grafts are usually available and have fewer rejection concerns. However, grafts prolong the surgical time and increase morbidity due to another surgical site.

Knowledge of the anatomy of the harvesting regions and the appropriate technique for the placement of grafts achieve safe and effective results.

Acknowledgements Mariana Meirelles, MD (drawings).

Juliana Grilo Telles, MD (video edition).

Maria A. G. Nascimento, MD (photo).

References

1. Berggren J, Tenland K, Ansson CD, et al. Revascularization of free skin grafts overlying modified hughes tarsoconjunctival flaps monitored using laser-based techniques. Ophthalmic Plast Reconstr Surg. 2019;35(4):378–82.
2. Rathore DS, Chickadasarahilli S, Crossman R, Mehta P, Ahluwalia HS. Full thickness skin grafts in periocular reconstructions: long-term outcomes. Ophthalmic Plast Reconstr Surg. 2014;30(6):517–20.
3. Adams DC, Ramsey ML. Grafts in dermatologic surgery: review and update on full-and split-thickness

skin grafts, free cartilage grafts, and composite grafts. Dermatol Surg. 2005; 31(8 Part 2):1055–67.
4. Mai C, Bertelmann E. Oral mucosal grafts: old technique in new light. Ophthalmic Res. 2013;50(2):91–8.
5. Grixti A, Malhotra R. Oral mucosa grafting in periorbital reconstruction. Orbit. 2018;37(6):411–28.
6. Segal KL, Nelson CC. Periocular reconstruction. Facial Plast Surg Clin North Am. 2019;27(1):105–18.
7. Henderson HWA, Collin JRO. Mucous membrane grafting. Dev Ophthalmol. 2008;41:230–42.
8. Patel BC, Patipa M, Anderson RL, McLeish W. Management of postblepharoplasty lower eyelid retraction with hard palate grafts and lateral tarsal strip. Plast Reconstr Surg. 1997;99(5):1251–60.
9. Mackay DR, Manders EK, Saggers GC, Schenden MJ, Zaino R. The fate of dermal and dermal-fat grafts. Ann Plast Surg. 1993;31(1):42–6.
10. Baroody M, Holds JB, Vick VL. Advances in the diagnosis and treatment of ptosis. Curr Opin Ophthalmol. 2005;16:351–5.
11. Sagoo MS, Olver JM. Autogenous temporalis fascia patch graft for porous polyethylene (Medpor) sphere orbital implant exposure. Br J Ophthalmol. 2004;88(7):942–6.
12. Fan J. Frontalis suspension technique with a temporal-fasciae-complex sheet for repairing blepharoptosis. Aesthetic Plast Surg. 2001;25:147–51.
13. Jovanovic N, Carniciu AL, Russell WW, Jarocki A, Kahana A. Reconstruction of the orbit and anophthalmic socket using the dermis fat graft: a major review. Ophthalmic Plast Reconstr Surg. 2020;36(6):529–39.
14. Hardy TG, Joshi N, Kelly MH. Orbital volume augmentation with autologous micro-fat grafts. Ophthalmic Plast Reconstr Surg. 2007;23(6):445–9.

Fundamentals of Eyelid and Facial Flaps

7

Stephanie H. Noh, Shijun Sung, and Lilangi S. Ediriwickrema

Abstract

A flap is tissue transferred from one site (donor) to another (recipient) while maintaining its own blood supply. In oculofacial surgery, defects occur due to congenital anomalies, infiltrative and inflammatory processes, traumatic injuries, or iatrogenic causes. In this chapter, the authors describe fundamentals and the various classifications of flaps used for eyelid or periorbital reconstruction.

Keywords

Periocular reconstruction · Eyelid flaps · Facial flaps

Introduction

The eyelids provide essential structural and functional support for the eye. They form a barrier for the globe against trauma, regulate light influx, and maintain the tear film. Defects of the eyelids and periocular tissue can occur from congenital anomalies, infiltrative and inflammatory processes, traumatic injuries, or iatrogenic causes (i.e., surgery or radiation). Partial-thickness eyelid defects involve skin and superficial muscles (anterior lamellar defect), whereas full-thickness defects extend from the skin through the conjunctiva. Oculofacial reconstructive surgery aims to optimize visual function and protection of the ocular surface while preserving/restoring facial expression provided by periocular muscles.

Eyelid reconstruction should be guided by the size and depth of the defect while carefully considering eyelid, orbital, and lacrimal anatomy. Anterior lamella defects can be well reconstructed by transferring neighboring tissue (flaps) which have similar histology, texture, and thickness. If there is insufficient adjacent tissue, full-thickness skin grafts from the upper lid, inner upper arm, pre or postauricular region, or supraclavicular area may be used. Because the face has good vascular supply, myocutaneous flaps play an integral role in eyelid and periocular reconstruction. The surgeon should consider periorbital and eyelid anatomy, aesthetic units of face, and appearance of the final scar to select the reconstructive approach that optimizes both functional and aesthetic outcome.

Flaps should be considered in periocular reconstruction when direct closure, secondary

Supplementary Information The online version contains supplementary material available at https://doi.org/10.1007/978-3-031-63178-8_7.

S. H. Noh · S. Sung
University of California, Irvine, Irvine, CA, USA

L. S. Ediriwickrema (✉)
Division of Oculofacial Plastic and Orbital Surgery, University of California, Irvine, Irvine, CA, USA
e-mail: rlorn@hs.uci.edu

J. Tao (ed.), *Efficient Oculofacial Surgery*, https://doi.org/10.1007/978-3-031-63178-8_7

intention, or skin grafting could produce an unfavorable cosmetic or functional result. Because the flap is adjacent to the defect, the flap will heal with similar color and texture to the surrounding tissue. Another advantage is rich vascular supply which allows for optimal healing and a decreased propensity for tissue contraction. There are several types of myocutaenous flaps, but some of the most common types of flaps utilized in oculoplastic surgery include sliding, advancement, rotation, and transposition flaps.

In advancement flaps, the flap is moved directly forward into the defect with no lateral or rotational movement (a single vector). Sliding flaps are even simpler and involve undermining adjacent tissue to allow for primary closure. In rotational flaps, the flap rotates along the edge of the flap around a pivot point and is positioned into an adjacent defect. Examples of rotational flaps include the semicircular (Tenzel) flap and larger cheek (Mustarde) rotational flap. In contrast, a transposition flap is transposed around a pivot point across an intervening segment of normal tissue into a nonadjacent defect.

With any flap, care should be taken to minimize wound tension and preserve vascular supply. In this chapter, the authors delineate the basic types of tissue flaps. Several specific oculofacial flaps are introduced in this chapter and detailed in other chapters.

Sliding and Advancement Flaps

Sliding flaps are the most fundamental type of flap and involve undermining local tissue in order to allow for primary closure. In advancement flaps, the flap is advanced in one direction into the defect (without any lateral movement or rotation). Advancement flaps are utilized when primary closure of a defect may result in excessive tension. An example of an advancement flap is demonstrated in the initial steps of the Cutler-Beard procedure (composite lower to upper eyelid flap) in reconstructing a large upper eyelid defect. A lower eyelid rectangular flap is advanced superiorly into the full thickness upper eyelid defect to reconstruct the anterior lamella.

Rotation Flaps

Rotation flaps are typically elevated using a semicircular or arcuate incision. If necessary, the primary defect should be enlarged into a triangular shape to allow for the ideal closure. In rotation flaps, tension is mostly distributed perpendicular to the arc of the incision. Back cuts and triangular resections (a.k.a., Burrow's triangles) can be created at the distal end of the arc to gain additional rotational tissue recruitment. Specific rotation flaps used in oculoplastic surgery include the semicircular (Tenzel) flap and the cheek (Mustardé) rotational flap. The semicircular (Tenzel) advancement flap (Fig. 7.1, Video 7-1) is used for larger eyelid defects that affect approximately one-third to two-thirds of the eyelid. In this technique, a lateral semicircular myocutaneous flap is created after first performing a canthotomy and cantholysis. Within the flap, the skin and orbicularis are carefully undermined, and then advanced to close the lid margin defect. The cheek (Mustardé) rotational

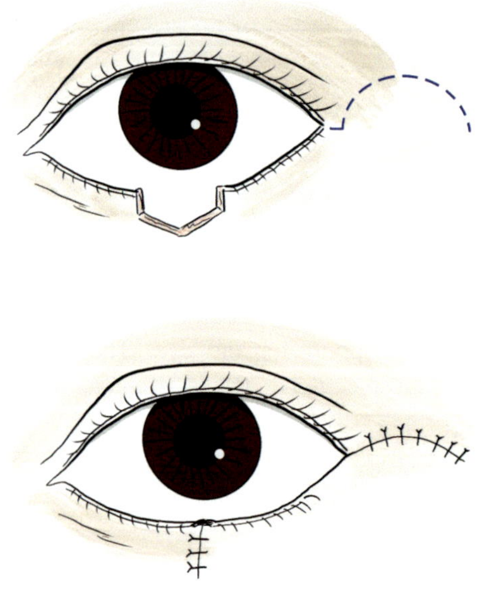

Fig. 7.1 Semicircular flap (Tenzel flap). A lateral myocutaneous flap (marking shown in dotted blue line) is created after performing a canthotomy and cantholysis. The flap is advanced medially to close the eyelid margin defect

flap (Fig. 7.2) is used to repair anterior lamellar defects of the lower eyelid and cheek. A subciliary incision is made extending laterally from the defect to the lateral canthus, then curves superiorly into the temple region and then inferiorly towards the preauricular space, like that of a facelift incision. When undermining the lateral aspect of the flap (lateral to the lateral canthus), care is taken to remain in the subcutaneous plane so as not to damage the branches of the facial nerve. Extensive dissection may need to be performed to minimize tension on the flap and skin. The flap is then rotated medially to close the defect.

Transposition Flaps

In transposition flaps, the flap is transposed across an intervening segment of normal tissue into a defect. Some common examples of transposition flaps include the Z-plasty and rhomboid flap, and specialized transposition flaps include the glabellar V to Y flap, paramedian forehead flap, forehead transposition flap (Fricke flap), and Tripier flap.

The Z-plasty (Fig. 7.3) is a basic transposition flap that involves transposing two triangular flaps adjacent to each other. Common indications for this flap include scar contractures or when working around webs/folds of tissue. Z-plasties allow for increased tissue and relaxation along the primary axis of the Z. It shortens/tightens perpendicular to this primary axis. The McGregor flap (Fig. 7.4) is like the Tenzel flap but also utilizes a lateral Z-plasty, allowing for horizontal tissue recruitment. A modified Z-plasty may be indicated for medial epicanthoplasty or medial web reduction (Figs. 7.9, 7.10, 7.11, 7.12, 7.13, 7.14 and 7.15, Video 7-2). A specific modification includes the jumping man flap, which combines a V-Y advancement flap with two lateral Z-plasties (Fig. 7.16).

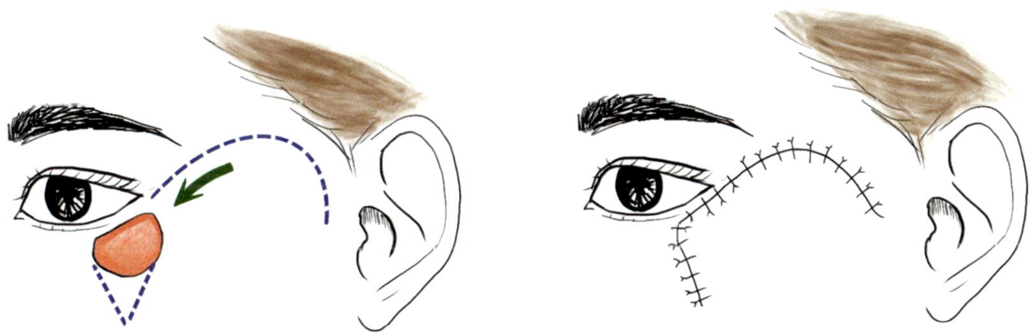

Fig. 7.2 Cheek rotational flap

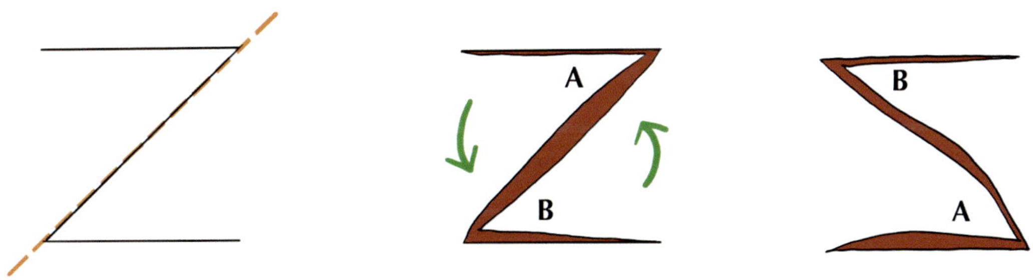

Fig. 7.3 Z-plasty flap

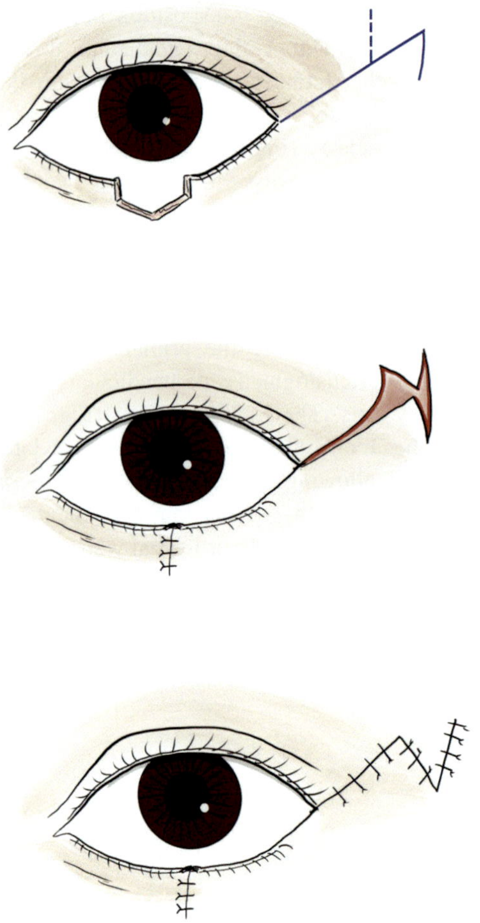

Fig. 7.4 McGregor flap. Similar to the semicircular Tenzel flap but utilizes a lateral Z-plasty as shown

The rhomboid flap (Fig. 7.5, Video 7-3) is another commonly used transposition flap for small to medium defects that is simple, effective, and modifiable. The defect is enlarged into a parallelogram and the flap is transposed along the short axis, ideally within the relaxed skin tension lines.

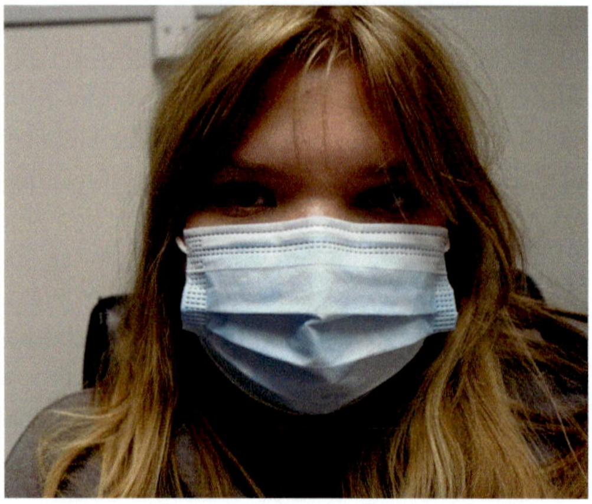

Fig. 7.5 Patient with a disfiguring right medial canthal web after trauma

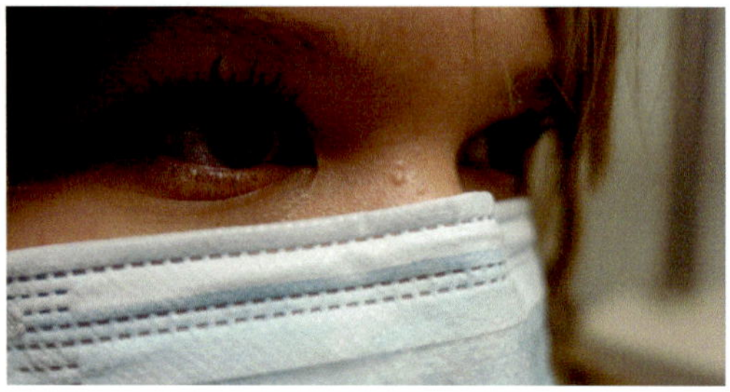

Fig. 7.6 Oblique view of right medial canthal web

The glabellar V to Y flap (Fig. 7.6, Video 7-1) is used to reconstruct medial canthal defects. This technique involves creating an inverted V incision in the glabellar area adjacent to the defect. The flap is then undermined and rotated into position.

The paramedian forehead transposition flap (Fig. 7.7) is used for large defects involving the medial canthus and lower eyelid. This is a two-stage procedure in which a rotational regional skin flap is harvested from the contralateral forehead. The pedicled flap obtains its vasculature

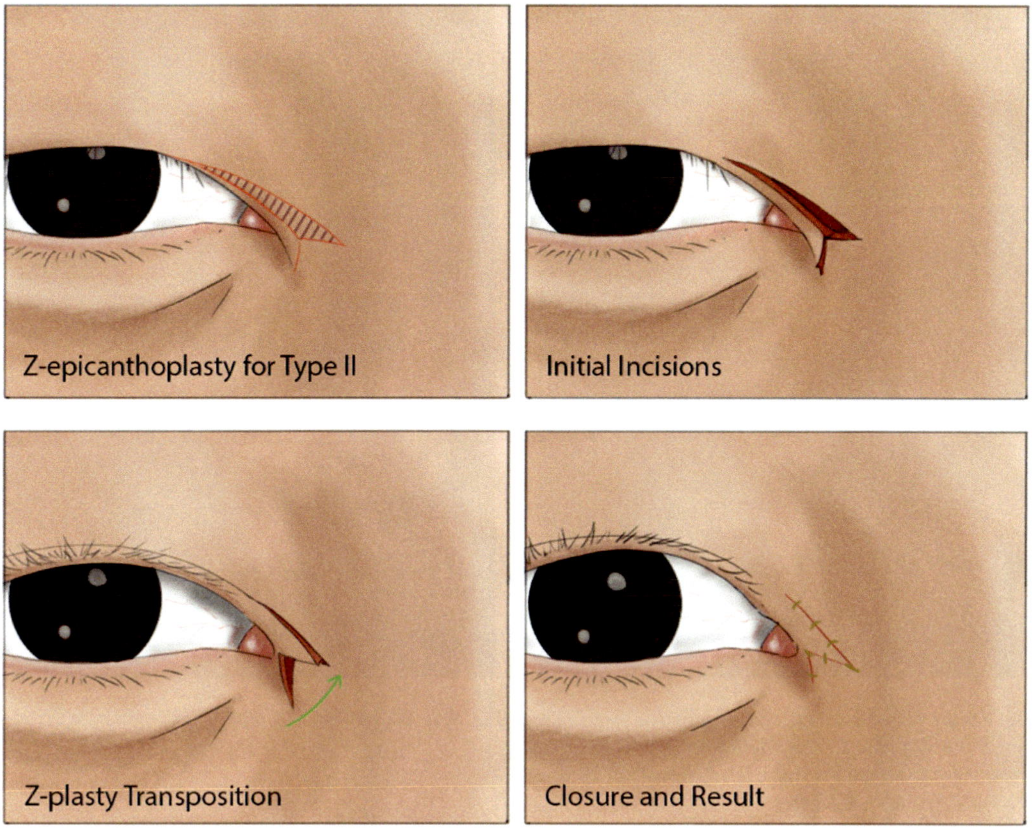

Fig. 7.7 Z-plasty design to soften a medial canthal web or prominent epicanthal fold

from the supraorbital/supratrochlear neurovascular bundle. After the flap is incised, dissection is carried out anterior to the periosteum of the frontal bone. The flap is then rotated to cover the defect and care should be taken to avoid excessive tension during closure to prevent flap necrosis. The donor site may need extensive undermining to approximate the wound edges for direct closure, but residual defects can also be repaired with a skin graft or left to granulate. In the second stage of the procedure, the pedicle is divided several weeks later, and the flap may be further thinned and sculpted.

The forehead transposition flap (also known as Fricke flap) (Fig. 7.8) is a lateral forehead skin flap advanced from the upper brow that is used to reconstruct upper and lower eyelid defects. Disadvantages of this flap include relatively thick skin in comparison to eyelid skin, and postoperatively, the patient may have asymmetric brow elevation due to excising tissue from the supraciliary region (Figs. 7.9, 7.10, 7.11, 7.12, 7.13, 7.14, 7.15 and 7.16).

The Tripier flap is a transpositional pedicle flap in which the skin and orbicularis from the upper eyelid is used to reconstruct a lower eyelid defect.

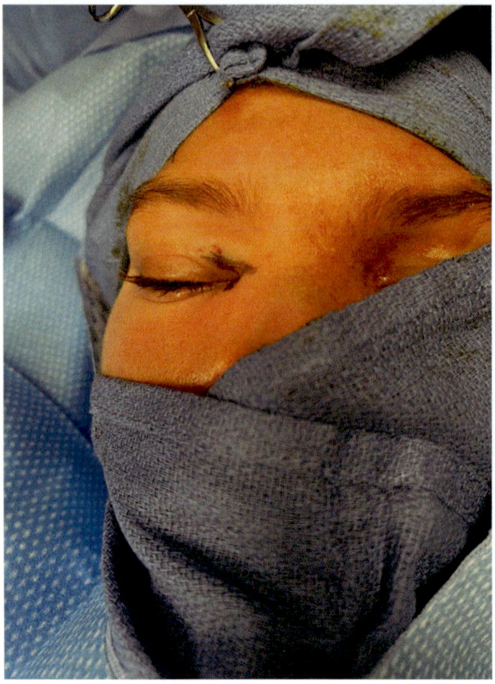

Fig. 7.8 Z plasty marked with methylene blue. The primary axis of the Z plasty follows the web from the crease. One transposition flap is created with an incision extending medially from superior aspect of the primary axis (a small ellipse is excised off the superior axis of this wound to further alleviate the web). The other transposition flap is created with an incision extending superolaterally off the inferior aspect of the primary axis

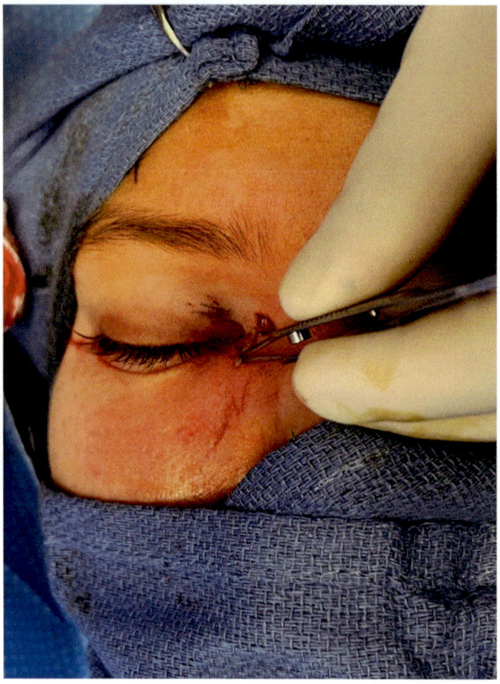

Fig. 7.9 Flaps dissected free

The flap can be unipedicled or bipedicled. The bipedicle flap can reconstruct a total lower eyelid defect, whereas the unipedicle flap can reconstruct one-third to one-half of the eyelid length. Of note, this flap is limited in vertical height as it recruits excess skin and orbicularis from the upper eyelid.

Post-operative Management and Pearls

Postoperative instructions for periocular reconstructive flaps include rest, smoking avoidance, hydration, keeping the head of the bed elevated as tolerated, as well as topical/oral antibiotic and analgesics as indicated. It is important to avoid excessive icing, and bolsters and patches should be left in place as directed.

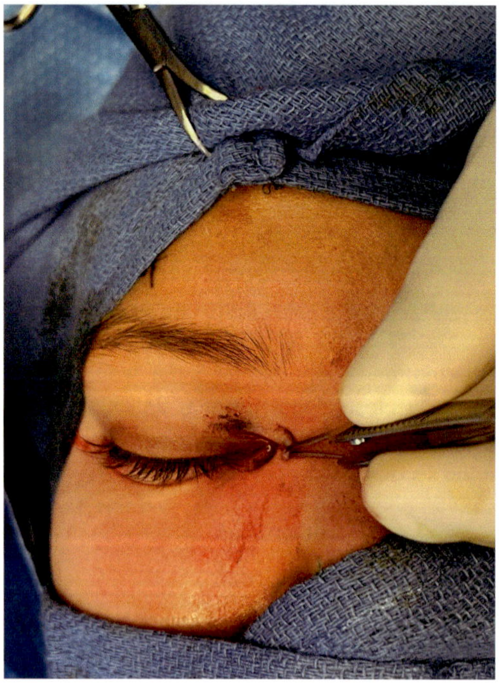

Fig. 7.10 Flaps transposed

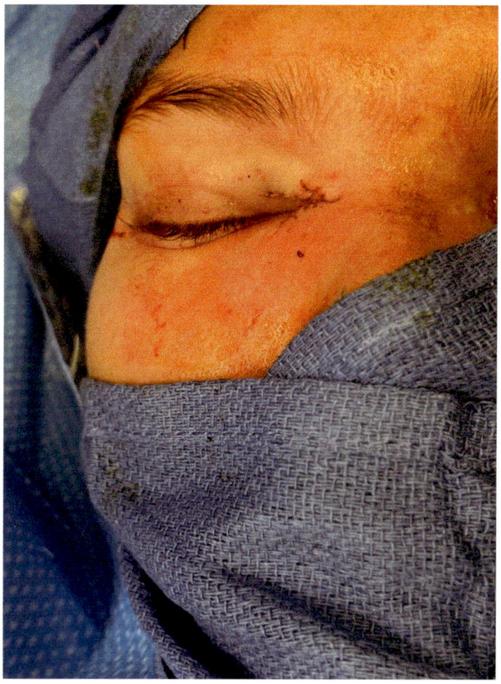

Fig. 7.11 Flaps sewn into place

Scar Optimization and Healing

To promote healing and scar optimization, the patient should be advised to minimize manipulation and movement (no lifting or vasovagal procedures) for several weeks postoperatively. Additionally, the patient should use all topical ointment as prescribed. Other environmental factors include avoiding sun exposure and maintaining a balanced diet for adequate nutrition. For any resulting scars, further options include steroids, laser, antimetabolites, and/or surgical intervention.

Conclusions

A variety of tissue flaps are utilized in oculofacial surgery. Owing to the complex contours and variable skin types in the periocular region, proper flap selection and design are important to achieve favorable results.

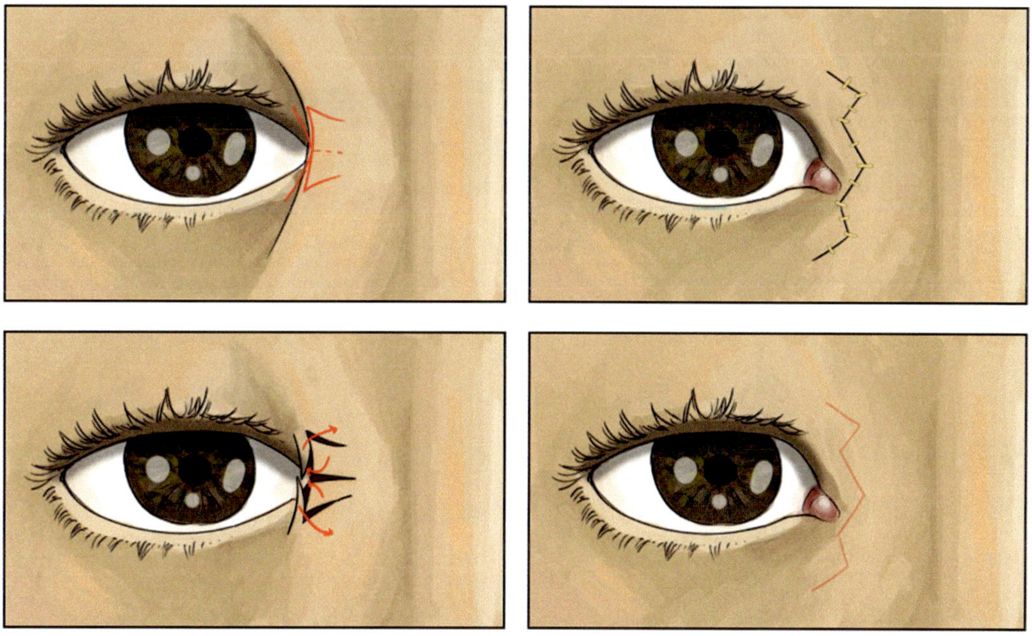

Fig. 7.12 Jumping man apposing Z-plasty design

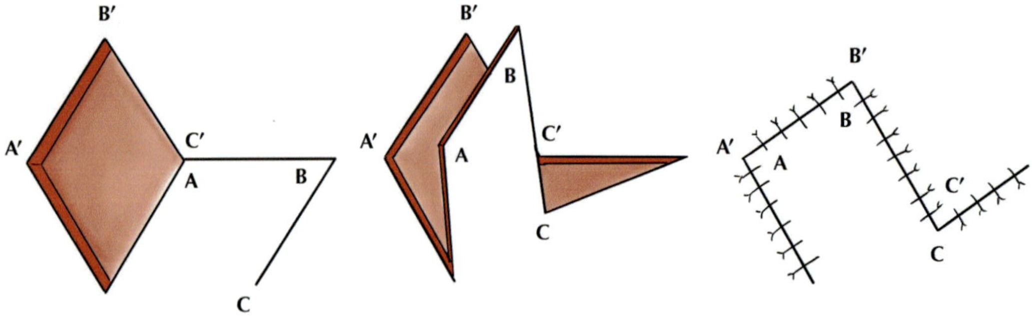

Fig. 7.13 Rhomboid flap

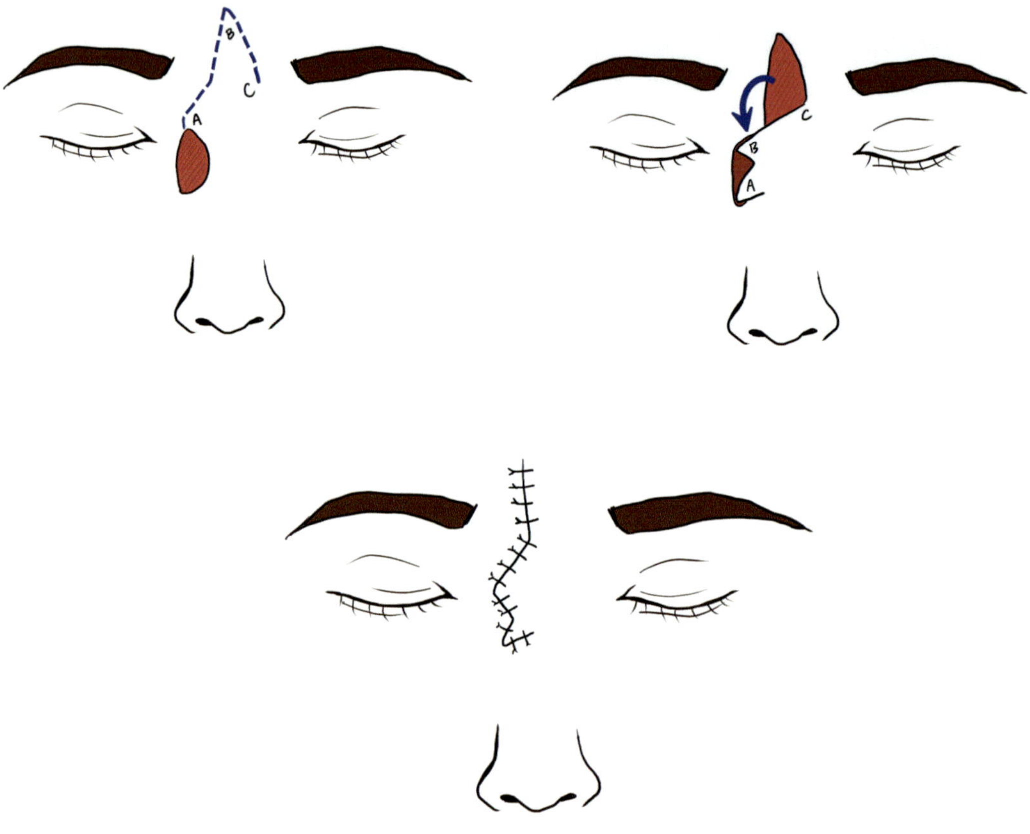

Fig. 7.14 Glabellar V to Y flap

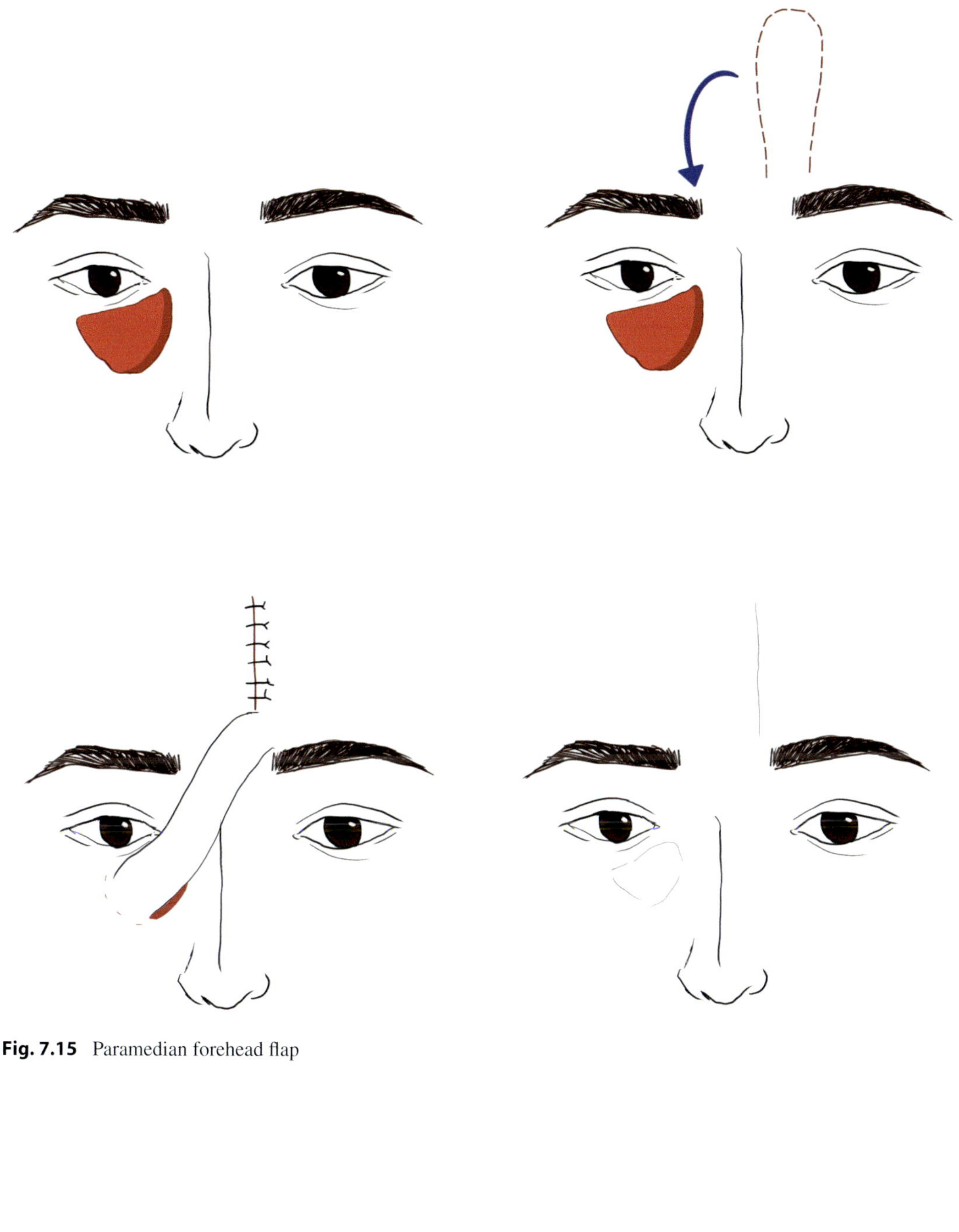

Fig. 7.15 Paramedian forehead flap

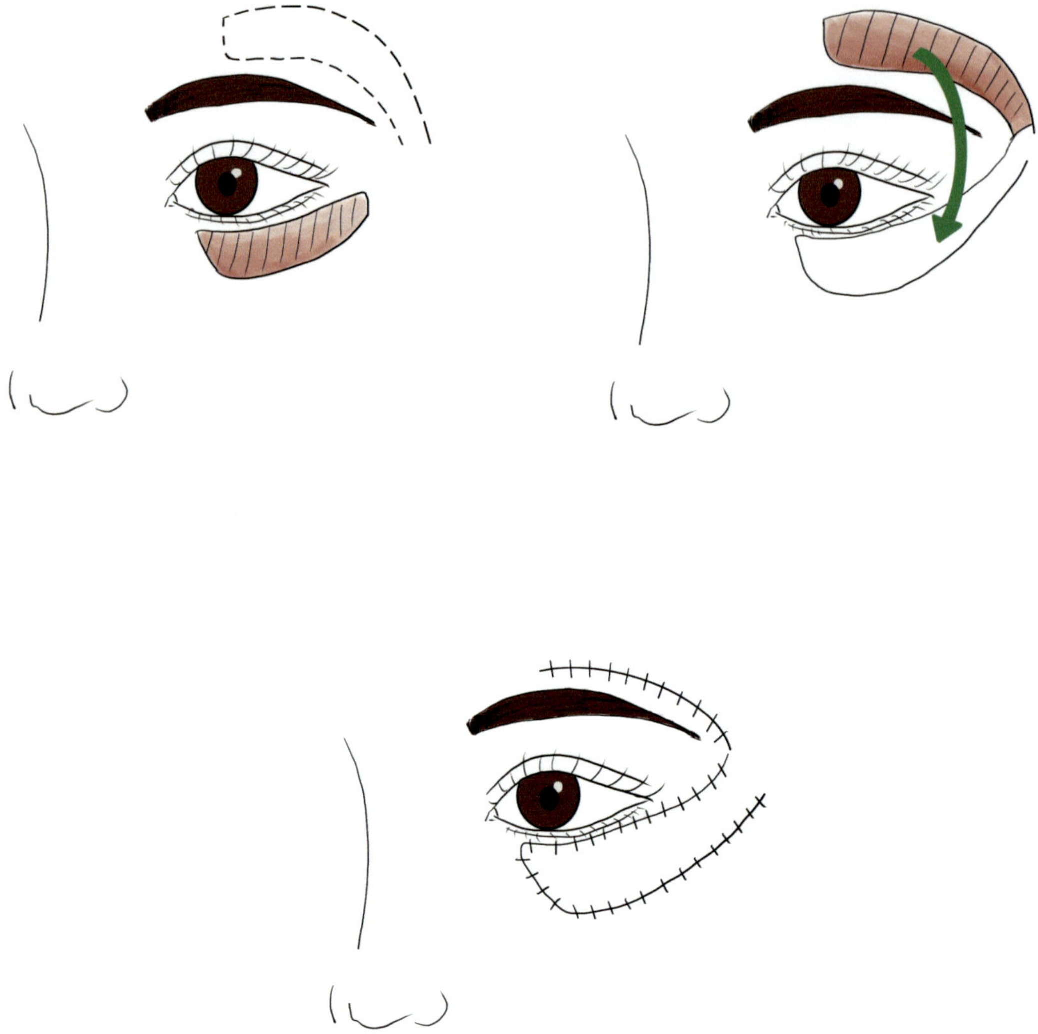

Fig. 7.16 Fricke flap

References

1. Sand JP, Zhu BZ, Desai SC. Surgical anatomy of the eyelids. Facial Plast Surg Clin North Am. 2016;24(2):89–95 (in English).
2. Segal KL, Nelson CC. Periocular reconstruction. Facial Plast Surg Clin North Am. 2019;27(1):105–18 (in English).
3. Holds JB. Lower eyelid reconstruction. Facial Plast Surg Clin North Am. 2016;24(2):183–91 (in English).
4. Hayano SM, Whipple KM, Korn BS, Kikkawa DO. Principles of periocular reconstruction following excision of cutaneous malignancy. J Skin Cancer. 2012:438502.
5. Alghoul MS, Kearney AM, Pacella SJ, Purnell CA. Eyelid reconstruction. Plast Reconstr Surg Glob Open. 2019;7(11):e2520 (in English).
6. Espinoza GM, Prost AM. Upper eyelid reconstruction. Facial Plast Surg Clin North Am. 2016;24(2):173–82 (in English).
7. Ang TW, Juniat V, O'Rourke M, et al. The use of the paramedian forehead flap alone or in combination

with other techniques in the reconstruction of periocular defects and orbital exenterations. Eye. 2022.
8. Machado WL, Gurfinkel PC, Gualberto GV, Sampaio FM, Melo ML, Treu CM. Modified tripier flap in reconstruction of the lower eyelid. An Bras Dermatol. 2015;90(1):108–10.
9. Mustardé JC. Surgical treatment of malignant tumours of the upper lid. Chirurgia plastica. 1971;1(1):25–33.
10. Yan Y, Fu R, Ji Q, et al. Surgical strategies for eyelid defect reconstruction: a review on principles and techniques. Ophthalmol Ther. 2022;11:1383–408.

Repair of Full Thickness Upper Eyelid Defects

8

Jordan Miller O'Dell and Jason A. Sokol

Abstract

Repair of full thickness upper eyelid defects is indicated to restore ocular protective functions and cosmesis. While small defects may be closed primarily, larger defects often require flaps or grafts or both. While the anterior lamella may be replaced by skin, mucous membrane is required for the internal posterior lamella lining of the eyelid to maintain ocular surface health and comfort. This chapter details a systematic approach for reconstruction of upper eyelid defects.

Keywords

Upper eyelid repair · Upper eyelid flap · Upper eyelid defect · Upper eyelid graft · Upper eyelid reconstruction · Cutler-beard flap · Sliding tarsoconjunctival flap

Supplementary Information The online version contains supplementary material available at https://doi.org/10.1007/978-3-031-63178-8_8.

J. M. O'Dell (✉) · J. A. Sokol
University of Kansas, Kansas City, MO, USA
e-mail: jordanemiller09@gmail.com

J. A. Sokol
e-mail: jsokolmd@gmail.com

Introduction

Defects of the upper eyelid pose unique reconstructive considerations. Both the mechanics and form of the eyelid must be restored. Unlike the lower eyelid, the upper eyelid must be able to fully cover the ocular surface during a blink and clear the visual axis when the eyelid is open. This is not only important cosmetically, but ensures the cornea and globe are protected [1]. Often, repair must be done urgently [2]. This chapter will describe a systematic approach for reconstruction of the upper eyelid, beginning with small, simple defects and progressing to more complex reconstructions.

Anatomic Considerations

The upper eyelid is composed of two lamellae. The anterior lamella consists of the skin and orbicularis, and the posterior lamella consists of the tarsus and conjunctiva. Determining which lamella is involved in a defect is important in selecting a reconstructive technique.

The tarsus provides structure to the upper eyelid; it is approximately 29 mm long, 10 mm tall centrally and tapers toward the ends, and 1 mm thick. In addition to providing structure, it contains the meibomian glands, which secrete the lipid component of the tear film. The orbicularis provides eyelid closure and gets its

J. Tao (ed.), *Efficient Oculofacial Surgery*, https://doi.org/10.1007/978-3-031-63178-8_8

innervation from the temporal and zygomatic branches of the facial nerve. The levator, and, to a lesser degree, Muller's muscle, are responsible for eyelid opening and receive innervation from cranial nerve III and sympathetic branches, respectively (Fig. 8.1). Most of the blood flow to the upper eyelid comes from the marginal and peripheral arcades. The marginal arcade is located between pretarsal orbicularis and tarsus, 2–3 mm above the eyelid margin. The peripheral arcade is located between levator and Muller's muscle, just superior to the tarsus. The anterior lamella drains into the angular vein medially and the superficial temporal vein laterally, while the posterior lamella drains into the deeper orbital vein, anterior facial vein, and pterygoid plexus. The lymphatic drainage is an important consideration in the case of tumor resection; the lateral two-thirds of the upper eyelid drains into preauricular nodes, and the medial one-third drains into submandibular nodes [1].

Prior to proceeding with repair, a thorough history should be taken to assess for prior radiation, smoking history, or diabetes. These are important considerations when performing a flap, as adequate blood flow is needed for successful healing [2].

Direct Closure

Direct closure may be considered for some small upper eyelid defects. In young patients who have taut skin, defects up to one third the upper eyelid margin may be repaired directly. In older patients with more tissue laxity, defects up to one half of the eyelid may tolerate direct closure. This may, however, require lateral cantholysis to relieve tension on the wound [2, 3]. In general, when repairing the eyelids, horizontal tension is better tolerated than vertical tension, as the latter may produce cicatricial changes resulting in retraction and exposure keratopathy [1].

When closing any defect involving the eyelid margin, it is important to avoid eyelid notching. A notch is not only conspicuous but risks ocular surface exposure. Generally, in pediatric cases or those with uncertain follow up, absorbable suture should be used [2].

The tarsal edges are trimmed perpendicular to the eyelid margin and made full thickness through the tarsus (Fig. 8.2). A 6-0 silk or polyglactin is used to approximate the gray line, and the ends of the suture are left long (Fig. 8.3). If the wound is under significant tension, a lateral cantholysis is performed with a

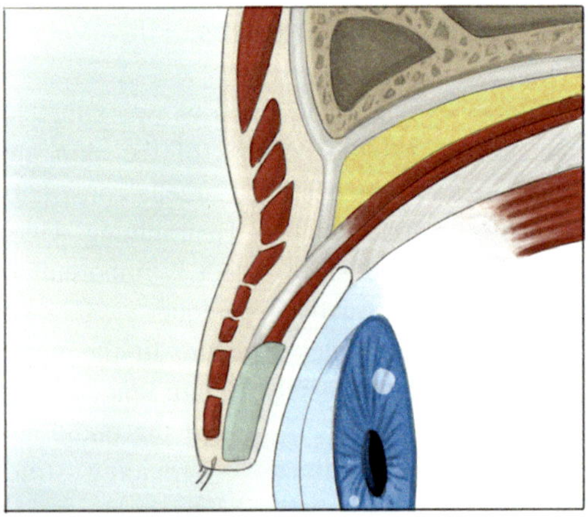

Fig. 8.1 Upper eyelid cross-section, courtesy of Michael Han MD

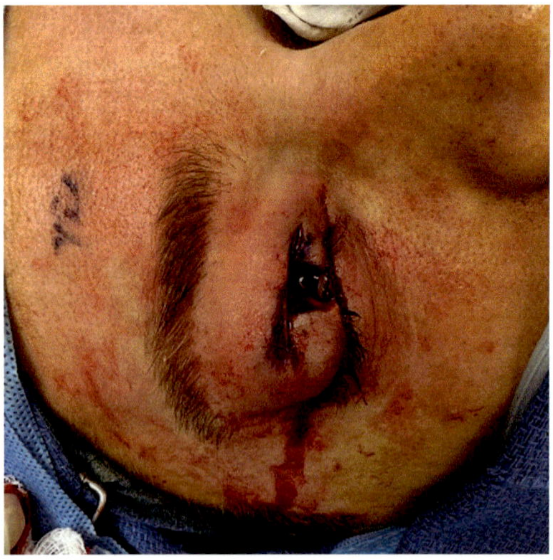

Fig. 8.2 Small upper eyelid defect

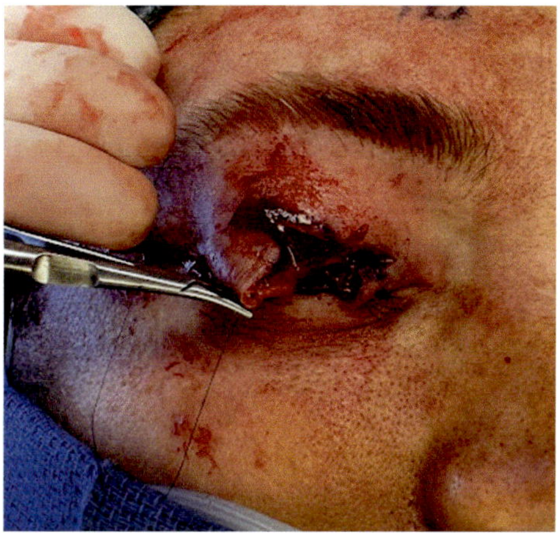

Fig. 8.3 Approximate the gray line

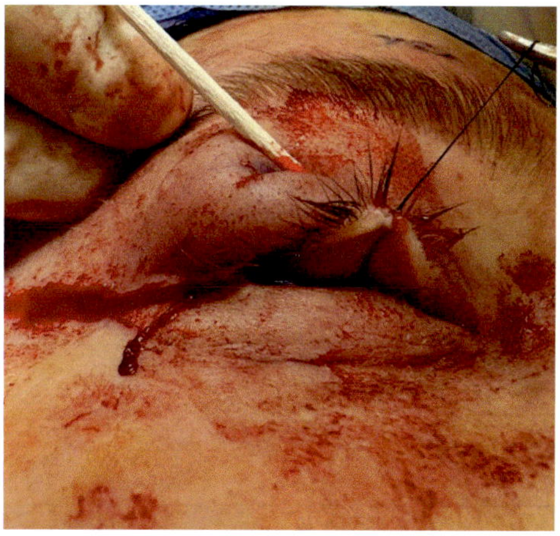

Fig. 8.5 Eyelid everted

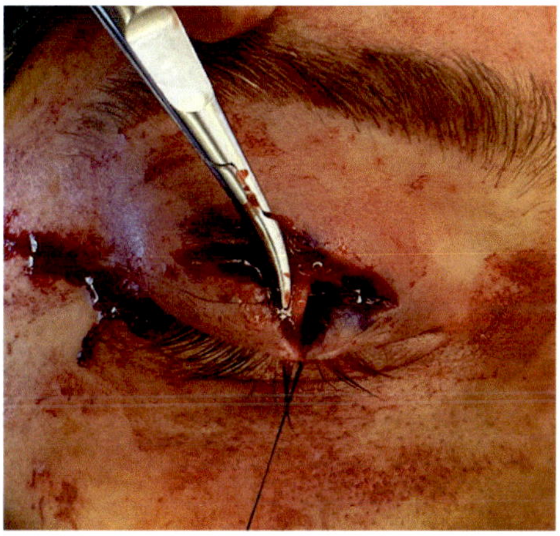

Fig. 8.4 Approximate the tarsus

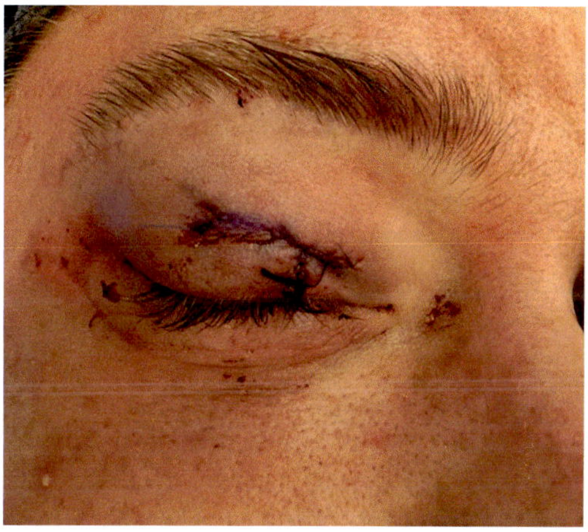

Fig. 8.6 Skin closure

15-blade used to incise through the skin at the lateral canthus and scissors are used to release the superior ramus of the lateral canthal tendon. The tarsus is then re-approximated with three interrupted partial thickness bites using 6-0 polyglactin or 7-0 silk suture (Fig. 8.4). Next, a 6-0 silk or polyglactin is placed at the lash margin, with the ends left long (Fig. 8.5). The skin is then closed using 6-0 or 7-0 silk or plain gut in a running fashion (Fig. 8.6). The long ends of the lash margin and gray line sutures are then pulled superiorly and taped to the upper eyelid or brow to prevent irritation of the ocular surface (Fig. 8.7). Ointment can be applied three times daily for a week, and permanent sutures removed at the one to two-week post-operative visit [1–3]. Varying degrees of ptosis may be present following repair and should simply be observed for six months prior to revision as this will usually improve [4].

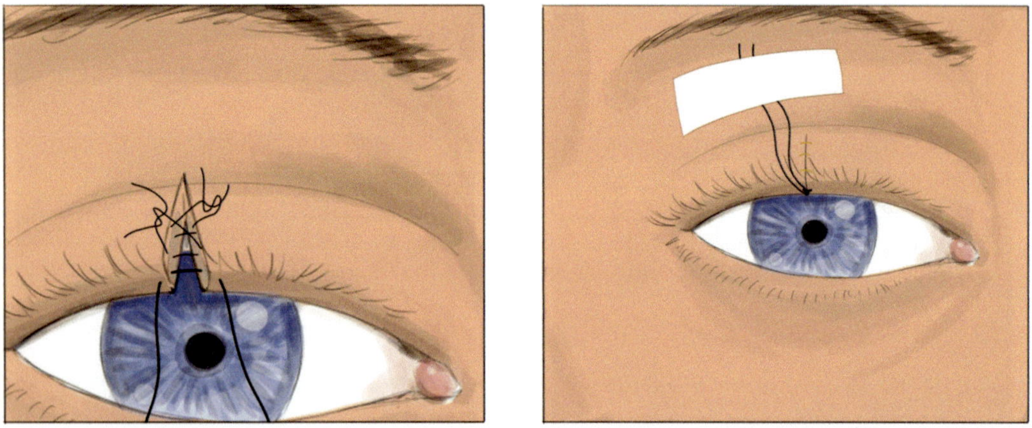

Fig. 8.7 Direct closure, courtesy of Michael Han MD

Cantholysis and Semicircular Flap

Defects up to 40% of the eyelid margin for which direct closure is not feasible may be treated with a semicircular flap formed at the lateral canthus. A curved line is marked starting from the edge of the lateral canthus and extending inferiorly and laterally before curving upward with a diameter of approximately 20 mm. The length of the semicircular flap depends on the amount of needed tissue recruitment and is usually commensurate or slightly larger than the size of the eyelid defect to be repaired. This line is incised using a 15-blade through the musculocutaneous layer. The superior ramus of the lateral canthal tendon must be released, and the tissue sufficiently undermined, so the flap can be rotated into the upper eyelid defect. Undermining is performed in a sub-orbicularis or subcutaneous plane. The eyelid margin is closed as described in the previous section, taking care not to take full thickness bites to avoid suture rubbing against the ocular surface. The lateral most aspect is secured to the periosteum of the lateral orbital rim to recreate the canthal angle and ensure the eyelid contour is abutting the globe [1]. If no periosteum is available, the lateral canthus may be reconstructed by suturing through drill holes placed in the lateral orbital rim [2]. The conjunctiva can be advanced to the eyelid margin and closed with running 6-0 or 7-0 polyglactin or plain gut. The musculocutaneous incision is closed in two layers, with 5-0 polyglactin in the subcutaneous layer and 6-0 silk or plain gut cutaneous suture (Fig. 8.8).

Sliding Tarsoconjunctival Flap

A sliding tarsoconjunctival flap is useful when the defect cannot be repaired directly. First, the eyelid is everted (over cotton tip applicators or a Desmarres retractor), and a 15-blade is used to make an incision in the tarsal plate 4–5 mm above the eyelid margin, approximately the width of the defect. The flap is then dissected to the superior border of the tarsus and the Mullers muscle is dissected away from the flap. The tarso conjunctival flap is rotated into the defect and the edge is attached to the periosteum or lateral canthal tendon with 5-0

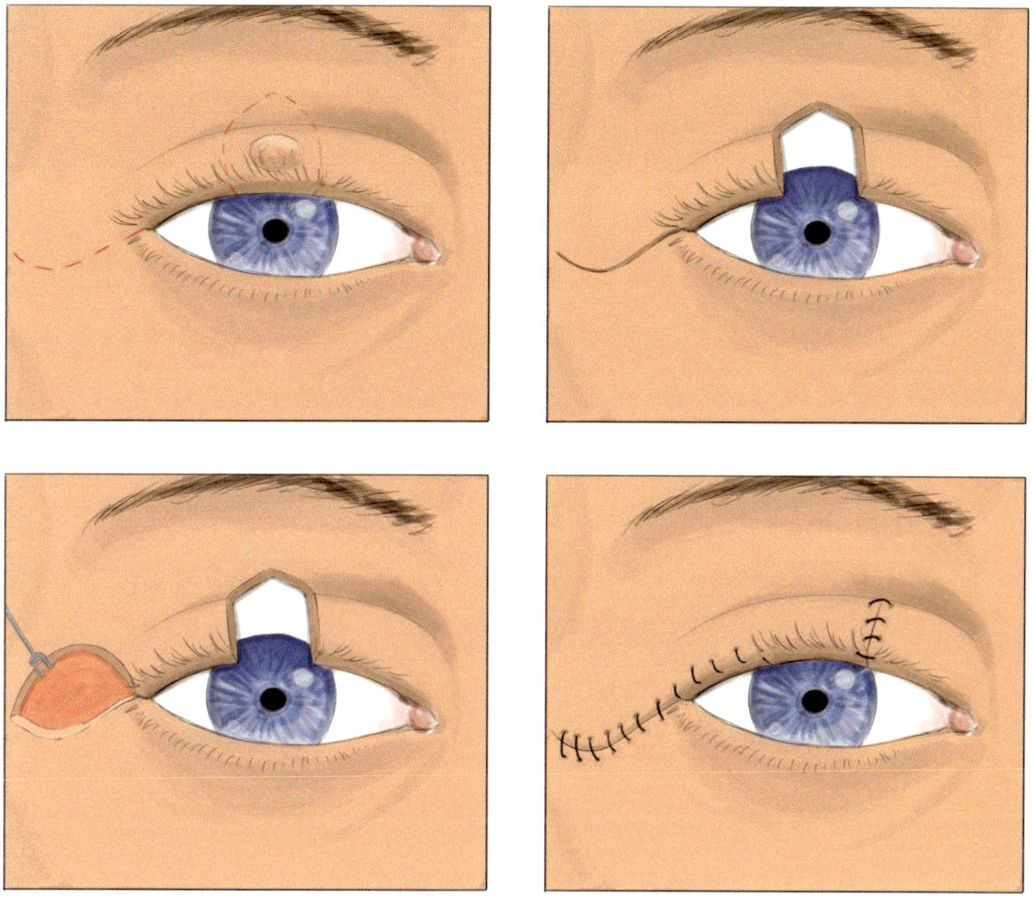

Fig. 8.8 Semicircular flap, courtesy of Michael Han MD

polyglactin suture. 6-0 polyglactin or 7-0 silk is used to place lamellar bites at the residual tarsal edge of the defect and approximate the lash margin. A full thickness skin graft from the retro-auricular area, opposite eyelid, or medial upper arm is placed over the tarsoconjunctival flap and secured with interrupted 6-0 or 7-0 silk or plain suture, being careful not to rotate the skin under the eyelid margin. When using a full thickness skin graft, it is important to make sure the skin chosen is free of hair to prevent keratopathy. A temporary tarsorrhaphy or F rost suture is placed with a 4-0 silk to place the eyelid on stretch while it heals for one week and the area is covered with a pressure patch over a non-adherent pad (Fig. 8.9) [2].

Split-Level Eyelid Grafts for Cicatricial Upper Eyelid Retraction

Cicatricial changes to the upper eyelid, such as those resulting from burns or radiation, lead to vertical shortening of the upper eyelid. These full-thickness defects may be repaired by employing a split-level graft where the anterior lamella is replaced with retro-auricular or opposite eyelid skin graft, and the posterior lamella is

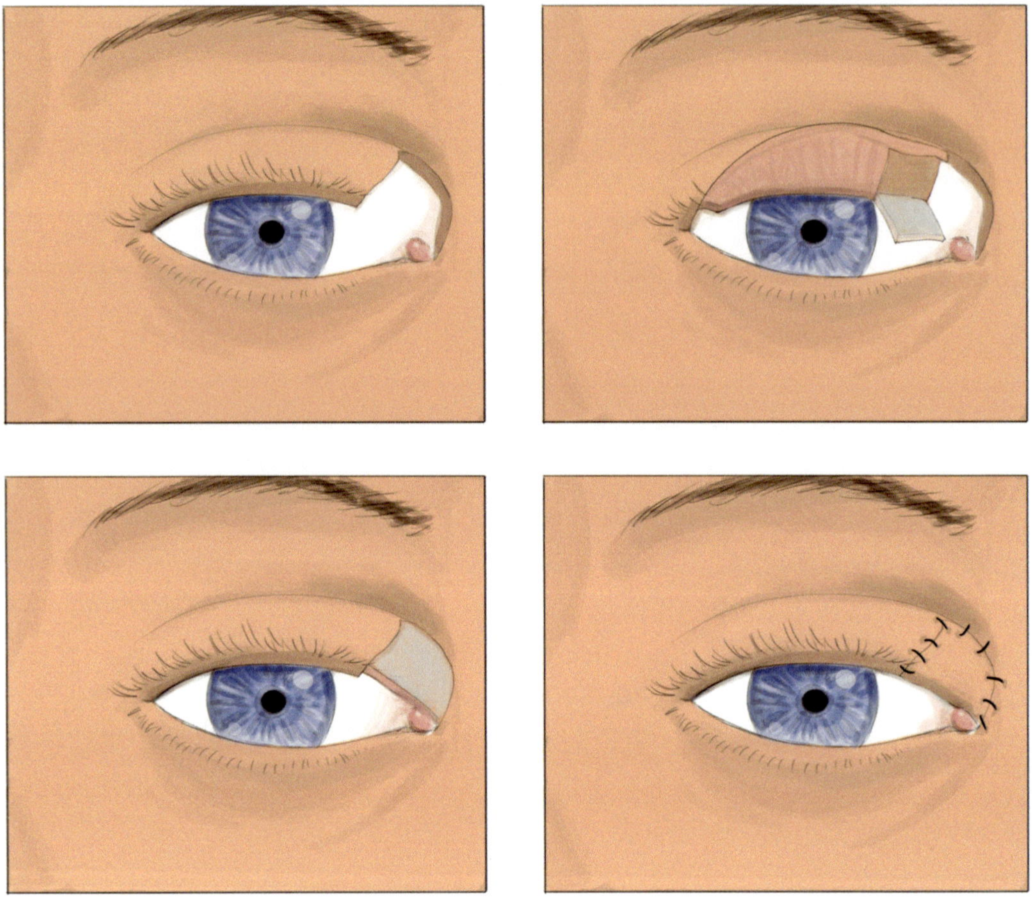

Fig. 8.9 Sliding flap, courtesy of Michael Han MD

replaced with buccal mucosal graft. These grafts are placed at split vertical positions so that each has its own vascular supply, and the split nature of the graft allows for vertical lengthening of the contracted eyelid. This technique begins much like the sliding flap technique. The upper eyelid is everted over a Desmarres retractor, and a horizontal incision is made through the tarsus approximately 4–5 mm superior to the eyelid margin. The retractor is removed, and the eyelid is retracted inferiorly with a 4-0 silk suture. A horizontal incision is made through the skin at the superior edge of the tarsus. Westcott scissors are used to undermine the skin superiorly and inferiorly. The eyelid is then everted again, and a buccal mucosal graft is sutured between the edges of the tarsal conjunctiva with a running 6-0 plain or fast gut suture. The eyelid is then retracted inferiorly, and a full thickness retroauricular or opposite upper eyelid skin graft is sutured between the cut skin edges with 6 or 7-0 silk or plain suture (Fig. 8.10). A temporary tarsorrhaphy with pressure patch is placed [2, 3].

Medial and Temporal Forehead Flaps

When there is extensive loss of tissue and no other technique is possible, a medial or temporal forehead flap can be used. However, this recruits

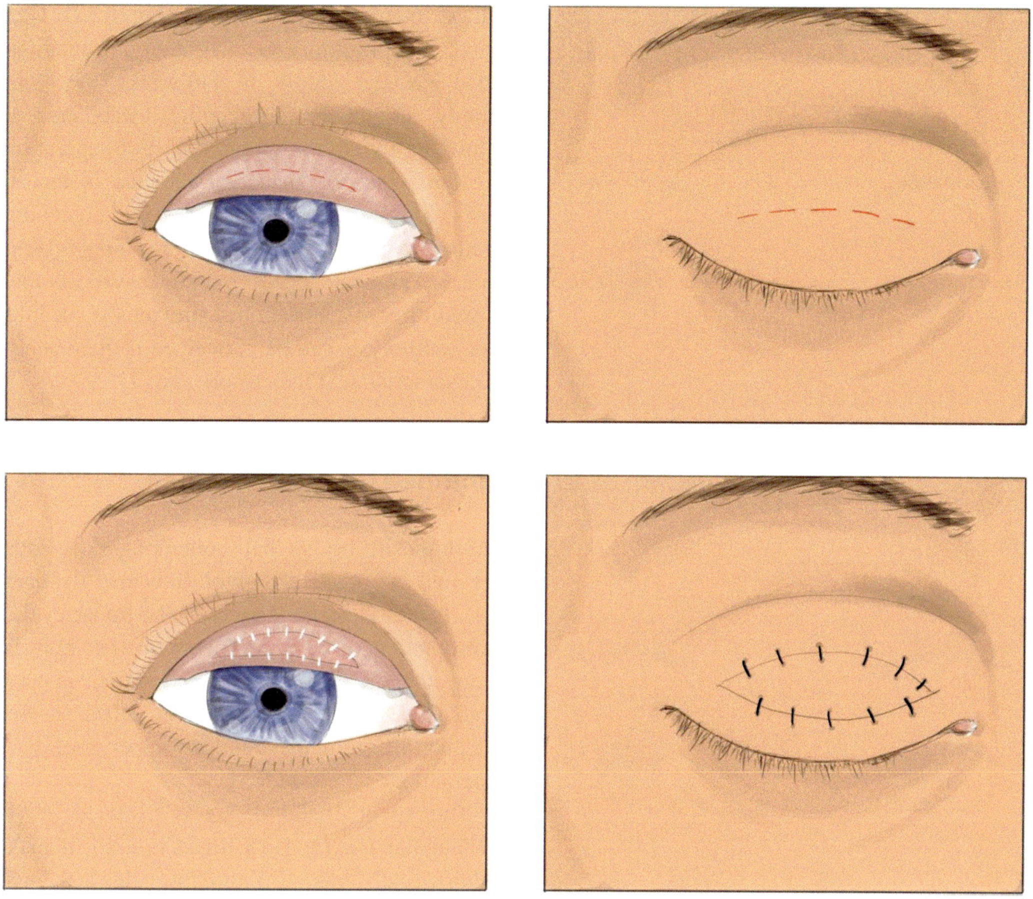

Fig. 8.10 Split-level graft, courtesy of Michael Han MD

tissue that is significantly thicker than eyelid skin, and thus often requires revision to achieve a better outcome.

For a medial forehead flap, a vertical flap no taller than five times its width is incised, using one of the epitrochlear vessels for best chances of survival. A temporal forehead flap includes the superficial temporal artery. Both are incised using a 15-blade and undermined sufficiently to allow for rotation into the defect. When undermining the temporal forehead flap, care must be taken to avoid the superficial facial nerve. The underside of the flap must be lined with a mucous membrane, ideally from the adjacent conjunctiva, but alternatively from a free buccal mucosal graft. If using conjunctiva from the lower eyelid, this can be separated in two weeks. The flap is then attached to the levator with 6-0 silk mattress sutures through the flap to help achieve some mobility of the new upper eyelid. The lateral edge of the flap is attached to the lateral canthal tendon, or its remnants, using 5-0 polyglactin suture. The graft site is closed in two layers, with 5-0 polyglactin in the subcutaneous layer and 6-0 fast or plain gut cutaneous suture (Fig. 8.11). Revision surgery can be performed as early as 6–8 weeks and after sufficient vascularization of the flap. These may be to create a eyelid crease or to release the temporal or medial base of the flap [1–3].

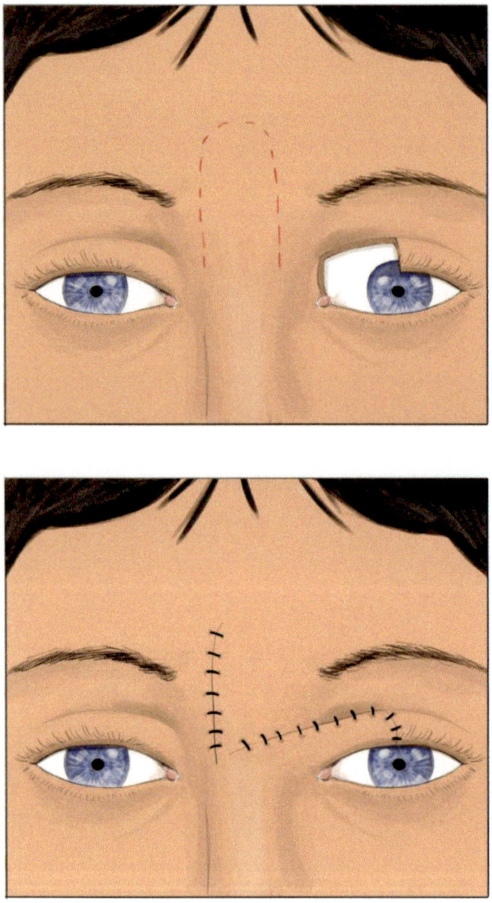

Fig. 8.11 Median forehead flap, courtesy of Michael Han MD

Lower Eyelid Pedicle Flap

When there exists a shallow upper eyelid margin defect, a lower eyelid pedicle flap may be indicated. The chief advantage is the reconstructed eyelid has lashes, albeit thinner and shorter than native upper eyelid lashes. A pedicle is taken from the center of the lower eyelid including the entire thickness of the tarsus and marginal artery, and therefore must be approximately 5 mm in width. This is then rotated superiorly into the upper eyelid defect and secured with 7-0 silk or 6-0 polyglactin suture (Fig. 8.12). Care is taken to minimize electrocautery, to maintain good vascular supply. In 4–6 weeks, the blood supply should be sufficiently established to allow for separation of the flap. For separation, the most inferior aspect of the flap is incised and then rotated into the upper eyelid defect and secured in place using 7-0 silk or 6-0 polyglactin suture. The lower eyelid margin incision is then closed directly as described previously. An inferior cantholysis can be performed if there is significant tension at the closure site [2].

Modified Cutler-Beard Flap

A composite bridge flap containing skin, muscle, and conjunctiva may be indicated to repair full thickness, large defects of the upper eyelid. Entropion may be a complication that may be reduced with the use of an additional support graft (e.g., autogenous auricular cartilage, free tarsal graft from the opposite upper eyelid, or scleral donor grafts) [2, 3].

The upper eyelid defect is trimmed into a rectangular shape. A 15-Blade is used to make a horizontal incision 5 mm from the lash margin of the lower eyelid approximately the same width as the upper eyelid defect. A vertical incision is placed at either end of the horizontal incision on the conjunctival side down to the most inferior part of the fornix and the skin is undermined to the level of the malar eminence. Westcott scissors are used to dissect the conjunctiva away from the flap, and the conjunctiva is then passed under the lower eyelid margin into the upper eyelid defect. This is then sutured into place using a 6-0 plain gut suture. Autologous ear cartilage, free tarsal graft, or donor sclera is fashioned to fit the defect and serve as the tarsus for the upper eyelid and sutured into place with a 7-0 silk, attaching superiorly to the levator aponeurosis or muscle

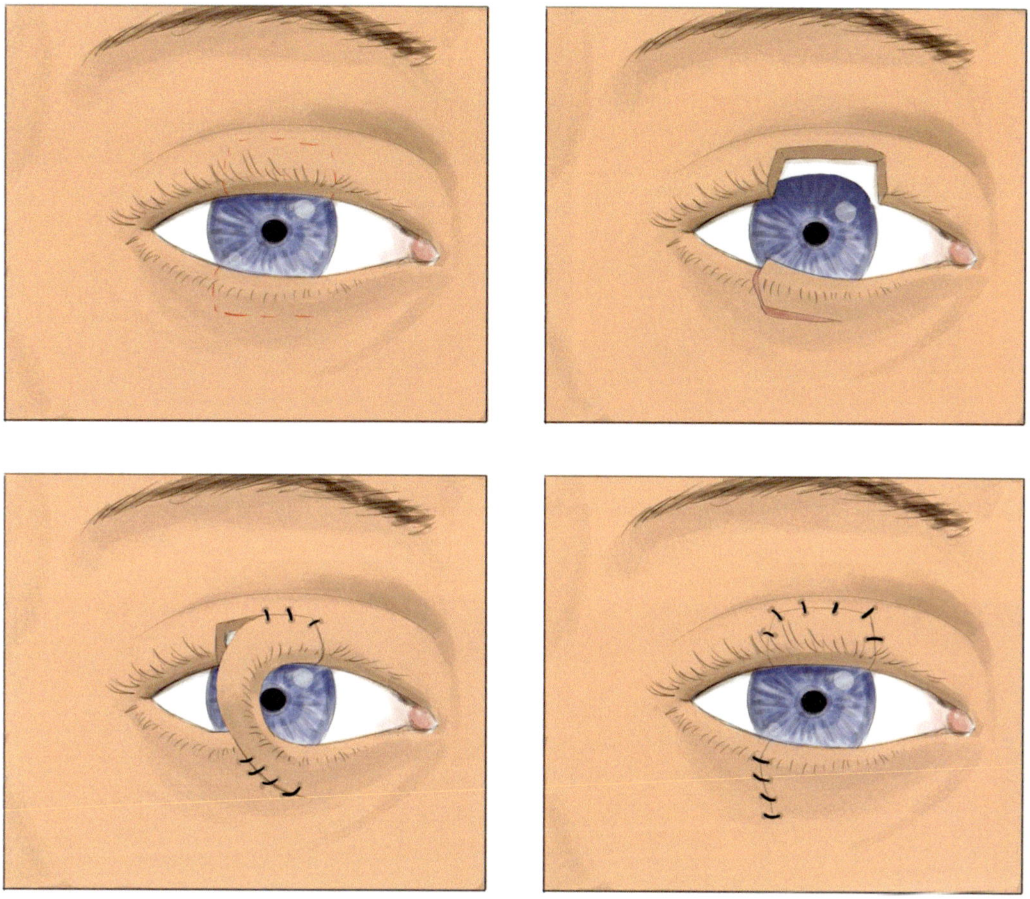

Fig. 8.12 Lower eyelid pedicle flap, courtesy of Michael Han MD

(Figs. 8.13, 8.14, 8.15, 8.16, 8.17, 8.18, 8.19, 8.20, 8.21, 8.22 and 8.23). This step can be skipped, although aforementioned, there exists a slight greater risk for entropion. Alternatively, a similar technique may be used where the remaining tarsus and conjunctiva from the upper eyelid is connected to the tarsoconjunctival flap

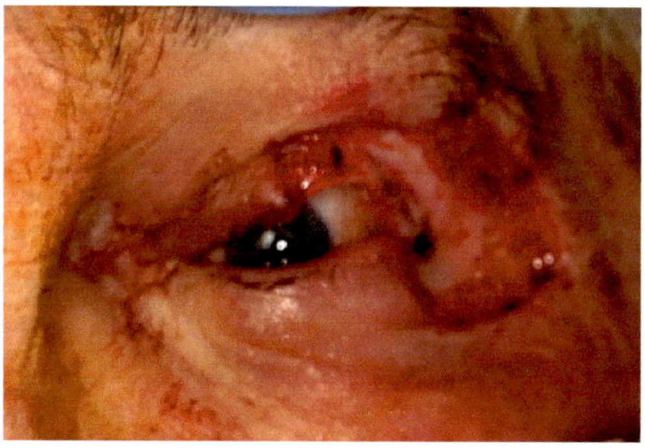

Fig. 8.13 Upper eyelid defect following Mohs

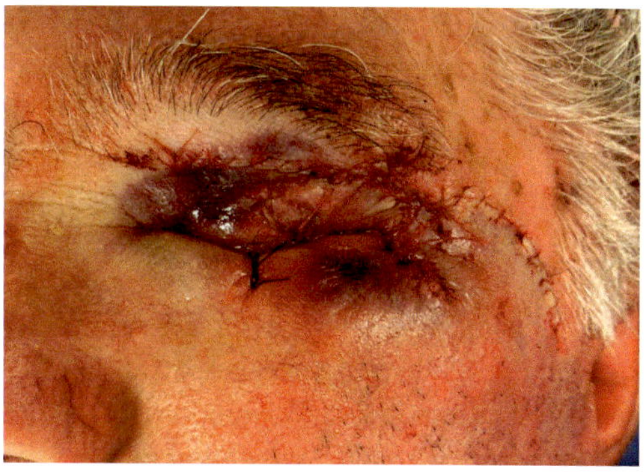

Fig. 8.14 Patient in Fig. 8.13 after reconstruction with a composite lower eyelid flap and lateral musculocutaneous flap

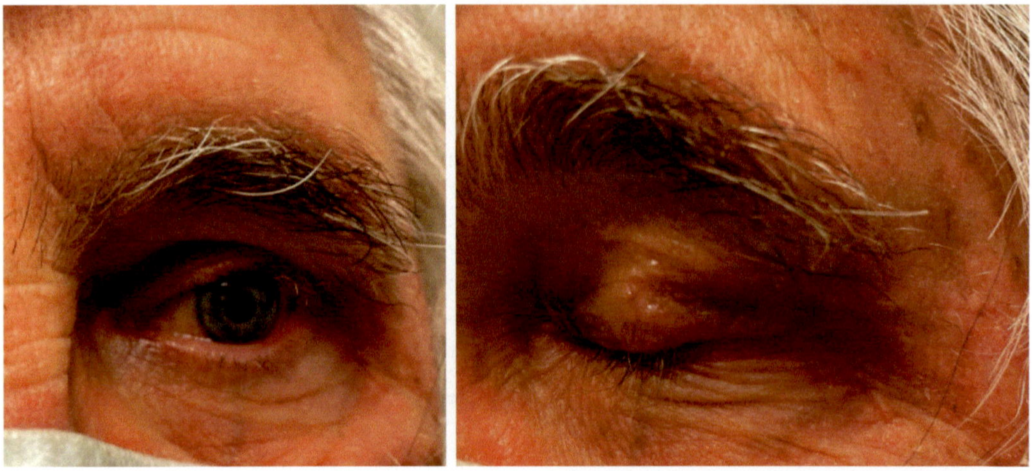

Fig. 8.15 Patient in Fig. 8.13 t hree months post-operative after a composite flap from the lower eyelid

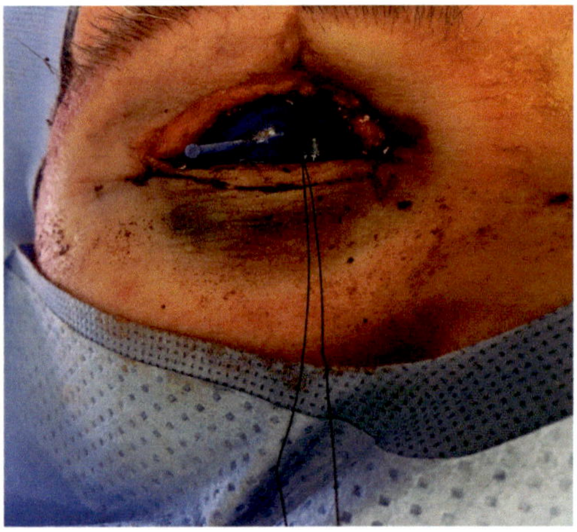

Fig. 8.16 Upper eyelid full thickness defect

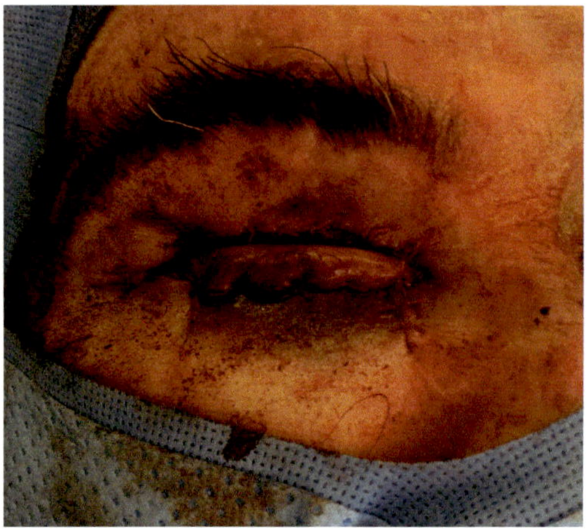

Fig. 8.17 Reconstruction of patient in 8.16 with a composite lower eyelid flap

from the lower eyelid. The additional step helps provide stability to the reconstructed upper eyelid and helps prevent skin and hair from growing toward the ocular surface [4]. The musculocutaneous portion of the flap is then passed under the eyelid margin and sutured to the skin edges of the upper eyelid defect with 7-0 interrupted silk. This is allowed to vascularize for approximately 6–8 weeks prior to separation.

For the second stage (separation of the flap), a 15-blade or scissors are used to incise the skin 2 mm inferior to the desired location of the new upper eyelid margin, and scissors are used to incise the remaining thickness of the flap. (Video 8-1) The conjunctiva is rotated anteriorly to cover the eyelid margin. The lower eyelid margin is then de-epithelialized at the most inferior aspect, and the skin is sutured together using 7-0 silk or 6-0 plain suture. Permanent sutures can be removed in two weeks. Once healed, eyelid notches can be removed by excising the notched area and closing directly, as

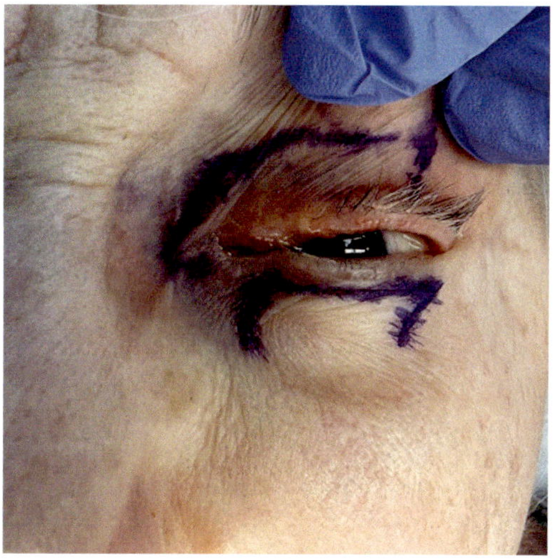

Fig. 8.18 Upper eyelid lesion markings

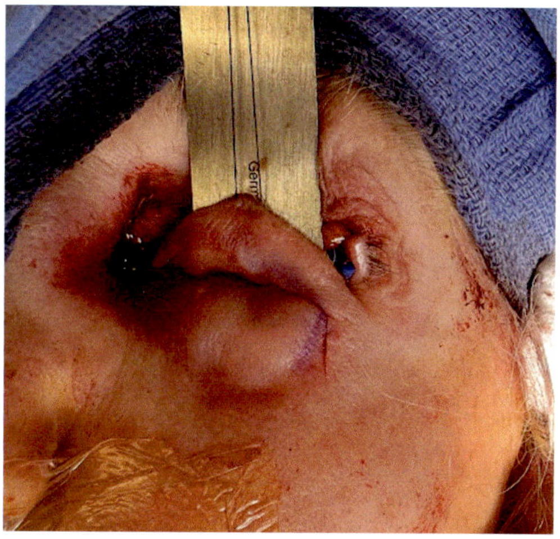

Fig. 8.20 Lower eyelid dissection

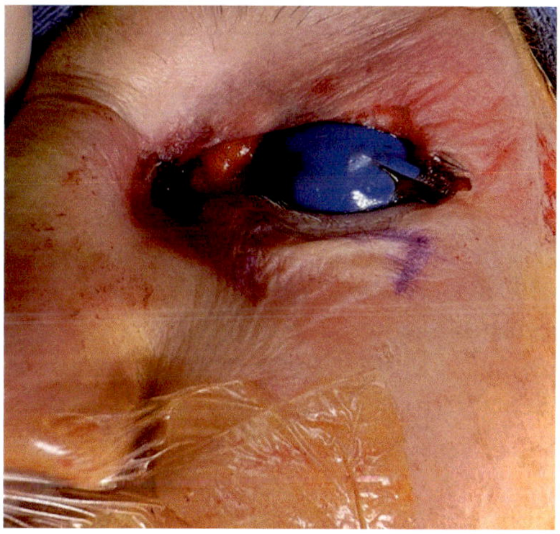

Fig. 8.19 Large upper eyelid defect

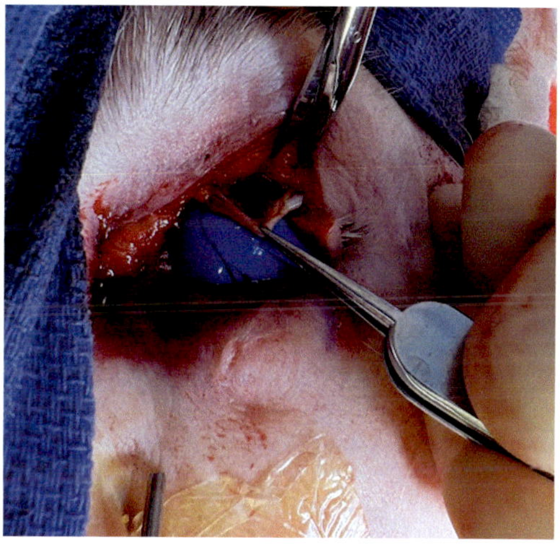

Fig. 8.21 Tarsoconjunctival flap

described in the first section of this chapter. If corneal irritation occurs due to skin hairs this can be treated with cryotherapy [2, 3].

Complications of bridging flaps include entropion, instability of the lower eyelid, post-operative scarring, and disruption of the lower eyelid retractors. Patients who are monocular may not be candidates as one must remain occluded for 4–8 weeks [2, 5].

Medial Canthal Reconstruction

When reforming the medial canthal area, diamond-shaped defects are the easiest to close, and, when excising a lesion or cancer, this shape should be utilized if possible. The skin can be closed either directly, with a free full-thickness skin graft, with a glabellar forehead flap, or with simple granulation tissue. In some instances, allowing the area to granulate (a.k.a. laissez faire

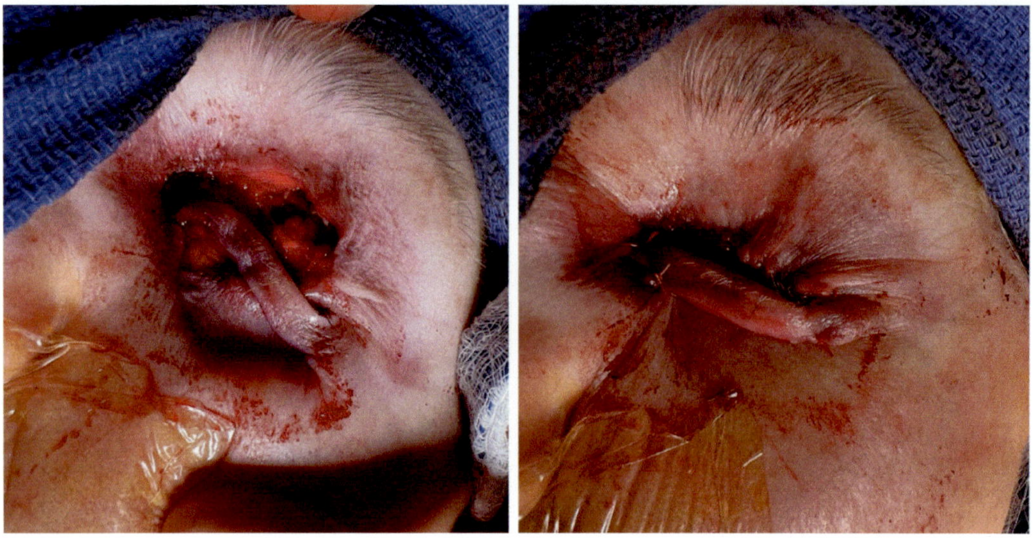

Fig. 8.22 Musculocutaneous flap

technique) will result in a suitable aesthetic outcome. If a graft or flap is pursued, care should be taken to secure this to the posterior aspect of the medial canthal tendon. This helps facilitate a normal and aesthetic contour, as well as future placement of a Jones tube. A half-circle ME-2 or P-2 needle is useful for this step. These techniques should only be performed if clear margins have been obtained following removal of a cancerous or suspicious lesion [1, 3]. Often, it is appropriate to delay repair of the lacrimal system.

Conclusions

Upper eyelid defects require thoughtfulness in repair since the ocular surface is at risk. While small defects can be repaired primarily, larger ones require various local flaps or grafts. The best options recreate an eyelid that protects the ocular surface and has minimally conspicuous scarring.

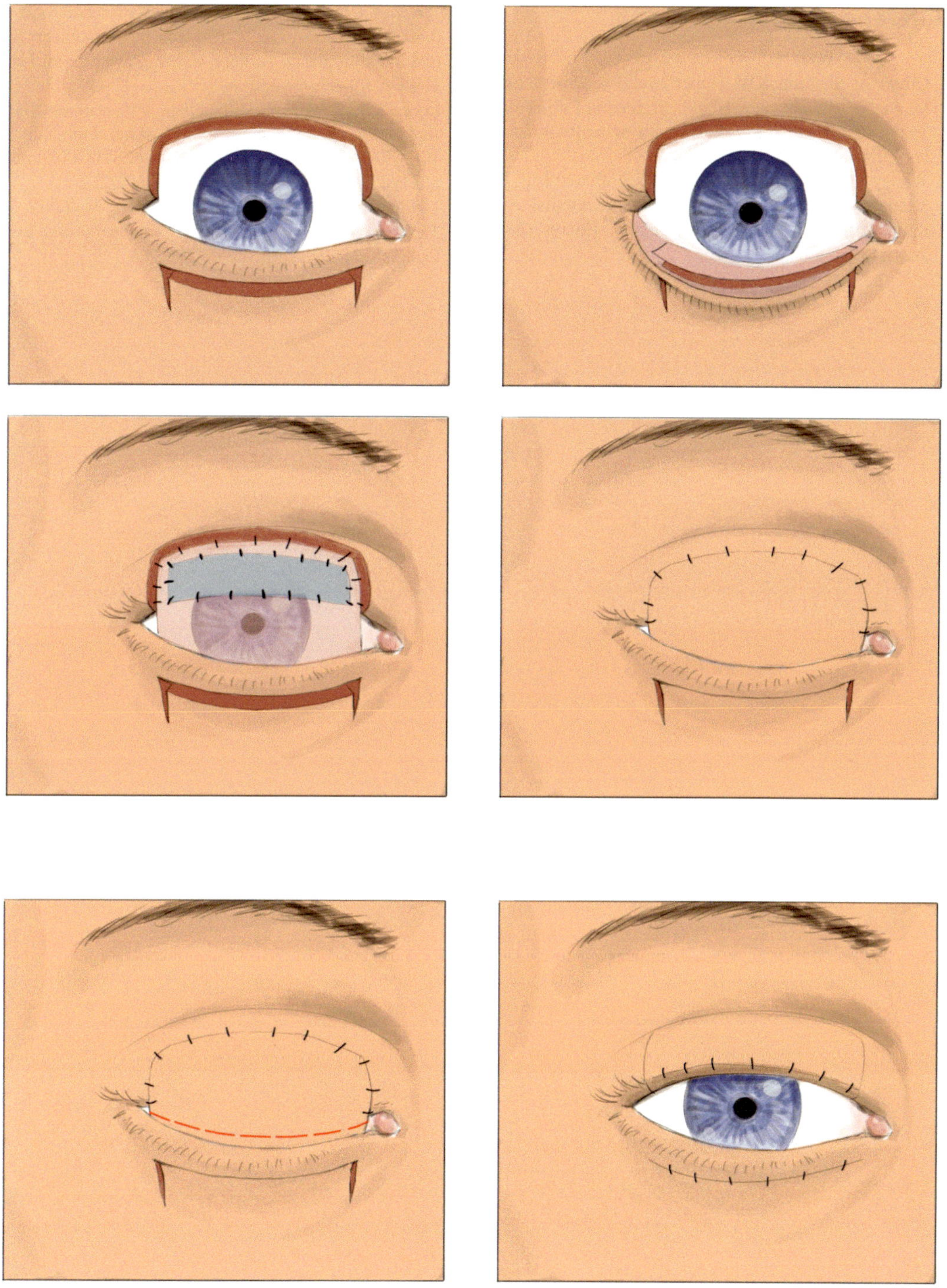

Fig. 8.23 Modified Cutler-Beard composite flap technique, courtesy of Michael Han MD

References

1. Omari A, Shaheen KW. Upper eyelid reconstruction. In: StatPearls. Treasure Island: StatPearls Publishing; 2021. Available from https://www.ncbi.nlm.nih.gov/books/NBK551694/.
2. Wesley RE, McCord CD, Nunery WR, Tanenbaum M. Reconstruction of the upper eyelid and medial canthus, 3rd ed. In: Oculoplastic surgery. Essay, Raven Press, Ltd.; 1995. p. 99–116.
3. McCord CD, Nunery WR. System of repair of full thickness eyelid defects, 3rd ed. In: Tanenbaum N, editor. Oculoplastic surgery. Essay, Raven Press, Ltd.; 1995. p. 85–97.
4. Leone CR Jr. Tarsal-conjunctival advancement flaps for upper eyelid reconstruction. Arch Ophthalmol. 1983;101(6):945–8. https://doi.org/10.1001/archopht.1983.01040010945019. PMID: 6860211.
5. Morley AM, deSousa JL, Selva D, Malhotra R. Techniques of upper eyelid reconstruction. Surv Ophthalmol. 2010;55(3):256–71.

9 Repair of Full Thickness Lower Eyelid Defects

Lalita Gupta, Mark A. Prendes, and Peter J. Timoney

Abstract

The repair of full thickness defects of the lower eyelid varies based on the size, location, and configuration. The posterior lamella should be replaced with mucous membrane—namely conjunctiva, if available. The anterior lamella may be reconstructed with skin flaps or grafts. The goal of repair is to restore structure and function. A properly reconstructed eyelid should achieve comfort, reasonable cosmesis, and, importantly, protection of the ocular surface. This chapter describes a systematic approach to lower eyelid reconstruction.

Keywords

Lower eyelid defects · Tarsoconjunctival flap · Hughes flap · Hewes flap · Mustarde flap · Tenzel flap · Semicircular flap · Bilobed flap · Glabellar flap

Supplementary Information The online version contains supplementary material available at https://doi.org/10.1007/978-3-031-63178-8_9.

L. Gupta · P. J. Timoney
Department of Ophthalmology,
University of Kentucky, Lexington, KY, USA

M. A. Prendes (✉)
Department of Ophthalmology and Visual Sciences,
Case Western Reserve University, Cleveland, OH, USA
e-mail: markprendes@gmail.com

Introduction

Lower eyelid defects compromise structure and function of the eyelid, if not repaired correctly. The choice of approach for reconstruction of a full thickness lower eyelid defect depends on the size, location and depth of the defect. To reduce the risk of eyelid malposition or impaired eyelid closure, inferior tension on the eyelid must be minimized. Also, one must consider the eyelid's bilamellar structure. The posterior lamella should be mucous membrane to line the ocular surface. The anterior lamella should consist of skin. One of the lamellae should provide a blood supply and should be a flap since a graft-on-graft construct will fail. Mobility of the tissue and resultant scars may influence choice of advancement flap.

Full-Thickness Marginal Defects

The size of the defect guides the approach. The following details a systematic approach to selecting specific reconstruction techniques according to defect size.

Small Defects

Defects of 33% or less of the horizontal width of the lower eyelid, can usually be closed directly

J. Tao (ed.), *Efficient Oculofacial Surgery*, https://doi.org/10.1007/978-3-031-63178-8_9

(Fig. 9.1). If there is greater laxity such as in older patients, defects involving up to 40% of the lower eyelid can be closed directly as well. A lateral canthotomy and cantholysis can be used to further mobilize tissue.

Direct Closure (Video 9-1)

Steps:

1. A 6-0 polyglactin or silk suture is first passed through the grey line of the eyelid margin in a vertical mattress fashion. This suture can be left long, draped anteriorly. Slight vertical tension on this suture can help expose internal structures that need to be secured.
2. The tarsus is closed with 6-0 polyglactin suture passed partial thickness. 6-0 polyglactin may also be used to close the orbicularis oculi muscle.
3. An additional 6-0 suture is used at the lash line then skin in an interrupted fashion.

The grey line and lash line sutures may be left long (5–10 mm), pulled anteriorly, and secured under the skin sutures to keep the sutures away from the cornea.

Moderate-Large Defects

Full thickness lower eyelid defects involving 33–50% of the eyelid margin can be repaired by advancing a semicircular rotational flap based at the lateral canthus (Fig. 9.2) [1, 2]. Freeing the septum, lower eyelid retractors and conjunctiva, can further mobilize the flap to close defects involving more than 60% of the lower eyelid [3].

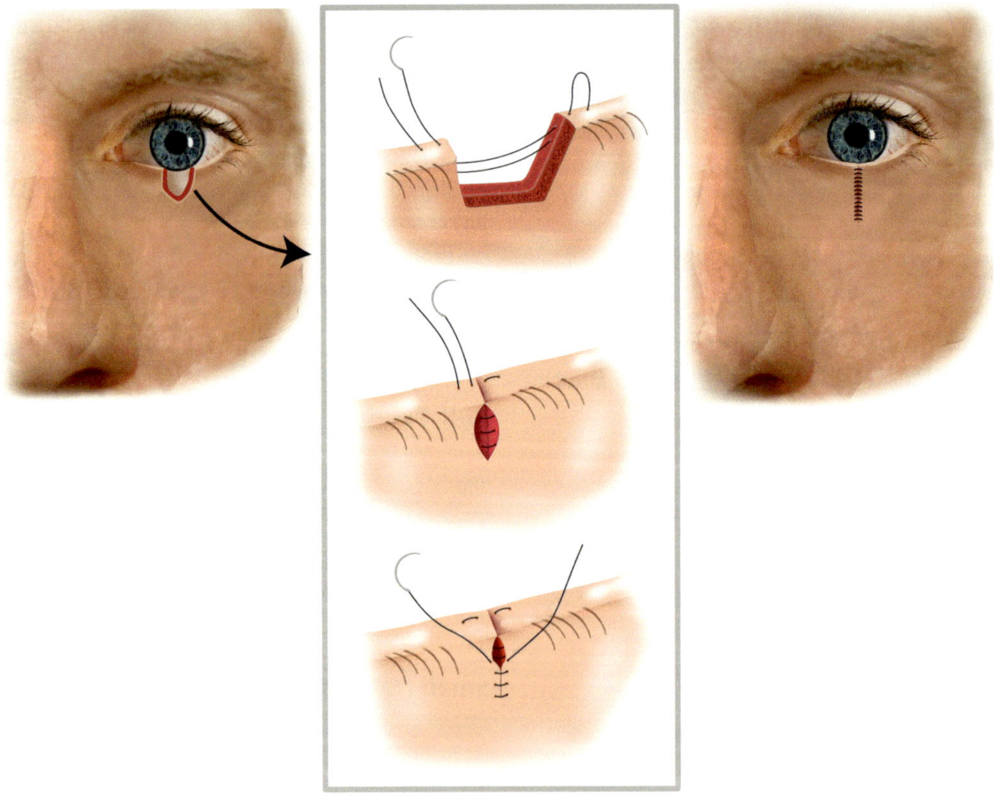

Fig. 9.1 Direct closure

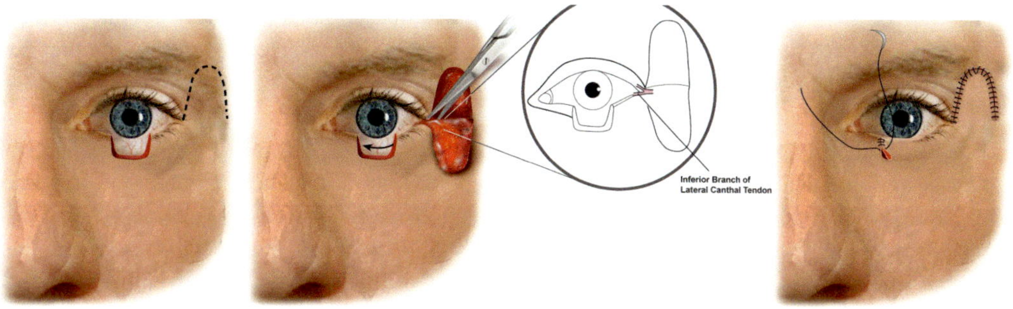

Fig. 9.2 Semicircular rotational flap

Semicircular rotational flap (Video 9-2)

Steps

1. A lateral canthotomy and inferior cantholysis is performed. From this canthal wound, a semicircular skin incision is made arching superiorly and temporally. The flap is undermined and elevated. The authors generally start with a small, 1–3 cm flap design that is extended laterally if more tissue recruitment is needed.
2. The lateral edge of the defect can then be mobilized to meet the medial edge of the defect and the edges of the defect are closed directly as above.
3. To reform the lateral canthus, a 5-0 polyglactin suture is used to secure the flap to the periosteum of the lateral orbital rim.
4. The skin is closed with 6-0 plain or silk suture.
5. The newly constructed lateral lower eyelid may be left bare, especially if only a small flap was required or may be covered with a tarsoconjunctival flap from the lateral upper eyelid, to reconstruct the posterior lamella.

Tarsoconjunctival Flap (Video 9-2)

A tarsoconjunctival advancement flap is frequently used for lower eyelid reconstruction [4–12]. These flaps are advanced from the ipsilateral upper eyelid and form the posterior lamella of the reconstructed lower eyelid.

The initial incision for the flap is commonly 4 mm above the superior eyelid margin on the central eyelid to avoid destabilizing the upper eyelid. Lateral tarsoconjunctival flaps may be constructed slightly closer to the margin since the canthal attachments help maintain stability. Attachments to Muller's muscle and the levator are often severed to reduce the risk of upper eyelid entropion or retraction. A skin or skin and muscle flap of the cheek or temple is useful for the anterior lamella (as described above) [8]. A full thickness skin graft is also an option [13]. Skin grafts may have the disadvantage of more scarring and graft to host mismatch. The tarsoconjunctival flap is generally taken down after a minimum of 6 weeks, and if a skin graft was used, after necessary collateral vascularization has formed. If the tarsoconjunctival flap is attached to a skin and muscle flap, division may be performed within weeks since each layer has its own blood supply [14–17].

First stage

Steps

1. After placing a traction suture through the upper eyelid margin, the eyelid is everted over a Desmarres retractor or cotton tip applicator. A #15 blade incision is made horizontally approximately 4 mm from the eyelid margin with a width corresponding to the defect. Vertical incisions at the medial and lateral aspect of the horizontal tarsal incision are made.

2. The flap is then created by first dissecting anterior to tarsus until the superior border of tarsus. Then dissection is continued superiorly. Leaving Muller's muscle intact may increase vascularity of the flap, but separation may be more difficult, and Muller's muscle may need to be recessed at the second stage to prevent upper eyelid retraction [13].
3. The tarsoconjunctival flap is advanced inferiorly and sutured to the inferior fornix conjunctiva and retractor muscle layer with 6-0 polyglactin suture. It is also sutured to the remaining tarsus and if needed, the internal aspect of the lateral orbital rim periosteum.
4. A full thickness skin graft or an advancement flap is used for the anterior lamella.

Second stage (tarsoconjunctival flap takedown; Video 9-3)

Steps

1. The tarsoconjunctival flap is divided at the new lower eyelid margin using scissors.
2. Recession of the retractors of the upper eyelid or release of any apparent contracture is performed to prevent upper eyelid retraction.
3. 6-0 or 7-0 polyglactin sutures are used to suture the conjunctiva to reform the eyelid margin. In some instances, no sutures are required.

Side effects include lower eyelid erythema which can be prevented by cutting the flap flush with lower eyelid margin and avoiding excessive anterior draping the mucosal tissue over the margin [11, 18]. Flap dehiscence has been reported but left to heal without surgical intervention with satisfactory outcomes [16]. Lower eyelid laxity can be prevented by proper sizing of the flap [11]. Upper eyelid entropion or retraction can be prevented by severing attachments to Muller's muscle and the levator. Tarsal kinking of the upper eyelid after flap division has been reported but can be treated surgically [19].

Large Defects

For large full thickness lower eyelid defects involving more than 50% of eyelid margin, placing the tarsoconjunctival flap over the pupil is sometimes necessary, (Fig. 9.3). Many patients poorly tolerate this occlusion of vision. Occluding vision in young children places them at risk of amblyopia. The technique of rotation of the remnant lateral eyelid medially (with canthotomy and semicircular flap) and placing a tarsoconjunctival flap laterally obviates central vision occlusion concerns. The resultant scar configuration may also more likely conform to facial tension lines and be less conspicuous than other techniques such as skin graft.

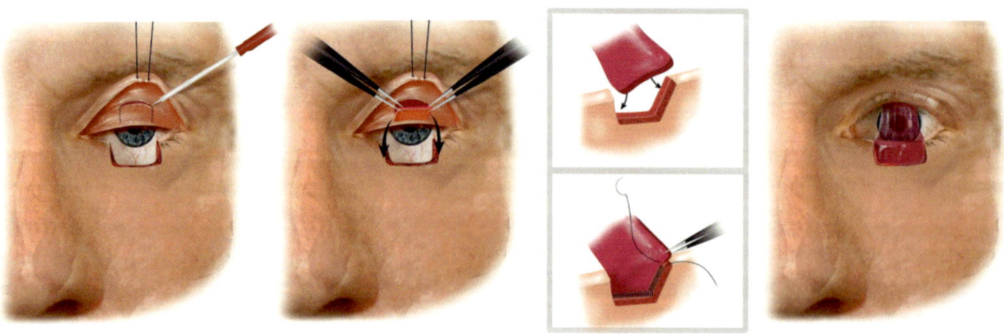

Fig. 9.3 Modified Hughes tarsoconjunctival flap

Horizontal pedicle tarsoconjunctival flap

This tarsal transposition flap is designed horizontally and hinged laterally and is sometimes referred to as a Hewes flap. It is used for shallow, lateral defects and requires only one stage (Fig. 9.4) [20]. This design obviates temporary vision occlusion requirements of large tarsoconjunctival flaps bridged down vertically. The chief disadvantage is that the flap only repairs shallow defects, and the reconstructed lower eyelid lacks significant upwards traction making the new lower eyelid more prone to retraction.

Steps

1. A 4-0 silk suture is placed through the gra y line for traction and the eyelid is everted over a Desmarres retractor.
2. A laterally based tarsoconjunctival flap from the upper eyelid, hinging at the lateral canthal tendon, is created. A #15 blade is used to make an incision through the conjunctiva and tarsus and a second parallel incision superior to the attachment of the levator palpebrae superioris, leaving 4 mm of tarsus. The medial edge of the flap should extend 2 mm lateral to the edge of the lower eyelid defect to prevent excessive laxity once secured in place. Westcott scissors are used to dissect the tarsus from the levator aponeurosis and Muller's muscle. Laterally, the lateral canthal tendon and adjacent orbicularis are left intact and form the proximal edge of the flap.
3. The tarsoconjunctival flap is then transposed to the lower eyelid to reconstruct the posterior lamella. The flap is sutured into place using a 5-0 or 6-0 polyglactin suture. Medially the flap is secured 1–2 mm higher than the eyelid margin. Laterally, the flap is fixated to the lateral orbital rim with 5-0 polyglactin suture. Inferiorly, the flap is sutured to the conjunctiva.
4. An advancement flap or a full thickness skin graft form the anterior lamella. Leone used a skin-muscle flap from the upper eyelid [21]. If a full thickness skin graft is used, care is taken to recess the top of the graft from the top of the tarsoconjunctival flap with horizontal mattress 6-0 chromic sutures to prevent contact between keratinized epithelium and the ocular surface. The skin graft is sutured into place with 6-0 plain suture. A bolster is placed on the lower eyelid over a nonadherent dressing (e.r., Telfa™) and a temporary tarsorrhaphy is sometimes performed.

The technique may be modified depending on the location of the defect. For a defect involving the lateral canthus, a higher-based tarsoconjunctival flap not involving the lateral canthal tendon is used and fixated to the periosteum. For

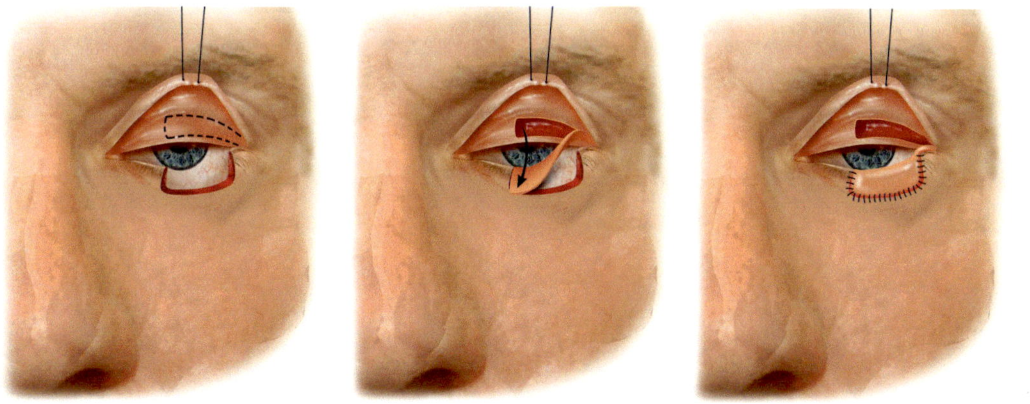

Fig. 9.4 Hewes tarsal transposition flap

a medial defect, a lateral cantholysis and rotational cheek flap is performed, and the Hewes flap is used for the new lateral defect.

Free tarsoconjunctival graft

A free tarsoconjunctival graft can be used to recreate the posterior lamella (Fig. 9.5) [22–25]. A unipedicled or bipedicled myocutaneous advancement flap can then be used for the anterior lamella [26, 27]. If a full thickness skin graft is used, an orbicularis flap can be advanced and sandwiched in between the two grafts [28, 29].

Steps

1. Attention is directed to the contralateral upper eyelid for obtaining the tarsoconjunctival graft. A 4-0 silk suture is placed through the grey line for traction and the eyelid is everted over a Desmarres retractor or cotton tip applicator. A #15 blade is used to make a horizontal incision through the conjunctiva and tarsus 4 mm above the eyelid margin. The width of the graft depends on the defect size. Care is taken to leave at least 4 mm of tarsus behind to maintain stability of the upper eyelid. Westcott scissors are used to dissect the tarsus from the levator aponeurosis and Muller's muscle. An extra 2 mm fringe of conjunctiva may be taken to help form the eyelid margin. The graft is placed in saline until it is used.
2. The graft is sutured into place using a 5-0 or 6-0 polyglactin suture and 1–2 mm higher the eyelid margin medially due to possible contraction. It is fixated to the periosteum of the lateral orbital rim using 5-0 polyglactin suture. It is also sutured to the conjunctiva.
3. A skin muscle flap can be rotated from the upper eyelid for the anterior lamella and sutured into place with 6-0 plain gut. The top of the skin-muscle flap is recessed from the top of the tarsoconjunctival flap with horizontal mattress 6-0 chromic sutures to prevent contact between the keratinized epithelium and the ocular surface.

Complications may include eyelid retraction, wound dehiscence, cicatricial ectropion and lower eyelid laxity, trichiasis and notching of the eyelid margin [22, 24, 30].

A sliding tarsal flap can be created from residual tarsus for a shallow tarsal defect. The inferior border of the tarsus is freed from septal attachments and an incision is made through residual tarsus into the retractors [31]. The two remnants of tarsus are attached to each other. Advancement flaps or full thickness skin grafts can be used for the anterior lamella [32]. Complications may include entropion, eyelid retraction, notching, trichiasis [31–33].

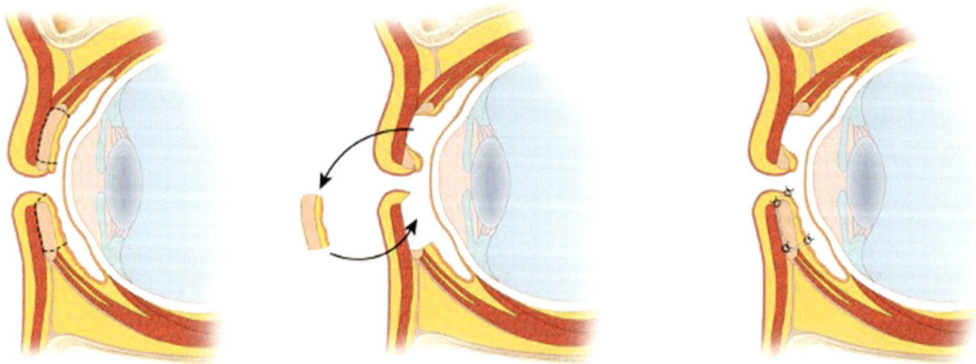

Fig. 9.5 Free tarsoconjunctival graft

Semicircular facial flap (Video 9-4)

For large lower eyelid defects, an advancement or rotational flap can be used for the anterior lamella, such as a Mustarde flap, a Tripier flap or bipedicle flap of upper eyelid skin and muscle, the temporal forehead (Fricke) flap, or a superiorly directed skin and orbicularis oculi muscle advancement flap [33–35]. A tarsal substitute may then be used for the posterior lamella such as hard palate or buccal mucosa, nasal or ear cartilage, sclera or homologous tarsus [36–38]. Mustarde described a large myocutaneous cheek flap with nasal chondromucosa (Fig. 9.6) [39].

Steps

1. A curvilinear incision is made with a #15 blade from the lateral canthus arching laterally and superiorly extending higher than the brow and then turning inferiorly 1–1.5 cm anterior to the tragus. The inferior crus and attachments to the orbital septum are cut.
2. The flap is elevated with blunt dissection. Care is taken to avoid dissection deep to the subcutaneous tissue to avoid damage to the facial nerve.
3. The flap is then rotated, and advanced medially.
4. A graft is used for the posterior lamellar defect. Mustarde originally used a composite graft of nasal chondromucosa. Other mucous membrane or cartilaginous grafts can be considered but a tarsoconjunctival flap, if available, may be preferable.
5. The myocutaneous cheek flap is secured into place. After fixating the flap to the periosteum of the lateral orbital rim, it is anchored with deep 5-0 polyglactin sutures. The skin is closed with 6-0 suture.

Lower eyelid eyelid retraction and ectropion may occur but can be prevented by using a high-arched flap and anchoring the flap to the lateral orbital rim periosteum and lateral canthal tendon [40]. A tarsoconjunctival flap from the upper eyelid, if used, provides an excellent upwards vector for the tissues recruited for eyelid construction.

Lateral Canthal Defects

If the lateral canthus is involved, fixating the lower eyelid to the periosteum of the lateral orbital rim helps forestall ectropion. A periosteal flap or temporalis fascia can also be used for additional support [41–45]. Some have made slings using temporalis fascia or the palmaris longus tendon to provide stronger support at the lateral canthus [44, 46, 47].

Periosteal strip

Steps

1. After dissecting down to the periosteum, the flap is constructed by incising a rectangular strip of periosteum with a #15 blade and then peeling it off with a periosteal elevator [43]. Various dimensions have been

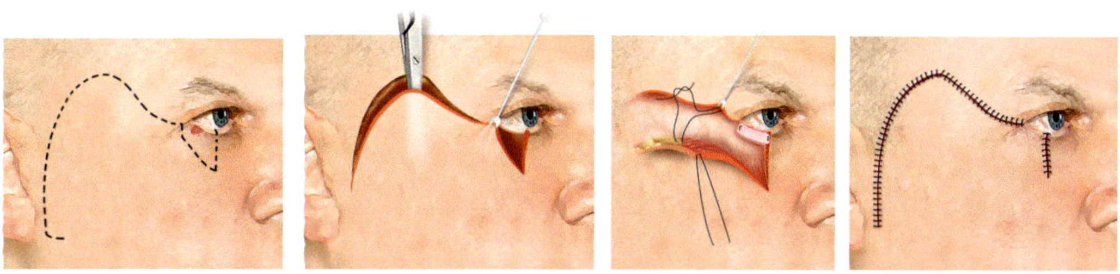

Fig. 9.6 Mustarde flap

used. Incising just above the level of the lateral canthal angle, a strip with a width of 5–10 mm and a length based on the length needed, usually 1 cm, can be developed [41, 45]. Temporalis fascia may be used to supplement the strip.
2. The strip is elevated and attached to the tarsus of the eyelid. Conjunctiva can also be advanced.

Two periosteal strips can be created and overlapped if both the upper and lower eyelid require reconstruction [41, 42]. Complications of the periosteal strip may include notching, dehiscence, ectropion, or rounding of the lateral canthal angle [41].

Medial Canthal Defects

For medial canthal defects, spontaneous granulation, a.k.a. the "laissez faire" technique is an option, but healing may take a long time and cicatricial complications may ensue [48]. An attempt at direct closure is generally preferable. A full thickness skin graft can be used for small shallow defects. Also, advancement and transposition flaps can be used. A lateral canthotomy and cantholysis or semicircular rotational flap can help reduce tension. Also, multiple flaps can be combined [49–51].

The approach to achieve posterior fixation of the eyelid medially depends on presence of the medial canthal tendon and the periosteum. If there are remnants of the medial canthal tendon, the eyelid can be attached directly to the tendon (Video 9-4). If the medial canthal tendon is absent, the eyelid can be fixated to the periosteum of the posterior lacrimal crest. If periosteum is not intact, the eyelid can be fixated to a titanium miniplate fixated to bone [52]. Trans nasal wiring has been used to create an anchor fixation point for the medial canthus but introduces hardware risks [53].

If the lacrimal apparatus is lost, reconstruction must wait until one can ensure that there is no recurrence of tumor. Primary repair with a silicone stent can be used. However, if the canaliculus does not remain, a conjunctivodacryocystorhinostomy with a Pyrex® Jones tube may be necessary.

Bilobed flap

A bilobed flap is a local transposition flap used primarily for the reconstruction of small to moderate-sized cutaneous defects, especially those of the lateral nose. The bilobed flap is a double transposition flap wherein the first lobe serves fills the primary defect, and a second lobe fills the defect created from formation of first lobe (the secondary defect) (Fig. 9.7) [54].

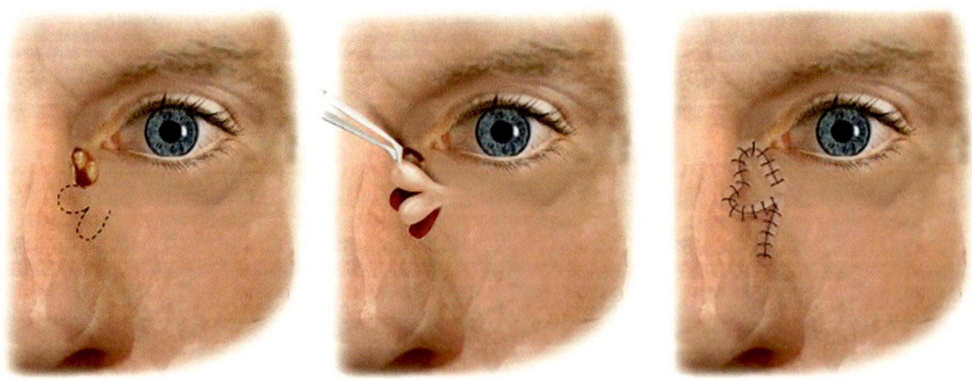

Fig. 9.7 Bilobed flap

Steps

1. The flap is based superior and medial to the defect to avoid inferior tension that may cause eyelid retraction. The sizes, angles, and tissues recruited for the lobes have vary, but typically the first lobe slightly smaller than the defect and the second lobe slightly smaller than the first lobe [55–57]. An angle of 90° between the lobes is used with the axes along relaxed skin tension lines as much as possible. After marking out the two lobes, a #15 blade is used to create the incision and undermine the flaps.
2. The first flap is mobilized. The first lobe is rotated into the primary defect while the second lobe is rotated into the secondary defect. The tertiary defect is closed directly. The flap is anchored into place with deep buried 5-0 or 4-0 polyglactin sutures in an interrupted fashion.
3. The skin is closed with 6-0 suture such as prolene.

Glabellar flap (Video 9-4)

For deep defects, a glabellar flap can be used. It is usually performed as an inverted V-Y (Fig. 9.8) [58]. Cosmesis may be limited by the thickness of the skin, the scar, and a reduction in the distance between the brows. Some excise excess skin from the flap may serve as a skin graft to fill the defect and minimize the narrowing of the distance between the brows [59].

Steps

1. The flap is constructed such that one arm of the V arises from the defect. The size of the flap depends on the defect size, depth, and distance from the glabellar region. One may also consider the prominence of the nasal bridge and relationship between the medial canthus and the nose. The forehead skin is generally advanced only to the lateral nasal base since its thickness is not ideal for use to reconstruct eyelids. After marking, an inverted V incision is made with a #15 blade. The flap is undermined and dissected and then rotated across the nasal bridge into the defect.
2. The flap is sutured into place with 5-0 or 4-0 polyglactin suture. The brow defect is closed with 4-0 polyglactin suture. The skin is closed with 6-0 polypropylene.

A paramedian forehead flap can be used in some very large deep defects [60]

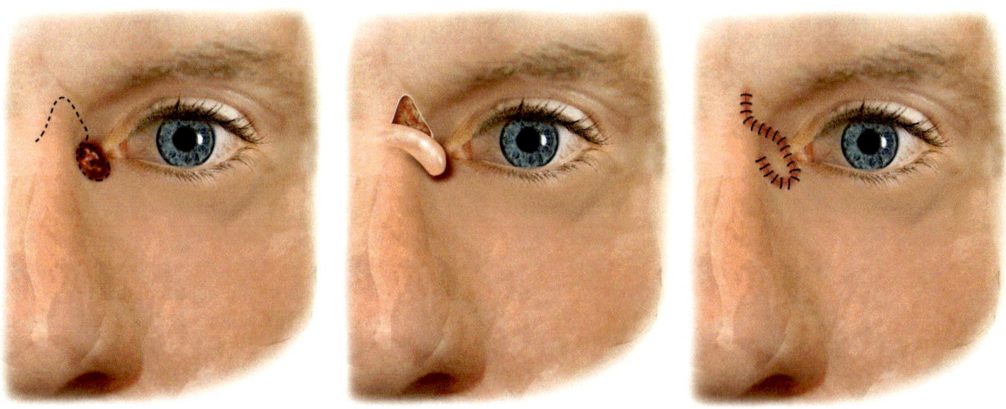

Fig. 9.8 Glabellar flap

Nonmarginal Defects

Full thickness skin grafts can be used from the upper eyelid, preauricular skin, retroauricular area, supraclavicular fossa or inner upper arm and aim to match the color, thickness, and texture of the eyelid skin. Of note, one must consider possible risks to not only the recipient site but also the donor site.

In contrast with grafts, flaps generally have better cosmesis, less contraction, and provide their own blood supply derived from the dermal-subdermal plexus [61]. Most flaps used in oculofacial surgery are random pattern skin flaps instead of axial pattern skin flaps. The periorbital skin flaps have been categorized as sliding flaps which move over to close a defect, advancement flaps which have three sides and are advanced to cover an adjacent defect, rotational flaps which rotate about a pivot point, and transposition flaps which are transposed to a nonadjacent defect [61]. Prior surgery, radiation, tobacco use, and vasculopathies can compromise viability of a flap.

Conclusion

The size, location and depth of a lower eyelid defect drive the reconstruction approach. Each reconstruction is customized to the patient. In general, flaps and grafts that leave scars in the relaxed facial tension lines, as well as those that do not place inferior traction on the eyelid, are preferred to forestall ectropion or retraction. Tarsoconjunctival flaps from the upper eyelid are often the first choice for constructing the posterior lamella of larger defects. When possible, tarsoconjunctival flaps should be placed lateral to the visual axis, since many patients do not tolerate visual occlusion.

References

1. Tenzel RR. Reconstruction of the central one half of an eyelid. Arch Ophthalmol. 1975;93(2):125–6.
2. Tenzel RR, Stewart WB. Eyelid reconstruction by the semicircle flap technique. Ophthalmology. 1978;85(11):1164–9.
3. Levine MR, Buckman G. Semicircular flap revisited. Arch Ophthalmol. 1986;104(6):915–7.
4. Reifler D, editor. The American Society of ophthalmic plastic and reconstructive surgery (ASOPRS). The first twenty-five years: 1969–1994. History of ophthalmic plastic surgery: 2500 BC-AD 1994. Winter Park, FL: ASOPRS/Norman; 1994.
5. Köllner H. Verfahren für den plastischen Ersatz des Unterlides. Munch Med Wochenschr. 1911;41: 2166–8.
6. Dupuy-Dutemps LJBMSFO. Refection d'une paupiere detruite dans toute don epaisseur par greffe cutanee et tarso-donjonctivale prise a l'autre paupiere autoplastie palpebro-palpebrale integrale. 1927;40:262–71.
7. Cirincione GJCO. Sulla blefaroplastica. 1901;2:449–73.
8. Hughes WL. A new method for rebuilding a lower lid: report of a case. 1937;17(6):1008–17.
9. Hargiss JL. Bipedicle tarsoconjunctival flap. Ophthalmic Plast Reconstr Surg. 1989;5(2):99–103.
10. Moss AL, Cooper MA, Lendrum J, Hiles RW. The sanctity of the upper lid in lower eyelid reconstruction questioned. A modification of a lid sharing procedure with a long-term follow-up. Br J Plast Surg. 1987;40(3):246–57.
11. Hughes WL. Total lower lid reconstruction: technical details. Trans Am Ophthalmol Soc. 1976;74:321–9.
12. Custer PL, Maamari RN. The Kollner Tarsoconjunctival Flap for Lower Eyelid Reconstruction: Historical Perspective and Surgical Outcomes of 140 Cases. Ophthalmic Plast Reconstr Surg. 2021.
13. Hishmi AM, Koch KR, Matthaei M, Bolke E, Cursiefen C, Heindl LM. Modified Hughes procedure for reconstruction of large full-thickness lower eyelid defects following tumor resection. Eur J Med Res. 2016;21(1):27.
14. McNab AA. Early division of the conjunctival pedicle in modified Hughes repair of the lower eyelid. Ophthalmic Surg Lasers. 1996;27(6):422–4.
15. Leibovitch I, Selva D. Modified Hughes flap: division at 7 days. Ophthalmology. 2004;111(12):2164–7.
16. Bartley GB, Messenger MM. The dehiscent Hughes flap: outcomes and implications. Trans Am Ophthalmol Soc. 2002;100:61–5; discussion 5–6.
17. McNab AA, Martin P, Benger R, O'Donnell B, Kourt G. A prospective randomized study comparing division of the pedicle of modified hughes flaps at two or four weeks. Ophthalmic Plast Reconstr Surg. 2001;17(5):317–9.
18. Bartley GB, Putterman AM. A minor modification of the Hughes' operation for lower eyelid reconstruction. Am J Ophthalmol. 1995;119(1):96–7.
19. Custer PL. Tarsal kinking after Hughes flap. Ophthalmic Plast Reconstr Surg. 1998;14(5):349–51.

20. Hewes EH, Sullivan JH, Beard C. Lower eyelid reconstruction by tarsal transposition. Am J Ophthalmol. 1976;81(4):512–4.
21. Leone CR Jr, Van Gemert JV. Lower eyelid reconstruction with upper eyelid transpositional grafts. Ophthalmic Surg. 1980;11(5):315–8.
22. Hawes MJ, Grove AS Jr, Hink EM. Comparison of free tarsoconjunctival grafts and Hughes tarsoconjunctival grafts for lower eyelid reconstruction. Ophthalmic Plast Reconstr Surg. 2011;27(3):219–23.
23. Leone CR Jr, Hand SI Jr. Reconstruction of the medial eyelid. Am J Ophthalmol. 1979;87(6):797–801.
24. Stephenson CM, Brown BZ. The use of tarsus as a free autogenous graft in eyelid surgery. Ophthalmic Plast Reconstr Surg. 1985;1(1):43–50.
25. LvJO B. Über Totalplastik des unteren Lides. Bildung einer hinteren Lidplatte durch Transplantation eines Tarsus und Bindehautstreifens aus dem Oberlide. 1918;40:222–7.
26. Katz TL, Pennington TE, Yohendran J, Ghabrial R. One-step reconstruction of large lower eyelid defects: technique and outcomes. Clin Exp Ophthalmol. 2014;42(9):889–92.
27. Leone CR Jr, Van Gemert JV. Lower lid reconstruction using tarsoconjunctival grafts and bipedicle skin-muscle flap. Arch Ophthalmol. 1989;107(5):758–60.
28. Paridaens D, van den Bosch WA. Orbicularis muscle advancement flap combined with free posterior and anterior lamellar grafts: a 1-stage sandwich technique for eyelid reconstruction. Ophthalmology. 2008;115(1):189–94.
29. Naugle TC, Levine MR, Carroll GS. Free graft enhancement using orbicularis muscle mobilization. Ophthalmology. 1995;102(3):493–500.
30. Hawes MJ, Jamell GA. Complications of tarsoconjunctival grafts. Ophthalmic Plast Reconstr Surg. 1996;12(1):45–50.
31. deSousa JL, Malhotra R, Davis G. Sliding tarsal flap for reconstruction of large, shallow lower eyelid tarsal defects. Ophthalmic Plast Reconstr Surg. 2007;23(1):46–8.
32. Custer PL, Neimkin M. Lower eyelid reconstruction with combined sliding tarsal and rhomboid skin flaps. Ophthalmic Plast Reconstr Surg. 2016;32(3):230–2.
33. Skippen B, Hamilton A, Evans S, Benger R. One-stage alternatives to the hughes procedure for reconstruction of large lower eyelid defects: surgical techniques and outcomes. Ophthalmic Plast Reconstr Surg. 2016;32(2):145–9.
34. Manchester WM. A simple method for the repair of full-thickness defects of the lower lid with special reference to the treatment of neoplasms. Br J Plast Surg. 1951;3(4):252–63.
35. Wilcsek G, Leatherbarrow B, Halliwell M, Francis I. The 'RITE' use of the fricke flap in periorbital reconstruction. Eye (London). 2005;19(8):854–60.
36. Beyer CK, Albert DM. The use and fate of fascia lata and sclera in ophthalmic plastic and reconstructive surgery. Ophthalmology. 1981;88(9):869–86.
37. Suga H, Ozaki M, Narita K, Kurita M, Shiraishi T, Ohura N, et al. Comparison of nasal septum and ear cartilage as a graft for lower eyelid reconstruction. J Craniofac Surg. 2016;27(2):305–7.
38. Jordan DR, Tse DT, Anderson RL, Hansen SO. Irradiated homologous tarsal plate banking: a new alternative in eyelid reconstruction. Part II. Human data. Ophthalmic Plast Reconstr Surg. 1990;6(3):168–76.
39. Mustarde JC. The use of flaps in the orbital region. Plast Reconstr Surg. 1970;45(2):146–50.
40. Callahan MA, Callahan A. Mustarde flap lower lid reconstruction after malignancy. Ophthalmology. 1980;87(4):279–86.
41. Weinstein GS, Anderson RL, Tse DT, Kersten RC. The use of a periosteal strip for eyelid reconstruction. Arch Ophthalmol. 1985;103(3):357–9.
42. Leone CR Jr. Lateral canthal reconstruction. Ophthalmology. 1987;94(3):238–41.
43. Leone CR Jr. Periosteal flap for lower eyelid reconstruction. Am J Ophthalmol. 1992;114(4):513–4.
44. Holt JE, Holt GR, van Kirk M. Use of temporalis fascia in eyelid reconstruction. Ophthalmology. 1984;91(1):89–93.
45. Smith B, English FP. Techniques available in reconstructive surgery of the eyelid. Br J Ophthalmol. 1970;54(7):450–5.
46. Holt JE, Holt GR, Van Kirk M. Use of temporalis fascia in eyelid reconstruction. Arch Otolaryngol. 1985;111(3):165–7.
47. Wang W, Meng H, Yu S, Liu T, Shao Y. Reconstruction of giant full-thickness lower eyelid defects using a combination of palmaris longus tendon with superiorly based nasolabial skin flap and palatal mucosal graft. J Plast Surg Hand Surg. 2021;55(3):147–52.
48. Lowry JC, Bartley GB, Garrity JA. The role of second-intention healing in periocular reconstruction. Ophthalmic Plast Reconstr Surg. 1997;13(3):174–88.
49. Harris GJ, Logani SC. Multiple aesthetic unit flaps for medial canthal reconstruction. Ophthalmic Plast Reconstr Surg. 1998;14(5):352–9.
50. Motomura H, Taniguchi T, Harada T, Muraoka M. A combined flap reconstruction for full-thickness defects of the medial canthal region. J Plast Reconstr Aesthet Surg. 2006;59(7):747–51.
51. Lee BJ, Elner SG, Douglas RS, Elner VM. Island pedicle and horizontal advancement cheek flaps for medial canthal reconstruction. Ophthalmic Plast Reconstr Surg. 2011;27(5):376–9.
52. Howard GR, Nerad JA, Kersten RC. Medial canthoplasty with microplate fixation. Arch Ophthalmol. 1992;110(12):1793–7.
53. Peter H, Freihofer M. Experience with transnasal canthopexy. J Maxillofac Surg. 1980;8(2):119–24.

54. Esser JFS. Gestielte lokale Nasenplastik mit zweizipfligem Lappen, Deckung des sekundären Defektes vom ersten Zipfel durch den zweiten. Deutsche Zeitschrift für Chirurgie. 1918;143(3):385–90.
55. Meadows AE, Rhatigan M, Manners RM. Bilobed flap in ophthalmic plastic surgery: simple principles for flap construction. Ophthalmic Plast Reconstr Surg. 2005;21(6):441–4.
56. Sullivan TJ, Bray LC. The bilobed flap in medial canthal reconstruction. Aust N Z J Ophthalmol. 1995;23(1):42–8.
57. Perry JD, Taban M. Superiorly based bilobed flap for inferior medial canthal and nasojugal fold defect reconstruction. Ophthalmic Plast Reconstr Surg. 2009;25(4):276–9.
58. Maloof AJ, Leatherbarrow B. The glabellar flap dissected. Eye (London). 2000;14(Pt 4):597–605.
59. Meadows AE, Manners RM. A simple modification of the glabellar flap in medial canthal reconstruction. Ophthalmic Plast Reconstr Surg. 2003;19(4):313–5.
60. Price DL, Sherris DA, Bartley GB, Garrity JA. Forehead flap periorbital reconstruction. Arch Facial Plast Surg. 2004;6(4):222–7.
61. Patrinely JR, Marines HM, Anderson RL. Skin flaps in periorbital reconstruction. Surv Ophthalmol. 1987;31(4):249–61.

Repair of Canalicular Trauma

10

Benyam Kinde and Seanna R. Grob

Abstract

Injury to the nasolacrimal drainage system is common after periocular trauma. Early detection and intervention are important to prevent canalicular dysfunction and persistent epiphora. Herein, we review the etiology, preoperative evaluation, surgical management, and potential complications of canalicular trauma. In this chapter, the authors describe three common surgical approaches for canalicular trauma repair.

Keywords

Canalicular trauma · Canalicular laceration · Canaliculus · Canalicular repair · Repair of canaliculus · Tear drain trauma

Supplementary Information The online version contains supplementary material available at https://doi.org/10.1007/978-3-031-63178-8_10.

B. Kinde
Oculofacial Plastic and Orbital Surgery, Byers Eye Institute, Stanford University, Palo Alto, CA, USA

S. R. Grob (✉)
Oculofacial Plastic and Orbital Surgery, Gavin Herbert Eye Institute, University of California, Irvine, Irvine, CA, USA
e-mail: seannagrob@gmail.com

Introduction

Canalicular injury is among several urgent issues in the periocular trauma patient. Canalicular injury in children is most often secondary to eyelid avulsion secondary to dog bites, while in adults, injury more commonly occurs in the setting of assault or motor vehicle or bike accidents [1, 2]. In the elderly, falls represent the most common cause of canalicular injury [3]. The majority of canalicular injuries occur in males (74.8%) across a broad age range [3].

It has been proposed that most canalicular injuries occur secondary to indirect trauma (i.e. physical assault with a fist, car accident) resulting in avulsion of the eyelid and associated canaliculi rather than direct trauma (i.e. penetrating injury from foreign object) [4]. More recent work has suggested that penetrating trauma may represent a larger fraction of total canalicular injuries [5], though this has been debated [6].

Lacrimal Drainage System Anatomy

The superior and inferior puncta and canaliculi represent the initial entry point for tears into the nasolacrimal drainage system [7]. The puncta are located 5 mm lateral to the medial canthal tendon and extend vertically into the eyelid approximately 2 mm. From the puncta,

J. Tao (ed.), *Efficient Oculofacial Surgery*, https://doi.org/10.1007/978-3-031-63178-8_10

tears then enter the canaliculus, which extends 8 mm medially. In about 90% of patients, the superior and inferior canaliculi form a common canaliculus prior to entering the lacrimal sac. In the remaining 10% of patients, the superior and inferior canaliculi drain separately into the lacrimal sac, though a more recent cadaveric study suggests that this percentage is likely much lower [8]. The lacrimal sac lies in the lacrimal sac fossa and is surrounded by the anterior and posterior limbs of the medial canthal tendon. The sac is 10–15 mm in length and about 2 mm in width (range 1–4 mm). From the lacrimal sac, tears drain though the nasolacrimal duct for approximately 15 mm before draining into the inferior meatus in the nose [7].

Clinical Examination and Pre-operative Assessment

In the setting of trauma, any life-threatening injuries should be ruled out first. Then, a thorough periocular and ophthalmic exam should be performed. This includes evaluation of the globe. It is imperative to rule out more serious ocular injuries, such as an open globe. Up to 20% of canalicular lacerations are associated with globe injury [9], and ruling out and managing globe trauma is a priority over significant periocular manipulation to diagnose or repair other periocular trauma. Pressure on the globe during eyelid evaluation may cause extrusion of intraocular fluid or contents or precipitate a choroidal hemorrhage.

Once the globe is deemed stable, a complete evaluation of the periocular area should be completed. Sometimes the eyelids need to be cleaned of dried blood to fully evaluate for trauma and lacerations. Any laceration or injury medial to the puncta on the upper or lower eyelid should prompt a high suspicion for canalicular trauma. This may also include avulsion of the upper or lower eyelid or both from the medial canthus. The eyelids may need to be gently manipulated and tissues separated to visualize a laceration. Probing of the canalicular system should be performed if a canalicular injury is suspected, but not definitively visualized. After dilating the upper and lower puncta with a punctal dilator, a lacrimal probe is inserted through the punctum initially perpendicular to the eyelid margin for about 2 mm. The probe is then rotated horizontally or more parallel to the eyelid margin (approximately 90°) and aimed medially with lateral traction of the eyelid. These maneuvers follow the natural anatomic trajectory of the canaliculi. A hard stop after inserting the probe approximately 8–12 mm indicates the probe has contacted the nasal bone. Visualization of the leading edge of the probe along this path suggests canalicular injury (Fig. 10.1).

Computed tomography (CT) imaging of the face and orbits should be obtained if ocular or orbital trauma (such as an orbital fracture or foreign body) is suspected. If orbital fat is visualized externally, orbital imaging is warranted, as this suggests penetration or disruption of the orbital septum. Mechanism of injury can play a role in determining potential risk of orbital or ocular foreign body (i.e., projectile foreign bodies) as well as risk of fracture. Prophylactic antibiotics should be considered in the setting of animal bites or dirty wounds and a tetanus booster should be administered if vaccination status is remote or unknown.

Surgical Approach to Canalicular Repair

Ideally, canalicular repair should be repaired urgently or as soon as possible since delay and tissue contracture may make identifying the cut ends of the injured canaliculus more difficult. The authors prefer repair in the operating room and placement of bicanalicular tubes, owing to greater stability of the tube. However, bedside repair with a monocanalicular system (e.g., Mini Monoka, FCI Ophthalmics, Pembroke, MA) is also an option and obviates the need for systemic anesthesia.

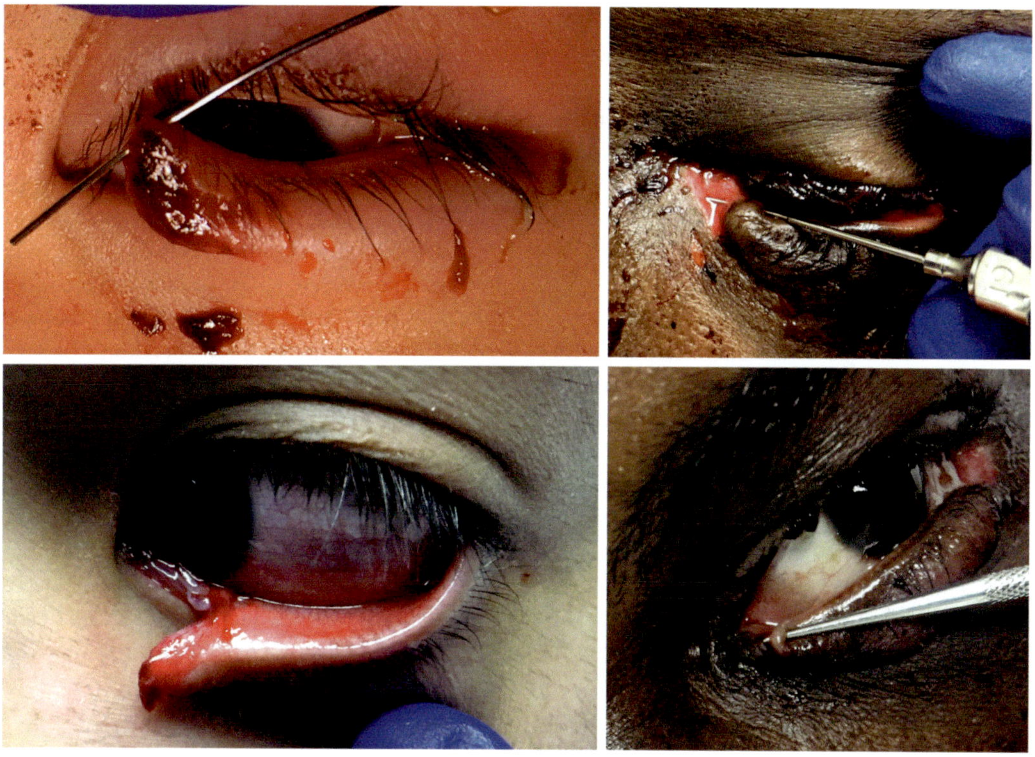

Fig. 10.1 Examples of canalicular injury showing eyelid injuries nasal to the punctum with exposure of a canalicular probe at the location of the discontinuous canaliculus in several of the images

The wounds should be thoroughly cleaned and explored. The surgical field should be prepped using an appropriate antiseptic agent such as povidone iodine. Local anesthesia is then injected into the affected eyelids and periocular area.

The objectives of canalicular injury repair are to reapproximate the cut ends of the canaliculus to promote a patent pathway for tears to flow from the ocular surface to the nose. First, the cut ends of the canaliculus need to be identified. Identifying the cut end of the canaliculus can be challenging. In sharp, clean lacerations closer to the punctum, identifying the canaliculus may be easier. However, if the eyelid is torn or avulsed, especially closer to the medial canthus, identifying the distal end can be more challenging. Using forceps or fine skin hooks to gently separate the tissues can sometimes expose an otherwise less visible, collapsed canaliculus. Exploration with cotton-tip applicators can also be helpful to avoid iatrogenic trauma. Additional headlight or overhead room light illumination can be helpful as can magnification with loupes. Following the anatomy and trajectory of the normal canaliculus (if one is present) by placing a Bowman lacrimal probe, can also help direct you to the possible location of the distal cut canaliculus. Alternatively, irrigating air under balanced salt solution or sterile water, or fluorescein-dyed balanced salt solution through the uninjured canaliculus to look for regurgitation in the wound may help highlight the distal injured canaliculus[10, 11]. A pigtail probe can be placed through the uninjured canaliculus and gently rotated with the probe handle perpendicular to the patient to identify the injured canaliculus.

Once the two ends of the canaliculus have been identified, repair can be achieved via a bicanalicular (e.g., Crawford stent) or monocanalicular (e.g. mono-Crawford or Mini Monoka™

stent) approach, which are described in detail below. However, a bi-canalicular intubation and retrieval of the stent under the turbinate in the nose is the gold standard to ensure not creating a false passage.

Bicanalicular Approach to Repairing Canalicular Trauma (Video 10-1)

The chief advantage of the bicanalicular intubation approach is stability of the stent and complete canalization of both the upper and lower canalicular system. Especially in the setting of extensive injury to the upper and lower eyelids, eyelid avulsion, or bicanalicular injury, a stable, bicanalicular stent can aid in aligning other anatomic structures. The chief limitation is that placement of bicanalicular stents usually requires the patient to be under general anesthesia in the operating room.

A bicanalicular stenting system, such as Crawford stents (FCI Ophthalmics, Pembroke, MA), is the authors' preference. The first step involves identifying the cut ends of the canaliculus. Once identified, the stent should be passed through the punctum and out of the cut end and then advanced through the distal cut end of the canaliculus (Fig. 10.2). The stent should then be advanced down the nasolacrimal duct and retrieved in the nose using a Crawford hook. In a similar manner, the other end of the stent is passed through the opposite canaliculus and retrieved in the nose (Fig. 10.2). With a very medial canalicular laceration or a laceration at the common canaliculus, completing the pass from the hard stop down into the nasolacrimal duct can sometimes be challenging. Care should be taken to not create a false passage when probing or placing the stent. Once the stent is passed, deep, buried sutures are then placed in the pericanalicular tissues to help reapproximate the cut ends of the canaliculus, typically using 7-0 polyglactin suture (Fig. 10.2). The eyelid margin and the eyelid and periocular lacerations are then repaired (Fig. 10.3). The stent is then tied in the nose. The stent should not be tied with tension to forestall cheese-wiring of the punctum and canaliculus. The authors prefer to tie the arms of the tube loosely in the nare with one square knot. The tube can be removed in clinic after 3–6 months through the nose or the eyelids. The authors prefer removal through the canaliculus/eyelid. It is helpful to rotate the tube to expose the knot prior to cutting and removing the tube (Video 10-2). In rare instances, the tube will need to be removed through the nose using an endoscope or nasal speculum for visualization, or the patient can blow their nose to retrieve it after it has been cut.

In some instances, trauma to the canaliculus is iatrogenic or intended. A common condition for which the canaliculus needs to be incised is canaliculitis with a retained foreign sulfur granule. After canaliculotomy that allows removal of infectious, foreign material, the canaliculus is intubated with a Crawford silicone tube and repaired (Video 10-3).

Monocanalicular Approach to Repairing Canalicular Trauma

For easily visualized monocanalicular injuries, intubation of the damaged canaliculus using the monocanalicular approach can be considered. Two options include the Mono-Crawford stent or the Mini Monoka™ stent. The Mono-Crawford is inserted through the punctum and is passed through the nasolacrimal duct and is retrieved in the nose with similar techniques to the bicanalicular stent. It has a punctal flange that keeps it in position. Like bicanalicular intubation with stent retrieval in the nose, use of Mono-Crawford stents likely necessitates anesthesia and is not typically a suitable approach for a bedside procedure. In contrast, the Mini Monoka™ stent intubates the canaliculus and is held in place by a punctal flange. The Mini Monoka™ stent canalizes the canaliculus and ideally extends down into the lacrimal sac, but does not need to be retrieved in the nose. This makes the use of a Mini Monoka™ stent a good option for bedside or in-office repairs. The

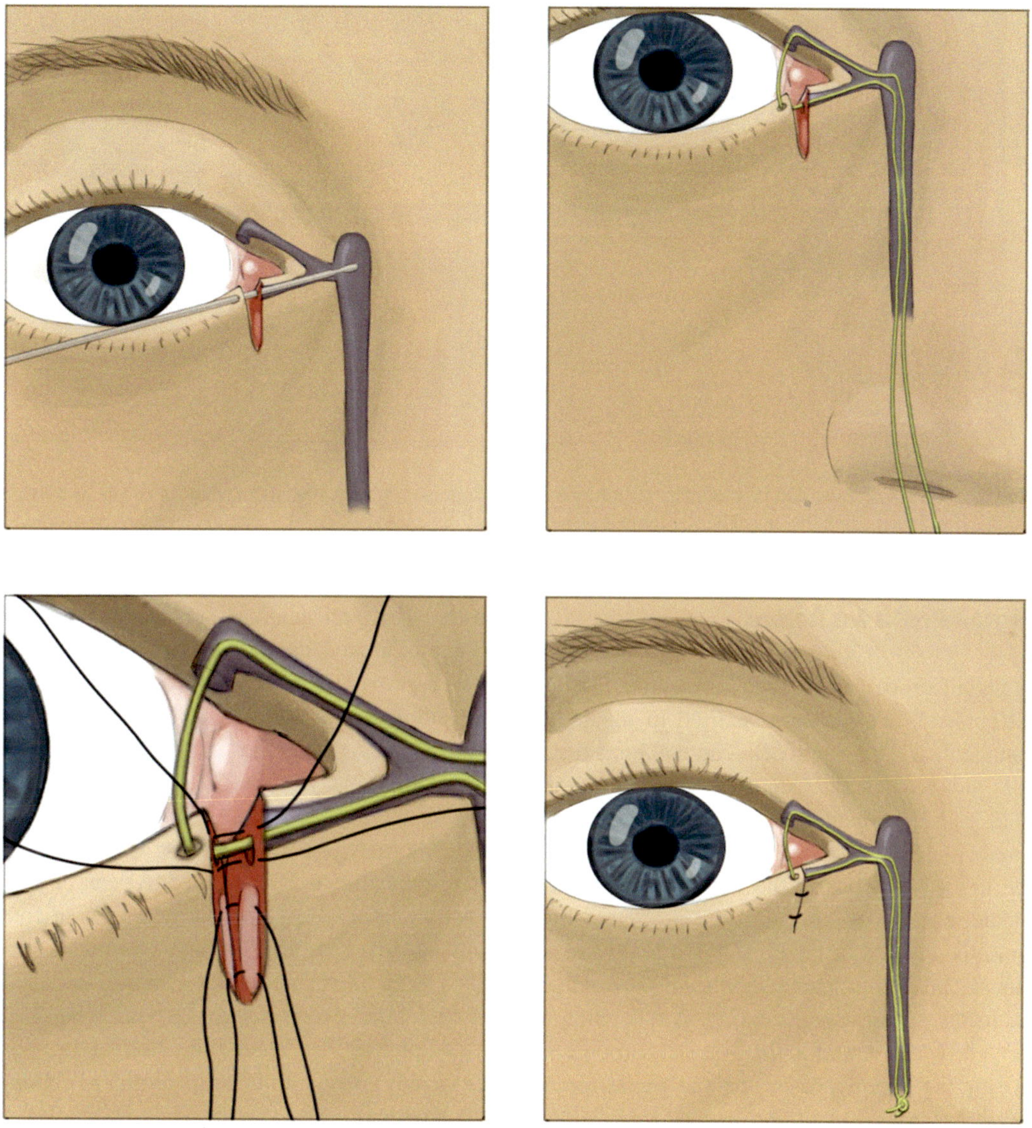

Fig. 10.2 Steps of canalicular repair. Top left, the stent is inserted into the punctum and then passed along canaliculus. The distal cut end of canaliculus is identified, and the probe is inserted and passed along the remainder of the canaliculus until a hard stop is identified and then the stent is rotated and passed down into the nose and is retrieved in the inferior meatus. Top right, the same procedure is completed to pass the other end of the lacrimal stent through the upper canaliculus and the stent is retrieved in the nose. Bottom left, sutures are then placed to approximate the cut ends of the canaliculus and then the eyelid margin laceration is repaired. Bottom right, the tube is then tied in the nose in one square knot taking care to not leave tension on the punctum. (Figure designed by Michael Han, MD at University of California, Irvine)

authors have found this technique most useful for monocanalicular lacerations closer to the punctum and for relatively linear, non-complex eyelid injuries. The primary disadvantage of monocanalicular intubation is the possibility of the stent becoming dislodged. In addition, the footplate at the eyelid margin can cause irritation to the ocular surface.

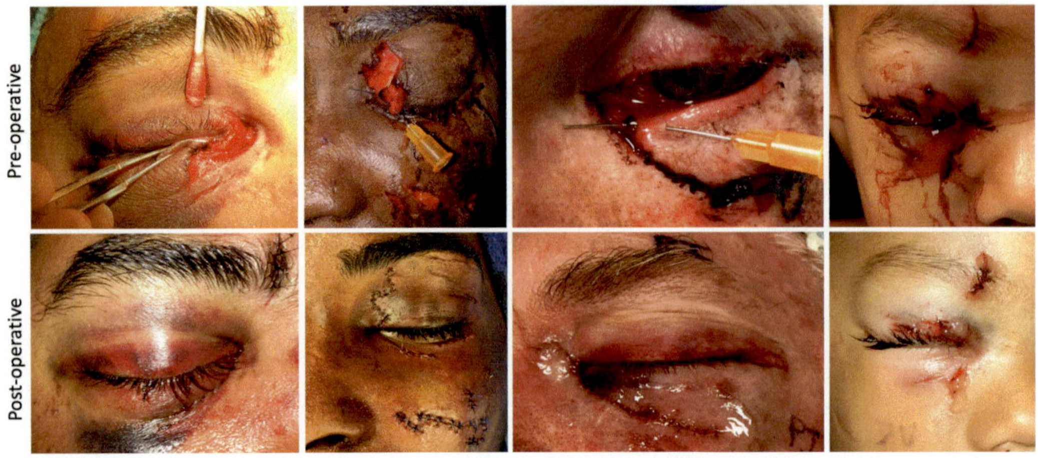

Fig. 10.3 Pre- (top row) and post-operative (bottom row) photographs showing canalicular injury before and immediately after repair using the bicanalicular intubation technique

Pigtail Probe for Repair

A pigtail probe can be used to identify the distal cut end, but can also be used to repair the canaliculus. This approach can be considered for monocanalicular injuries. Repair begins with passing a pigtail probe though the uninjured punctum and canaliculus and rotating the probe (posterior to the anterior limb of the medial canthal tendon) until the probe emerges from the cut end of the opposite, injured canaliculus. The probe handle should be perpendicular to the patient when rotating. A 6-0 nylon or polypropylene suture is then passed through the eye of the pigtail probe, and the pigtail probe is rotated back out of the normal canaliculus. The suture should then be passed through the remaining canaliculus and punctum. This can be done by hand, or the pigtail probe can be passed through the alternate punctum and the suture passed through the eye of the probe and then the probe is rotated back through the other punctum. The suture should now pass through the entire upper and lower canalicular system. A silicone stent can then be cut to size and then threaded over the suture, and the suture is pulled to guide the stent through the bicanalicular system. Sometimes a back-and-forth motion is necessary to help guide the silicone stent over the suture. The pericanalicular tissue should then be approximated using 7-0 polyglactin sutures to help provide support to the cut canaliculus. The suture within the lumen of the stent should now be tied, and the suture/stent complex rotated to avoid contact of the cut end of the silicone tubing and suture with the ocular surface. Alternatively, the Goldberg Cerclage stent (FCI Ophthalmics, Pembroke, MA) can be used which is a polypropylene suture with a silicone stent already combined, which eliminates having to thread a cut stent over a suture. Repair of the eyelid and eyelid margin laceration can now be completed. The chief limitation of the pigtail system is the significant potential to cause a false passage.

Postoperative Care and Complications

Topical antibiotic ointment should be applied to the wounds for 1 week after surgery. Stents are typically left in place for 3–6 months. The Crawford stents or stents placed using the pigtail probe method can be removed by cutting the stent between the upper and lower puncta and pulling the single arm of the stent out though a punctum. Of note, the bicanalicular stent can only be tied in one square knot to use this method and otherwise needs to be cut and retrieved in the nose. If the silicone tubing placed via the Crawford bicanalicular intubation method is not easily removed through the punctum, the patient can blow their nose and the stent recovered from the nose. Alternatively, an in-office endoscope or nasal speculum can be used to visualize and remove the stent.

The success rate of canalicular repair has been estimated to be as high as 85% [12]. The most common complication is obstruction of the canaliculus resulting in persistent epiphora, occurring in approximately 10% of cases [2]. Patients with combined upper and lower canalicular injury are at significantly greater risk of developing epiphora post-operatively, as were patients 30 years of age or greater [3]. While epiphora occurred more commonly among those where a stent was not placed, no difference in success rate has been appreciated among the different stent types [3]. In addition to persistent epiphora, other potential complications are listed in Table 10.1.

Symptomatic epiphora may require revision via dacryocystorhinostomy (DCR) if there is a patent canaliculus or via a conjunctivodacryocystorhinostomy (CDCR) if necessary. Prolapse of the stent and irritation of the ocular surface may also occur, which may necessitate premature stent removal.

Table 10.1 Potential complications from canalicular laceration repair

1	Persistent epiphora
2	Premature extrusion of the stent
3	Canalicular obstruction
4	Cheese-wiring of stent with elongation of punctum
5	Bleeding or epistaxis
6	Pain
7	Infection
8	Pyogenic granuloma
9	Scarring or poor healing
10	Eyelid malposition
11	Need for more surgery
12	Vision changes or loss

Conclusion

In the setting of periocular trauma, it is important to carefully evaluate for canalicular injury. When promptly identified and repaired, patients can have a greater potential for a functioning lacrimal drainage system and no epiphora symptoms. Several methods and lacrimal stents are available for repair, with the goal of intubating the cut canaliculus with a stent, approximating the cut canaliculus, and repairing the eyelid laceration or avulsion.

References

1. Murchison AP, Bilyk JR. Pediatric canalicular lacerations: epidemiology and variables affecting repair success. J Pediatr Ophthalmol Strabismus. 2014;51(4):242–8. https://doi.org/10.3928/01913913-20140604-05.
2. Chu YC, Wu SY, Tsai YJ, Liao YL, Chu HY. Early versus late canalicular laceration repair outcomes. Am J Ophthalmol. 2017;182:155–9. https://doi.org/10.1016/j.ajo.2017.08.006.
3. Kennedy RH, May J, Dailey J, Flanagan JC. Canalicular laceration. An 11-year epidemiologic and clinical study. Ophthalmic Plast Reconstr Surg. 1990;6(1):46–53.
4. Wulc AE, Arterberry JF. The pathogenesis of canalicular laceration. Ophthalmology. 1991;98(8):1243–9. https://doi.org/10.1016/s0161-6420(91)32148-1.
5. Jordan DR, Ziai S, Gilberg SM, Mawn LA. Pathogenesis of canalicular lacerations. Ophthalmic Plast Reconstr Surg. 2008;24(5):394–8. https://doi.org/10.1097/IOP.0b013e318183267a.
6. Kersten RC. Re: "Pathogenesis of canalicular lacerations". Ophthalmic Plast Reconstr Surg. 2009;25(5):420–1; author reply 421. https://doi.org/10.1097/IOP.0b013e3181b398d6.
7. JONES LT. An anatomical approach to problems of the eyelids and lacrimal apparatus. Arch Ophthalmol. 1961;66:111–24. https://doi.org/10.1001/archopht.1961.00960010113025.
8. Zoumalan CI, Joseph JM, Lelli GJ, et al. Evaluation of the canalicular entrance into the lacrimal sac: an anatomical study. Ophthalmic Plast Reconstr Surg. 2011;27(4):298–303. https://doi.org/10.1097/IOP.0b013e31820d1f7b.
9. Singh S, Ganguly A, Hardas A, Tripathy D, Rath S. Canalicular lacerations: factors predicting outcome at a tertiary eye care centre. Orbit. 2017;36(1):13–8. https://doi.org/10.1080/01676830.2017.1279646.

10. Reifler DM. Management of canalicular laceration. Surv Ophthalmol. 1991;36(2):113–32. https://doi.org/10.1016/0039-6257(91)90125-y.
11. Kwitny A, Baker JD. Functional results of the surgical repair of a lacerated canaliculus in children. J Pediatr Ophthalmol Strabismus. 2011;48(2):117–9. https://doi.org/10.3928/01913913-20100518-02.
12. Lin CH, Wang CY, Shen YC, Wei LC. Clinical characteristics, intraoperative findings, and surgical outcomes of canalicular laceration repair with monocanalicular stent in Asia. J Ophthalmol. 2019;2019:5872485. https://doi.org/10.1155/2019/5872485.

Medial Canthal Reconstruction

11

Carolina P. B. Gracitelli, and Eliana A. Forno

Abstract

Medial canthal reconstruction is challenging owing to the complex anatomy. Moreover, tissue matching in color and thickness is sometimes not available. In this chapter, the authors describe techniques to reconstruct medial canthus defects that afford good functional and aesthetic results.

Keywords

Medial canthus · Canthoplasty · Canthopexy · Medial canthus reconstruction · Glabellar flap

Introduction

Many tumors affect the medial canthus with the most common malignancy being basal cell carcinoma, responsible for approximately 90% of the cancers of the periorbital region [1]. Malignant tumors rarely respect aesthetic facial subunits and may spread to adjacent tissues. As they grow at the medial canthus, they can infiltrate to one or both eyelids, the cheek, or nose. This area is also prone to cancer recurrences [1].

The medial canthus has a concave shape and has important structures within it, such as the lacrimal drainage apparatus and the medial canthal tendon. The latter gives support to both eyelids, necessary for eyelid function and protection of the globe [2].

Defects affecting the medial canthus may be superficial or deep. Reconstruction ranges from primary closure to skin grafts to flaps. Some resections may include bone removal, with no resultant tissue bed and require vascularized flaps.

The medial canthus has four aesthetic units: upper eyelid, lower eyelid, nasal sidewall above and nasal sidewall below the medial commissure. In general, adjacent tissues rotated to the medial canthus area achieve better aesthetic results than skin grafts from distant areas. The medial canthal tendon is an important anchor and it guides the reconstruction in most cases.

A variety of flaps and grafts may be used alone or in combination to achieve a satisfactory functional and aesthetic outcome. In this chapter, the authors describe techniques for the reconstruction of the medial canthus.

Supplementary Information The online version contains supplementary material available at https://doi.org/10.1007/978-3-031-63178-8_11.

C. P. B. Gracitelli (✉)
Federal University of Sao Paulo, Escola Paulist de Medicina (UNIFESP/EPM), Rua Botucatu, 821. Vila Clementino, Sao Paulo 04023-062, Brazil
e-mail: carolepm@gmail.com

E. A. Forno
University of São Paulo (USP), São Paulo, Brazil

J. Tao (ed.), *Efficient Oculofacial Surgery*, https://doi.org/10.1007/978-3-031-63178-8_11

Superficial Canthal Defects

1. **Second intention healing (*laissez faire* Technique)**

When a defect is superficial and very small, second intention healing, i.e., allowing spontaneous wound granulation, may be considered [3]. Small defects that are at or just superior to the medial canthal tendon may heal more favorably with this approach [4]. However, scar contraction may cause some loss in the concave shape and the wound bed fibrosis can cause canthal webbing [4]. Furthermore, deeper defects can take long periods to epithelialize and a chronic open sore may be problematic for patients [4–6].

2. **Direct closure**

In some cases, direct closure of a small defect in the medial canthal area is acceptable. Care must be taken to avoid closure that would result in web formation. The concave configuration of the medial canthus makes it prone to vertical scar band formation. For this reason, flaps are often indicated to forestall web formation from tissue shortage and contracture [7].

3. **Full-thickness skin graft**

Simple, non-marginal superficial defects may be reconstructed using a simple full-thickness skin graft. Several anatomic sites serve as good donor areas. These include, the upper eyelid, retroauricular, inner brachial, or supraclavicular areas [8, 9]. Skin grafts to this region generally heal well owing to the rich vascular supply.

However, especially with the use of upper eyelid skin, skin thickness, texture and color are dissimilar to the native medial canthus. Other drawbacks of skin grafts to the medial canthus are hypertrophy, graft contraction, and graft failure. Graft contraction may also lead to eyelid retraction, ectropion, or webbing that may necessitate subsequent corrective surgery [8, 9].

Full-thickness skin grafts are nevertheless a reasonable option, especially with large defects where flaps cannot completely close the defect or where adjacent skin and tissues are poor (e.g., scar, sun-damage, or skin carcinoma) [3].

4. **Regional Flaps**

Due to risks of webbing or a conspicuous scar, even small medial canthus defects are better reconstructed with a local flap [10, 11]. Rotational and advancement flaps replace missing tissue with skin of similar color and compatible texture. The thickness of the flap can be controlled to match the depth of the defect by careful dissection of the subcutaneous tissue. If the medial eyelids are part of the defect, the eyelids may be rotated medially. It is important to ensure an excellent posterior fixation of the eyelid to ensure the eyelid hugs the globe (Video 11-1). A fixation point too anterior results in ectropion or eyelid tenting away from the ocular surface.

Flaps should be created to control skin tension vectors and prevent undesired tension on the eyelid margin [3]. A general rule is the most m obile region around the defect is the best donor area [10, 11]. In addition, flaps may be designed so that resultant scars are hidden in normal facial tension lines. If a defect is large enough that only one flap is not sufficient to cover the defect, it is possible to use two or even three flaps from different skin units of the face. Subsequent sections of this chapter will describe particulars of different flaps of several sizes and depths.

4.1 **Rhomboid flap**

The rhomboid flap is a versatile and simple flap used for repair of small to medium size medial canthal defects [12–14]. The flap can be modified to accommodate different shapes, size and depth of the defect [15].

Rhomboid flap design begins with considering a defect as a diamond or rhomboid shape with a long axis and a short axis. From the short axis tip, a line is extended and a subsequent line drawn parallel to the rhomboid side is formed as a "V" the size, depending on the amount needed to fill the defect [3]. With a diamond/rhomboid defect, f our different possible rhomboid flaps are possible. The two optimal flaps are those whose subsequent scar lines fall within relaxed facial skin tension lines (parallel to the lines of maximum extensibility). Of these two possible flaps, it is usually very easy to select the one that lies farthest from a critical structure to be avoided during surgery, such as the eyebrow or eyelid margin [3]. The flap does not need to be perfectly proportioned, so long as the flap fills the defect area and the donor site can be closed.

A scalpel is used to incise the flap and dissection is performed with scissors to create a flap of the desired thickness to match the depth of the defect. The pedicle of the flap brings the blood supply. Then the flap is rotated to the area of the defect. A central mattress suture anchored to periosteum may help maintain the concavity of the medial canthus. Usually, a light pressure patch is maintained for one to two days after the surgery.

4.2 Bilobed rotational flap

For moderate and large sized defect, bilobed rotational flap may be a good option. This earliest technique utilized two similar sized flaps oriented 90 and 180° from the defect [16] Various modifications have been described including making narrower angles between flaps to decrease deformation, tension, and the required size of the second flap lobe. Usually, the flap is created in the glabellar area above the medial canthal defect to provide upward traction on the reconstructed area and prevent lower eyelid traction [3].

In designing this flap, the lobe to be rotated into the defect should be about 80% of the area of the defect, and the second flap about 50% of the area of the first flap. The angle of the flaps is determined by the location of the defect and the surrounding anatomy. Orienting the second flap to align with the vertical glabellar furrow results in satisfactory camouflage of the incision scar.

During the dissection, preservation of a supraorbital or supratrochlear artery will allow for good blood supply to the flap. When the flaps are developed, the tissue surrounding the flaps and the defect should be undermined to allow for optimal tissue transposition. When the flaps are rotated and localized into the right position, an anchor suture may be performed to attach the center of the flaps to the periosteum of the underlying bone to match the concavity of the region [3].

Judicious placement of buried subcutaneous suture is implemented to decrease tension along the edges of the flaps. Lastly, either interrupted or running suture is used to align the skin edges along the entire perimeter of the flaps. It is crucial to pay attention in the depth of suture placement to line up the top surface of the flap to that of the recipient edge. A light pressure dressing applied several days allows for good apposition of the flap to the defect base promoting good healing [3].

Bilobed rotational flaps may be also used in combination with other different flaps when defects are large or involve different anatomic areas. The chief advantage of this technique is that the tension is divided by the broad area involving both flap lobes [17, 18].

4.3 Mid forehead flap

Kazajian, in 1944, described this flap as a wide pedicle (based on bilateral supratrochlear arteries), but this design was limited in the reach of the flap [19]. Many modifications to the mid forehead flap have been described. The paramedian forehead flap is centered over one supratrochlear artery and hence has a narrower pedicle and more maneuverability with a better arc of rotation. A tunneled de-epithelized pedicle is one modification [20]. A glabellar flap has also been combined with orbicularis oculi myocutaneous advancement flap for relatively large medial canthal defects involving upper/inferior eyelid [21].

The mid forehead flap is a hybrid of these flaps involving a midline forehead centered flap using the blood supply of just one supratrochlear artery plus mid forehead collaterals from the angular artery [22, 23]. The preservation of the supratrochlear artery may allow for a richly vascular flap on a narrow pedicle which can support a long flap that is pliable and can reach distant areas [3]. The mid forehead flap is useful for large, deep defects in the medial canthal area, especially those extending downward into the lower eyelid and tear trough. It may also be useful in situations where smaller regional flaps have been previously utilized, and additional surgery is required in the region.

Limitations of this technique include a temporary mound of redundant skin and subcutaneous tissue at the medial brow and the need for a secondary procedure several weeks later to debulk this area. In addition, eyebrow distortion is possible.

In the design, this flap is centered on the forehead midline and extends to the hairline. The area width should not exceed about two centimeters to allow for primary closure of the donor site defect. The flap should be long enough to reach the desired location. The pedicle of the flap should be the contralateral medial brow, allowing good length to bend the flap over a bridge of intact skin to feed the defect. The supratrochlear artery should be preserved.

The plane of dissection may be subperiosteal, preperiosteal, or subdermal, depending on the desired flap thickness and defect depth. This vertical forehead incision is closed in layers, with consideration of vertical mattress sutures superficially to allow for maximal wound edge eversion. Later, the flap is rotated over the intact bridge of skin as pedicle. It is anchored into position with subcutaneous sutures to reduce wound tension and then cutaneous running or interrupted sutures to align the skin edges. After 6 weeks, a second procedure to debulk the pedicle may be performed [3]. Modifications such as a tunneled flap can obviate the need for a secondary procedure [20].

4.4 Island flap or V–Y flap

The V to Y glabellar flap combines the location and donor site closure technique of a mid-forehead flap (but does not extend as far superiorly to the hairline) with the rotational technique of a rhomboid flap.

The width of the flap should be equal to the width of the defect and the length of each flap should be double the defect length. The movement vectors of the flaps should be parallel to skin tension lines.

At the glabellar area, incisions are designed to fall in the relaxed facial skin tension lines. At the medial canthus inferiorly, incisions are made at the nasofacial sulcus so that the scar lines are hidden at the boundaries of the facial aesthetic units. Incisions are made on both sides deep to the muscle plane in order to permit its movement at the direction of the defect.

In this technique, flap pedicles can be thinned to avoid tension and to allow its further advancement. At the periorbital region, especially at the inner canthus, even small pedicles are possible because of the rich blood supply, but in general, the flap is designed to capture the contralateral supraorbital blood supply.

In this type of flap reconstruction, it is important to fixate the deep dermis of the flap to deep tissues such as the periosteum or the anterior crus of the medial canthal tendon. A 5-0 suture (polyglactin, braided polyester, or polypropylene) is placed to avoid traction on the lower eyelid, and resultant ectropion or webbing. It is also important to aim to recreate the natural concave shape at the medial canthus. After the flap is properly fixed at the desired position, 5-0 absorbable sutures are placed at the sides and tail of the flap at the subcutaneous plane. Skin closure can be made with a 6-0 nonabsorbable suture, such as 6-0 silk or nylon. The resultant wound will form an inverted Y-shaped patterned scar (Fig. 11.1, Video 11-2).

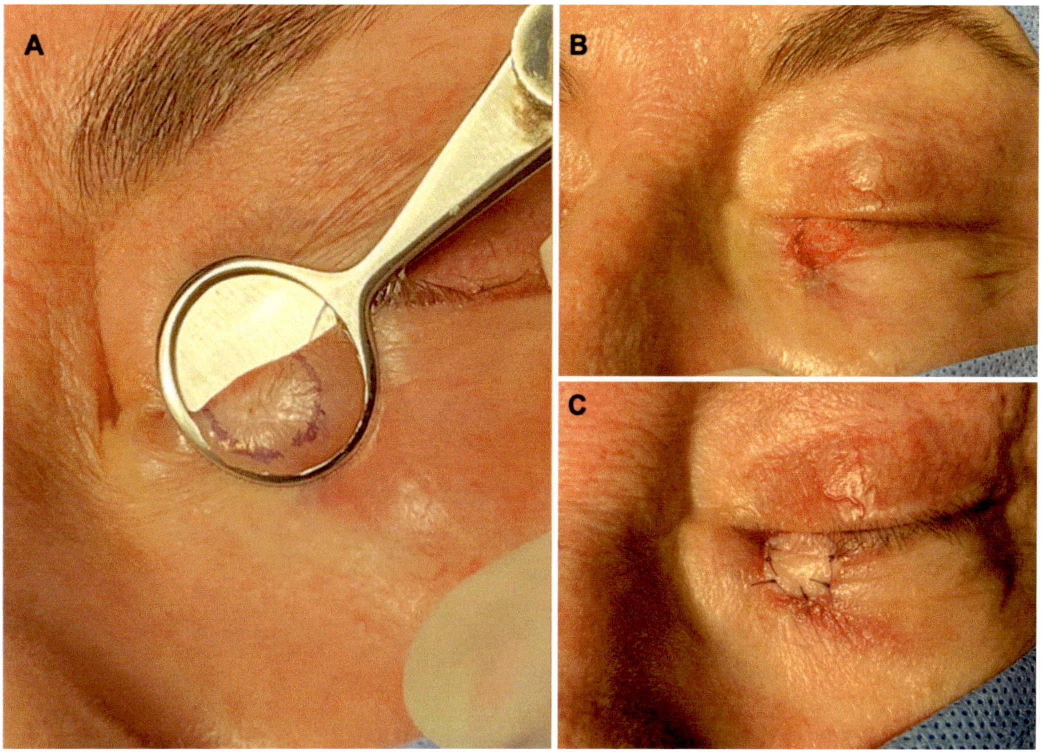

Fig. 11.1 (A) Example of a patient with a small superficial lesion of the medial lower eyelid near the canthus; (B) lesion excised with a partial thickness incision, sparing the tarsal plate; (C) the defect reconstructed with a small skin graft

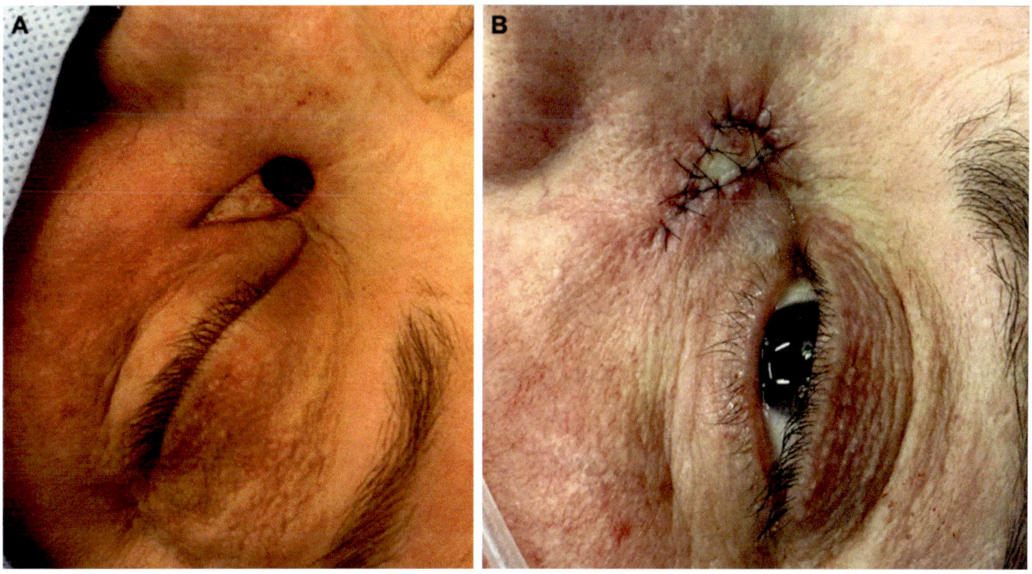

Fig. 11.2 (A) A small canthal defect at the medial canthus; (B) reconstruction with a small island flap

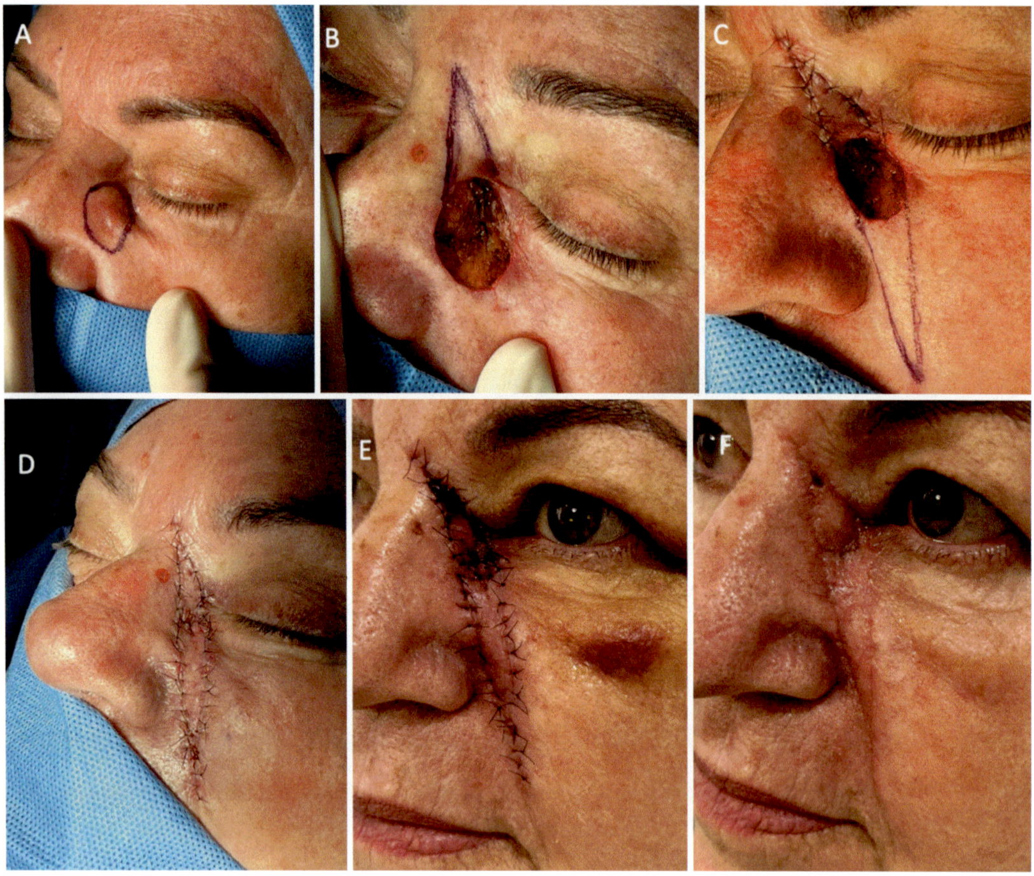

Fig. 11.3 (A) Basal cell carcinoma with the planned resection margins inked (eyelid margins and lacrimal drainage apparatus were spared); (B-C) superior and inferior flaps were advanced and sutures; (D) appearance after the flaps were advanced and sutured; (E) appearance after 5 days; (F) appearance after 20 days

This advancement flap has some advantages. In terms of match, these adjacent flaps have good color and texture match. In addition, they have excellent blood supply with very low probability of necrosis or graft failure. In addition, compared to a forehead flap, this technique avoids a bridge of tissue over intact skin, that requires a second surgery to correct. Moreover, the vertical forehead scar is shorter (Figs. 11.2, 11.3, 11.4, 11.5, 11.6 and 11.7).

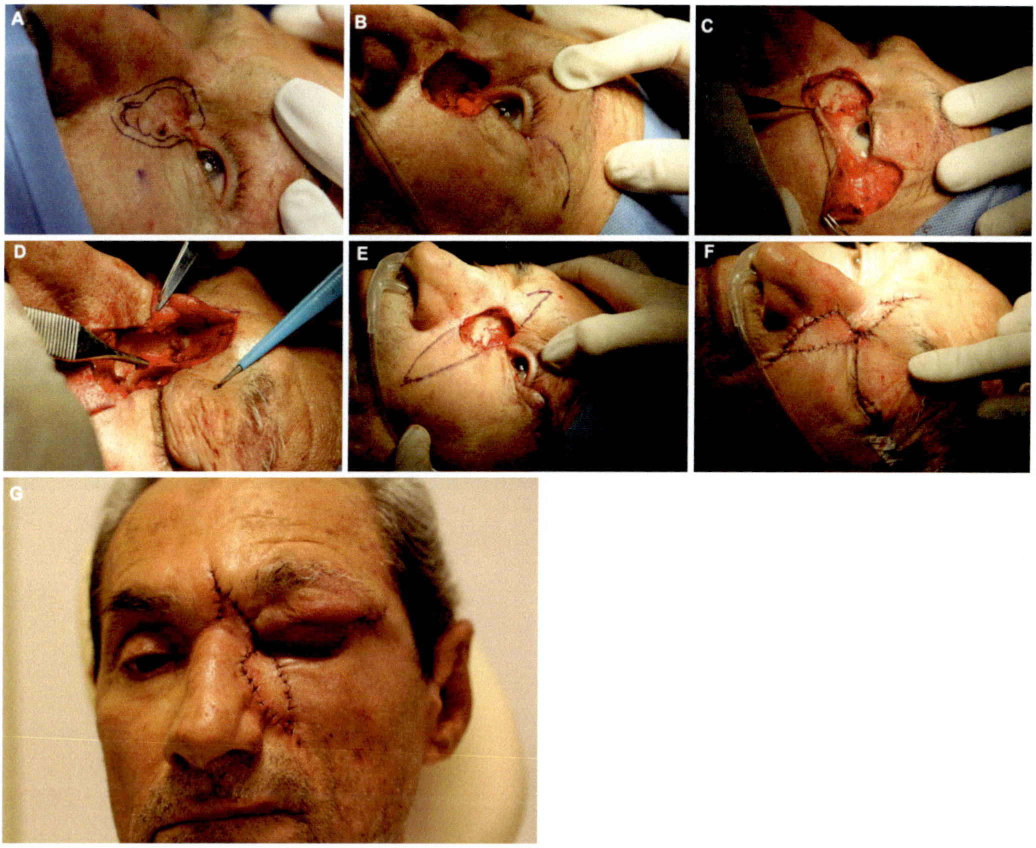

Fig. 11.4 (A) Basal cell carcinoma of the inner canthus and the planned resection margins inked; (B) defect after complete removal of the tumor; (C) semicircular flap dissected. (D) Medial tarsus fixed at the medial orbit periosteum as posteriorly as possible; (E) planned island V–Y pedicle flaps marked. Superior flap is dissected from the glabellar area and the inferior flap from the nasofacial sulcus area; (F) final result after combining 3 flaps showing the total coverage of the defect; (G) after 1 week

Complications and Other Procedures

This area is a high-risk site for webbing of the skin after reconstruction that may be due to both cicatrization and inadequate deep fixation of tissue into the medial canthal hollow. Sometimes, excision or release of the cicatrix, with or without further skin grafts or flaps may be necessary. Scar revision with Z plasty can help flatten webs. Epiphora is also possible due to injury to the underlying lacrimal drainage apparatus or eyelid malposition or both. Tear drain surgery may be necessary [24–26].

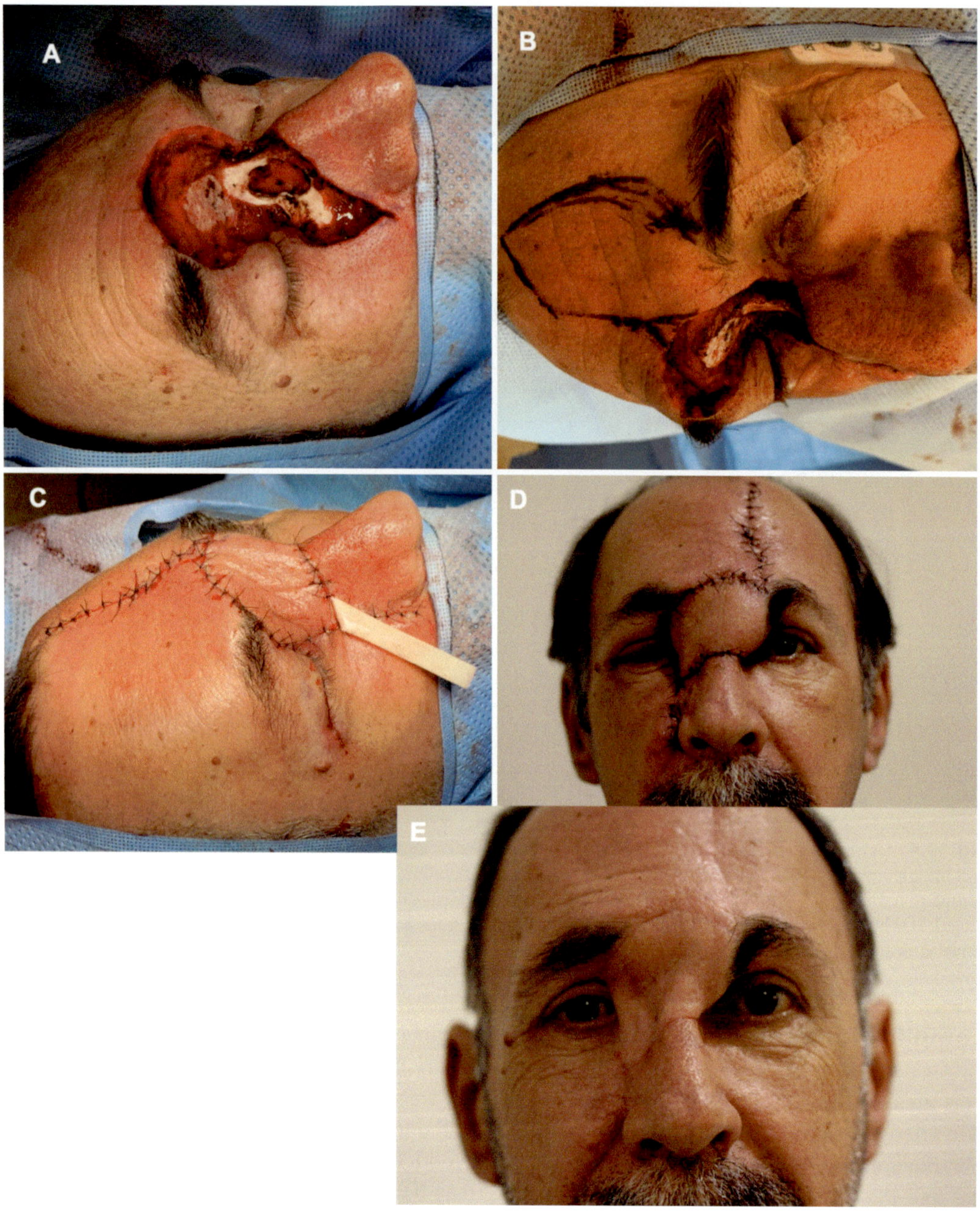

Fig. 11.5 (A) Large, deep glabellar area, nasal base and nasofacial sulcus defect after removal of a dermatofibrosarcoma; (B) reconstruction was planned with a large glabellar flap preserving the supra orbital and supratrochlear vessels of the contralateral side; (C) flap sutured. (D) Post operative after 10 days; (E) after 4 months

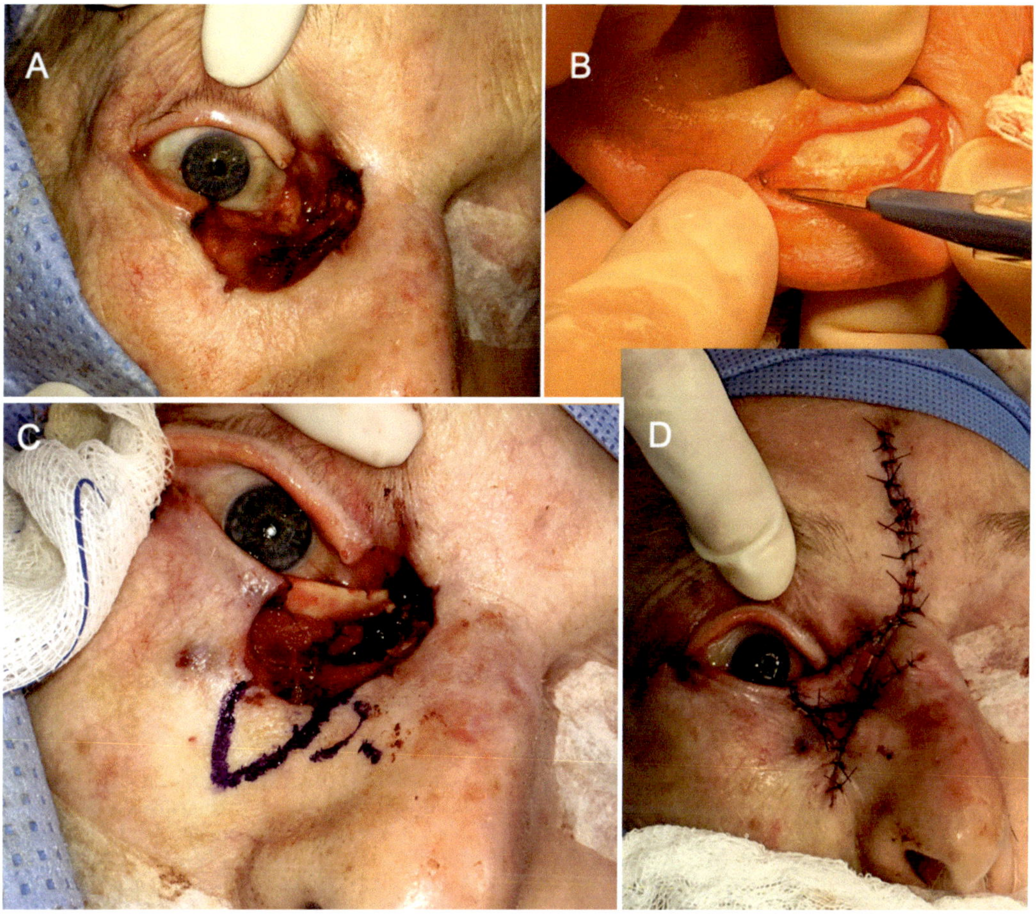

Fig. 11.6 (A) Medial canthus and lower eyelid defect after basal cell carcinoma excision; (B) ear cartilage graft harvested to reconstruct the posterior lamella of lower eyelid; (C) ear cartilage sewn to recreate the eyelid posterior lamella; (D) immediate postoperative appearance after a paramedian forehead flap and a small nasofacial flap

Conclusion

Repair of defects in the medial canthus require planning due to the complex anatomy that involves the lacrimal system, canthal tendons, eyebrows, and neurovascular bundles. The different reconstruction options described in this chapter offer good final aesthetic and functional results. Keys to repair are suitable posterior medial canthal tendon anchoring and tissue

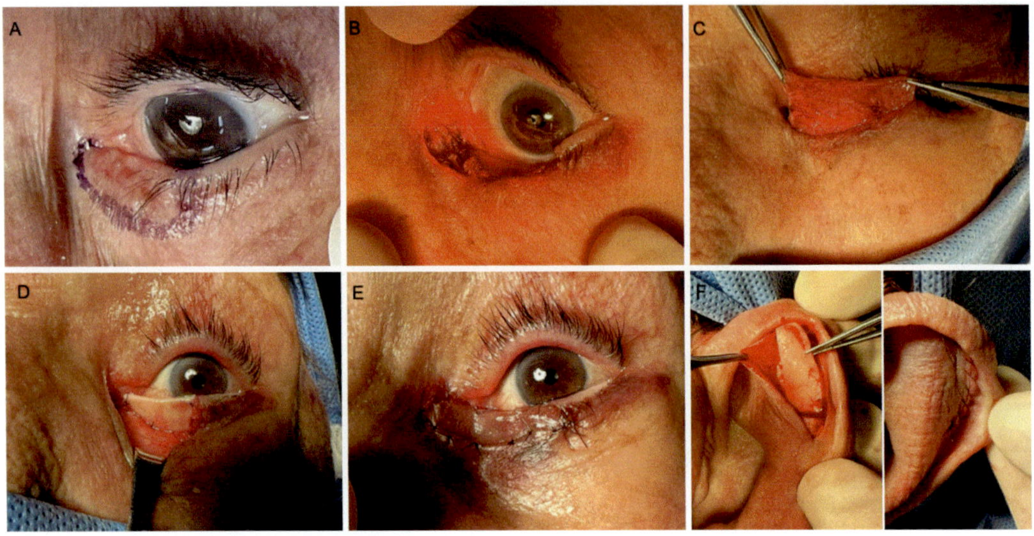

Fig. 11.7 Sandwich technique for eyelid reconstruction (**A**) Basal cell carcinoma affecting the lower eyelid and medial canthus; (**B**) defect after excision; **C** remnant orbicularis oculi muscle dissected and pulled superiorly; (**D**) ear cartilage sewn into the defect, posterior to the muscle flap for reconstruction of the posterior lamella; (E) skin graft anterior to the orbicularis oculi muscle forming the anterior lamella (**F**) ear cartilage ear graft was harvested from the pinna through an anterior incision

rearrangement or graft procedures that respect aesthetic units of the face.

References

1. Czyz CN, Cahill KV, Foster JA, Michels KS, Clark CM, Rich NE. Reconstructive options for the medial canthus and eyelids following tumor excision. Saudi J Ophthalmol. 2011;25:67–74.
2. Ogino A, Onishi K, Okada E, Nakamichi M. Medial canthal reconstruction with multiple local flaps. JPRAS Open. 2018;15:4–9.
3. Freitag SK, Lee NG, Lefebvre DR, Yoon MK. Eyelid reconstruction. Thieme. 2020;42–59.
4. Lowry JC, Bartley GB, Garrity JA. The role of second-intention healing in periocular reconstruction. Ophthalmic Plast Reconstr Surg. 1997;13:174–88.
5. Fox SA, Beard C. Spontaneous lid repair. Am J Ophthalmol. 1964;58:947–52.
6. Harrington JN. Reconstruction of the medial canthus by spontaneous granulation (Laissez-Faire): a review. Ann Ophthalmol. 1982;14:956–960, 963–956, 969–970.
7. Thaller VT, Then KY, Luhishi E. Spontaneous eyelid expansion after full thickness eyelid resection and direct closure. Br J Ophthalmol. 2001;85:1450–4.
8. Ratner D. Skin grafting. From here to there. Dermatol Clin. 1998;16:75–90.
9. Leibovitch I, Huilgol SC, Hsuan JD, Selva D. Incidence of host site complications in periocular full thickness skin grafts. Br J Ophthalmol. 2005;89:219–22.
10. Jordan DR, Anderson RL, Nowinski TS. Tarsoconjunctival flap for upper eyelid reconstruction. Arch Ophthalmol. 1989;107:599–603.
11. deSousa JL, Malhotra R, Davis G. Sliding tarsal flap for reconstruction of large, shallow lower eyelid tarsal defects. Ophthalmic Plast Reconstr Surg. 2007;23:46–8.
12. Limberg AA. Mathematical principles of local plastic procedures on the surface of the human body. Medgis, Leningrad, Russia; 1944.
13. Limberg AA. Modern trends in plastic surgery. Design of local flaps. Mod Trends Plast Surg. 1966;2:38–61.
14. Limberg AA. Design of local flaps. Mod Trends Plast Surg. 1966;2:38–61.
15. Bullock JD, Koss N, Flagg SV. Rhomboid flap in ophthalmic plastic surgery. Arch Ophthalmol. 1973;90:203–5.
16. Esser JFS. Gestielte locale nasenplastik mit zweizipfligen lappen, decking des sekunderen defektes vom ersten zipfel durch den zweiten. Deutsch Z Chir. 1918;143:385.
17. McGregor JC, Soutar DS. A critical assessment of the bilobed flap. Br J Plast Surg. 1981;34:197–205.
18. Sullivan TJ, Bray LC. The bilobed flap in medial canthal reconstruction. Aust N Z J Ophthalmol. 1995;23:42–8.

19. Kazanjian VH. The repair of nasal defects with the median forehead flap; primary closure of forehead wound. Surg Gynecol Obstet. 1946;83:37–49.
20. Mombaerts I, Gillis A. The tunneled forehead flap in medial canthal and eyelid reconstruction. Dermatol Surg. 2010;36:1118–25.
21. Chao Y, Xin X, Jiangping C. Medial canthal reconstruction with combined glabellar and orbicularis oculi myocutaneous advancement flaps. J Plast Reconstr Aesthet Surg. 2010;63:1624–8.
22. Harris GJ, Logani SC. Multiple aesthetic unit flaps for medial canthal reconstruction. Ophthalmic Plast Reconstr Surg. 1998;14:352–9.
23. Onishi K, Maruyama Y, Okada E, Ogino A. Medial canthal reconstruction with glabellar combined Rintala flaps. Plast Reconstr Surg. 2007;119:537–41.
24. Rose GE, Welham RA. Jones' lacrimal canalicular bypass tubes: twenty-five years' experience. Eye (London). 1991;5(Pt 1):13–9.
25. Welham RA, Guthoff R. The Lester-Jones tube: a 15-year follow-up. Graefes Arch Clin Exp Ophthalmol. 1985;223:106–8.
26. Lim C, Martin P, Benger R, Kourt G, Ghabrial R. Lacrimal canalicular bypass surgery with the Lester Jones tube. Am J Ophthalmol. 2004;137:101–8.

Upper and Lower Blepharoplasty

12

Filipe José Pereira

Abstract

Classically, blepharoplasty is the removal of excess skin, muscle, and fat from the eyelids. Indications for upper or lower blepharoplasty include enhancing the patient's appearance. Upper eyelid blepharoplasty may be indicated to improve superior field vision. Whether the indication is functional or aesthetic, a natural appearing result is desired. Outcomes can be enhanced by recognizing eyelid pathology, including malposition or laxity. Concomitant procedures encompass blepharoptosis repair, canthal tightening of the eyelids, fat transposition, or brow procedures, among many others. This chapter details surgical technique and other aspects of upper and lower blepharoplasty surgery.

Keywords

Blepharoplasty · Dermatochalasis · Eyelid lift

Supplementary Information The online version contains supplementary material available at https://doi.org/10.1007/978-3-031-63178-8_12.

F. J. Pereira (✉)
Clínica Catarinense de Pálpebras e Olhos, Florianopolis, Brazil
e-mail: filipe@ccpo.com.br

Introduction

The eyelid and surrounding structures are a spotlight of facial beauty. The periocular region is key in the appearance of aging as well as expression [1].

With aging, the upper and lower eyelids loosen and skin becomes redundant, described as dermatochalasis. Other important factors, including genetic influences, sun exposure, and smoking, hasten changes to the eyelids.

Blepharoplasty is the surgical correction of excess eyelid skin and other changes. Blepharoplasty can address cosmetic concerns and can expand the field of vision [2].

Blepharoplasty

Blepharoplasty is one of the most common aesthetic surgeries performed worldwide. Many patients undergo blepharoplasty for functional indications as well.

The assessment begins with understanding a patient's complaints. A useful tactic is to ask the patient point out the areas of concern in a mirror. Old photos of the patient's face may further allow the surgeon to observe for some important pre-existing characteristics, such as asymmetries, proptosis, ptosis, or eyelid retraction, among other pathologies.

J. Tao (ed.), *Efficient Oculofacial Surgery*, https://doi.org/10.1007/978-3-031-63178-8_12

Goals should be reasonable and it is important to screen for psychological disturbances, especially body dysmorphic disorder. In some instances, expectations may not align with what is possible with surgery and further discussion or aborting surgical intervention may be necessary [3]. Ophthalmologic history is important especially corneal diseases and dry eyes. Incomplete blink, lagophthalmos, and irregularities of the corneal-conjunctival surface at biomicroscopy are important details that should be considered. Associated eyelid problems, including blepharoptosis, eyebrow ptosis or eyelid retraction should be considered, since they can be repaired concomitantly [4–7].

With lower eyelid assessment, it is important to identify retraction, sagging or midface ptosis. Poor lower eyelid tone impairs the tear pump function during blinks [8]. Eyelid laxity should be tested prior to surgery with the distraction test, snap back test, and assessing the lower margin to reflex distance (MRD 2).

In the distraction test, the skin of the middle of the lower eyelid is pulled in the anterior direction. Up to 8 mm of movement of the eyelid away from the ocular surface is considered normal.

In the snap back test, the lower eyelids are pulled down and released. If the eyelids immediately return to the original position of contact with the ocular surface the test is considered negative for eyelid laxity. A positive test can be divided into: mild sagging (returns slowly), moderate (returns incompletely but totally when blinking), and severe (return is incomplete even after blinking).

The lower eyelid margin-reflex distance (MRD 2) measures, the distance between the corneal light reflex and the lower eyelid margin, with the head in neutral position and the eyeball in a straight-ahead gaze.

Differential Diagnosis

Blepharoptosis and eyebrow ptosis may confound dermatochalasis. In moderate to severe blepharoptosis, the relaxed structures of the posterior lamella "unfold" the eyelid and the amount of dermatochalasis may be less apparent. Many patients undergoing blepharoptosis repair without skin excision note excess upper eyelid skin postoperatively. In eyebrow ptosis, the apparent amount of upper eyelid skin may be exaggerated. The normal position of the eyebrow is, in general, slightly above the upper orbital edge, but there is a difference in the position of the eyebrow between men (straighter, lower, and thicker) and women (more temporally arched and thinner). In cases of severe eyelid ptosis, the eyebrows are generally more elevated, with contraction of the frontal muscle as a compensatory mechanism. In cases of paresis/paralysis of the frontal part of the facial nerve, the forehead is smoother and the eyebrow is lower.

Procedure Details

Blepharoplasty may be performed awake or with intravenous sedation or general anesthesia. No matter the type of systemic anesthesia, local anesthetic infiltration is an initial step. Typically, lidocaine or bupivacaine or both, with epinephrine are administered. The use adjunctive tranexamic acid (TXA) in the local admixture may help decrease postoperative ecchymosis. (The editor combines equal parts of 1% lidocaine with 1:100,000 epinephrine, 0.5% bupivacaine, and TXA 100 mg/ml.)

Upper Blepharoplasty (Video 12-1)

First, the skin to be removed is marked in the upright position in neutral gaze with the brow relaxed (Fig. 12.1a). Preference is given to maintaining the existing upper eyelid crease (Fig. 12.1b). The crease is usually located 8 to 10 mm above the eyelid margin but varies according to race or ethnicity. In general, the crease is much lower in Asian patients. An atraumatic forceps is used to perform a pinch test to determine the amount of skin to be excised (Fig. 12.1c), respecting the minimum

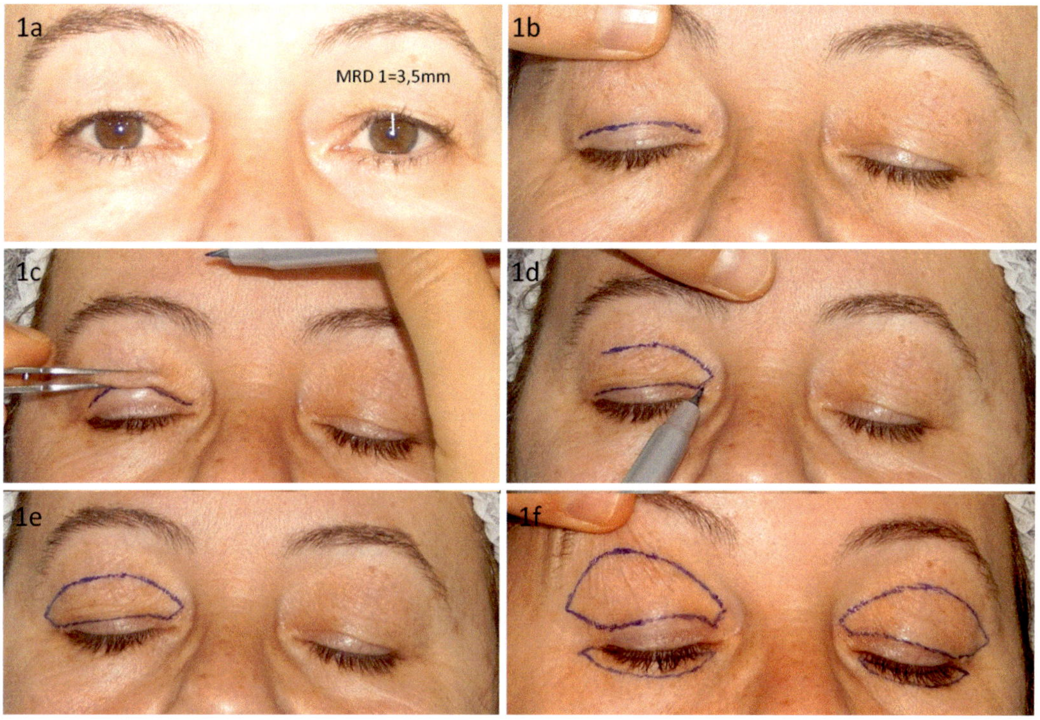

Fig. 12.1 Sequence of demarcation of upper blepharoplasty

of 10 mm from the inferior border of the brow, so as not to include any brow skin. If there is an excess of skin in the most medial portion, a triangle of skin in the super-nasal direction of about 6–8 mm is removed, embedded in the primary demarcation (Fig. 12.1d). Laterally, the lower incision curves superiorly for 10–15 mm (Fig. 12.1e). In cases of upper and lower blepharoplasty a minimum gap of 5 mm between the upper and lower incisions laterally is preserved (Fig. 12.1f).

Skin markings are incised with a no. 15 blade (Fig. 12.2a), the excess skin is resected with scissors or a scalpel. In patients with orbicularis hypertrophy, a small amount of preseptal orbicularis muscle is excised. The pretarsal orbicularis is generally preserved to preserve eyelid closure strength. In the upper eyelid the nasal portion of the septum is opened with sharp dissection and the orbital fat is resected (Fig. 12.2b), avoiding excessive traction. Gentle posterior compression of the eyeball facilitates fat pad prolapse for its identification (Fig. 12.2c). Generally, only nasal orbital fat is resected in the upper eyelids and it is removed conservatively to avoid a hollowed appearance. There is generally no temporal fat in the upper eyelid; protrusions in this area are usually caused by the prolapsed lacrimal gland. If the gland is prolapsed, it may be reposited into its native position posterior to the orbital rim, suturing it to inner rim periosteum. Hemostasis measures must be taken because minimal postoperative bleeding provides a shorter recovery, better appearance and less potential for serious complications. For skin closure, continuous suture with nylon 6-0 (Fig. 12.2d—immediate postoperative) is used. If more definitive crease formation is desired, eyelid closure includes deep passes that engage epitarsus or the levator aponeurosis.

Lower Blepharoplasty

External lower blepharoplasty is associated with a high incidence of eyelid malposition complications. Risk factors include a negative vector morphology or any cicatricial changes, among

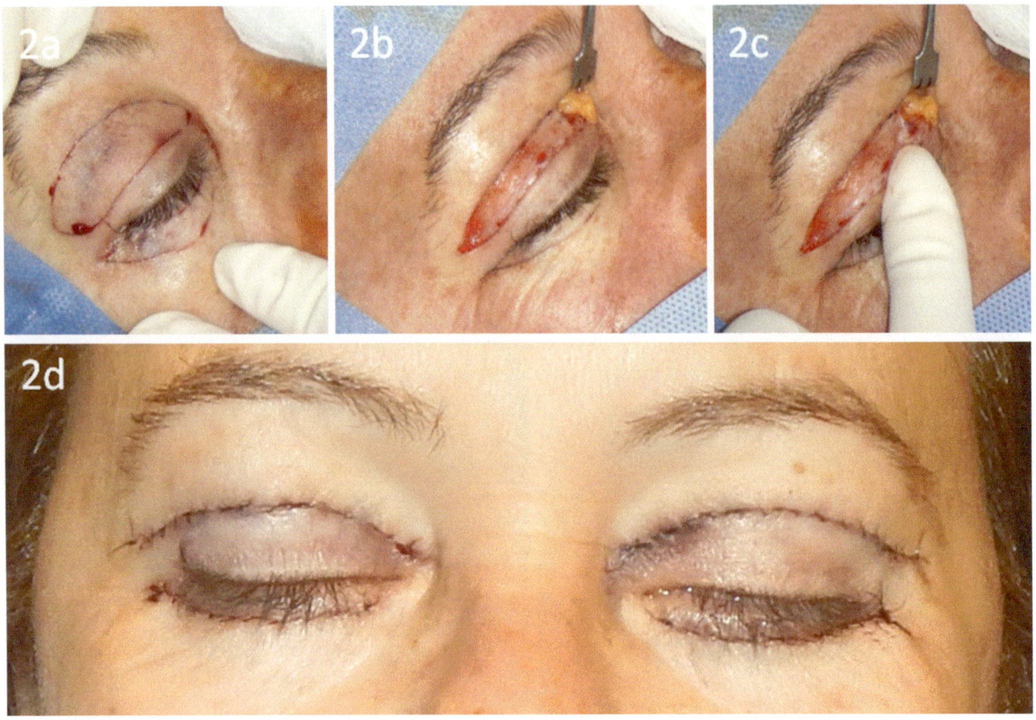

Fig. 12.2 Upper blepharoplasty sequence

others. In general, external blepharoplasty is less favored than transconjunctival or midface lift approaches, and should be reserved for patients without risk factors for eyelid retraction.

In external blepharoplasty (Fig. 12.3a), the skin resection is between a sub ciliary line from the lacrimal punctum extending laterally to the external commissure. The amount of resection varies, but should be conservative. To quantify the amount of redundant skin that is safe to resect, the patients can be asked to look up and open their mouth while performing a pinch test maneuver (Fig. 12.3b).

Resection of excess skin is performed with a scalpel and scissors. In patients with orbicular hypertrophy, resection of some preseptal muscle is included (Fig. 12.4a). The septum is dissected and resection of the fat is performed with care to preserve the inferior oblique muscle (Fig. 12.4b). An external suture at the lateral canthus that engages the lateral rim periosteum is useful to forestall eyelid retraction.

Anterior lamella tissues may alternatively be resected in triangles, the first being the redundant tissues past the lateral canthus. This skin and muscle flap is secured to the lateral rim periosteum just lateral to the lateral eyelid commissure. The second triangle is formed by the redundant tissues in the subciliary zone. For skin closure, continuous suture is used with 6-0 nylon or 6-0 plain sutures.

Transconjunctival Lower Blepharoplasty (Video 12-2)

In patients who only have prominent fat pads or whose skin sagging is mild, resection of the bags via a transconjunctival approach may be appropriate. In addition to fat resection, fat repositioning to fill a deepened orbitomalar groove and tear trough may be performed.

The transconjunctival approach is performed through a conjunctival incision that extends

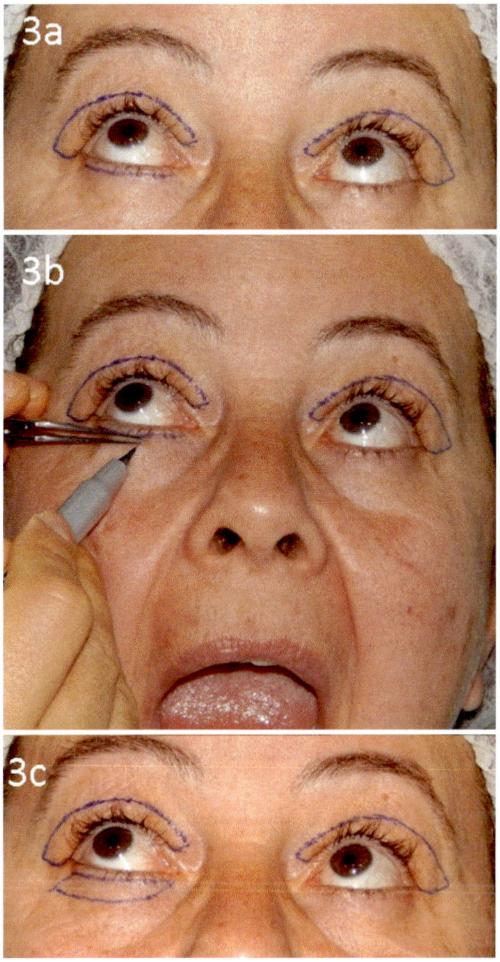

Fig. 12.3 Sequence of external lower blepharoplasty

from the lacrimal punctum to the lateral corner or 3 isolated small incisions done directly on the medial, central, and lateral fat pads. A canthotomy and inferior cantholysis can be performed to aid in exposure as well as in preparation for canthoplasty in patients needing eyelid tightening. The posterior lamellar incision is ideally placed between the inferior tarsal border and fornix. A 4-0 silk suture can be placed to engage the conjunctiva-retractor complex for superior traction that improves exposure. The slight compression of the eyeball helps in the identification and quantification of the fat to be removed. The fat is resected carefully (Fig. 12.5). Special care must be taken to avoid injury to the inferior oblique muscle, visible between the central and medial fat pads. The conjunctiva may be left unsutured or two to three plain gut sutures may be placed (Fig. 12.6).

Complications

Complications in blepharoplastyare usually mild and self limited [9, 10]. Common adverse effects are outlined here.

Eye discomfort. Burning, conjunctival hyperemia, and foreign body sensation are usually related to eye surface dryness or keratitis due to ocular exposure to antiseptic products used prior to surgery. In the immediate postoperative period, the intense lubrication with eye drops

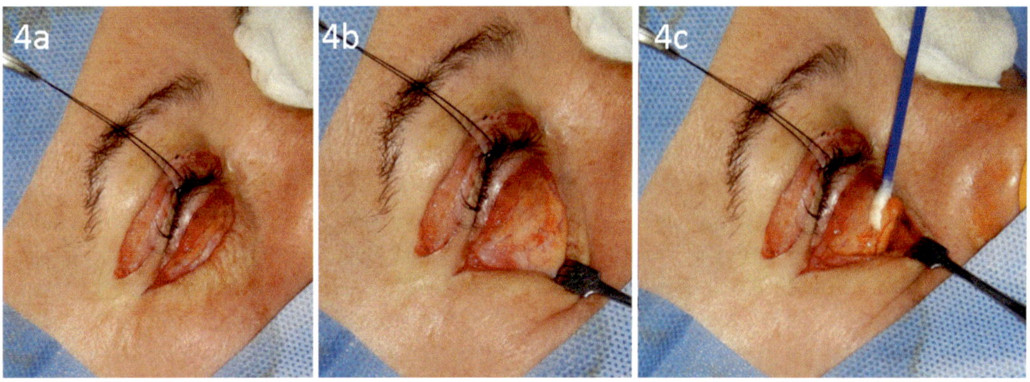

Fig. 12.4 Inferior blepharoplasty sequence

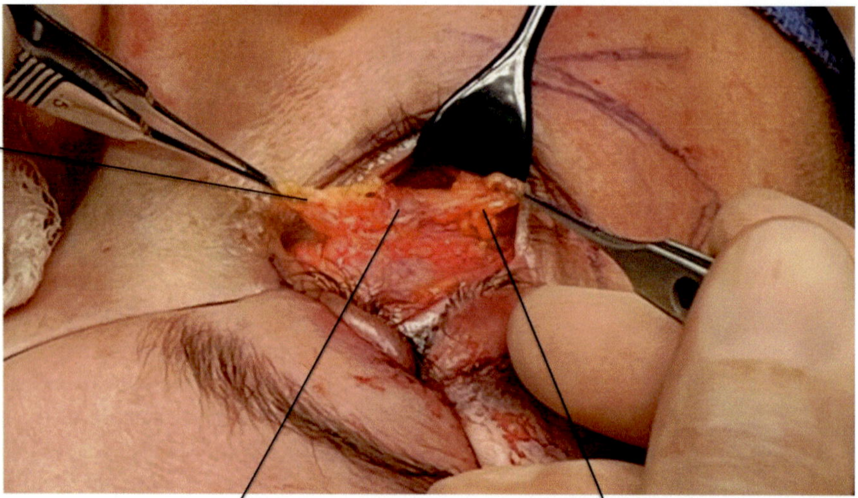

Fig. 12.5 Intraoperative photo during transconjunctival inferior blepharoplasty with orbital fat compartments identified

or lubricating gels is advised. In case of intense eye discomfort or lack of response to the above measures, a bandage contact lens can be helpful.

Alternatively, occlusion of the eye after applying antibiotic ointment or asking the patient to keep their eyes closed may hasten ocular surface recovery. In cases of small epithelial defects of the cornea, reepithelialization is rapid, rarely recovering within hours to one day. Severe pain and discomfort that persists many hours after the above measures especially with significant vision deterioration demands immediate evaluation.

Dry eyes. One of the most common complaints to ophthalmologists, dry eye can worsen in patients who undergo blepharoplasty. Lubricant eye drops are the foundation of therapy for the treatment of dry eye syndrome, stabilizing the tear film and providing relief of symptoms. Other forms of treatment are warm compress therapy, topical corticosteroids food supplementation with omega-3, autologous serum eye drops and, in severe cases, tear outflow occlusion through plugs or surgical closure of the lacrimal canal [10–12].

Lagophthalmos. An inability to close the eyelids may be on spontaneous blink or with volitional forceful closure. Lagophthalmos alters the distribution of the tear film on the ocular surface. Symptoms may be simple irritation to corneal ulcer. It may be caused by excessive removal of skin or muscle, scarring, or rarely paresis (Fig. 12.7). The initial treatment of the lagophthalmos is eye lubricating eye drops or gels, therapeutic contact lenses, or moisture chamber eye patch. Closure of the lacrimal ducts by placing plugs, may also help. Massaging with corticosteroid ointments provides partial to total improvement. At the appropriate time, usually months later, surgical treatment may be indicated to restore eyelid function.

Retraction. Related to lagophthalmos, retraction is vertical displacement of the eyelid margin with increase of the MRD so the palpebral aperture is widened. Treatment includes the aforementioned medical interventions for dry eye and lagophthalmos. Surgical repair may be necessary if medical management fails or the eyelid retraction is disfiguring. These are described in detail in other chapters. Briefly, upper eyelid

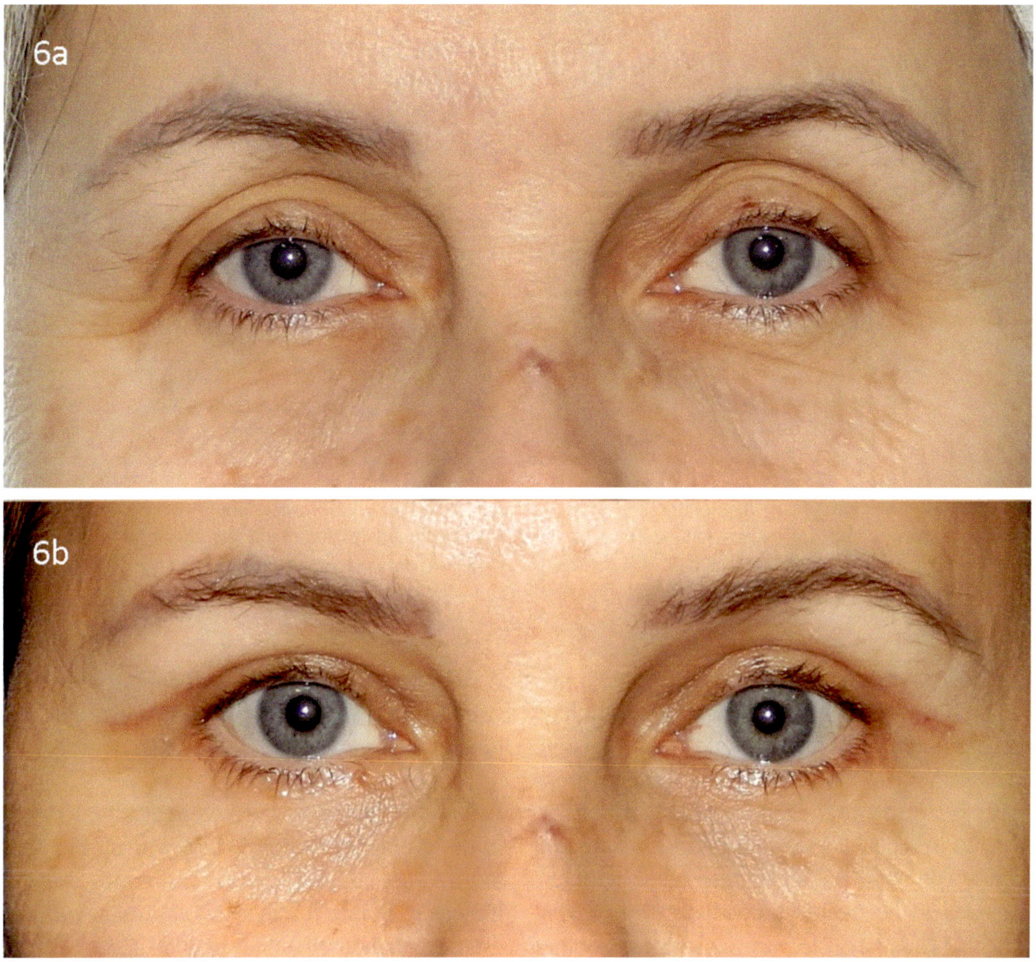

Fig. 12.6 Patient before and after upper blepharoplasty with concomitant lateral canthopexy and a minimal ptosis repair posterior approach

retraction is commonly repaired through levator recession. Inferior eyelid retraction is commonly repaired with spacer grafts or lateral canthal anchoring or suspension procedures (Fig. 12.8). Skin grafts are sometimes required for eyelid retraction but are generally avoided in patients still seeking an aesthetically sound result.

Ectropion: Ectropion is the eversion of the eyelid away from the ocular surface, which can occur after excessive skin is resected in blepharoplasty. Ectropion is detailed in another chapter, but mild forms may be treated with canthoplasty (Fig. 12.9). Skin grafting is necessary in many cases.

Eyelid hematoma. Ecchymosis is to be expected after blepharoplasty. Mild to moderate hematoma can form as well, especially in patients with poor clotting parameters or those who are on anticoagulant or antiplatelet medications. So long as the hematoma is superficial, full recovery is to be expected with no effect on vision or the result. Tranexamic acid use in the local admixture may decrease ecchymosis and hematoma formation, although there is insufficient evidence.

Orbital hematoma. One of the most serious complications is an orbital hematoma, also known as a retrobulbar hematoma, which

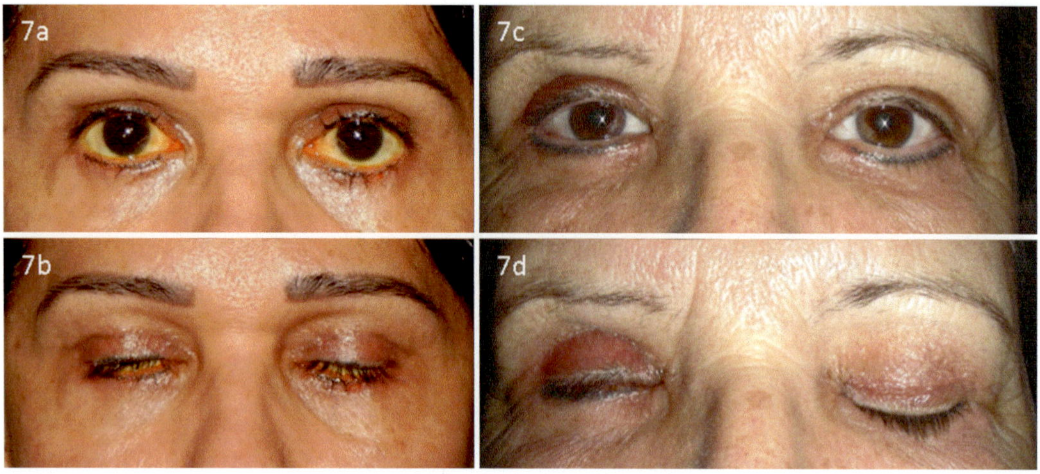

Fig. 12.7 Post-blepharoplasty lagophthalmos due to excessive skin resection (a) patient with eyes open and (b) attempted eyelid closure with sclera still exposed; post-blepharoptosis right lagophthalmos due to septal incarceration. (c) Different patient (than in a and b) with eyes open and (d) attempted eye closure with sclera still exposed

can cause orbital compartment syndrome. Symptoms are usually severe and include pain, nausea, vomiting, and decreased vision. Findings include tense, firm eyelids and/or proptosis. Restricted or frozen extraocular motility, elevated intraocular pressure, loss of vision, and an afferent pupillary defect are other features. This should be treated immediately to prevent permanent damage to the optic nerve, other cranial nerves and the retina. Surgical wounds should be opened and a lateral canthotomy and cantholysis should be performed. Blood should be evacuated and any actively bleeding vessels should be stopped (i.e., with cautery, ligation, or hemostasis aids such as methylcellulose sponges). If these measures are inadequate, orbital bone decompression is a therapeutic option. Intraocular pressure lowering eye drops or systemic medicines (e.g., IV mannitol) have a limited or no role and should not be used in lieu of the prior steps (Fig. 12.10).

Diplopia. Injury of the superior oblique muscle or trochlea during upper blepharoplasty or inferior oblique muscle in lower blepharoplasty may cause a small percentage of cases of symptomatic diplopia. Edema is another potential cause of diplopia. Most cases of diplopia after blepharoplasty are self-limited and resolve with time. A very small percentage of patients may need strabismus evaluation and management that may include prism spectacles or strabismus surgery.

Infection. Owing to the excellent blood supply to the eyelids, infection is rare with sterile technique. Topical or systemic antibiotics may be indicated. In rare instances of abscess formation, drainage and debridement may be necessary.

Chemosis. Conjunctival edema affects a small percentage of blepharoplasty patients. Risk factors are conjunctivochalasis, excessive surgical manipulation or direct compromise to lymphatic drainage. It may resolve spontaneously in weeks or months. The use of lubricants and topical corticosteroids may hasten recovery. A moisture chamber (an adherent film dressing such as Tegaderm™ or Glad Press N Seal™ work well). In rare instances, a suture tarsorrhaphy may be indicated.

Epicanthal folds. This is due to excessive skin resection in the medial part to the upper lacrimal punctum, usually in severe dermatochalasis. It is prevented by ensuring the blepharoplasty incision does not extend onto the medial canthus. For its correction, classical techniques such as Y-V or apposing z-plasties may be indicated.

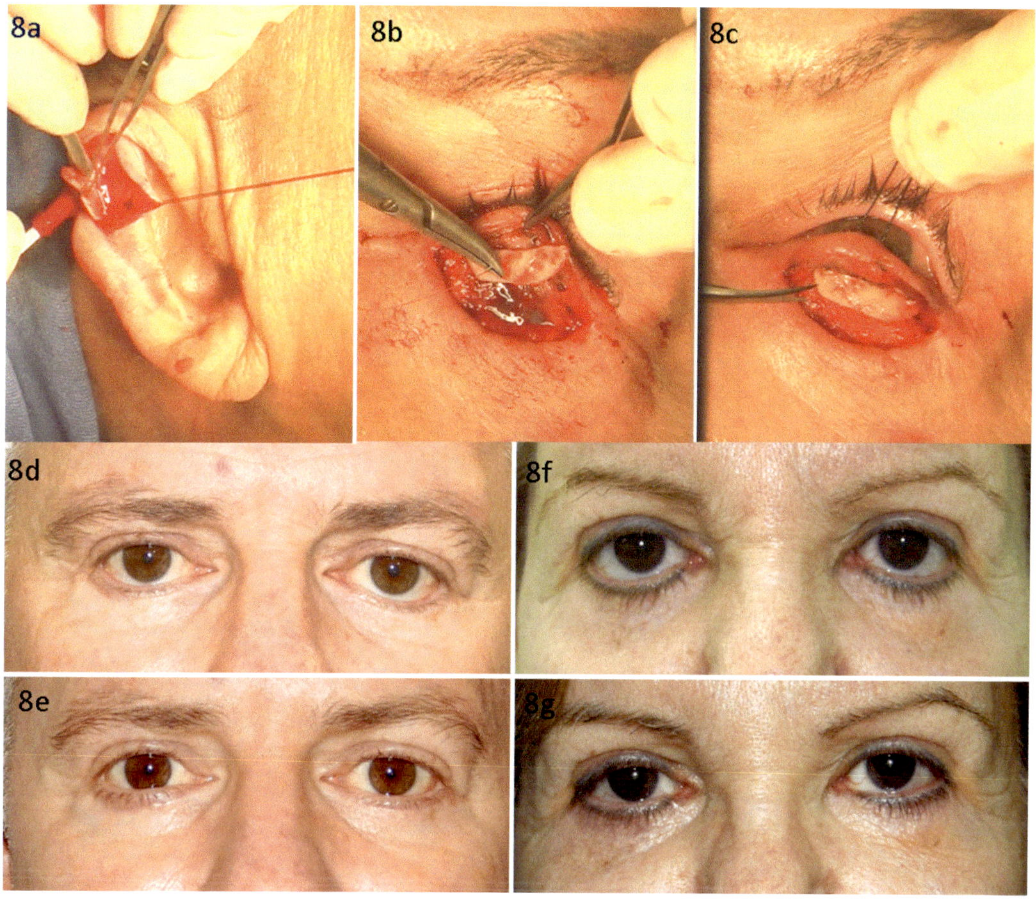

Fig. 12.8 (a) Removal of cartilage from the scapha in the proportion of 2 mm cartilage for each 1 mm of desired lower eyelid elevation, recession of the retractors and (b & c) suturing the cartilage to the posterior lamella. (d) A patient before; and (e) after retraction repair with a posterior lamella cartilage graft; (f) a patient before; and (g) after retraction repair with a posterior lamella cartilage graft

Residual skin or excess fat. Under correction is possible and revision surgery may be necessary. Resection of excess skin and/or fat can be performed again and it is useful to remind patients that under correction is preferable to overcorrection, since the latter is more difficult to treat and can cause serious injury.

Hypertrophic scar. Owing to the eyelid skin being the thinnest of the body, scarring is rare. Importantly, one should not conflate the proliferative phase of healing in the early weeks and months after surgery with permanent features. Patients should be reassured. Topical silicone gel or corticosteroid ointment can be prescribed. Corticosteroid or 5 fluorouracil injections may hasten scar softening as well.

Conclusion

Blepharoplasty remains one of the most common oculofacial surgeries. The benefits include improved facial appearance and improved field vision. Concomitant blepharoptosis, brow ptosis, or eyelid malposition or laxity should be addressed. Attention to these factors and good technique offer safe and effective results, although it is important to recognize and manage complications that occur in a minority of cases.

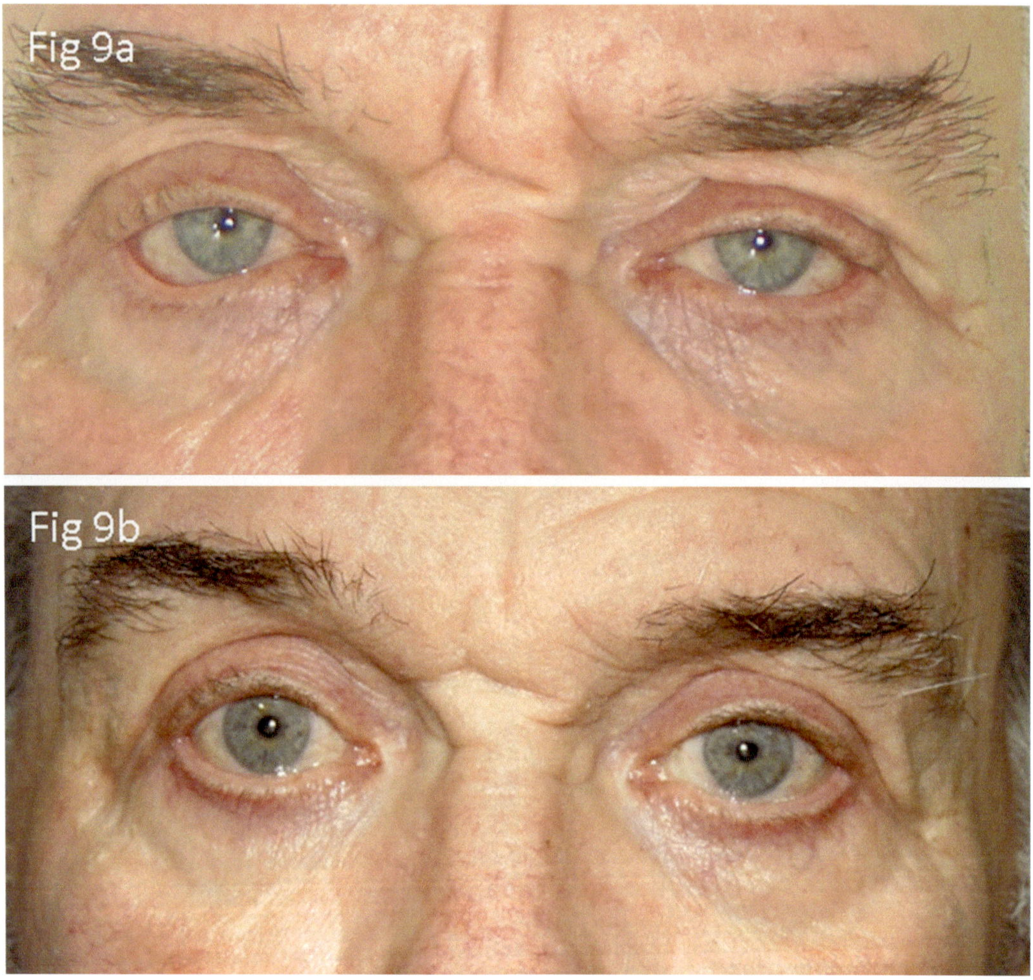

Fig. 12.9 (a) Pre and; (b) postoperative photos of a patient treated with lateral tarsal strip for iatrogenic ectropion after blepharoplasty (patient had concomitant upper blepharoplasty with bilateral posterior ptosis repair)

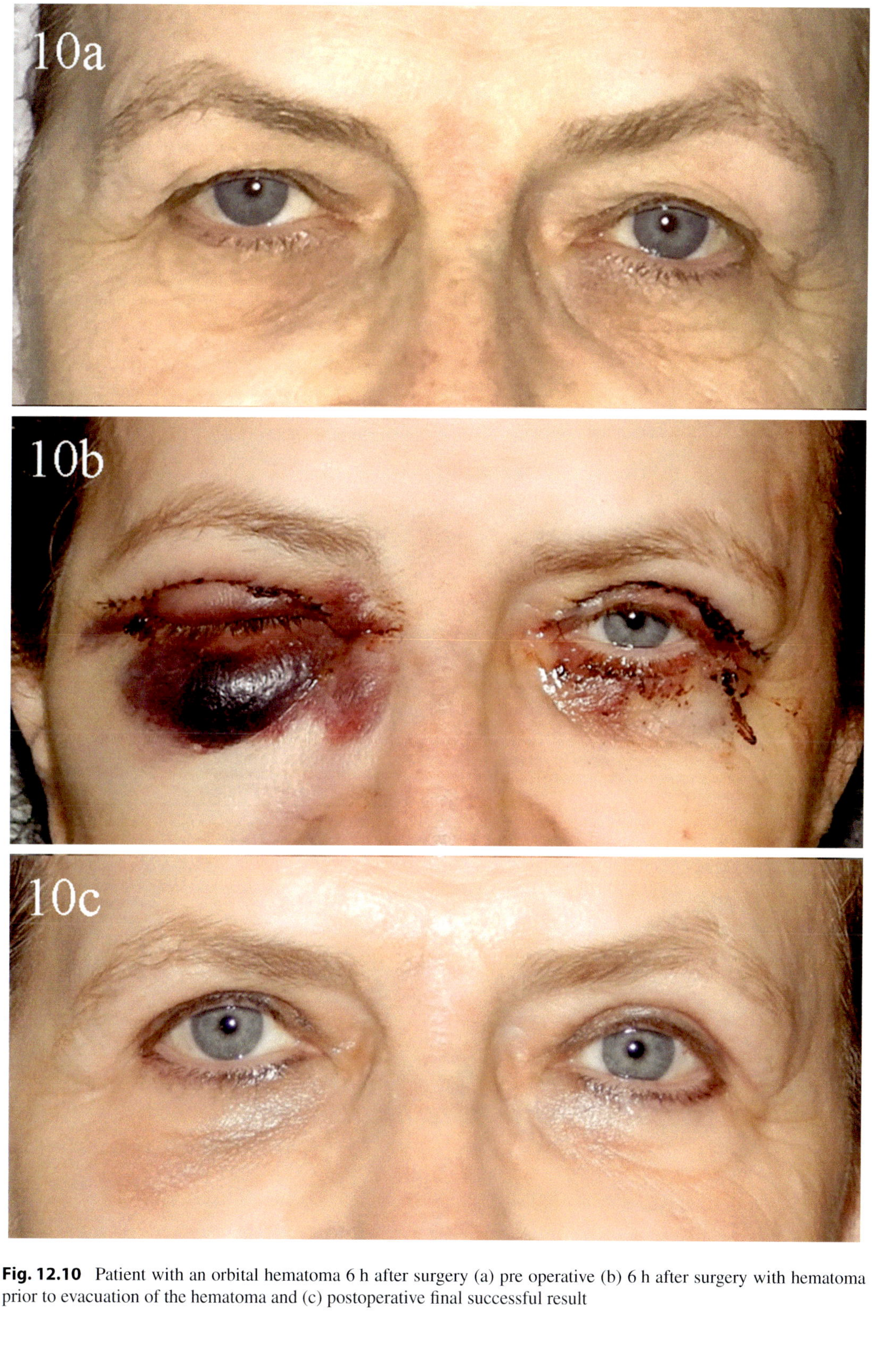

Fig. 12.10 Patient with an orbital hematoma 6 h after surgery (a) pre operative (b) 6 h after surgery with hematoma prior to evacuation of the hematoma and (c) postoperative final successful result

References

1. Nguyen HT, Isaacowitz DM, Rubin PA. Age- and fatigue-related markers of human faces: an eye-tracking study. Ophthalmology. 2009;116(2):355–60.
2. Jindal K, Sarcia M, Codner MA. Functional considerations in aesthetic eyelid surgery. Plast Reconstr Surg. 2014;134(6):1154–70.
3. Smith BC, Della Rocca RC, Nesi FA, Lisman RD. Blepharoplastic. Ophthalmic plastic and reconstructive surgery. vol. 1. The C. V. Mosby Company; 1987. p. 703–43 [chapter 34].
4. Lew H, Goldberg RA. Maximizing symmetry in upper blepharoplasty: the role of microptosis surgery. Plast Reconstr Surg. 2016;137(2):296e–304e.
5. Brown MS, Putterman AM. The effect of upper blepharoplasty on eyelid position when performed concomitantly with Müller muscle-conjunctival resection. Ophthalmic Plast Reconstr Surg. 2000;16(2):94–100.
6. Golbert M, Pereira FJ, Garcia DM, Cruz AAV. Contour symmetry of the upper eyelid following bilateral conjunctival-Müller's muscle resection. Aesthet Surg J. 2017;37(3):269–75.
7. Putterman AM, Urist MJ. Müller's muscle-conjunctival resection ptosis procedure. Ophthalmic Surg. 1978;9(3):27–32.
8. Zoumalan IC, Roostaeian J. Simplifying blepharoplasty. Plast Reconstr Surg. 2016;137(1):196e–213e.
9. Morax S, Touitou V. Complications of blepharoplasty. Orbit. 2006;25(4):303–18.
10. Hartstein ME, Kikkawa D. How to avoid blepharoplasty complications. Oral Maxillofac Surg Clin North Am. 2009;21(1):31–41.
11. Floegel I, Horwath-Winter J, Muellner K, Haller-Schober EM. A conservative blepharoplasty may be a means of alleviating dry eye symptoms. Acta Ophthalmol Scand. 2003;81(3):230–2.
12. Lima CG, Siqueira GB, Cardoso IH, Sant'Anna AE, Osaki MH. Evaluation of dry eye in the preoperative and postoperative period of blepharoplasty. Arq Bras Oftalmol. 2006;69(3):377–82.

Upper Blepharoplasty in East Asian Patients

13

Susan Ruyu Qi and Patrick T. Yang

Abstract

Upper blepharoplasty in Asian patients is unique, owing to differences in anatomy and goals. A desired surgical outcome may be a higher crease or "double eyelid" but this should not be confounded with a Western or Caucasian eyelid. Special care must be taken for surgical planning that is individualized to each patient's eyelid anatomy and objectives. This chapter describes Asian eyelid anatomy, surgical techniques, and the pearls for a successful Asian blepharoplasty.

Keywords

Asian blepharoplasty · East Asians · Asian lids · Double eyelid surgery · Epicanthoplasty

Introduction

The goals of Asian blepharoplasty may be functional (i.e., to improve upper field vision) or aesthetic. Importantly, most patients desire a natural appearance. Compared to blepharoplasty in other races or ethnicities, Asian blepharoplasty may be more prone to dissatisfaction with a resultant high crease. Upper blepharoplasty in the Asian patient, therefore, requires careful preoperative discussion, specific surgical planning, and appropriate surgical techniques with an understanding of the anatomic differences in the Asian eyelid.

Anatomy

In the Caucasian eyelid, the orbital septum fuses with the levator aponeurosis 5–10 mm above the superior tarsal border to form the eyelid crease [1]. The Asian eyelid, on the other hand, has a lower fusion point where the orbital septum fuses with the levator aponeurosis a few millimeters below the superior tarsal border [1]. This lower fusion point results in an inferior descent of the preaponeurotic fat pad and about 50% of Asians do not have an upper eyelid crease with the other 50% having at least some form of crease [2]. This is a significant anatomic difference to the non-Asian eyelid that has a defined crease, often in a semi-lunar configuration and typically located higher than in the Asian eyelid.

Supplementary Information The online version contains supplementary material available at https://doi.org/10.1007/978-3-031-63178-8_13.

S. R. Qi · P. T. Yang (✉)
University of British Columbia, Vancouver, Canada
e-mail: Patrick.Yang@islandhealth.ca

J. Tao (ed.), *Efficient Oculofacial Surgery*, https://doi.org/10.1007/978-3-031-63178-8_13

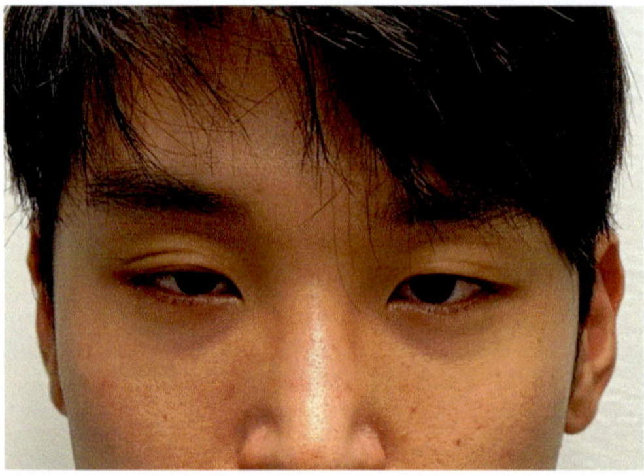

Fig. 13.1 Patient with complaints of crease asymmetry

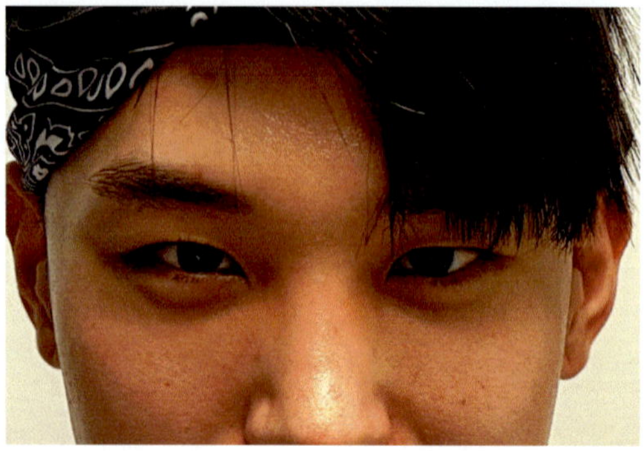

Fig. 13.2 Patient in Fig. 13.1 one week after posterior blepharoptosis repair to the right side only and with excellent correction of eyelid crease asymmetry. Photo credit: Jeremiah Tao

Assessment

For many younger East Asian patients, blepharoplasty is their first cosmetic operation. Careful preoperative discussion is crucial. Patients often desire a well-defined symmetric upper eyelid crease, also known as a "double eyelid". It is believed that the upper eyelid crease gives the impression of a larger eye-opening, even when the palpebral fissure is the same. A false impression is that most Asian eyelids are absent of a crease. In fact, about half of those of Asian descent will have a natural upper eyelid crease, albeit usually lower than compared to the typical non-Asian eyelid [2]. The goal of the surgery is to create a natural, usually low, Asian upper eyelid crease rather than trying to emulate eyelids of other races or ethnicities. Moreover, patients should be assessed for blepharoptosis when assessing the eyelid crease. In many instances slight levator dehiscence causes crease elevation and eyelid asymmetry can be addressed with blepharoptosis repair and direct crease surgery (Figs. 13.1 and 13.2).

Surgical Techniques

Suture Ligation Method

The tarsal plate height is measured and noted first by eyelid eversion pre-operatively. 3 mm linear marks (nasal, central, and lateral) are made at the desired eyelid crease height (Fig. 13.3), usually corresponding to the measured height of the tarsal plate. Small doses of local anesthetic using Lidocaine 1–2% with epinephrine are injected to the previous markings. A number 15 Bard-Parker blade is used to fashion 3 mm stab incisions at the prior crease markings. A 7-0 polyglactin suture is passed into the incision and through the eyelid full thickness and retrieved from the conjunctival side of the eyelid. The suture is placed back through the palpebral conjunctiva, exiting through the previous skin incision. This suture is then tied with the knot buried to invert the wound. The skin can be closed with an interrupted 6-0 nylon suture. Identical sutures are placed at the remaining two stab incision sites to complete a total of three buried sutures. Skin sutures are not always necessary to close the stab incisions; if used, they are removed in one week.

External Incision Method (Video 13-1)

The authors favor an incision method with supratarsal fixation, for a more durable result than with crease formation using the previously described suture ligation method.

Scanning electron microscopy studies have shown that the palpebral crease in the double eyelid is formed by a fibrous link between levator aponeurosis and the upper eyelid skin [3]. As such, double-eyelid procedures should aim to establish a stable attachment between levator aponeurosis and the eyelid skin.

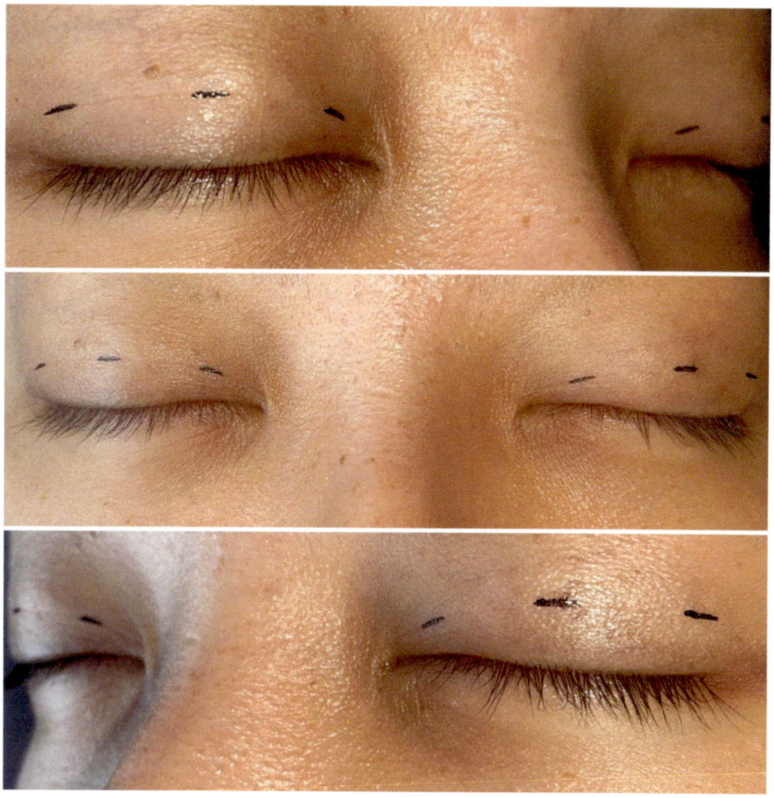

Fig. 13.3 Surgical "stab incision" markings of suture ligation method

The location of the upper eyelid crease must be planned carefully. In the Caucasian eyelid, the crease is often located at a height of 8–10 mm from the lash margin, however this would be abnormally high for most Asian eyelids. Furthermore, in Asians, the upper tarsus is often shorter in height, and the distance between the eyebrow and the upper eyelid margin is proportionately less in comparison to the Caucasian eyelid [4]. In addition, the design and curvature of the upper eyelid crease in an Asian patient should follow these three principles for natural results: (1) the nasal aspect tapers into the epicanthal fold or remain parallel to the eyelid margin; (2) the lateral aspect of the eyelid crease remains parallel to the eyelid margin or flares slightly superiorly, and (3) the crease between the nasal and lateral ends must be parallel with the eyelid margin and not overly-arched (Fig 13.6).

Especially in older patients, it is appropriate to perform a pinch test to assess for redundant skin amount that is marked for resection (Figs. 13.4, 13.5 and 13.6). Once symmetrical eyelid creases are marked, local anesthetic is infiltrated to the markings. Care is taken to avoid an excessive volume of anesthetic. Next, a number 15 Bard-Parker blade is used to incise exactly along the markings. Westcott scissors are used to remove skin and to dissect through the subcutaneous layer down to the level of the tarsal plate. A small, 1–2 mm thick strip of pretarsal orbicularis oculi muscle is resected to further encourage crease formation. Sometimes, medial or central orbital fat is removed for eyelids if it is herniated. However, this step must be taken carefully, as excessive pretarsal dissection and fat debulking can lead to multiple or abnormal crease formation. Hemostasis is achieved with electrocautery. Next, skin closure with or without crease formation sutures are placed. The skin incision edge can be secured deeply to the tarsal plate or the levator aponeurosis. The

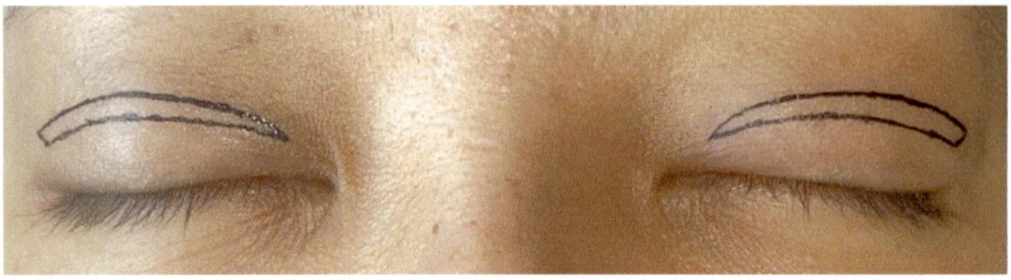

Fig. 13.4 External incision technique markings

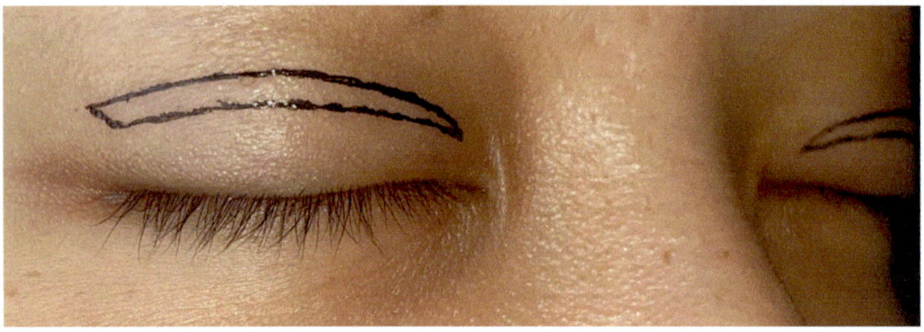

Fig. 13.5 External incision technique markings (three-quarter angle view, marking tapered nasally with a parallel tail)

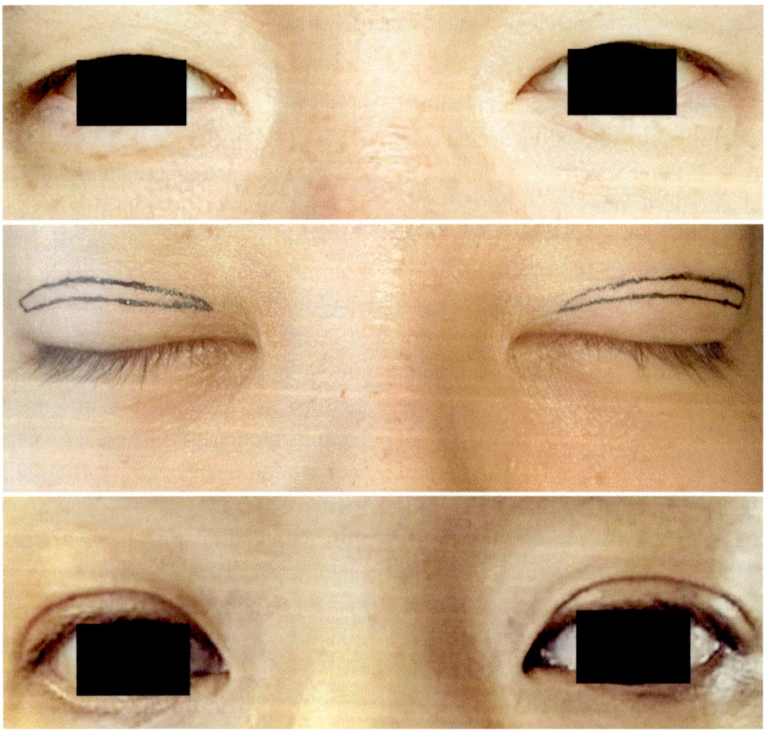

Fig. 13.6 Upper blepharoplasty by external incisional technique in an East Asian patient

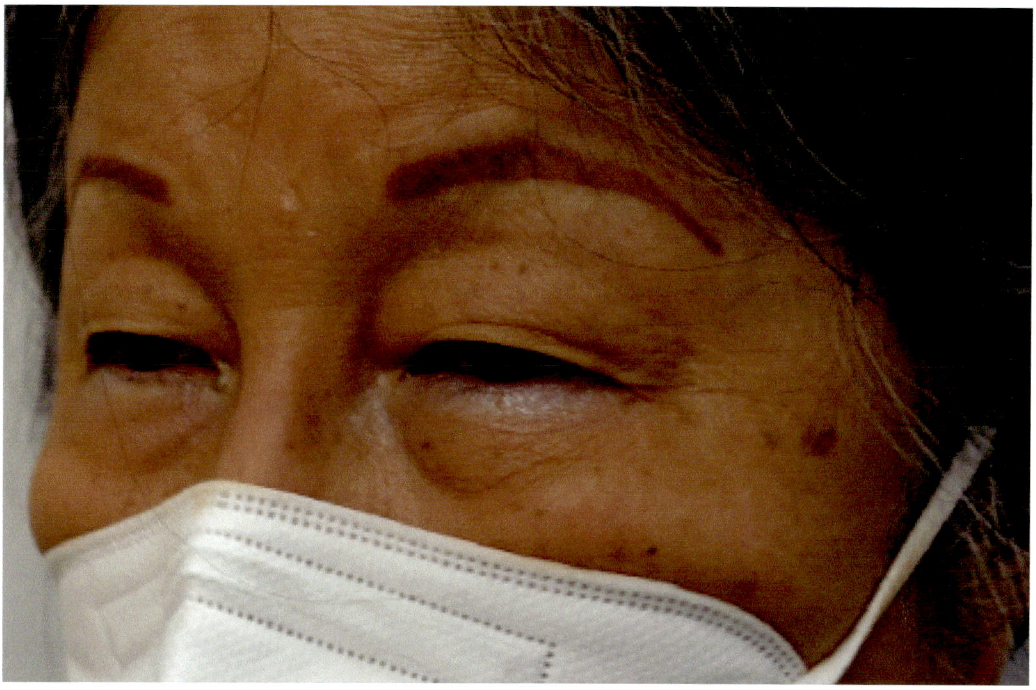

Fig. 13.7 Dermatochalasis and skin hooding in an Asian patient

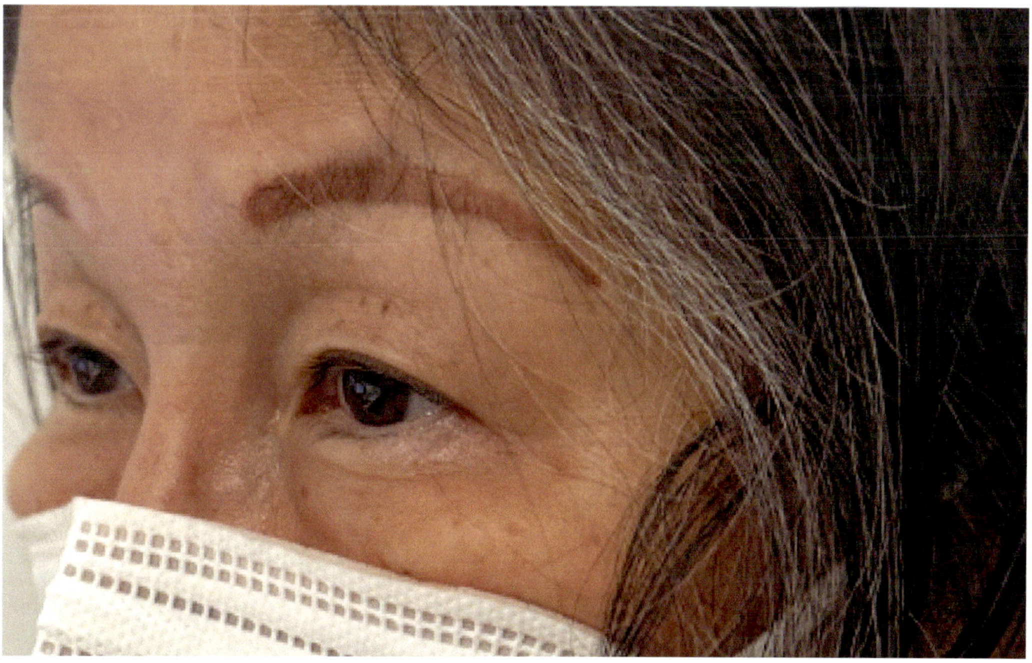

Fig. 13.8 Patient Fig. 13.7 after blepharoplasty with a desirable, low crease. Photo credit: Jeremiah Tao

authors prefer to form the crease using multiple interrupted 6-0 prolene sutures with inverting needle passes through the skin edges and central deep passes. The deep fixation is to the levator aponeurosis just superficial to the tarsal plate. These sutures are repeated both medially and laterally along the skin incision to form the crease. Finally, the skin incision is closed with a running 6-0 prolene or silk suture. Skin sutures are removed between 5–8 days postoperatively.

Epicanthoplasty (Video 13-2)

In some Asian patients, dermatochalasis may be associated with a prominent epicanthal fold. This fold obscures the caruncle and medial bulbar surface. There exist a variety of tissue rearrangement techniques to treat the epicanthal fold. Many Z plasty techniques are associated with visible scars.

For moderate severity epicanthal folds, the authors recommend a Z-epicanthoplasty as described by Park et al. [5]. This technique is usually concomitant to blepharoplasty (Fig. 13.9). The technique involves a triangle-shaped pretarsal skin resection medially with transposition of the epicanthal fold into this defect in a Z-plasty tissue rearrangement. This lengthens skin along the epicanthal to soften the fold. The excision and rearrangement also pull skin superiorly and medially to subtly expose the underlying canthus and caruncle.

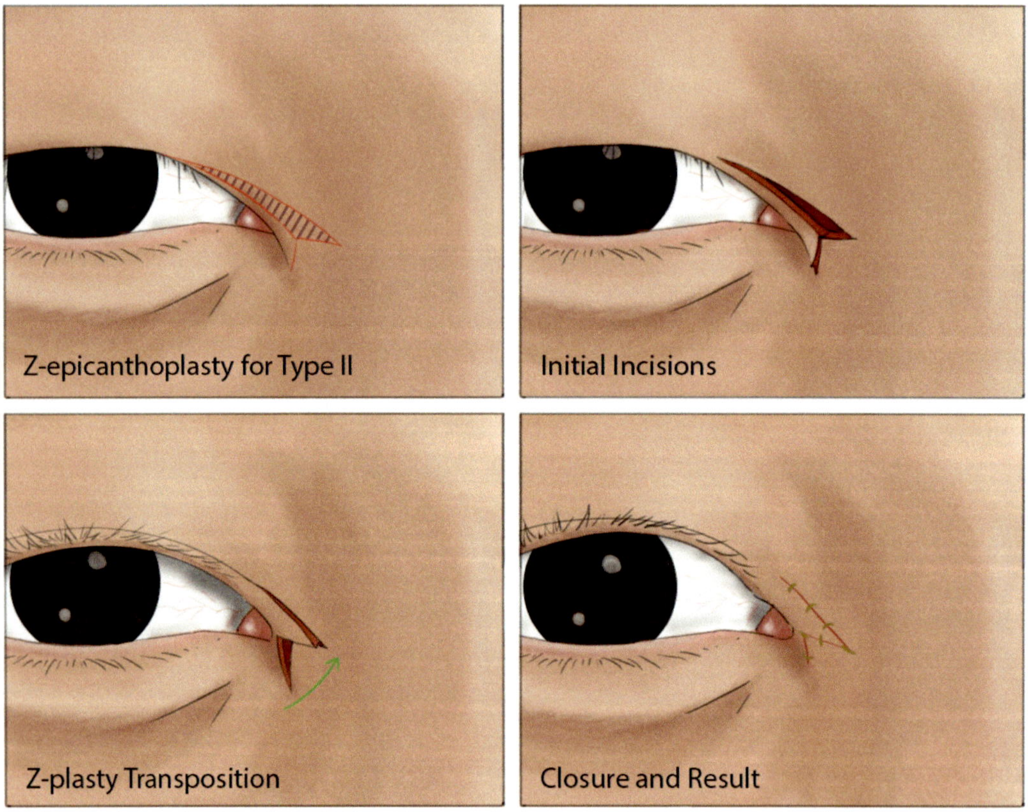

Fig. 13.9 Z-epicanthoplasty for mild-moderate epicanthal fold

Conclusion

Blepharoplasty in Asians has key differences with traditional eyelid surgery in Western eyelids. Chiefly, the design is a well-formed crease that is low, often just millimeters above the lash line (Figs. 13.7 and 13.8). Most durable techniques involve deep suture fixation of cut skin edges to the tarsus or inferior levator aponeurosis. Epicanthoplasty is sometimes a useful adjunct.

References

1. Song HM, Tran KN. Incisional blepharoplasty for the Asian eye. Facial Plast Surg Clin North Am [Internet]. 2021;29(4):511–22. Available from: https://pubmed.ncbi.nlm.nih.gov/34579834/ [cited 2022 Sep 19].
2. Saonanon P. Update on Asian eyelid anatomy and clinical relevance. Curr Opin Ophthalmol [Internet]. 2014;25(5):436–42. Available from: https://pubmed.ncbi.nlm.nih.gov/24852200/ [cited 2022 Sep 19].
3. Cheng J, Xu FZ. Anatomic microstructure of the upper eyelid in the Oriental double eyelid. Plast Reconstr Surg [Internet]. 2001;107(7):1665–8. Available from: https://pubmed.ncbi.nlm.nih.gov/11391182/ [cited 2022 Sep 19].
4. Chen WP-D, Preceded by: Chen WP-D. Asian blepharoplasty and the eyelid crease.
5. Park JI, Park MS. Park Z-Epicanthoplasty. Facial Plast Surg Facial N Am. 2007;15:343–52.

Browpexy

14

Roberto Murillo Limongi
and Marisa Novaes de Figueiredo Rassi

Abstract

Brow position and brow fullness are important considerations in oculofacial surgery. Brow ptosis can aggravate upper eyelid dermatochalasis. Additionally, fullness at the brow-eyelid junction may be a desirable aesthetic result. While some patients require brow lifting (e.g. direct or post trichial incisions), others may benefit from the less invasive approach of an internal browpexy during upper blepharoplasty. In this chapter, the authors describe a browpexy procedure to stabilize the brow and add fullness to the lateral brow-eyelid region.

Keywords

Browpexy · Brow lift · Brow contour · Blepharoplasty

Supplementary Information The online version contains supplementary material available at https://doi.org/10.1007/978-3-031-63178-8_14.

R. M. Limongi (✉) · M. N. de Figueiredo Rassi
Division of Oculoplastic Surgery,
Department of Ophthalmology,
Federal University of Goiás, Goiás, Brazil
e-mail: rmurillousp@hotmail.com

Introduction

Loss of the three-dimensional contour due to tissue laxity and fat atrophy is important in facial aging and should be considered during upper blepharoplasty planning. There are numerous techniques for correction of the eyebrow ptosis, but for minimal brow droop, eyelid surgery alone will not help and potentially worsen brow ptosis. In addition to mechanical vectors pulling the brow down due to skin resection of blepharoplasty, some patients lose frontalis recruitment after eyelid lifting.

Zarem described a variant of eyebrow pexy in which the lateral orbicularis muscle was suspended to the upper arcus marginalis as an adjunct technique for blepharoplasty. Goldberg and collaborators modified the technique and described these procedures in terms of brassiere sutures that secure the orbicularis muscle adjacent to the superior blepharoplasty wound edge to the periosteum of the superolateral orbit rim. These sutures suspend the retro orbicularis oculi fat (ROOF) that not only stabilizes the brow but may promote improved contour and projection of the lateral eyebrow. Importantly, these do not increase the height of the eyebrow but rather avert inferior descent. These procedures may add volume that contribute to a more youthful appearance.

Upper eyelid blepharoplasty remains one of the most common facial plastic surgeries

J. Tao (ed.), *Efficient Oculofacial Surgery*, https://doi.org/10.1007/978-3-031-63178-8_14

performed in the world. In the past, the upper blepharoplasty procedure was largely subtractive and focused on the removal of excess skin, muscle, and fat. Current paradigms suggest that a more youthful and rejuvenated appearance is achieved with tissue preservation or even augmentation of certain areas. The lateral upper eyelid and brow is one anatomical zone where this is relevant (Fig. 14.1).

Surgical Technique (Video 14-1)

The planned upper skin resection outline should use a marking pen in a standard skin pinch technique for upper blepharoplasty. Next each eyelid is infiltrated with 3–4 cc of local anesthesia. The skin incision is fashioned with a number 15 scalpel blade. Next, a 3–4 mm width strip of orbicularis oculi muscle is removed using scissors or an electrosurgical unit. Hemostasis is achieved with electrocautery. At the superior wound edge laterally, a 6-0 polyglactin suture is passed through the orbicularis oculi muscle deep to skin to the periosteum at the superolateral rim. Additional identical sutures may be placed medial or lateral to the first suture depending on the desired breadth of brow fixation. The blepharoplasty incision is closed with 6-0 polypropylene or nylon sutures to the skin. The deep browpexy sutures may induce slight upper eyelid ectropion or lagophthalmos that resolve within days to weeks. The patient should be instructed to aggressively lubricate the eyes in the early postoperative period (Figs. 14.2, 14.3, 14.4 and 14.5).

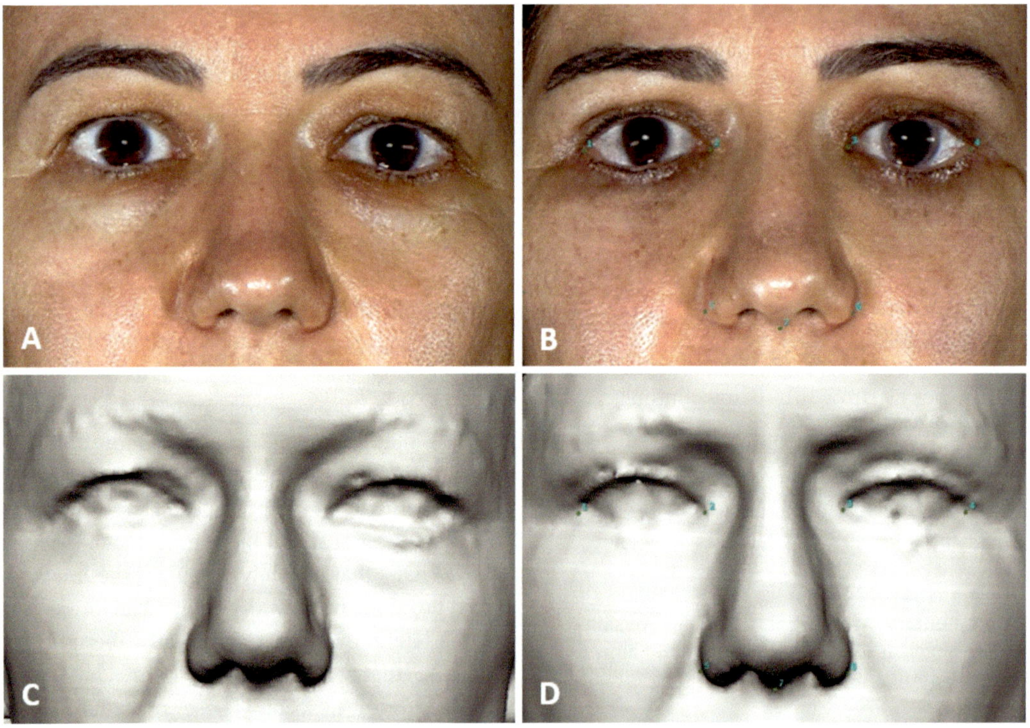

Fig. 14.1 (**A**) Preoperative 3D image of a 47-year-old patient who underwent browpexy intervention; (**B**) postoperative 3D image at 14 months; (**C**) corresponding preoperative untextured image; (**D**) corresponding postoperative untextured image

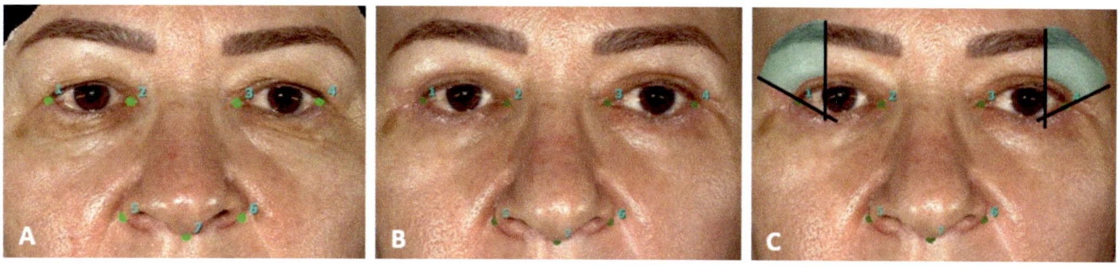

Fig. 14.2 (**A**) Preoperative; (**B**) postoperative 3D image of a patient who underwent browpexy intervention; (**C**) lateral brow-eyelid complex shaded in green

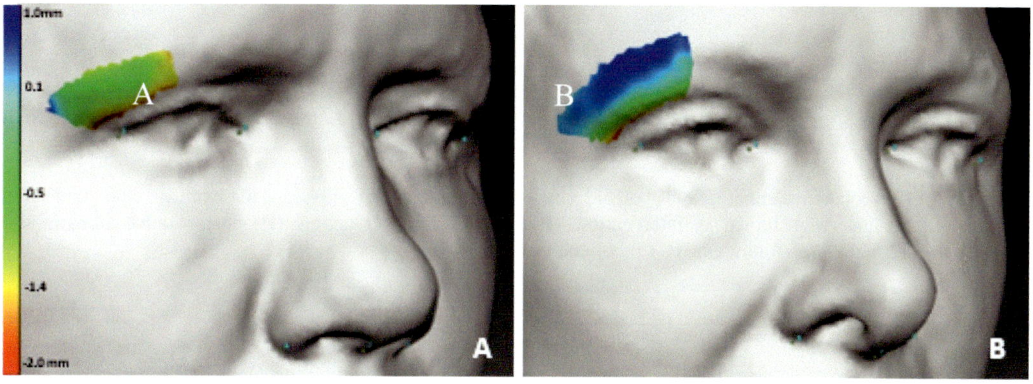

Fig. 14.3 (**A**) 3D colorimetric analysis of a patient who underwent traditional blepharoplasty; (**B**) patient who underwent browpexy showing areas of volume (blue) at 18-month of follow-up. Blue represents increased volume green denotes no change, and red denotes loss of volume

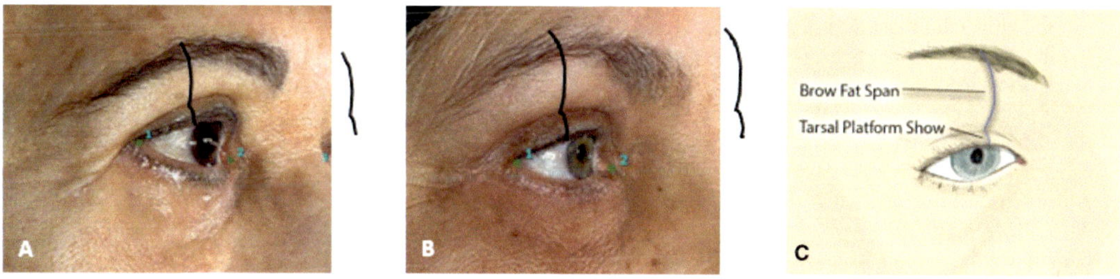

Fig. 14.4 (**A**) Traditional blepharoplasty flatter convexity; (**B**) showing double convexity, higher inferior convexity and increase in tarsal platform show. The black line emphasizing the postoperative contour change; (**C**) drawing representing the lateral brow-eyelid contour

Conclusion

Adjunctive browpexy sutures during blepharoplasty can stabilize the brow and increase the volume of the upper and lateral brow and create a double-convexity contour of the lateral brow-eyelid complex. These findings, while subtle, are efficient and easy to add as adjuncts to upper blepharoplasty to achieve volume and contour enhancements at the upper eyelid and lateral brow complex.

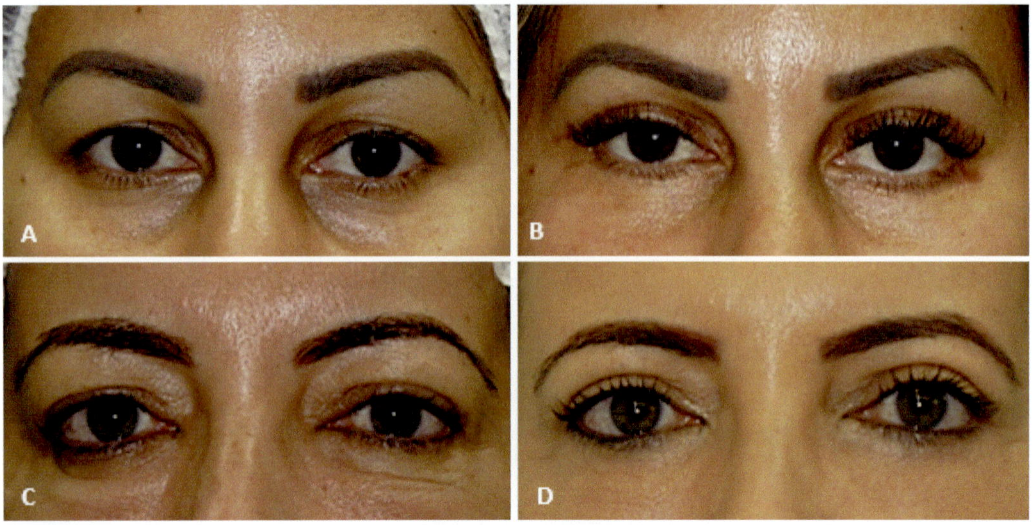

Fig. 14.5 (**A**) Preoperative photographs of 42-year-old woman who underwent browpexy intervention; (**B**) postoperative 12 months of follow-up; (**C**) preoperative photographs of 43-year-old woman who underwent browpexy intervention; (**D**) postoperative 14 months of follow-up

References

1. Knoll BI, Attkiss KJ, Persing JA. The influence of forehead, brow, and periorbital aesthetics on perceived expression in the youthful face. Plast Reconstr Surg. 2008;121(5):1793–802.
2. Fitzgerald R. Contemporary concepts in brow and eyelid aging. Clin Plast Surg. 2013;40(1):21–42.
3. Lambros V. Observations on periorbital and midface aging. Plast Reconstr Surg. 2007;120:1367–76.
4. Price KM, Gupta PK, Woodward JA, Stinnett SS, Murchison AP. Eyebrow and eyelid dimensions: an anthropometric analysis of African Americans and Caucasians. Plast Reconstr Surg. 2009;124(2):615–23.
5. Packiriswamy V, Kumar P, Bashour M. Photogrammetric analysis of eyebrow and upper eyelid dimensions in South Indians and Malaysian South Indians. Aesthet Surg J. 2013;33(8):1215.
6. Faigen S. Eyebrow analysis after blepharoplasty in patients with brow ptosis. Ophthal Plast Reconstr Surg. 1992;8(3):210–4.
7. Fagien S. Advanced rejuvenative upper blepharoplasty: enhancing aesthetics of the upper periorbita. Plast Reconstr Surg. 2002;110(1):278–91 [discussion 292].
8. Briceno CA, Zhang-Nunes SX, Massry GG. Minimally invasive surgical adjuncts to upper blepharoplasty. Facial Plast Surg Clin N Am. 2015;23:137–51.
9. Baker MS, Shams PN, Allen RC. The quantitated internal suture browpexy: comparison of two brow-lifting techniques in patients undergoing upper blepharoplasty. Ophthal Plast Reconstr Surg. 2016;32:204–6.
10. Zarem HA, Resnick JI, Carr RM, Wootton DG. Browpexy: lateral orbicularis muscle fixation as an adjunct to upper blepharoplasty. Plast Reconstr Surg. 1997;100(5):1258–61.
11. Zarem HA. Browpexy. Aesthet Surg J. 2004;24:368–72.
12. Eftekhari K, Peng GL, Landsberger H, Douglas R, Massry GG. The brow fat pad suspension suture: safety profile and clinical observations. Ophthalmic Plast Reconstr Surg. 2018;34(1):7–12.
13. Goldberg RA. Using a brassiere suture technique to define lateral tarsal platform and eyebrow fat contours. Paper presentation at: ASOPRS 2012 Fall Symposium.
14. Figueiredo MN, Tao J, Akaishi P, Limongi RM. Tarsal platform show after upper eyelid blepharoplasty with or without brassiere sutures. Arq Bras Oftalmol. 2017;80:6.
15. Stanek JJ, Fuller JC, Hilger PA. Brassiere suture technique in upper eyelid blepharoplasty. JAMA Facial Plast Surg. 2019;21(5):458–9.
16. Lambros V, Amos G. Three-dimensional facial averaging. Plast Reconstr Surg. 2016;138:980e–2e.
17. Lambros V. Facial aging: a 54-year, three-dimensional population study. Plast Reconstr Surg. 2020;145:921–8.
18. Camp MC, Wong WW, Filip Z, Carter CS, Gupta SC. A quantitative analysis of periorbital aging with three-dimensional surface imaging. J Plast Reconstr Aesthet Surg. 2011;64(2):148–54.

15 Upper Eyelid Ptosis Repair—Anterior Levator Approach

Sayyada Hyder, Victoria S. North, and Gary J. Lelli

Abstract

Blepharoptosis repair via an anterior approach is commonly preferred for the ability to treat more profound blepharoptosis and because skin and fat excess can be treated concomitantly. From an anterior surgical approach, the levator aponeurosis can be advanced or resected to elevate the eyelid. Muscle disinsertion causes aponeurotic ptosis. External levator advancement is primarily reserved for aponeurotic ptosis, in the setting of normal levator function and includes re-approximation of the dehisced levator muscle to the tarsus. In levator resection, the muscle is reinserted followed by removal of the excess levator tissue. In this chapter, the authors detail principles and techniques of anterior approach to blepharoptosis.

Supplementary Information The online version contains supplementary material available at https://doi.org/10.1007/978-3-031-63178-8_15.

S. Hyder · G. J. Lelli (✉)
Department of Ophthalmology, Weill Cornell Medicine, New York Presbyterian Hospital, New York, NY, USA
e-mail: gary.lelli@gmail.com

V. S. North
Department of Ophthalmology, Tufts Medical Center, Boston, MA, USA

Keywords

Blepharoptosis · External levator advancement · Levator resection · Anterior ptosis surgery · Aponeurotic ptosis · Congenital ptosis

Introduction

Blepharoptosis repair may be indicated for functional or cosmetic indications. External levator advancement or resection are classic surgical approaches. Levator tuck, as first described by Everbush in 1883, is the tightening of the levator palpebrae muscle via sutures, bringing the dehiscence or disinserted part of the levator back to its natural insertion on the tarsus [1]. Levator resection as described by Blaskovics in 1923 has been a long-standing approach to correct blepharoptosis with moderate levator function. This procedure has seen several modifications [2]. This chapter details techniques of levator resection or advancement.

Indication

The primary indication for anterior ptosis repair is visual impairment due to the ptotic eyelid, though these techniques may also be used for aesthetic correction and restoration of eyelid

J. Tao (ed.), *Efficient Oculofacial Surgery*, https://doi.org/10.1007/978-3-031-63178-8_15

symmetry. External levator advancement is primarily utilized for aponeurotic ptosis with normal, or moderately reduced, levator function.

Though the choice of whether to repair ptosis via an anterior versus posterior approach is largely surgeon preference, the anterior approach has several advantages. It can easily be combined with an upper eyelid blepharoplasty, as aponeurotic ptosis often coexists with dermatochalasis. It avoids manipulation or disruption of the conjunctiva, important in patients with ocular surface disease or glaucoma drainage devices. Moreover, posterior approaches may be insufficient for higher degrees of blepharoptosis. Finally, the eyelid contour or crease can be directly adjusted via an external approach that is especially useful in revision surgery. Levator resection may also be considered in the setting of congenital ptosis with moderate or fair levator function. Congenital ptosis with poor or absent levator function is corrected via frontalis suspension or a frontalis flap that bypasses a dysfunctional levator entirely and are described in other chapters.

Preoperative Evaluation

History is important to rule out alternative diagnoses. Duration of symptoms, unilateral versus bilateral involvement, evolution of symptoms during the day, weakness involving other muscle groups, diplopia, difficulty swallowing, and speech changes should be investigated. Any history of trauma to the eye and prior surgical procedures should also be documented. Clinical evaluation starts with an external exam to assess for lagophthalmos, Bell phenomenon, frontalis activation, and presence of concomitant dermatochalasis or brow ptosis. Levator function, marginal reflex distance, and eyelid crease height should be measured. Berke offered a guidelines to group levator function based on upper eyelid excursion as follows: 0–5 mm (poor), 6–11 mm (fair/moderate) and 12 mm or greater (good) [3]. The upper eyelid excursion and degree of ptosis direct the amount of resection [3, 4]. Eyelid crease height varies based on ethnicity and sex of the patient; normal ranges are 8–12 mm above the eyelid margin for females, 7–9 mm for males, and 4–6 mm for patients of Asian ethnicity [5]. A thorough exam also includes assessment of pupil size and reactivity, extra ocular motility, and exophthalmometry (especially for unilateral ptosis) [6]. Patients with unilateral ptosis should be evaluated for Hering's phenomenon in the contralateral eye.

Relevant Anatomy

The levator palpebrae superioris muscle originates from the lesser wing of the sphenoid bone, coursing superior-anteriorly towards the superior aspect of the orbit. It then distally forms the tendon sheath known as the levator aponeurosis. The tendon sheath starts at the level of the Whitnall's ligament, which is a transverse suspensory ligament. Medially and laterally, the levator aponeurosis has attachment points to the medial and lateral canthal ligament respectively. Anteriorly, it attaches to the upper eyelid skin, forming the natural eyelid crease, and inferiorly to the tarsal plate (Fig. 15.1) [7]. In aponeurotic ptosis, stretching and/or disinsertion of this levator aponeurosis occurs. Comparatively, congenital ptosis arises from internal muscle dysgenesis with replacement with adipose tissue and fibrous material [8].

The upper eyelid has a dual vascular supply from the internal carotid artery by means of the ophthalmic artery (branching to supra-orbital and lacrimal artery) and the facial artery branching from the external carotid artery (angular and temporal). Together, these form two major collateral circulation systems: the marginal arcade and peripheral arcade. The marginal arcade lies 2 mm superior to the eyelid margin anterior to the tarsus. The peripheral arcade is located superior to the tarsus, between Muller's muscle and levator aponeurosis [9].

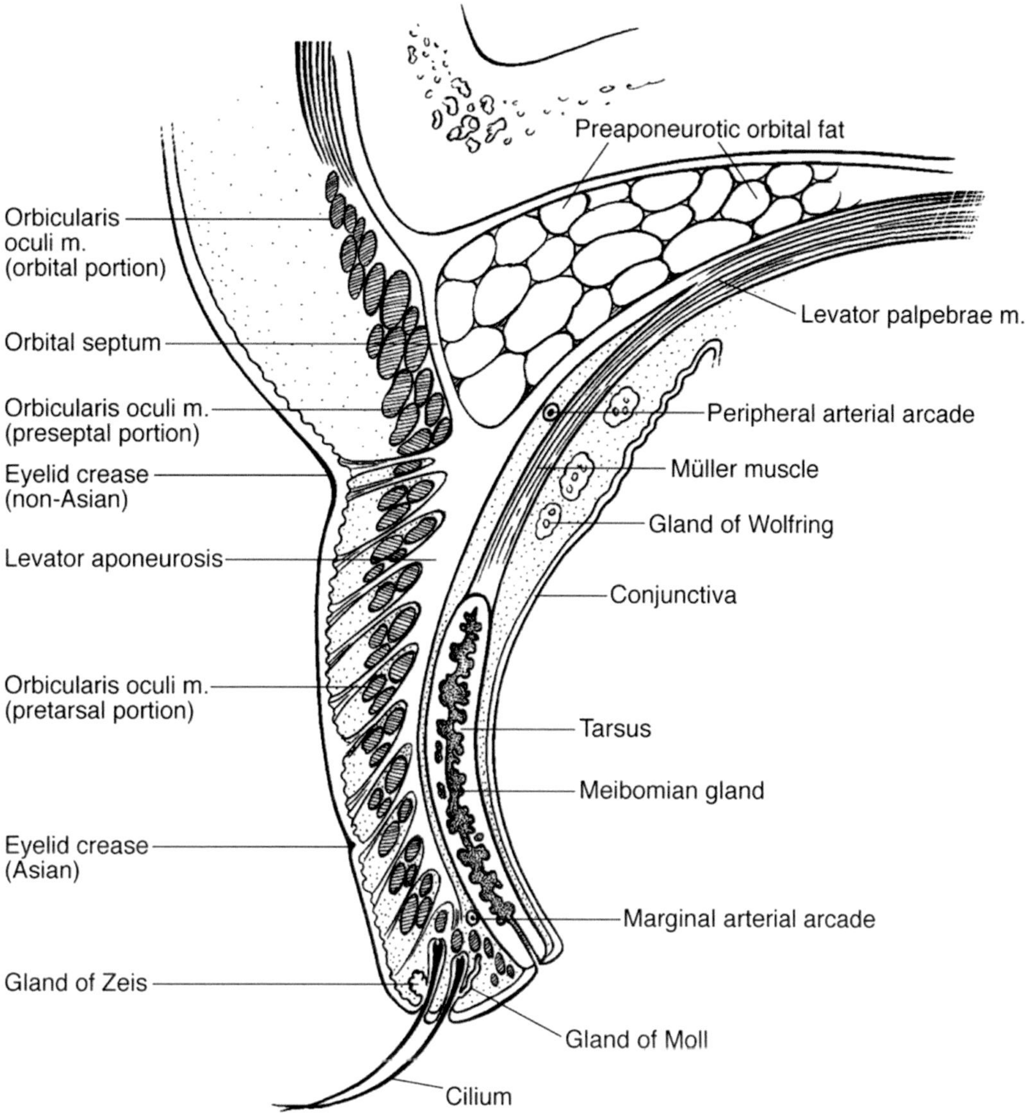

Fig. 15.1 **Transverse section of upper eyelid anatomy**. Demonstrating insertion of levator aponeurosis on the anterior surface of the tarsus (illustration by Christine Gralapp—reproduced with permission from AAO.org)

Surgical Technique—External Levator Advancement (Video 15-1)

Surgery in adults is usually performed under local anesthesia or monitored anesthesia care, which allows for intraoperative patient participation. First, an upper eyelid crease incision is marked—generally this will be at the patient's natural eyelid crease unless the crease has migrated and needs to be reset. If blepharoplasty is also performed, the desired excision should be planned at this stage. Once marked, the upper eyelid is instilled with local anesthetic. Care must be taken to inject a small amount of volume, as well as limited epinephrine to minimize eyelid position change due to infiltration or Muller's muscle stimulation [10].

The skin is incised along the pre-marked areas using a #15 blade. If a concomitant blepharoplasty is performed, the skin muscle flap is dissected off its base with scissors or cautery. Inferiorly, dissection is carried down to expose the superior aspect of tarsus. Superior dissection is performed through septum and preaponeurotic fat to expose the dehisced levator aponeurosis (Fig. 15.2A). The dehisced levator is then re-approximated to tarsus with one or more sutures passed in a horizontal mattress fashion (Fig. 15.2B). The authors use 6-0 or 7-0 silk, though polyglactin, polypropylene or nylon are also options. The first suture is passed in a partial-thickness manner through the superior edge of tarsus at a central location that gives the most natural eyelid contour. The eyelid should be everted to ensure the suture pass is not full thickness. Next the suture ends are passed through the levator aponeurosis and tied in a temporary fashion. The height can be adjusted with the patient's cooperation and with or without the patient moved to an upright seated position to account for gravitational vectors. If adrenaline in the local anesthetic admixture is thought to be inducing Mueller's muscle contraction, the eyelid margin should be set to a slightly overcorrected position. Additional sutures may be needed to achieve the desired height and contour. Once finalized, the sutures are tied in a permanent position. Finally, the skin is closed with 6-0 nylon or similar suture, and the eyelid crease can be enhanced if needed.

Surgical Technique—External Levator Resection

External levator resection begins in a similar fashion to levator advancement with a skin incision or skin resection if a concomitant blepharoplasty is performed. After the tarsus and levator aponeurosis are exposed, the levator muscle is carefully dissected free from the upper border of the tarsus and from the underlying Muller's muscle. This is accomplished with a gentle "stripping" technique using Wescott scissors with or without a prior incision through the aponeurosis with a #15 blade. It is helpful to place the eyelid on stretch with use of an assistant or traction sutures. Dissection is carried superiorly, generally to Whitnall's ligament or just beyond (Fig. 15.3). Care is taken to avoid disrupting the conjunctiva or the peripheral arcade.

Next, one or more double-armed sutures are passed in a horizontal mattress fashion from the superior aspect of the tarsus through levator according to the above technique. Typically, 6-0 or 7-0 silk is used, though some surgeons may prefer polyglactin, polypropylene or nylon. The technique differs from levator advancement in the height of the horizontal mattress—in advancement, the suture is passed through the edge of levator aponeurosis, which restores the native configuration of the muscle. In

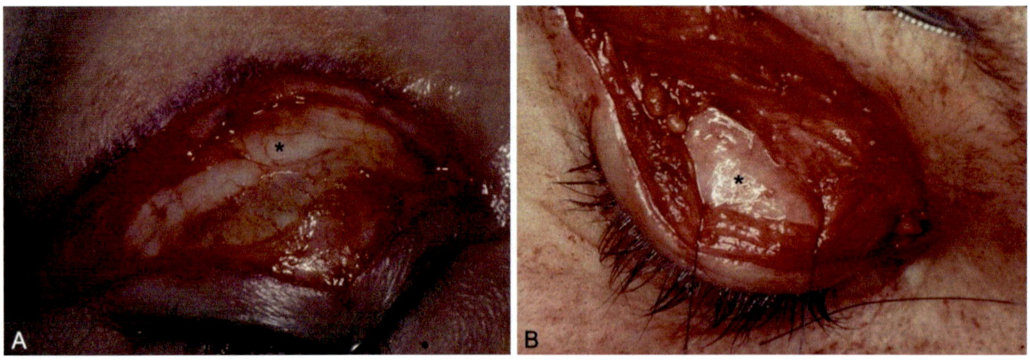

Fig. 15.2 Intraoperative view of external levator advancement. (A) Completed upper eyelid dissection showing the disinserted levator (*). (B) After levator (*) reinsertion onto tarsus using 6-0 silk sutures

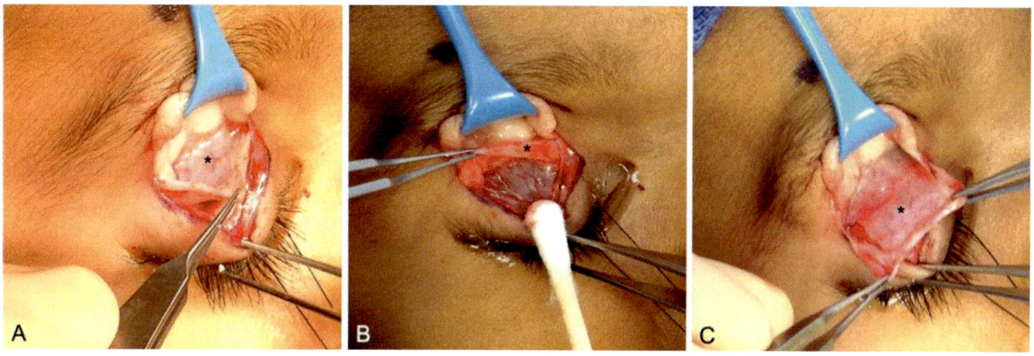

Fig. 15.3 Intraoperative view of levator resection for a case of congenital ptosis. (A) Initial upper eyelid dissection showing levator (*). (B) After the levator (*) is dissected off underlying Muller muscle and conjunctiva (beneath the cotton tip applicator). (C) Repositioning the dissected levator (*) toward tarsus in preparation to resect a portion of the muscle and re-attach the remaining portion to tarsus

levator resection, a much larger portion of levator must be incorporated with this suture. Once the desired height and contour are achieved, the sutures are tied permanently. The excess levator muscle is then resected with scissors to prevent undesirable bulk around the eyelid crease. The degree of levator resection can be estimated based on either the Beard or Berke guidelines, which consider the amount of ptosis and upper eyelid excursion. Finally, the eyelid crease is formed, if needed, with 7-0 polyglactin sutures passed from the inferior border of orbicularis to the levator aponeurosis. The skin is closed according to surgeon preference.

Complications

Under correction, over correction, and asymmetry are known complications of ptosis repair. Over correction can be especially problematic when it leads to lagophthalmos and exposure keratopathy. Post operatively, it can be managed with eyelid massage (lid pulling exercises to stretch or slightly dehisce the sutures), though surgical repair with levator tenotomy or recession may be needed. Abnormal eyelid contour may also occur—typically the contour is apparent at the time of the surgery, and care should be taken to optimize the appearance intraoperatively. Some surgeons recommend a standard approach with three sutures placed 3–4 mm apart, in the medial-mid pupillary-lateral positions, to minimize contour abnormalities [11]. However, if a suture breaks post-operatively, revision may be needed. Asymmetry can occur in unilateral or bilateral cases for several reasons and may require revision. In cases of unilateral ptosis, it is especially important to assess for Hering's law preoperatively [12]. In these cases, bilateral surgery can be considered to prevent postoperative asymmetry.

Conclusion

Levator advancement and levator resection are anterior surgical approaches to blepharoptosis repair. Surgical approach is dictated by the type of ptosis, levator function, and plan for combined blepharoplasty. Anterior ptosis repair achieves excellent, durable results when coupled with proper surgical technique and good understanding of the muscle and vascular anatomy (Fig. 15.4A and B). Overcorrection, under correction, contour abnormalities, and contralateral eyelid position changes due to Hering effects remain as complications and revision surgery is expected in a small percentage of patients.

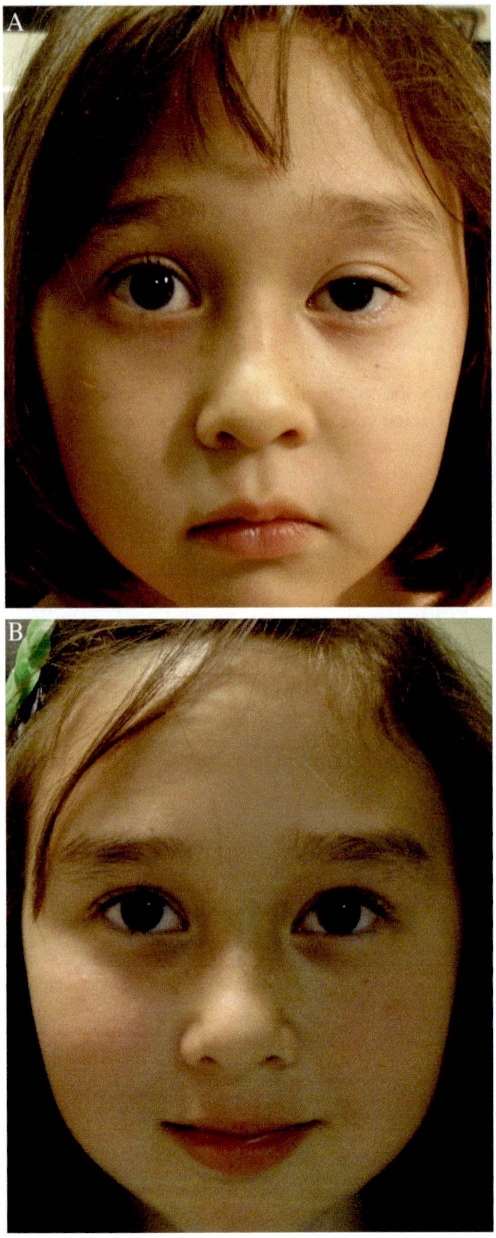

Fig. 15.4 **A** Pediatric patient with left upper eyelid blepharoptosis (moderate levator function). **B** Patient in (A) 3 months post left upper eyelid external levator resection blepharoptosis repair. Photo credit: Jeremiah Tao

References

1. Anderson RL. The levator aponeurosis. Arch Ophthalmol. 1977;95:1437.
2. Gonzalez M. The history of ptosis surgery. In: Evaluation and management of blepharoptosis. New York, NY: Springer; 2011. p. 5–11.
3. Berke RN. Results of resection of the levator muscle through a skin incision in congenital ptosis. Arch Ophthalmol. 1959;61:177–201.
4. Beard C. Congenital ptosis. In: Ptosis. CV Mosby Company. St. Louis, MO; 1976. p. 91–115.
5. Burkat C. External levator advancement and resection. In: Oculofacial, orbital, and lacrimal surgery. Cham: Springer; 2019. p. 29–39.
6. Burkat C. External (transcutaneous) levator advancement (resection) for ptosis. In: Oculofacial Plastic Surgery Education Center. AAO.
7. Knight B. Anatomy, head and neck, eye levator palpebrae superioris muscles. In: StatPearls. Treasure Island [FL]: StatPearls [Internet]; 2021.
8. Shukla UV, Patel BC. Congenital ptosis. In: StatPearls. Treasure Island [FL]: StatPearls [Internet]; 2022.
9. Orbit, eyelids, and lacrimal system. In: Basic and clinical science course, Section 7. San Francisco: American Academy of Ophthalmology. p. 170–1.
10. Bartley G. Results of levator-advancement blepharoptosis repair using a standard protocol: effect of epinephrine-induced eyelid position change. Trans Am Ophthalmol Soc. 1996;94:165–73.
11. Ahmed S, Della Rocca R. Blepharoptosis: evaluation, techniques, and complications. In: Facial plastic surgery. New York [NY]: Thieme Medical Publishers; 2007. p. 203–15.
12. Collin R. Ptosis. In: Fundamentals of clinical ophthalmology; plastic and orbital surgery. London: BMJ Publishing Group; 2001. p. 32–43.

Upper Eyelid Ptosis Repair—Posterior Approach

16

Sudarshan Srivatsan, Sruti S. Akella, Pete Setabutr, and Jeremiah P. Tao

Abstract

The posterior approach to surgical ptosis repair is useful for its predictability, good eyelid contour, and good symmetry. Other advantages include short procedure duration and fast recovery. In this chapter, the authors describe upper eyelid ptosis repair through a posterior approach.

Keywords

Blepharoptosis · Ptosis · Internal ptosis repair · Posterior ptosis repair · Müller's muscle-conjunctival resection (MMCR)

Figures 16.1 and 16.2 illustrated by Lauren Kalinoski, MS, CMI, Director of Biomedical Communications, University of Illinois at Chicago, Department of Ophthalmology, Chicago, IL 60623.

Supplementary Information The online version contains supplementary material available at https://doi.org/10.1007/978-3-031-63178-8_16.

S. Srivatsan
Department of Ophthalmology and Visual Sciences, John A. Moran Eye Center, University of Utah, Salt Lake City, UT 84132, USA

S. S. Akella
Department of Ophthalmology and Visual Sciences, The Ohio State University Wexner Medical Center, Columbus, OH 43212, USA

P. Setabutr (✉)
Department of Ophthalmology and Visual Sciences, Illinois Eye and Ear Infirmary, University of Illinois, Chicago, Chicago, IL 60623, USA
e-mail: Psetabut@uic.edu

J. P. Tao
Division of Oculofacial Plastic and Orbital Surgery, Department of Ophthalmology, University of California, Irvine, Irvine, CA, USA

Anatomy

The two muscles responsible for elevating the upper eyelid are the levator palpebrae superioris and Müller's muscle [1]. The levator palpebrae superioris is a striated muscle that is innervated by the superior division of the oculomotor nerve and is the primary elevator of the upper eyelid [1]. It travels anteriorly from its origin at the orbital apex above the annulus of Zinn to the equator of the globe [1]. At this point it transitions from muscle to its fibrous insertion, the levator aponeurosis [1]. Whitnall's ligament also inserts here and serves to change the direction of force exerted by the levator complex from an anterior–posterior vector to a superior-inferior direction [1]. From Whitnall's ligament, the levator aponeurosis travels inferiorly to insert on the anterior surface of the tarsus [1].

In contrast, Müller's muscle is smooth muscle that is innervated by the sympathetic nervous

J. Tao (ed.), *Efficient Oculofacial Surgery*, https://doi.org/10.1007/978-3-031-63178-8_16

system. It originates from the undersurface of the levator superioris, inserts superiorly on the tarsal border, and is thought to elevate the upper eyelid by 1–2 mm [1].

Blepharoptosis

Blepharoptosis or eyelid ptosis, refers to descent of the upper eyelid margin [2]. When severe, it can obstruct the visual axis and cause vision loss [3]. Symptoms of blepharoptosis include decreased quality of vision, difficulty reading, and forehead fatigue and headache secondary to chronic compensatory frontalis muscle recruitment [2]. The most common cause of blepharoptosis is levator aponeurosis dehiscence or stretching, usually as a result of aging [4]. Other risk factors include eyelid rubbing and contact lens use through which repetitive traction on the eyelid causes the muscle to dehisce [5]. One study of forty-four upper eyelids of twenty-two patients with unilateral blepharoptosis determined that levator aponeurosis thickness in eyelids with aponeurotic ptosis is thinner than the levator aponeurosis in normal eyelids [6]. In another histopathological study of nineteen eyelids of patients with aponeurotic ptosis, 71% of slides showed disinsertion of the levator aponeurosis, 12% showed attenuation, and 13% showed inconclusive changes [7]. Blepharoptosis may be managed with pharmacologic agents such as oxymetazoline, but these only transiently elevate the eyelid and chronic adrenergic use may be associated with side effects such as rebound hyperemia, among others. The definitive treatment of blepharoptosis is surgical correction [1].

Blepharoptosis Repair

The surgical approach to ptosis can be either internal (posterior) or external. According to a recent survey of 208 members of the American Society of Ophthalmic Plastic and Reconstructive Surgery (ASOPRS), 74% perform posterior approach ptosis surgery [8]. The posterior approach has been shown to achieve good symmetry with low re-operation rates [2].

There are two main approaches to posterior ptosis repair, Müller's muscle-conjunctival resection (MMCR) and the Fasanella-Servat procedure [2]. In recent years, MMCR has gained popularity and will be the focus of this chapter.

Müller's Muscle-Conjunctiva Resection

Described by Putterman and Urist in 1975 [9], MMCR has advantages of predictability, efficiency, improved contour, and low revision rates [10]. MMCR has traditionally been reserved for patients with only mild blepharoptosis. Greater degrees of blepharoptosis often require an anterior approach, however recent studies support MMCR in cases of moderate or even severe blepharoptosis [11].

Candidates for MMCR are often chosen based on their response to the phenylephrine test. As originally described, the phenylephrine test consisted of the application of several drops of 10% phenylephrine into the superior fornix. The post-phenylephrine eyelid position was then measured after 5 min, and the amount of resection was based off the new MRD1 [9]. Today, most surgeons use 2.5% phenylephrine [8]. The authors use the following algorithm: if the post-phenylephrine eyelid position is at the desired height, an 8 mm resection is planned. If the post-phenylephrine eyelid position is slightly below the desired height, then an 8–10 mm resection can be performed including an additional small 1–2 mm tarsectomy.

Description of the Surgical Procedure (Fig. 16.1A–H; Video 16.1)

Optional Pre-operative Eyedrops

At least ten minutes prior to surgery, a drop of 2.5% phenylephrine is placed in the operative

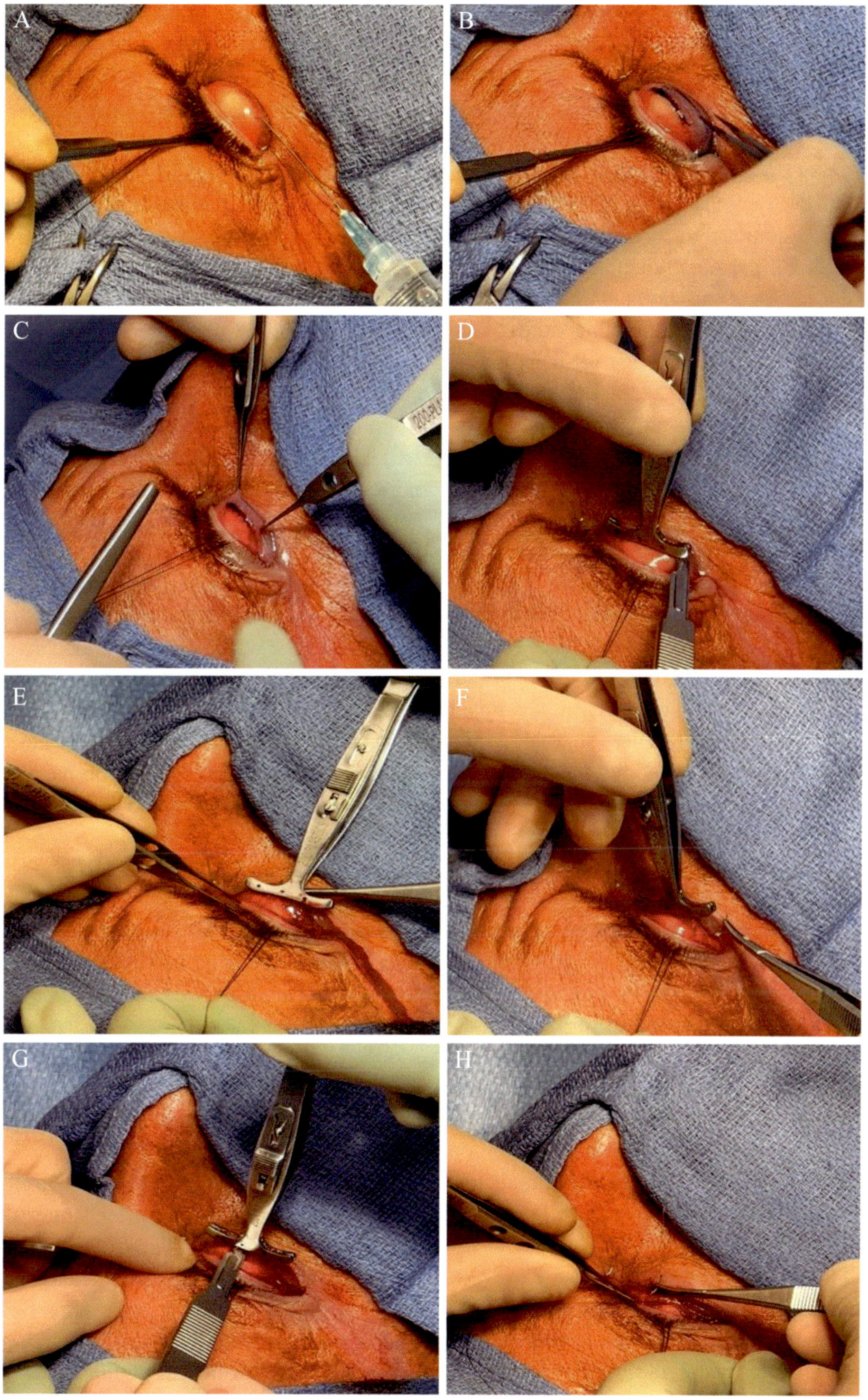

Fig. 16.1 **A** Upper eyelid everted with a Desmarres and a 4-0 silk suture passed through the margin and anesthesia. **B** Area of resection marked with methylene blue. **C** Conjunctiva grasped medially and laterally along areas marked with methylene blue. **D** Conjunctiva incised laterally for 4–8 mm. **E** Conjunctiva wound laterally for suture entry. **F** 6-0 plain suture passed into the lateral wound and then full thickness 2–3 mm away from the clamp back and forth through the posterior lamella tissues. **G** Conjunctiva and Muller's muscle resected with a scalpel, flush against the clamp. **H** Suture run back to approximate cut edges of conjunctiva and tied to itself buried within the lateral wound. Photo credit: Jeremiah Tao

eye. This optional step aims to blanch conjunctival vessels and reduce bleeding.

Step 1 [12]

The central upper eyelid margin and the upper eyelid crease are infiltrated with a small amount local anesthetic, typically 1% or 2% lidocaine with epinephrine. Additional injections can be made in the upper eyelid palpebral conjunctiva just superior to the tarsus at this point or later. Caution should be taken to avoid infiltrating excess fluid in this area and grossly distorting the conjunctival architecture. Additionally, excessive local anesthetic limits the ability to evert the eyelid.

Step 2 [12]

A 4-0 silk traction suture is passed through the tarsus at the central upper eyelid margin. The eyelid is everted over a Desmarres retractor or cotton tip applicators with slight tension on the traction suture. The upper eyelid tarsus and palpebral conjunctiva should now be exposed. Local anesthesia is administered in the upper eyelid palpebral conjunctiva just superior to the tarsus, if not yet done or additional anesthesia is needed. This injection to the upper posterior lamella also facilitates eyelid eversion.

Step 3 [12]

Calipers are used to measure half of the desired resection (i.e., calipers will be set at 4 mm for a desired 8 mm resection). A sterile marking pen or methylene blue are used to place marks superior to the superior border of tarsus. At each mark, the conjunctiva and Müller's muscle are grasped with forceps. Alternatively, 5-0 or 6-0 silk traction sutures may be placed. Traction on the suture or forceps will isolate the conjunctiva and Müller's muscle from the anterior lamella.

Step 4 [12]

With the conjunctiva and Müller's muscle held on traction, a Müller's muscle-conjunctival resection clamp grasps the tissues with the clamp aligned with the superior tarsal border. The clamp can also be placed to incorporate a small amount of tarsus (1–2 mm), if a greater lift is desired.

Step 5 [12, 13]

With the clamp held in the surgeon's non-dominant hand, a double-armed 6-0 plain gut suture is placed in a running horizontal mattress fashion, 1–2 mm below the inferior margin of the clamp. The suture should be far enough away from the clamp to avoid accidentally cutting the suture during the next step, but not so far as to rub on the cornea postoperatively. This suture can be placed from medial to lateral or lateral to medial, depending on surgeon's preference. An initial incision through 3–4 mm of the clamped conjunctiva laterally allows the first suture pass to enter within the wound (the last suture pass will also enter the wound so the knot and suture tails are buried to avoid eye irritation).

Step 6 [12, 13]

Next gentle traction is placed on each end of the suture to ensure that the plain gut is taut and intact. With the ptosis clamp elevated away from the globe, a #15 Bard-Parker blade is used to cut and therefore excise the tissues contained within the clamp (Fig. 16.2). The blade is beveled up towards the clamp, and metal-on-metal contact is maintained the entire time. This helps to avoid inadvertently cutting the suture.

Step 7 [12, 13]

The running suture is passed back toward the initial bite in a running fashion through conjunctiva and the ends are tied so that knot is buried in the conjunctival wound. Alternatively, using a double-armed 6-0 plain gut suture, both arms can be passed full-thickness through the eyelid to exit at the eyelid crease and tied externally (Fig. 16.3).

Antibiotic ointment is placed in the eye twice a day for one week after surgery. In the above description, the externalized or buried knot obviates the need for bandage contact lens placement. However, if a patient is complaining of localized foreign body sensation, a contact lens can be left in place for the first week postoperatively. The patient should be counseled to avoid rubbing the eye or sleeping on his or her stomach to avoid breaking the suture.

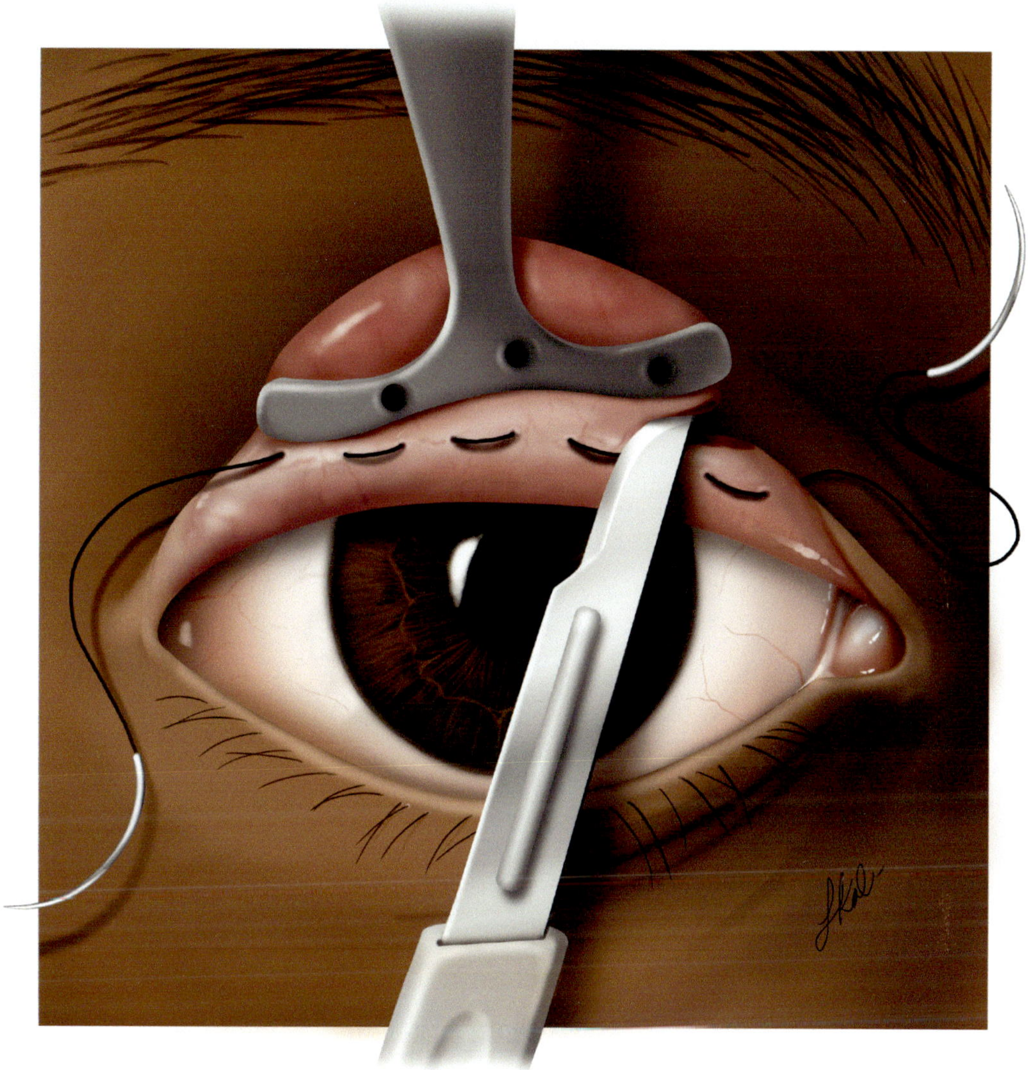

Fig. 16.2 The tissue within the ptosis clamp is elevated up and from the globe and a #15 Bard-Parker blade to excise the tissues contained within the clamp. The blade is beveled up towards the clamp, and metal-on-metal contact is maintained

Complications

The most common complication of a MMCR is inadvertently cutting or breaking the plain gut suture. This can result in a less predictable outcome, with either over- or undercorrection of ptosis. If the surgeon notes a broken suture immediately after excising the tissues held within the clamp, every attempt should be made to identify the severed end of the suture. Often the suture is cut in a single place, typically in the middle of the eyelid. An additional 6-0 plain gut suture can be tied to this severed end, and the needle can again be passed in the same running horizontal fashion through the wound edges and Müller's muscle.

If the patient breaks the externalized suture in the postoperative period, they should be

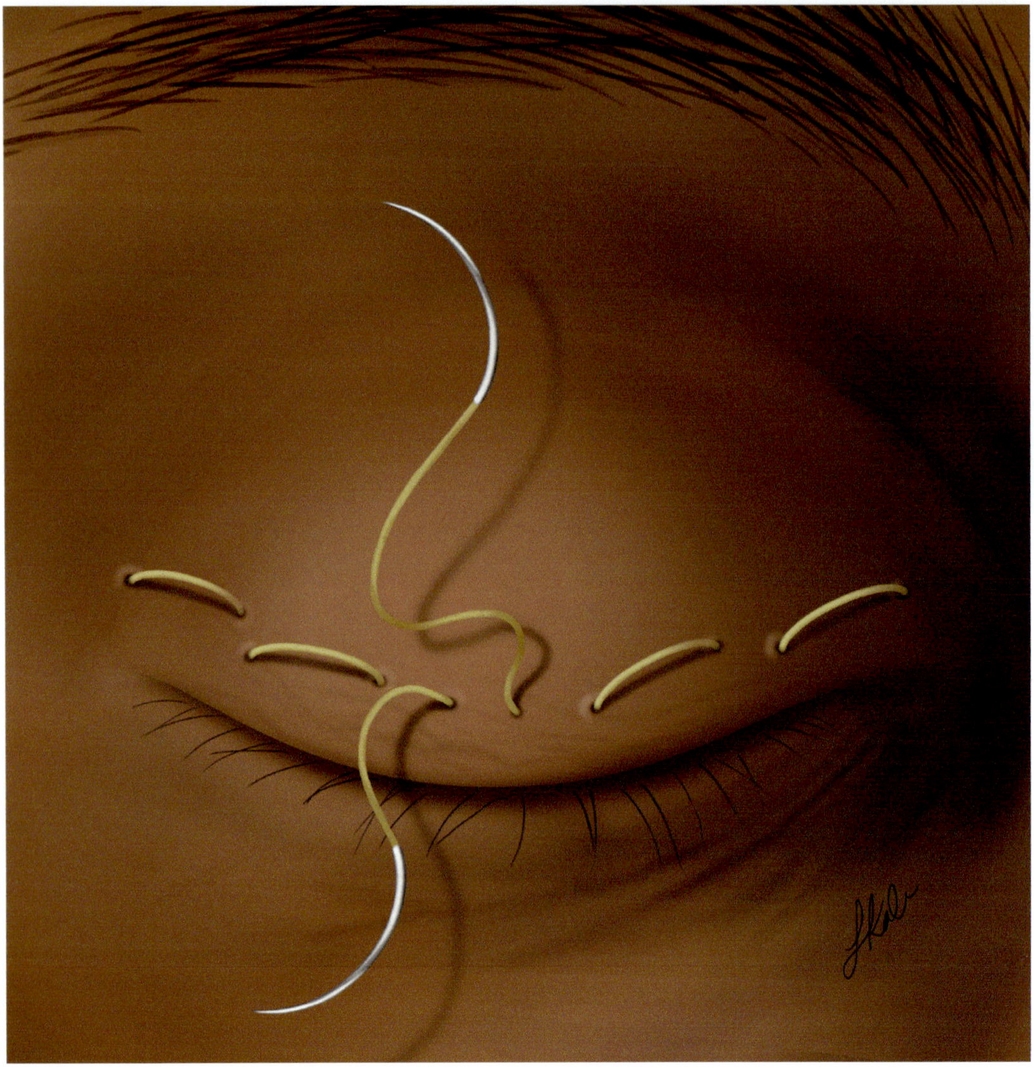

Fig. 16.3 Technique in which each pass of the 6-0 plain gut is full-thickness to exit at the eyelid crease just outside the wound. The ends are then passed subcutaneously towards the center and then tied externally

instructed to not rub or manipulate the upper eyelid further. Often, a good postoperative result can still occur, as the wound will contract slowly and elevate the eyelid. Importantly, it may take longer for the blepharoptosis to improve.

Another complication of posterior eyelid ptosis repair is corneal irritation and abrasion [12, 14]. Corneal irritation can occur due to exposed suture, suture that is placed too far below the ptosis clamp, and lagophthalmos. By externalizing or burying the suture, the risk of corneal irritation from an exposed suture knot is minimized; however, a bandage contact lens can still be placed as needed. Patients with lagophthalmos should be advised to use artificial tears and ointments; most lagophthalmos resolve within the first six weeks.

Over- or undercorrection can be seen in 3–10% of cases [14, 15]. In some cases, undercorrection can be caused by eyelid edema which should be observed until the eyelid position has stabilized. If undercorrection persists, further ptosis surgery may be required. In the case of overcorrection, downward massage or eyelid

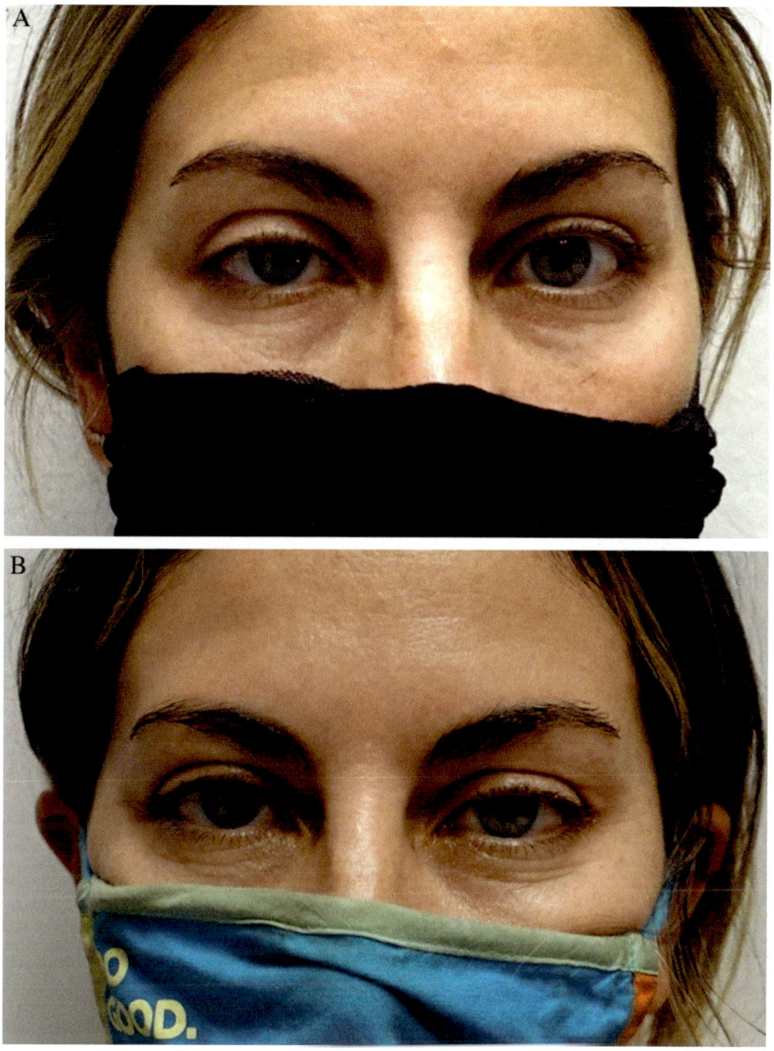

Fig. 16.4 **A** A patient with right upper eyelid blepharoptosis. **B** Same patient, status post right upper eyelid MMCR with subsequent mild left upper eyelid blepharoptosis due to Hering's effect. Photo credit: Jeremiah Tao

stretching exercises can be attempted in the immediate post-operative period [12]. If overcorrection persists, corrective surgery may be required.

Lastly, in unilateral cases, the contralateral eyelid may become ptotic after surgery (Fig. 16.4). This is known as Hering's effect and can be explained by the bilateral paired innervation of upper eyelids. When an eyelid is lifted after surgery, there may exist less feedback to the central nervous system that decreases tone not only to the operated eyelid, but also to the contralateral eyelid. Treatment may include blepharoptosis repair on the second eyelid.

MMCR has been performed safely in patients with glaucoma [16]. However, there have been cases of postoperative diplopia and symblepharon in glaucoma patients using topical intraocular pressure lowering agents [17]. The authors have not encountered any complications when using this technique in patients with previous filtering surgeries.

There can also be changes in corneal astigmatism in up to 72% of patients undergoing

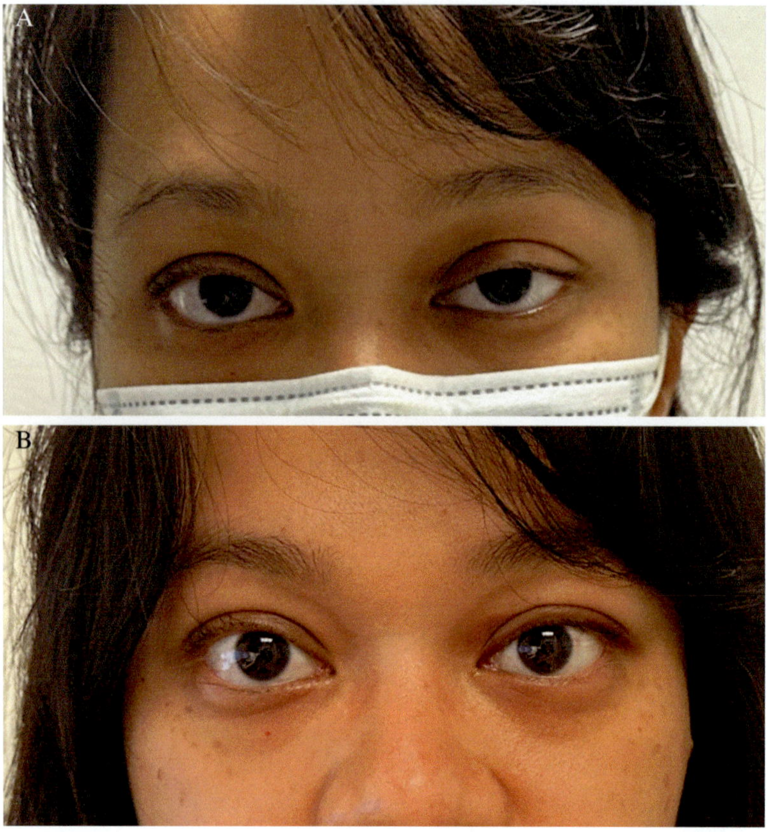

Fig. 16.5 **A** A patient with left upper eyelid blepharoptosis. **B** Same patient status post left upper eyelid MMCR with a good result. Photo credit: Jeremiah Tao

ptosis repair. However, in most cases, the astigmatism regresses back to pre-operative levels within a year [18].

It has also been postulated that the loss of palpebral conjunctival tissue and accessory lacrimal glands may cause worsening dry eye disease. However, studies have shown that there are no changes in tear composition, tear production, or subjective dryness following MMCR [19, 20].

Conclusion

Advantages of the MMCR procedure include its lack of an external scar, efficiency, short recovery, and the maintenance of the natural eyelid contour [11]. Additionally, MMCR is highly predictable, with the results of the phenylephrine test very closely mimicking the final outcome in the vast majority of cases [21]. It is a highly effective procedure and obviates inefficiencies of intraoperative adjustment inherent to many anterior ptosis repair techniques (Fig. 16.5A, B).

References

1. Finsterer J. Ptosis: causes, presentation, and management. Aesthetic Plast Surg. 2003;27(3):193–204. https://doi.org/10.1007/s00266-003-0127-5.
2. Liu CY, Chhadva P, Setabutr P. Blepharoptosis repair. Curr Opin Otolaryngol Head Neck Surg. 2018;26(4):221–6. https://doi.org/10.1097/MOO.0000000000000463.
3. Ho SF, Morawski A, Sampath R, Burns J. Modified visual field test for ptosis surgery (Leicester Peripheral Field Test). Eye. 2011;25(3):365–9. https://doi.org/10.1038/eye.2010.210.

4. Lim JM, Hou JH, Singa RM, Aakalu VK, Setabutr P. Relative incidence of blepharoptosis subtypes in an oculoplastics practice at a tertiary care center. Orbit Amst Neth. 2013;32(4):231–4. https://doi.org/10.3109/01676830.2013.788673.
5. Fujiwara T, Matsuo K, Kondoh S, Yuzuriha S. Etiology and pathogenesis of aponeurotic blepharoptosis. Ann Plast Surg. 2001;46(1):29–35.
6. Hoşal BM, Ayer NG, Zilelioğlu G, Elhan AH. Ultrasound biomicroscopy of the levator aponeurosis in congenital and aponeurotic blepharoptosis. Ophthal Plast Reconstr Surg. 2004;20(4):308–11. https://doi.org/10.1097/01.iop.0000129532.33913.e7.
7. Dortzbach RK, Sutula FC. Involutional blepharoptosis: a histopathological study. Arch Ophthalmol. 1980;98(11):2045–9. https://doi.org/10.1001/archopht.1980.01020040897022.
8. Aakalu VK, Setabutr P. Current ptosis management: a national survey of ASOPRS members. Ophthal Plast Reconstr Surg. 2011;27(4):270–6. https://doi.org/10.1097/IOP.0b013e31820ccce1.
9. Putterman AM, Urist MJ. Müller muscle-conjunctiva resection: technique for treatment of blepharoptosis. Arch Ophthalmol. 1975;93(8):619–23. https://doi.org/10.1001/archopht.1975.01010020595007.
10. How the Mueller muscle-conjunctival resection ptosis procedure: ophthalmic plastic and reconstructive surgery. https://journals.lww.com/op-rs/Fulltext/2016/03000/How_the_Mueller_Muscle_Conjunctival_Resection.24.aspx. Accessed 30 Mar 2022
11. Patel RM, Aakalu VK, Setabutr P, Putterman AM. Efficacy of Muller's muscle and conjunctiva resection with or without tarsectomy for the treatment of severe involutional blepharoptosis. Ophthal Plast Reconstr Surg. 2017;33(4):273–8. https://doi.org/10.1097/IOP.0000000000000748.
12. Sajja K, Putterman AM. Müller's muscle conjunctival resection ptosis repair in the aesthetic patient. Saudi J Ophthalmol. 2011;25(1):51–60. https://doi.org/10.1016/j.sjopt.2010.10.011.
13. Carruth BP, Meyer DR. Simplified Müller's muscle-conjunctival resection internal ptosis repair. Ophthal Plast Reconstr Surg. 2013;29(1):11–4. https://doi.org/10.1097/IOP.0b013e31826afb6b.
14. Putterman AM, Fett DR. Müller's muscle in the treatment of upper eyelid ptosis: a ten-year study. Ophthalmic Surg. 1986;17(6):354–60.
15. Thomas GN, Chan J, Sundar G, Amrith S. Outcomes of levator advancement and Müller muscle-conjunctiva resection for the repair of upper eyelid ptosis. Orbit. 2017;36(1):39–42. https://doi.org/10.1080/01676830.2017.1279650.
16. Georgescu D, Cole E, Epstein G, et al. Müller muscle-conjunctiva resection for blepharoptosis in patients with glaucoma filtering blebs. Ophthal Plast Reconstr Surg. 2007;23(4):285–7. https://doi.org/10.1097/IOP.0b013e318070d59d.
17. Lee WW, Portaliou D, Sayed MS, Kankariya S. Diplopia and symblepharon following Mueller's muscle conjunctival resection in patients on long-term multiple antiglaucoma medications. Ophthal Plast Reconstr Surg. 2017;33(3(3S)):S79–82. https://doi.org/10.1097/IOP.0000000000000760.
18. Holck DE, Dutton JJ, Wehrly SR. Changes in astigmatism after ptosis surgery measured by corneal topography. Ophthal Plast Reconstr Surg. 1998;14(3):151–8. https://doi.org/10.1097/00002341-199805000-00001.
19. Rymer BL, Marinho DR, Cagliari C, Marafon SB, Procianoy F. Effects of Muller's muscle-conjunctival resection for ptosis on ocular surface scores and dry eye symptoms. Orbit Amst Neth. 2017;36(1):1–5. https://doi.org/10.1080/01676830.2016.1243134.
20. Bautista SA, Wladis EJ, Schultze RL. Quantitative assessment of dry eye parameters after Müller's muscle-conjunctival resection. Ophthal Plast Reconstr Surg. 2018;34(6):562–4. https://doi.org/10.1097/IOP.0000000000001103.
21. Sweeney AR, Dermarkarian CR, Williams KJ, Allen RC, Yen MT. Outcomes after Müller muscle conjunctival resection versus external levator advancement in severe involutional blepharoptosis. Am J Ophthalmol. 2020;217:182–8. https://doi.org/10.1016/j.ajo.2020.04.039.

Upper Eyelid Ptosis Repair with Frontalis Flap

17

Tonya Lee, Nicole Topilow, and Catherine Y. Liu

Abstract

Frontalis flap advancement is an effective surgery for the correction of blepharoptosis with poor levator function. It obviates the need for a sling device or graft and other risks involved with frontalis sling procedures. This chapter describes indications, relevant anatomy, and technique of frontalis flap blepharoptosis repair.

Keywords

Blepharoptosis · Congenital ptosis · Myogenic ptosis · Frontalis advancement · Frontalis suspension · Frontalis flap

Introduction

Indications/Contraindications

The frontalis flap advancement is a surgical technique that involves the direct transfer of the frontalis muscle to the tarsus that thereby elevates the eyelid. It is indicated in cases of severe ptosis with poor levator palpebrae superioris function, as is seen in congenital ptosis [1–3]. The frontalis flap can also be used for patients who have failed prior levator advancement procedures [4]. Poor frontalis function due to facial nerve palsy or prior trauma is a contraindication to frontalis flap advancement [5]. This technique should also be avoided in patients with myasthenia gravis and those with pre-existing corneal disease who may be at risk of post-operative exposure keratopathy [5]. A careful ocular surface examination and evaluation for adequate Bell's reflex should be performed prior to surgery.

Supplementary Information The online version contains supplementary material available at https://doi.org/10.1007/978-3-031-63178-8_17.

T. Lee · N. Topilow · C. Y. Liu (✉)
University of California San Diego, San Diego, CA, USA
e-mail: catherine.liu@gmail.com

Brief History

Fergus et al. introduced direct transposition of the frontalis muscle onto the eyelid margin via a brow incision for treatment of eyelid ptosis in 1901 [6]. Song and Song subsequently reintroduced the concept in 1982 [7]. Variations in frontalis flap design have been described since then, with differences in skin incision, extent of dissection, and flap division [5, 8–12].

The frontalis flap advancement technique described in this chapter is performed with minimal dissection in the preseptal plane and through a single eyelid crease incision. No flap division or posterior dissection under the flap is

J. Tao (ed.), *Efficient Oculofacial Surgery*, https://doi.org/10.1007/978-3-031-63178-8_17

required, as the loose areolar attachments of the frontalis muscle to the periosteum differ from its firm subcutaneous attachments to the dermis.

Pros and Cons

One advantage of the frontalis flap advancement is that it avoids risks associated with various implants used in frontalis suspension procedures, including sling extrusion, infection, and granuloma formation around alloplastic materials [13–15]. The frontalis flap achieves substantial lift in eyelid height, and can be performed through one aesthetically pleasing incision at the eyelid crease, thus avoiding additional autogenous graft donor site morbidity [4, 16]. Because frontalis muscle matures earlier than fascia lata, frontalis flap advancement can be performed at an earlier age without waiting for sufficient fascia lata to be available for autogenous sling use (usually around 3 years of age) [14].

Successful frontalis flap advancement requires recruitment of the frontalis muscle to raise the eyelid. If the patient does not recruit the frontalis pre operatively, surgical success may be limited. Another limitation to this technique is that postoperative reversal or adjustment is more technically challenging than with a silicone frontalis sling [5]. There is potential for injury to the temporal branch of the facial nerve if dissection is taken too far supero laterally [4] (Fig. 17.1). In the technique described, dissection is limited to the subcutaneous (above the rim) and preseptal (below the rim) planes, thereby minimizing the risk of injury to the temporal branch of the facial nerve.

Anatomic landmarks in frontalis surgery include sensory and motor innervation to the upper face. Laterally, the facial nerve branches

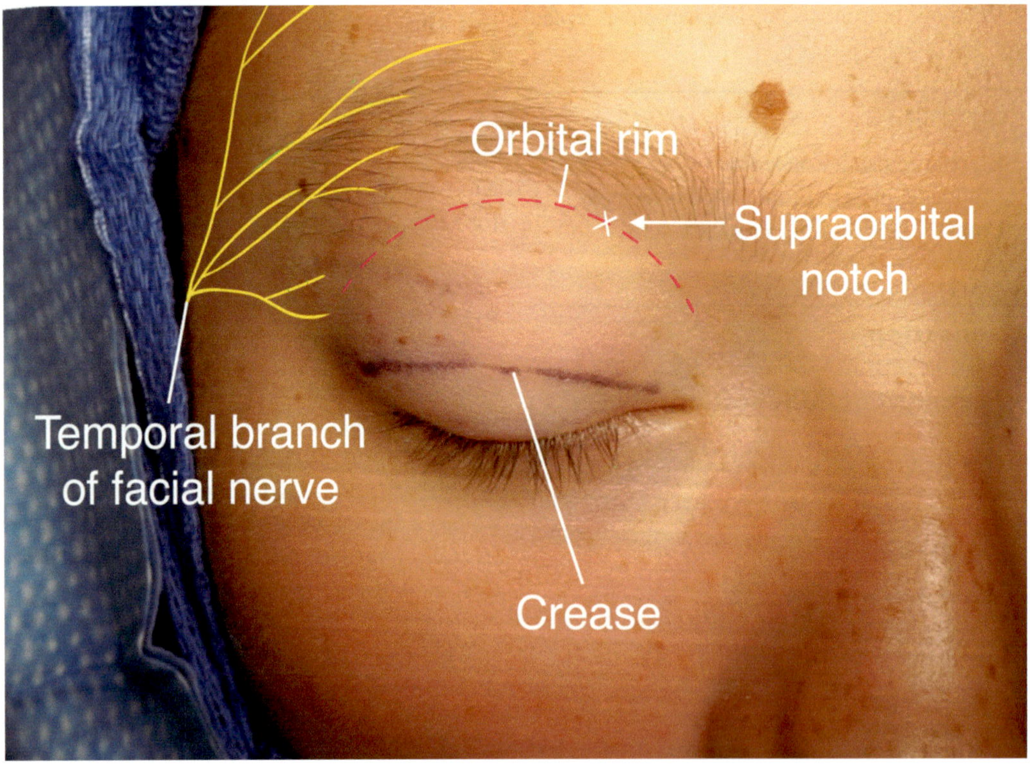

Fig. 17.1 Landmarks and overview. The supraorbital notch is palpated and may be marked. The eyelid crease is marked for incision. If the crease is ill-defined, the height of the contralateral eyelid may be measured with calipers and used as a reference

should be preserved at the lateral brow. At the medial brow lies the supraorbital sensory nerves that exit the supraorbital notch and run superiorly in the deep scalp (Fig. 17.1).

Surgical Technique

A small blepharoplasty skin incision is made with a #15 blade (Fig. 17.2). Dissection is carried superiorly in a sub-orbicularis, preseptal plane with scissors or cautery (Fig. 17.3). Sub-orbicularis dissection is carried superiorly to approximately 5 mm above the superior orbital rim (Fig. 17.4a). Here, dissection transitions to a subcutaneous plane (Fig. 17.4b).

The frontalis muscle is grasped with forceps to begin flap development. The frontalis muscle (white arrow) is identified anterior to the retro-orbicularis oculi fat (ROOF) pad (Fig. 17.5). Dissection is carried further superiorly in a subcutaneous plane to 1 cm above the brow using Stevens scissors (Fig. 17.6). Extreme care should be taken to avoid creating a buttonhole through the skin. Medially, the subcutaneous dissection should end lateral to the supraorbital notch. Laterally, the subcutaneous dissection should end medial to the lateral canthus (Fig. 17.7). Vertical relaxing incisions can be made at each end of the flap but are often unnecessary and may increase the risk of facial nerve branch injury.

Using scissors, the orbicularis oculi muscle is dissected off the superior tarsal border and the anterior tarsal surface is exposed (Fig. 17.8). The frontalis flap is advanced inferiorly and affixed to the superior 1/3 of the tarsus with two 6-0 polypropylene horizontal mattress sutures passed in a partial thickness, lamellar fashion through the tarsus and tied temporarily with slip knots (Fig. 17.9a and b). The eyelid should have a natural contour with a slightly nasal peak and should sit approximately 1–2 mm below the superior limbus (Fig. 17.10). Once the desired

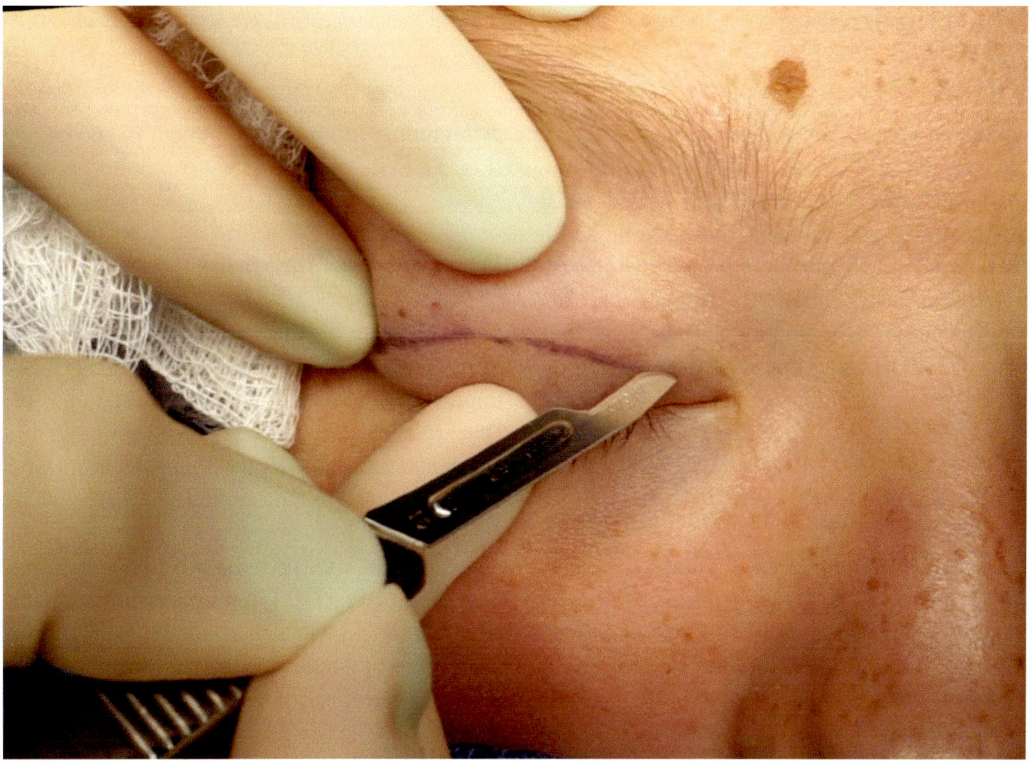

Fig. 17.2 **Skin incision.** The skin incision is performed with a #15 blade along the eyelid crease marking

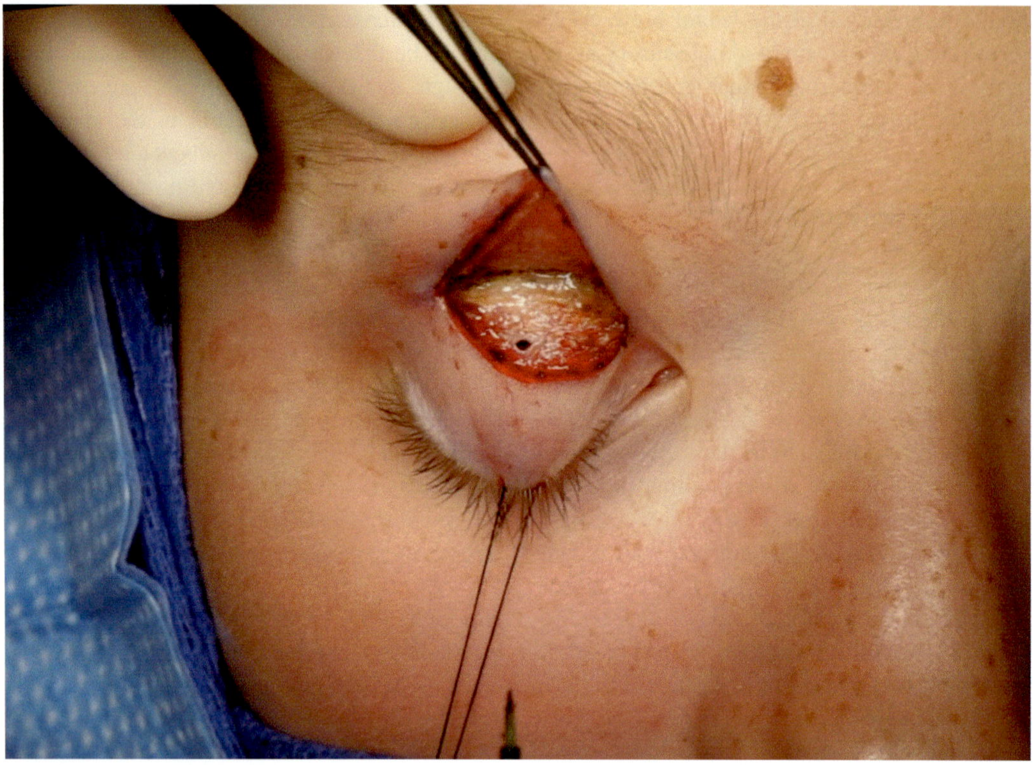

Fig. 17.3 Pre-septal dissection. Dissection is carried superiorly in a sub-orbicularis, pre septal plane with scissors or cautery

height and contour are achieved, the sutures are tied permanently. Three eyelid crease-forming 7-0 polyglactin 910 sutures are placed medially, centrally, and laterally; these are passed in an interrupted fashion through the orbicularis at the superior incision edge, the frontalis flap, and the orbicularis at the inferior incision edge. The incision is closed in a running fashion using 6-0 fast absorbing gut suture (Fig. 17.11).

Postoperative Care

Postoperatively, ice packs should be carefully applied to the upper eyelid (20 min on, 20 min off) for about 72 h. Antibiotic ointment should be applied to the incision twice daily for 2 weeks. Acetaminophen may be used as needed for pain. Frequent use of artificial tears as well as nighttime lubricating ointment is encouraged (Fig. 17.11).

Potential Complications

Lagophthalmos may occur following frontalis flap advancement but is typically well-tolerated and improves in the months following surgery [5, 17]. Dry eye secondary to increased corneal exposure can be treated with frequent application of lubricant eyedrops, gel, and ointment. Other possible complications include recurrent ptosis, entropion, and ectropion with separation of the eyelid from the corneal surface [1]. Intra-operatively, if ectropion is noted upon advancing the frontalis flap, the horizontal mattress suture can be shifted superiorly on the anterior tarsal surface and further dissection of the frontalis flap can be performed.

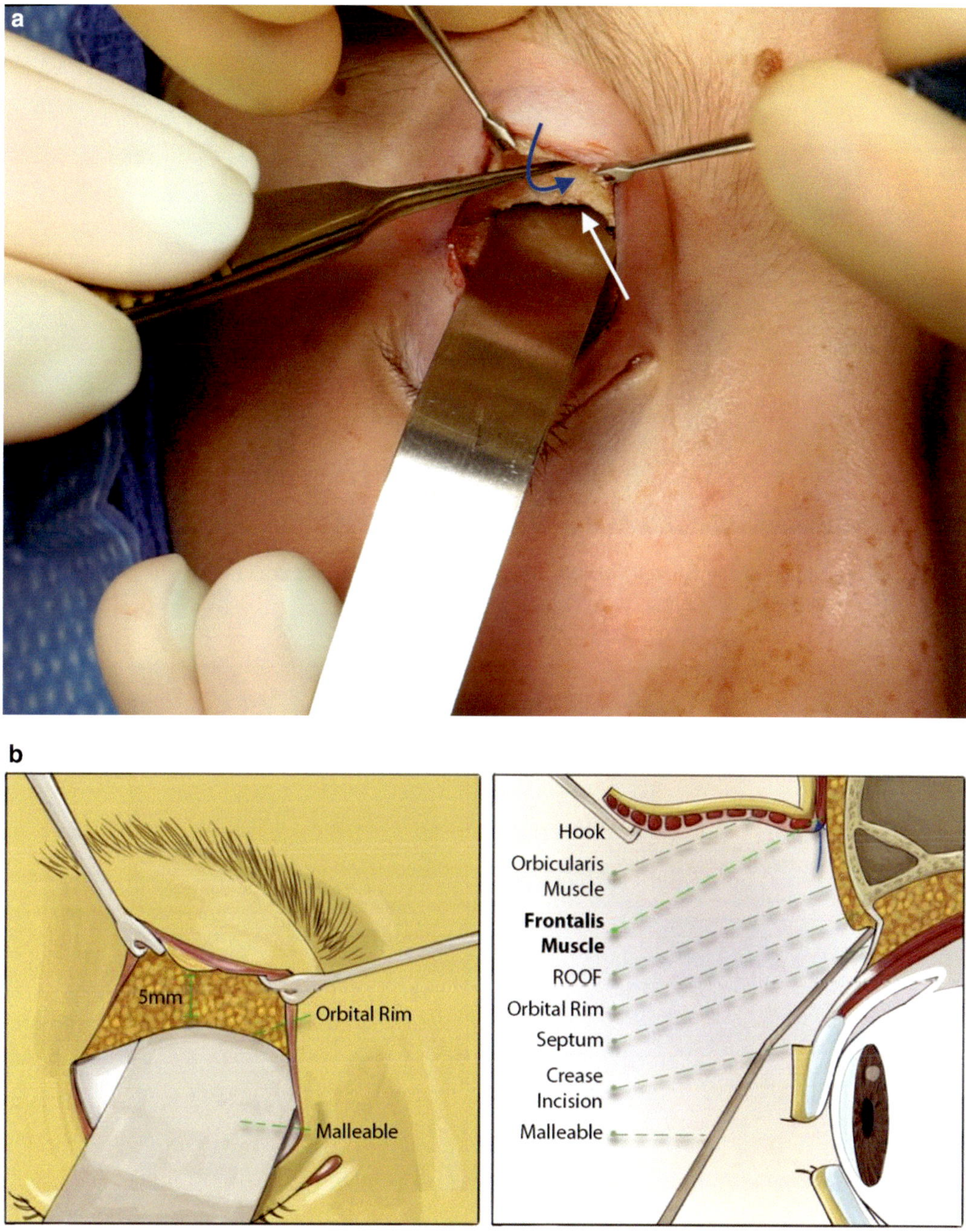

Fig. 17.4 a Superior extent of sub-orbicularis dissection. The sub-orbicularis dissection should be carried superiorly to approximately 5 mm above the superior orbital rim (straight white arrow). Here, dissection transitions to a subcutaneous plane (see illustration of planes in b). Forceps are shown here grasping the frontalis muscle to begin flap development (curved blue arrow). **b** Cross-section illustrating important tissue planes for flap development. The blue arrow denotes the transition of dissection to the subcutaneous plane approximately 5 mm above the orbital rim

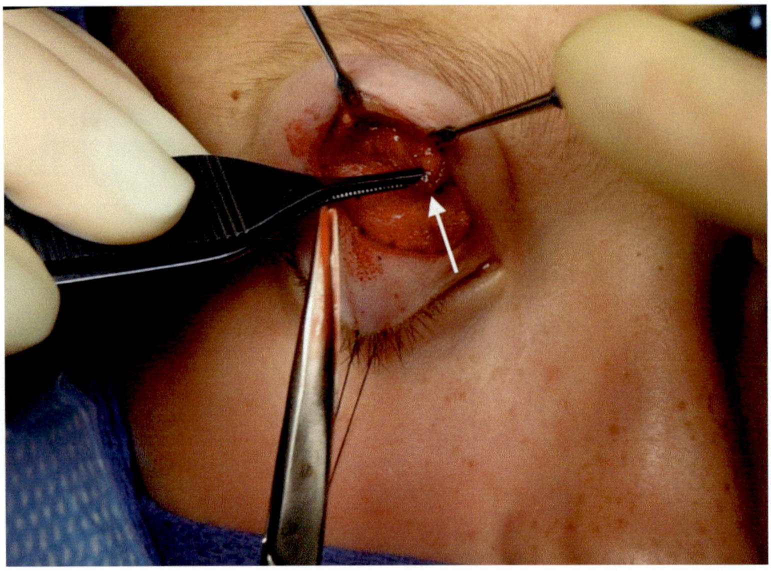

Fig. 17.5 Identification of the frontalis muscle. The frontalis muscle (white arrow) is identified anterior to the retro-orbicularis oculi fat (ROOF) pad

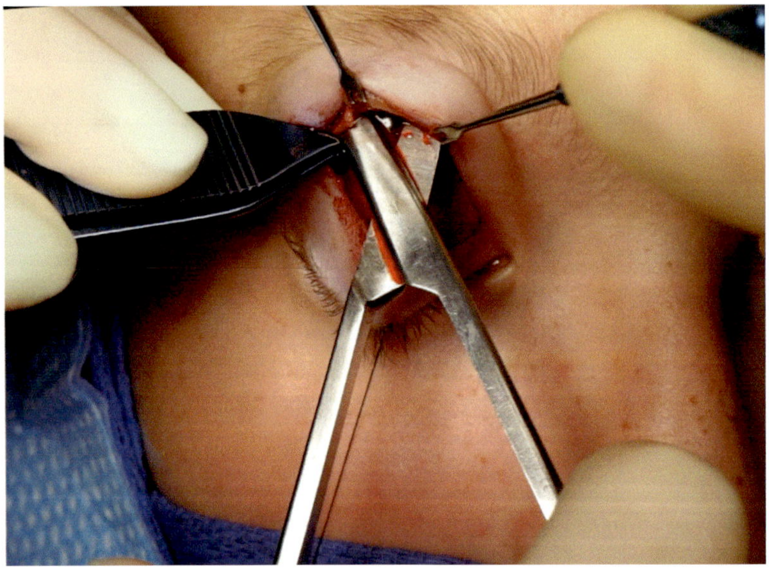

Fig. 17.6 Subcutaneous dissection. Dissection is carried further superiorly in a subcutaneous plane to 1 cm above the brow using Stevens scissors. Extreme care should be taken to avoid creating a buttonhole through the skin

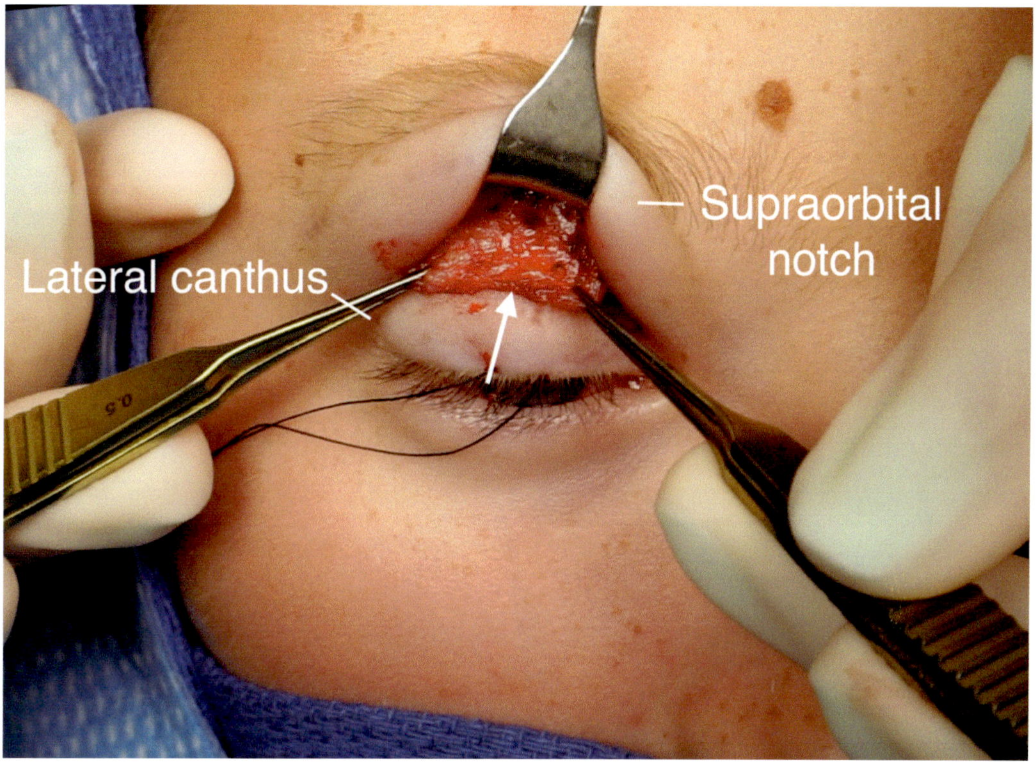

Fig. 17.7 Development of the frontalis flap. Medially, the subcutaneous dissection should end lateral to the supraorbital notch. Laterally, the subcutaneous dissection should end medial to the lateral canthus. Vertical relaxing incisions can be made at each end of the flap but are often unnecessary and may increase the risk of facial nerve branch injury

Conclusion

Frontalis flap advancement is an effective surgery for the correction of ptosis associated with poor levator function. It can be performed in infants and eliminates the need for a sling device or grafts required with frontalis sling procedures.

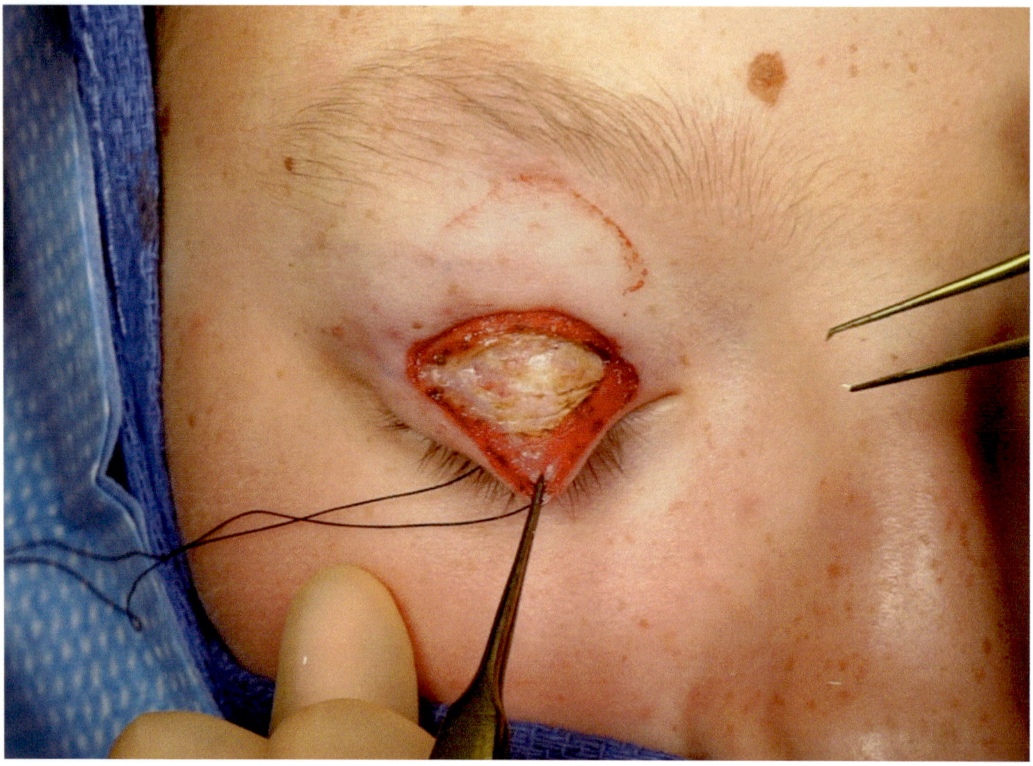

Fig. 17.8 Pre-tarsal pocket. Dissection is then carried inferior to the incision line in a sub-orbicularis plane using scissors. When the superior tarsal border is encountered, dissection is continued in a pre-tarsal plane to expose the anterior tarsal surface and create a pre-tarsal pocket for flap advancement

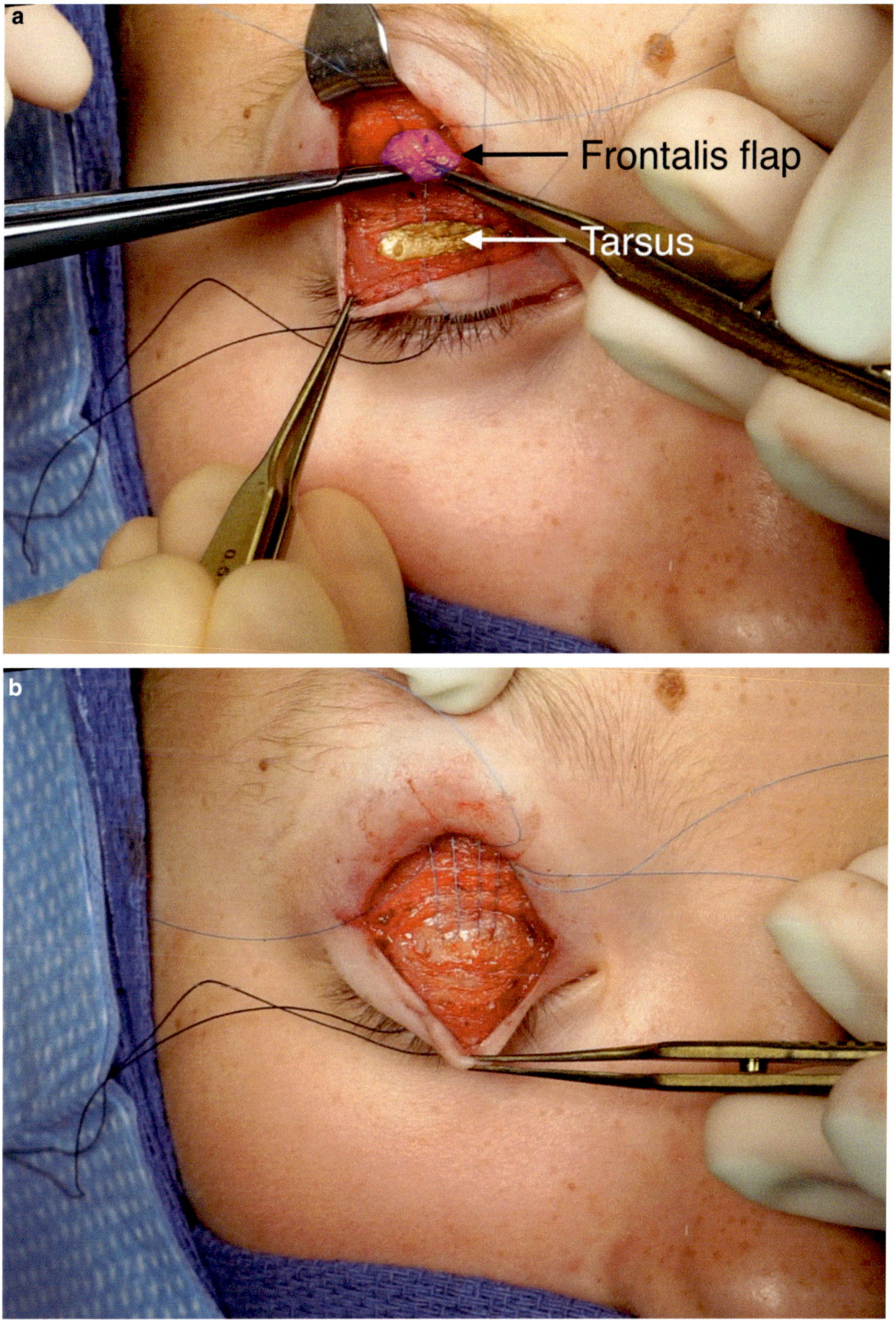

Fig. 17.9 a & b Frontalis flap advancement. The frontalis flap is advanced inferiorly and affixed to the superior 1/3 of the tarsus with two 6-0 polypropylene horizontal mattress sutures passed in a partial thickness, lamellar fashion through the tarsus and tied temporarily with slip knots

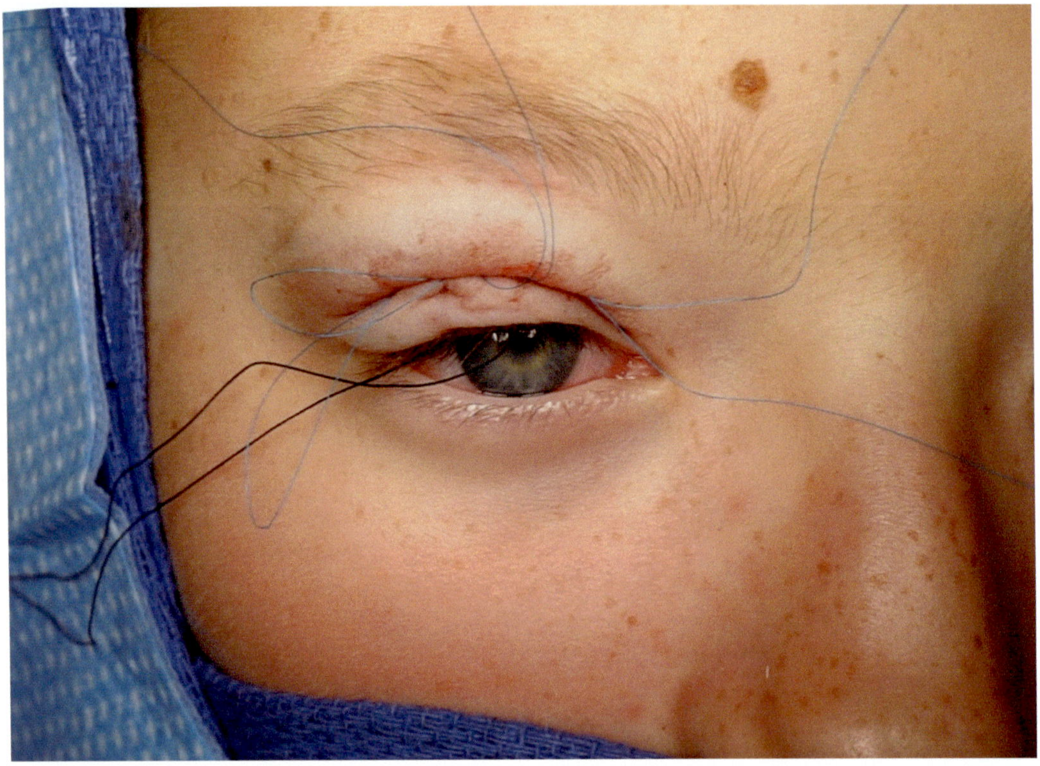

Fig. 17.10 **Assessment of eyelid height and contour.** The eyelid should have a natural contour with a slightly nasal peak and should sit approximately 1–2 mm below the superior limbus. If the eyelid sits too high, the tarsal suture can be shifted superiorly, and further dissection of the flap may be performed. Once the desired height and contour are achieved, the sutures are tied permanently

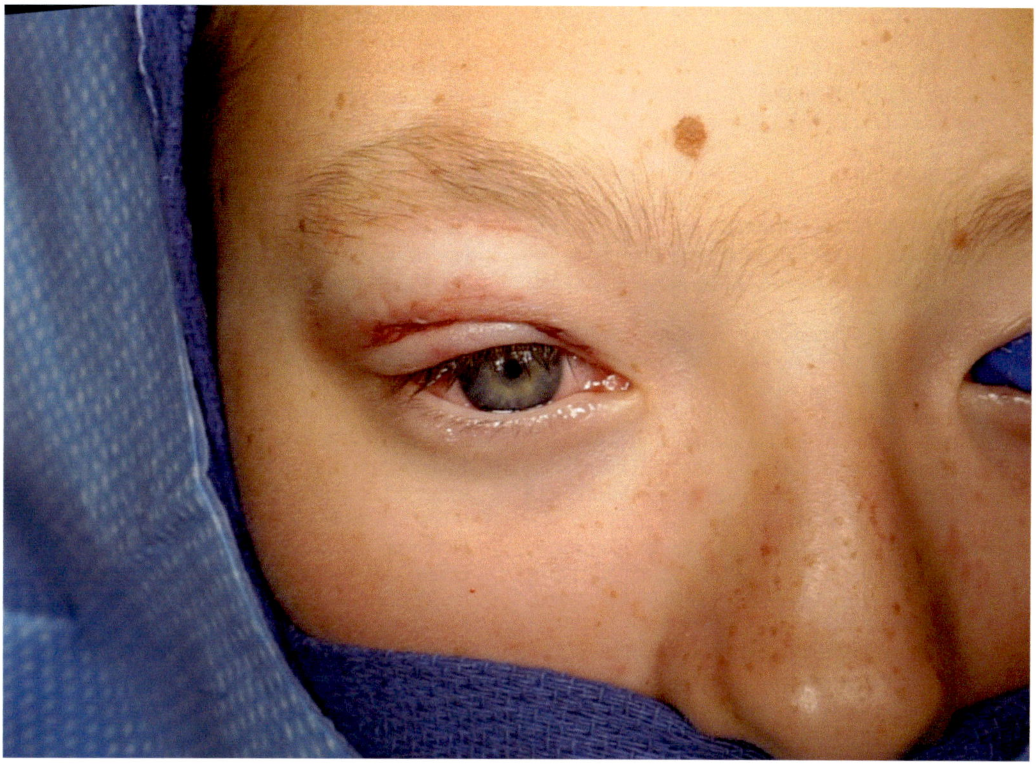

Fig. 17.11 **Soft tissue and skin closure.** Three eyelid crease-forming 7-0 polyglactin 910 sutures are placed medially, centrally, and laterally; these are passed in an interrupted fashion through the orbicularis at the superior incision edge, the frontalis flap, and the orbicularis at the inferior incision edge. The incision is closed in a running fashion using 6-0 fast absorbing gut suture

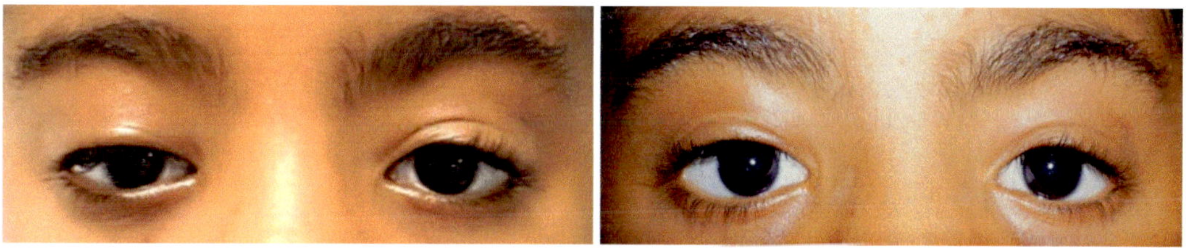

Fig. 17.12 (Left) Preoperative photo showing congenital ptosis of the right eyelid after a failed silicone sling procedure. (Right) Post-operative photo after the frontalis flap advancement procedure, demonstrating natural and symmetric eyelid position

References

1. Medel R, Vasquez L, Wolley Dod C. Early frontalis flap surgery as first option to correct congenital ptosis with poor levator function. Orbit. 2014;33(3):164–8. https://doi.org/10.3109/01676830.2014.881396.
2. Liu HP, Shao Y, Li B, Yu X, Zhang D. Frontalis muscle transfer technique for correction of severe congenital blepharoptosis in Chinese patients: an analysis of surgical outcomes related to frontalis muscle function. J Plast Reconstr Aesthet Surg. 2015;68(12):1667–74. https://doi.org/10.1016/j.bjps.2015.08.003.
3. Zhou M, Zhong M, Jin R, Li Q, Duan Y, Huang L, Li L, Yu D, Huang D. Frontalis muscle flap advancement for correction of severe ptosis under general anesthesia: modified surgical design with 162 cases in China. Aesthetic Plast Surg. 2014;38(3):503–9. https://doi.org/10.1007/s00266-014-0297-3.

4. Goldey SH, Baylis HI, Goldberg RA, Shorr N. Frontalis muscle flap advancement for correction of blepharoptosis. Ophthalmic Plast Reconstr Surg. 2000;16(2):83–93. https://doi.org/10.1097/00002341-200003000-00002.
5. Dallalzadeh LO, Park KS, Korn BS, Kikkawa DO, Liu CY. Minimal dissection direct frontalis muscle advancement flap for congenital ptosis repair. J Craniofac Surg. 2021;32(7):2358–61. https://doi.org/10.1097/SCS.0000000000007761.
6. Fergus F. An easy operation for congenital ptosis. Br Med J. 1901;1(2100):762. https://doi.org/10.1136/bmj.1.2100.762.
7. Song R, Song Y. Treatment of blepharoptosis. Direct transplantation of the frontalis muscle to the upper eyelid. Clin Plast Surg. 1982;9(1):45–8.
8. Cruz AAV, Akaishi APMS. Frontalis-orbicularis muscle advancement for correction of upper eyelid ptosis: a systematic literature review. Ophthalmic Plast Reconstr Surg. 2018;34(6):510–5. https://doi.org/10.1097/IOP.0000000000001145.
9. Han K, Kang J. Tripartite frontalis muscle flap transposition for blepharoptosis. Ann Plast Surg. 1993; 30(3):224–32. https://doi.org/10.1097/00000637-199303000-00005.
10. Kim WJ, Park DH, Han DG. Ten years of results of modified frontalis muscle transfer for the correction of blepharoptosis. Arch Plast Surg. 2016;43(2):172–80. https://doi.org/10.5999/aps.2016.43.2.172.
11. Medel R, Alonso T, Giralt J, Torres J, González-Candial M, Garcìa-Arumì J. Frontalis muscle flap advancement with a pulley in the levator aponeurosis in patients with complete ptosis and deep-set eyes. Ophthalmic Plast Reconstr Surg. 2006;22(6):441–4. https://doi.org/10.1097/01.iop.0000244514.66424.bd
12. Park DH, Ahn KY, Han DG, Baik BS. Blepharoptosis repair by selective use of superiorly based muscle flaps. Plast Reconstr Surg. 1998;101(3):592–603. https://doi.org/10.1097/00006534-199803000-00005.
13. Bleyen I, Hardy I, CodËre F. Muscle prolapse after harvesting autogenous fascia lata used for frontalis suspension in children. Ophthalmic Plast Reconstr Surg. 2009;25(5):359–60. https://doi.org/10.1097/IOP.0b013e3181b1e67a.
14. Carter SR, Meecham WJ, Seiff SR. Silicone frontalis slings for the correction of blepharoptosis: indications and efficacy. Ophthalmology. 1996;103(4):623–30. https://doi.org/10.1016/s0161-6420(96)30643-x.
15. Katowitz JA, Katowitz WR. Pediatric oculoplastics surgery. 2nd ed. New York: Springer; 2018.
16. Wheatcroft SM, Vardy SJ, Tyers AG. Complications of fascia lata harvesting for ptosis surgery. Br J Ophthalmol. 1997;81(7):581–3. https://doi.org/10.1136/bjo.81.7.581.
17. Medel R, Molina S, Vasquez LM, Visa J, Wert A, Wolley-Dod C. Frontalis muscle flap versus maximal anterior levator resection as first option for patients with severe congenital ptosis. Ophthalmic Plast Reconstr Surg. 2018;34(6):565–9. https://doi.org/10.1097/IOP.0000000000001105.

Frontalis Suspension Ptosis Repair

18

Alejandro M. Perez and Sanja G. Cypen

Abstract

Upper eyelid ptosis repair utilizing frontalis suspension is indicated for patients with moderate to severe ptosis due to impaired levator muscle function. In this procedure, the frontalis muscle is secured to the upper eyelid tarsal plate using a sling material, such as synthetic suture, silicone rod, or autogenous or cadaveric fascia lata. By elevating the upper eyelid in primary gaze, frontalis suspension improves both functional and aesthetic concerns in affected patients. In this chapter, the authors describe the surgical technique and highlight key considerations that contribute to achieving excellent patient outcomes and optimizing surgical efficiency.

Keywords

Ptosis · Congenital ptosis · Frontalis suspension · Frontalis sling · Surgical technique · Levator muscle · Eyelid

Supplementary Information The online version contains supplementary material available at https://doi.org/10.1007/978-3-031-63178-8_18.

A. M. Perez
Herbert Wertheim College of Medicine, Miami, FL, USA

S. G. Cypen (✉)
Center for Excellence in Eye Care, Miami, FL, USA

Introduction

Blepharoptosis is characterized by inferior displacement or drooping of the upper eyelid, thus posing functional and cosmetic concerns in affected patients. In cases of ptosis with preserved levator function an external or internal ptosis repair utilizing levator muscle advancement or conjunctival-Müller's muscle may be considered but these procedures are likely inadequate when there exists severe ptosis with poor levator function.

Frontalis suspension is a commonly performed for moderate to severe ptosis in cases of poor levator muscle function [1]. This procedure restores the upper eyelid position by utilizing a suspension band to connect the frontalis muscle to the upper eyelid tarsus, thus, improving the patient's visual field and appearance [2]. Poor levator function is most commonly due to dysgenesis of the muscle fibers during development or dystrophy of the fibers due to neuromuscular dysfunction from autoimmune disease or genetic disorder [3]. Indications for surgical repair include ptosis resulting in functional loss of the superior visual field, chronic neck pain secondary to chin up head positioning, risk of amblyopia in children, and cosmetic dissatisfaction. The specific indications for frontalis eyelid suspension include congenital ptosis with poor levator function (less than 5 mm), chronic progressive external ophthalmoplegia, muscular dystrophy,

J. Tao (ed.), *Efficient Oculofacial Surgery*, https://doi.org/10.1007/978-3-031-63178-8_18

traumatic ptosis, cranial nerve III palsy, blepharophimosis syndrome, myasthenia gravis, and Marcus Gunn jaw-wink phenomenon [1].

The technique for frontalis suspension was initially described by Payr [4] in 1909 and reintroduced by Wright [5] in 1922; it has been modified and refined over the years. Autogenous fascia lata has long been used due to its durability and host site acceptance [2]. However, limitations to autogenous fascia lata use include difficulty in harvesting quality tissue, donor site morbidity, inability to harvest sufficient length in children under 3 years of age, and prolonged surgical times [2]. Alloplastic suspension slings of silicone or Gore-Tex have been used to improve surgical efficiency and eliminate second surgical site morbidity. However, as with any implantable foreign body, there is a concern for implant extrusion and infection. Moreover, some of these devices can break or otherwise fail.

In addition to the several sling material options, various surgical techniques have been described. These include eyelid crease or stab incisions for fixation, lash margin rotation sutures, and suspension configurations, such as single loop, double pentagon, or rhomboid [1]. A frontalis muscle advancement flap (described in a separate chapter) is an alternative to traditional frontalis suspension techniques altogether [6].

Herein, the authors describe an open blepharoplasty surgical technique that utilizes one supra-brow stab incision through which the sling is secured. Notwithstanding, the need to procure a sling graft or device, the procedure is highly effective and efficient. The authors generally use autologous or donor fascia lata (Tutoplast™) or an alloplastic silicone rod.

Surgical Technique (Video 18-1)

The patient is brought to the operating room. General anesthesia is required for most pediatric patients while many adult may tolerate the procedure under monitored anesthesia care or local only. The upper eyelid is marked with methylene blue for a conservative blepharoplasty, even in pediatric patients to reduce dermatochalasis due to skin bunching after sling elevation of the eyelid (Fig. 18.1A). The eyelid and brow are anesthetized with local anesthesia. The face is then prepped and draped in the usual, standard, sterile fashion for oculofacial surgery, and corneal protectors are placed.

The upper eyelid skin is incised using a #15 blade, and the flap of skin is excised using Westcott scissors. A small segment of orbicularis muscle is removed separately with scissors exposing the anterior aspect of the upper tarsus. A single, horizontal supraciliary stab incision is then created at the mid-brow, and a small pre-frontalis muscle pocket is dissected using Stevens scissors.

If autogenous fascia lata selected for the sling, attention is turned to the lateral lower thigh. Local anesthetic is administered to the planned incision site. Flexion of the knee can aid in achieving a better harvest angle. A 4–6 cm incision is fashioned with a #15 blade and dissection is carried down to the tensor fascia lata band that appears glistening white and with striations parallel to the leg. Army-navy retractors are used to further expose the fascia. Using a facelift scissors, the tissues superficial to the fascia lata band are released up the lateral thigh. A strip of fascia 0.8–1.2 cm wide is developed with sharp dissection. The cut, rectangular leading edge of fascia is advanced into a fascia lata stripper. The distal end of the fascia is secured with hemostats. While pulling gently on the fascia, the stripper is pushed up the leg in the wound to develop a fascia lata strip of sufficient length (usually 11–16 cm). The stripper should be advanced parallel to the fascia striations. The distal end of the fascia strip is cut by activating the guillotine on the stripper and the fascia is removed from the leg. The fascia is then cleaned of extraneous fat and connective tissues. If bilateral ptosis repair is planned, the single strip is divided longitudinally with a #15 blade and scissors. With scissors, the fascia lata strips are tapered into a point to allow it the ends to

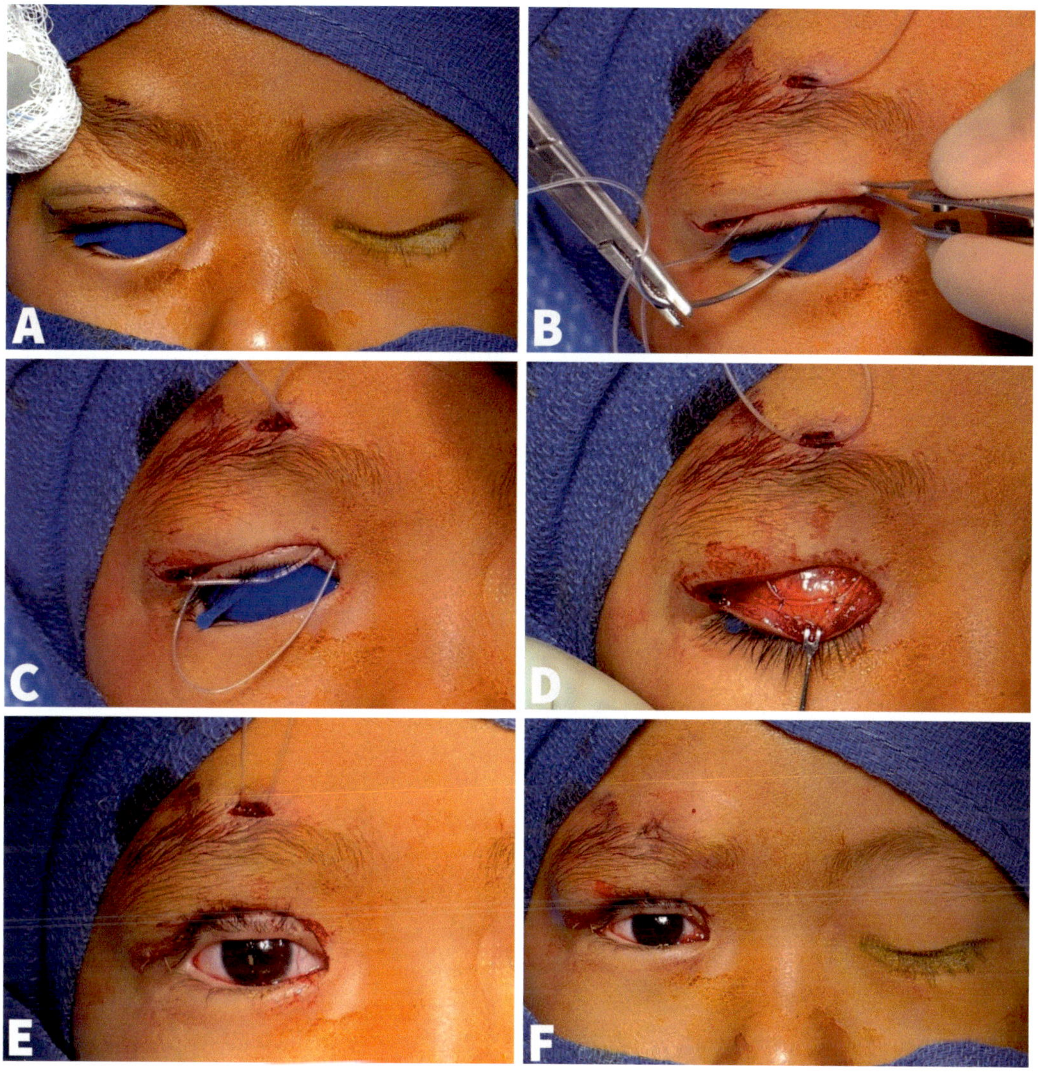

Fig. 18.1 (A) Crease marked for a conservative blepharoplasty; (B) frontalis sling (silicone shown) are introduced through the upper eyelid crease incision and advanced to the central stab incision at the brow with the aid of a free general surgery 1/2 circle needle; (C) the medial arm of the sling is secured to the superomedial orbital rim periosteum just anterior to the trochlea to forestall peaking of the eyelid margin contour due to sling tension from same superior vector; (D) the sling is sewn to the superior tarsal border anteriorly using two to three interrupted 6-0 polypropylene sutures; (E) the sling is tightened until adequate height, symmetry, and contour are achieved and then tied in a double knot; (F) immediate postoperative appearance

fit through a large general closure needle eyelet. The leg wound is closed with 3-0 polyglactin to the deep tissues and 5-0 chromic to the skin. Tissue glue (e.g. Dermabond™) is commonly used to reinforce the wound (Video 18-2).

The two ends of the frontalis sling (autologous or donor fascia lata or silicone) are introduced through the upper eyelid crease incision and advanced to the central stab incision at the brow with the aid of a free general surgery 1/2 circle needle (Fig. 18.1B). The medial arm of the sling is secured to the superomedial orbital rim periosteum just anterior to the trochlea to forestall nasal peaking of the eyelid margin contour (Fig. 18.1C). The lateral arm is advanced directly to the brow incision deep to the orbicularis muscle in the preseptal plane. The sling is then sewn to the superior tarsal border anteriorly using two to three interrupted 6-0 polypropylene sutures (Fig. 18.1D). Of note, care is taken to pass these sutures partial thickness to avoid cornea irritation. Several interrupted crease-forming 6-0 polyglactin sutures are placed through the cut edges of the upper eyelid skin incorporating superior tarsal tissue to form the eyelid crease. The rest of the skin incision on the upper eyelid is closed using interrupted 6-0 plain gut sutures. The sling is tightened until adequate height, symmetry, and contour are achieved and then tied in a double knot (Fig. 18.1E). The sling knot is then reinforced using a 6-0 polypropylene suture surrounding the knot. The tails of the knot are buried in the preformed deep tissue pocket, and the stab incision is closed using deep 6-0 polyglactin suture followed by 6-0 plain gut sutures to the skin. At the end of the case, the corneal protectors are removed, and antibiotic ophthalmic ointment is applied to the incisions (Fig. 18.1F). The patient is counseled on standard post-operative instructions and advised to continue frequent ocular surface lubrication, particularly in the early post-operative weeks. Figures 18.2 and 18.3 demonstrate a case of severe bilateral upper eyelid ptosis in a patient with chronic progressive external ophthalmoplegia who underwent successful ptosis repair with frontalis sling suspension.

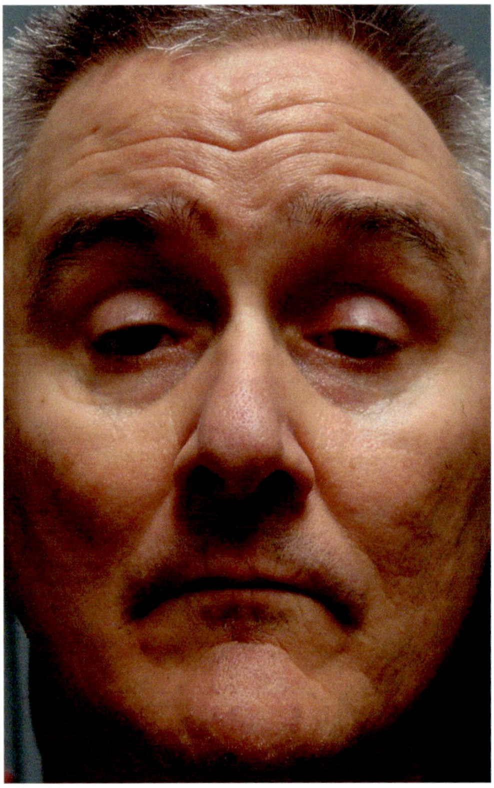

Fig. 18.2 Patient with bilateral poor levator function ptosis due to chronic progressive external ophthalmoplegia

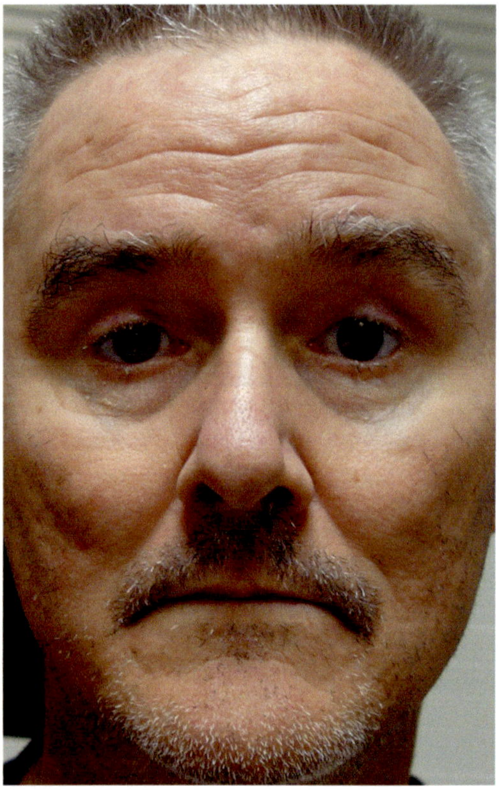

Fig. 18.3 Patient in Fig. 18.2 1-year status post bilateral frontalis suspension with a silicone rod with good improvement of blepharoptosis. Photo credit: Jeremiah Tao

Conclusion

Frontalis suspension ptosis repair is an effective surgical technique for patients with moderate to severe ptosis and poor levator function. The described open blepharoplasty with single brow incision technique achieves excellent functional and aesthetic results. Eyelid skin excision with skin anchoring may achieve a stronger eyelid crease without dermatochalasis than closed stab incision approaches. The single brow incision minimizes conspicuous forehead scars associated with other techniques. Autogenous fascia lata obviates cost or other complexities with procuring an alloplastic or donor device, but is associated with a second surgical site. Donor fascia lata or silicone are good off the shelf options, if available.

Financial Support The authors have no relevant sources of funding.

Conflicts of Interest The authors have no financial or conflicts of interest to disclose.

References

1. Sokol JA, Thornton IL, Lee HB, Nunery WR. Modified frontalis suspension technique with review of large series. Ophthalmic Plast Reconstr Surg. 2011;27(3):211–5.
2. Takahashi Y, Leibovitch I, Kakizaki H. Frontalis suspension surgery in upper eyelid blepharoptosis. Open Ophthalmol J. 2010;4:91–7.
3. Surve A, Sharma MC, Pushker N, Bajaj MS, Meel R, Kashyap S. A study of changes in levator muscle in congenital ptosis. Int Ophthalmol. 2019;39(6):1231–8.
4. Payr E. Plastik mittels freier Faszientransplantation bei ptosis. Dtsch Med Wochenschr. 1909;35:822.
5. Wright WW. The use of living sutures in the treatment of ptosis. Arch Ophthalmol. 1922;51:99–102.
6. Dallalzadeh LO, Park KS, Korn BS, Kikkawa DO, Liu CY. Minimal dissection direct frontalis muscle advancement flap for congenital ptosis repair. J Craniofac Surg. 2021;32(7):2358–61.

Lower Eyelid Ectropion Repair and Lateral Canthoplasty

19

Ian Patterson and Hassan Shah

Abstract

Ectropion is the outwards distraction of the eyelid away from the globe. This may cause ocular surface exposure and disfigurement. Ectropion may be due to involutional, mechanical, paralytic, or cicatricial etiologies. Treatment for ectropion varies according to the vector involved. This chapter will describe treatments for lower eyelid involutional ectropion that include horizontal tightening and lateral canthal anchoring.

Keywords

Ectropion · Involutional ectropion · Cicatricial ectropion · Paralytic · Canthoplasty · Canthopexy · Lateral tarsal strip · Medial spindle

Supplementary Information The online version contains supplementary material available at https://doi.org/10.1007/978-3-031-63178-8_19.

I. Patterson · H. Shah (✉)
Department of Ophthalmology and Visual Science, University of Chicago, Chicago, IL, USA
e-mail: hshah1@bsd.uchicago.edu

Introduction

Ectropion typically affects the lower eyelid and is one of the most frequently encountered eyelid malpositions [1, 2]. Clinically, it manifests as an everted eyelid, causing exposure of the conjunctiva and cornea and can result in chronic blepharitis, chronic conjunctivitis, and dry eye syndrome. Traditionally, ectropion is classified as either congenital or acquired, which includes involutional, paralytic, mechanical, and cicatricial etiologies. Involutional ectropion is the most common etiology and usually presents in older adults [1]. A number of factors contribute to its development, including laxity of the lateral and medial canthal tendons, orbicularis oculi degeneration, and disinsertion of the capsule-palpebral fascia and inferior tarsal muscle (lower eyelid retractors) [1]. It is generally thought that lateral canthal tendon laxity is the primary contributor to the development of involutional ectropion [2, 3]. A number of techniques exist for the surgical treatment of involutional ectropion.

Lateral Canthoplasty

The specific surgical objective is to rotate the out-turned eyelid so that it has good apposition to the globe. To tighten a lateral canthal tendon, the lower eyelid is disinserted, shortened, and reattached. There are variations, but almost all

J. Tao (ed.), *Efficient Oculofacial Surgery*, https://doi.org/10.1007/978-3-031-63178-8_19

techniques involve securing the lateral eyelid tarsus to the lateral orbital rim periosteum.

After administering local anesthetic to the lateral canthal region, a #15 Bard Parker blade scalpel is used to make an incision approximately 5 mm in length through the skin and orbicularis extending posteriorly from the lateral canthus. Cantholysis of the inferior ramus of the lateral canthal tendon is carried out with sharp dissection.

The lateral tarsal strip procedure, first described in 1979 by Anderson and Gordy, is a popular approach [2–4]. This procedure involves dissecting the lateral tarsus from the anterior lamella, excising these layers separately, and then using a double armed suture to anchor the tarsus to the lateral orbital wall periosteum (Fig. 19.1). Alternatively, a small lateral full thickness eyelid wedge resection and suturing the tarsus to periosteum (Bick procedure) can be performed (Video 19-1).

The exposed tarsus at the lateral eyelid is secured with 4-0, or 5-0 polyglactin, braided polyester, or polypropylene suture. This suture is then used to anchor the tarsus to the periosteum of the lateral orbital rim just inside the superior canthal tendon. Care is taken to make sure that the direction of the lower eyelid after re-anchoring is superior, posterior, and lateral. Once it is confirmed that the lower eyelid is in an appropriate position, the skin can then be closed in a simple interrupted fashion using 5-0 gut suture.

Possible complications of this procedure include overcorrection with inturning of the lateral eyelashes, suture related granuloma, and postoperative dehiscence of the lateral canthus.

Canthoplasty is an excellent option for most cases of ectropion. However, there are certain situations where a more robust attachment of the lateral canthal tendon to the lateral orbital periosteum is required. Medial ectropion sometimes mandates medial tightening procedures such as a medial spindle or retractor band tightening. Cases with concomitant eyelid retraction often require grafts to support the eyelid. In addition

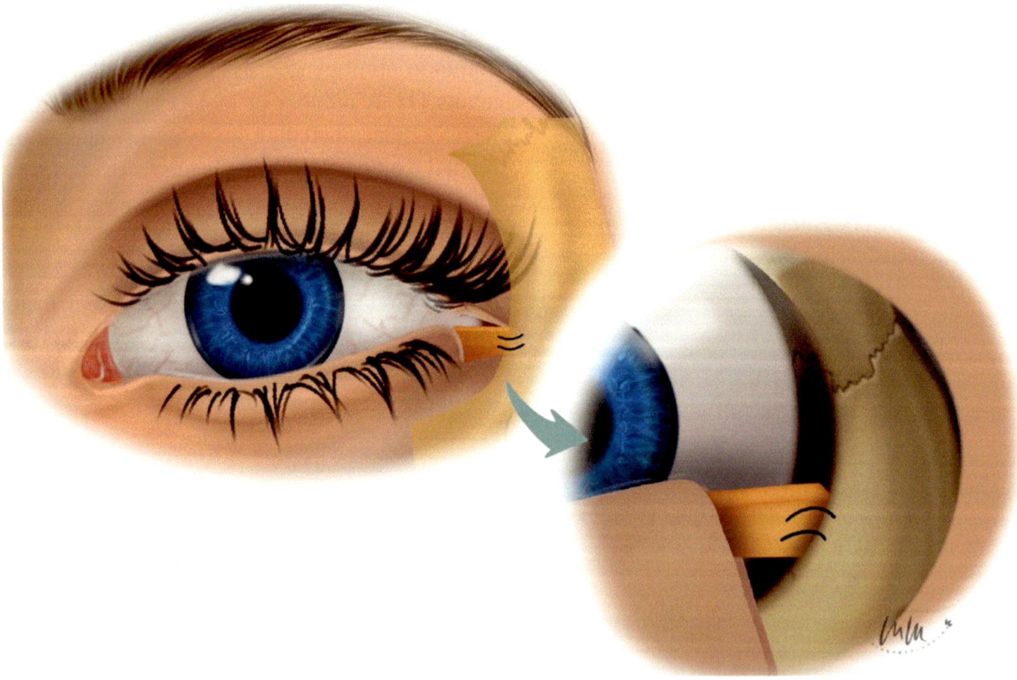

Fig. 19.1 Lateral tarsal strip illustration. Tarsal tongue is dissected then secures to the lateral orbital rim periosteum. *Image courtesy of Suzana Matayoshi, MD*

to grafts, a concomitant tarsoconjunctival flap to suspend the lower eyelid may be useful in the presence of lower eyelid retraction, especially due to paralytic vectors.

Lateral Drill Hole Canthopexy (Video 19-2)

When there are poor periosteal fixation options, a drill hole may be useful. After lateral canthotomy and cantholysis, the lateral orbital rim is exposed, incised and elevated to expose the lateral orbital rim bone. This dissection is carried out superiorly in the area where the transorbital holes will be created. These should ideally be placed 1 to 2 mm posterior and superior to the lateral orbital tubercle to create appropriate elevation and lateralization of the lower eyelid. Once the bone is exposed, one or two 1 mm holes are made through the lateral orbital rim. The globe should be protected with a malleable retractor during drill hole formation [5]. A non-absorbable 4-0 polypropylene or braided polyester suture is then used to secure the tarsus as described above. The 2 ends of the suture are then passed through the drill holes from internal to external. The suture ends are pulled to lateralize the lateral canthal tendon until the eyelid is in the correct position. The sutures are tied together on the external surface of the orbital rim. To obviate the suture knot being palpable at the rim, the sutures may be tied further lateral to the temporalis fascia. A temporalis fascial fixation point also requires only one drill hole, through which both arms can be passed. Closure of the canthotomy site is performed in a layered manner. Absorbable suture is used to close the periosteum and orbicularis. Finally, skin is closed in a simple interrupted fashion using 5-0 plain gut suture.

Lateral Periosteal Flap

In cases with tissue loss, the lateral periosteal flap offers another surgical alternative. Dryden and Edelstein and later, Korteweg described its applications for ectropion repair. Like the lateral transorbital canthopexy with drill holes, the lateral periosteal flap canthoplasty offers a durable fixation point for the lower lateral tarsus, theoretically lowering the risk of dehiscence [6, 7]. The periosteal flap is strong and when properly constructed, has a vector of action that mimics the natural lateral canthal tendon [7].

After completing a canthotomy and cantholysis, a periosteal elevator is used to expose the external orbital rim, elevating the orbicularis away from the periosteum so the periosteal flap can be created. The flap should be approximately 10 mm in length and 6 mm in height and should be medially based/hinged starting 2–3 mm inside the orbital rim. Once mobilized, the flap should be sutured to the denuded tarsus of the lower eyelid using a non-absorbable 5-0 polyglactin, braided polyester or polypropylene suture in an overlapping fashion (Fig. 19.2). The skin is then closed with 5-0 plain gut suture in a simple interrupted fashion [7].

Tarsoconjunctival Suspension Flap (Video 19-3)

In cases of ectropion with concomitant eyelid retraction, tarsoconjunctival suspension (a.k.a. onlay) flap (TCSF) may be useful. This is commonly combined with a horizontal tightening procedure such as a lateral tarsal strip. This achieves robust elevation of the lateral lower eyelid and a lateral tarsorrhaphy effect. Owing to the attachment site of the lower eyelid margin superior to the lateral (and posterior to) upper eyelid, the lower eyelid can be raised higher than with an intermarginal adhesion tarsorrhaphy.

The technique is described in detail in other chapters, but in brief, a temporary suture (e.g., 5-0 polyglactin or 4-0 silk) is passed through the upper eyelid margin and the upper eyelid is everted over cotton-tipped applicators or Desmarres retractor (Fig. 19.3). A lateral canthotomy and inferior cantholysis are performed with scissors and the lower eyelid is shortened 1–3 mm with or without developing a tarsal strip.

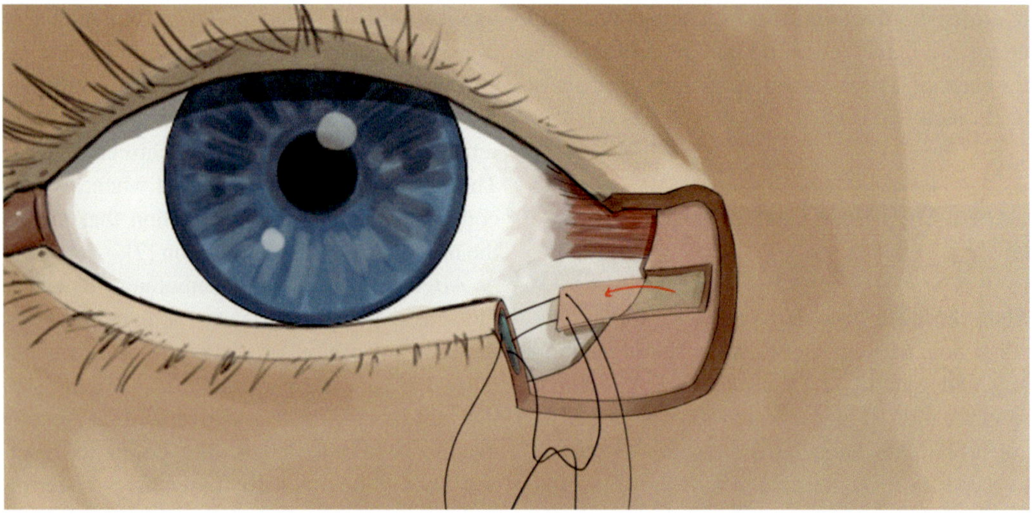

Fig. 19.2 Illustration depicting a periosteal flap developed at the lateral orbital rim

Methylene blue or a marker is used to delineate the tarsoconjunctival flap on the posterior lamella of the everted upper eyelid. Typically, a horizontal line is marked 2 to 4 mm superior to the upper eyelid margin from the far lateral canthus to the desired horizontal width of the flap. The horizontal width of the flap varies according to the amount of desired palpebral fissure narrowing but ranges from 3 to 10 mm. With smaller flaps, minimal or no tarsus may be included. The amount of vertical dissection is dependent on the amount of lower eyelid elevation desired; less dissection is associated with a greater lift. A vertical incision and dissection of 2 to 5 mm is usually sufficient. Using a 15-blade or scissors or both, the flap is developed along the desired markings. Hemostasis can be achieved with electrocautery.

With a 15-blade or scissors is used to denude epithelium posterior to the gray line of the lateral lower eyelid margin—the length of which corresponds with the size of the flap and extending medially from the inferior cantholysis. In some cases, the attachment site of the flap on the lower eyelid margin is placed slightly medial to the sagittal plane of the medial aspect of the flap origin to achieve some additional lower eyelid horizontal tightening.

The leading edge of the tarsoconjunctival flap is sewn to the denuded margin of the lower eyelid using a 5-0 polyglactin suture in an interrupted horizontal mattress fashion. The free lateral tarsus or tarsal strip is secured with 4-0 braided polyester suture and secured to the lateral rim periosteum. The result is a very stable lower eyelid that has strong fixation laterally (rim), and vertically (posterior lamella of the lateral upper fornix) that improves both ectropion and retraction (Figs. 19.4, 19.5, 19.6 and 19.7).

Medial Ectropion

In some cases of ectropion, lateral canthal tendon tightening may be inadequate. These cases may be better addressed with a *medial spindle procedure*. It can be a standalone procedure or an adjunct to horizontal eyelid tightening to further rotate the eyelid margin towards the globe. Using a blade or scissors, an excision from the posterior lamellae is fashioned in a diamond shape horizontally and vertically. Double armed 6-0 chromic gut or polyglactin sutures are then used engage the lower eyelid retractors, shorten the posterior lamella, and thereby rotate the medial eyelid margin against the globe. The sutures may be tied posteriorly and buried within the wound or passed and tied externally (Fig. 19.8).

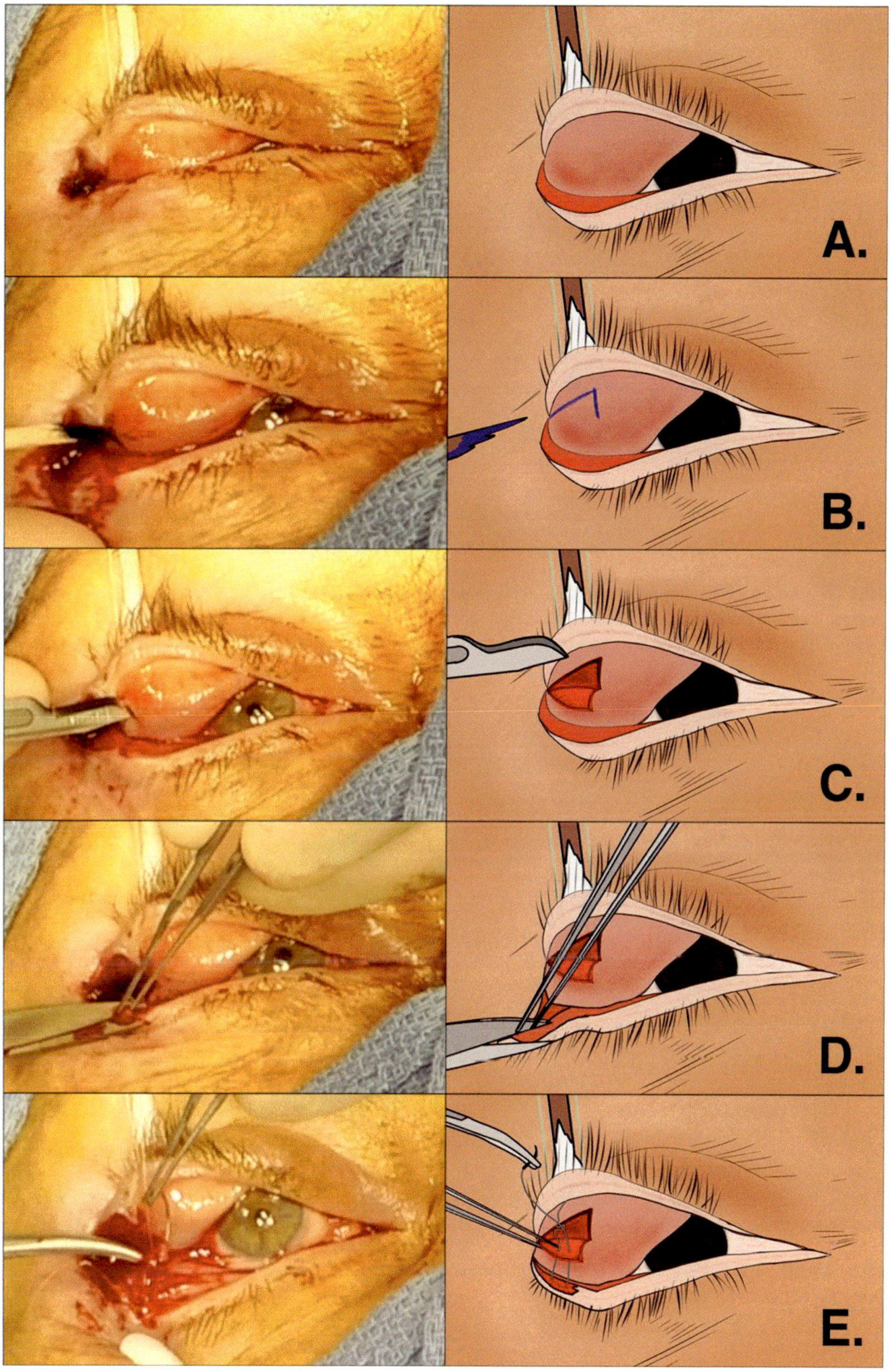

Fig. 19.3 Lateral tarsoconjunctival suspension flap surgical sequence with corresponding illustrations

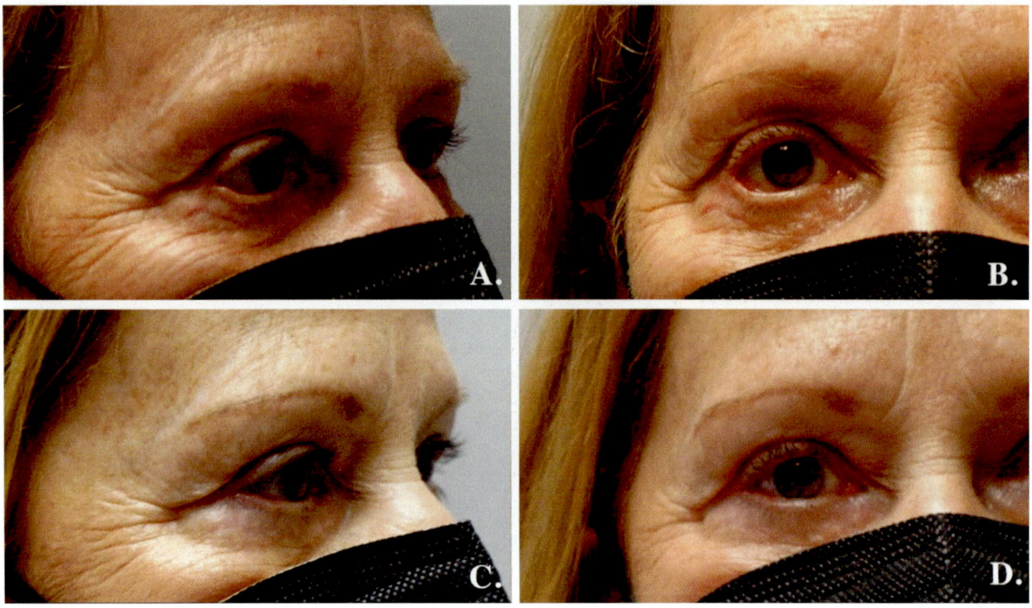

Fig. 19.4 Before (A, B) demonstrating cicatricial and involutional ectropion. Patient is status post cosmetic lower eyelid blepharoplasty as well as two prior attempts at lateral canthal anchoring alone elsewhere. After (C, D) lateral tarsoconjunctival suspension flap and lateral tarsal strip repair. Photo credit: Jeremiah Tao

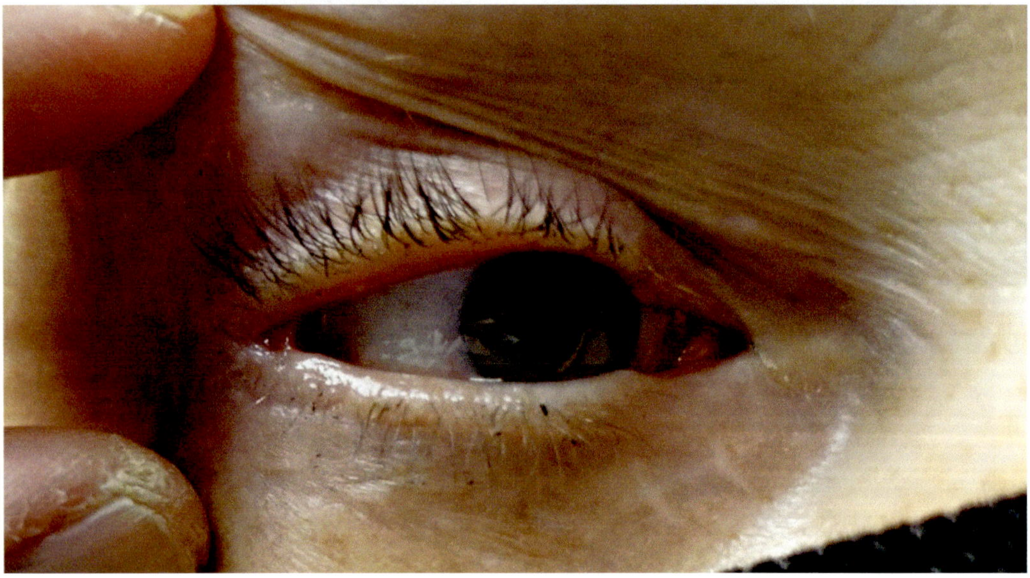

Fig. 19.5 Patient in Fig. 19.4 after ectropion and retraction repair with the tarsoconjunctival flap only visible with the upper eyelid manually elevated

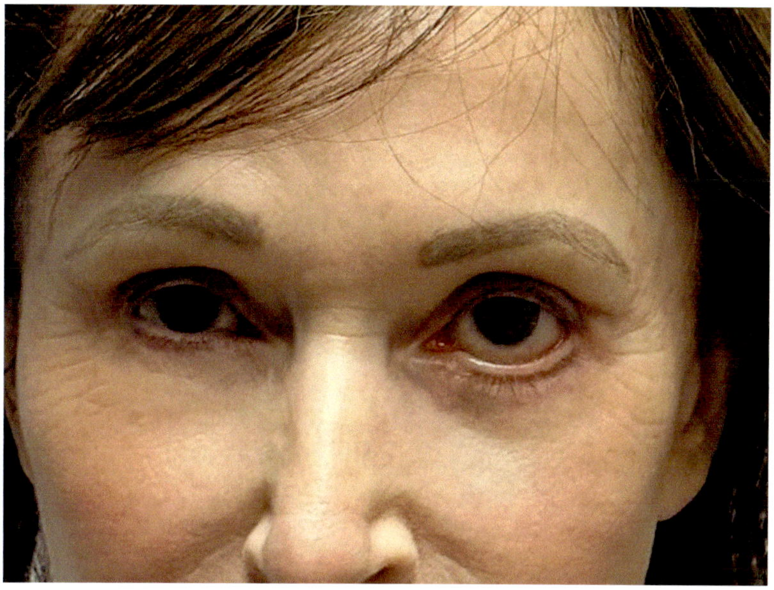

Fig. 19.6 Patient status post cosmetic lower eyelid blepharoplasty as well as two prior attempts at lateral canthal anchoring and posterior lamella acellular dermal matrix graft elsewhere

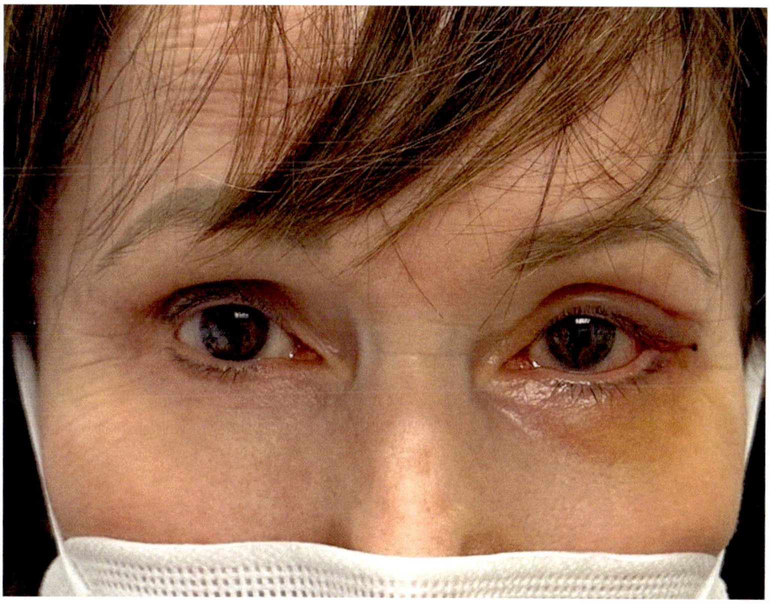

Fig. 19.7 Patient in Fig. 19.6 1-week status post lateral tarsoconjunctival suspension flap and lateral tarsal strip repair correction of lower eyelid ectropion and retraction. Photo credit: Jeremiah Tao

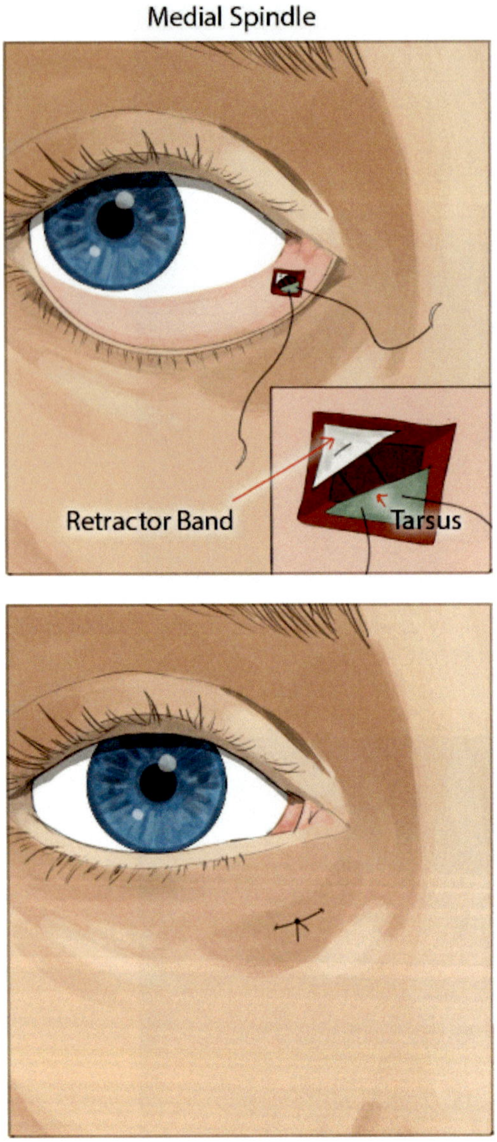

Fig. 19.8 Medial spindle procedure for medial ectropion

Conclusions

Ectropion is a common malposition of the lower eyelid that may result from involutional, cicatricial, paralytic, or mechanical vectors. Many cases of ectropion involve horizontal eyelid laxity. In these instances, a lateral canthal anchoring procedure such as the lateral tarsal strip is commonly used. Concomitant procedures such as a drill hole, suspension flap, or medial spindle may be useful in select cases.

References

1. Bedran EGM, Pereira MVC, Bernardes TF. Ectropion. Semin Ophthalmol. 2010;25(3):59–65.
2. Damasceno RW, Osaki MH, Dantas PEC, Belfort R. Involutional entropion and ectropion of the lower eyelid: prevalence and associated risk factors in the elderly population. Ophthalmic Plast Reconstr Surg. 2011;27(5):317–20.
3. Anderson RL, Gordy DD. The tarsal strip procedure. Arch Ophthalmol. 1979;97(11):2192–6.
4. Kam KYR, Cole CJ, Bunce C, Watson MP, Kamal D, Olver JM. The lateral tarsal strip in ectropion surgery: is it effective when performed in isolation? Eye. 2012;26:827–32.
5. Moe KS, Linder T. The lateral transorbital canthopexy for correction and prevention of ectropion: report of a procedure, grading system, and outcome study. Arch Facial Plast Surg. 2000;2(1):9–15.
6. Dryden RM, Edelstein JP. Lateral palpebral tendon repair for lower eyelid ectropion. Ophthalmic Plast Reconstr Surg. 1988;4(2):115–8. https://doi.org/10.1097/00002341-198804020-00012. PMID: 3154724.
7. Korteweg SF, Stenekes MW, van Zyl FE, Werker PM. Paralytic ectropion treatment with lateral periosteal flap canthoplasty and introduction of the ectropion severity score. Plast Reconstr Surg Glob Open. 2014;2(5): e151.

Cicatricial Ectropion Repair with Skin Graft

20

Jeremy Clark

Abstract

Cicatricial ectropion occurs when the eyelid is abnormally rotated outward due to shortening of the eyelid or midface skin. This eyelid malposition causes exposure of the ocular surface that can result in irritation, corneal dryness, conjunctival injection, and other visual complaints. Treatment typically involves replacement or recruitment of skin combined with lateral canthal anchoring procedures. This chapter describes lower eyelid ectropion repair with a skin graft.

Keywords

Skin graft · Cicatricial ectropion · Eyelid scarring

Introduction

Cicatricial ectropion is the abnormal rotation of the eyelid away from the ocular surface. It may be both disfiguring and medically significant. In addition to dry eye and ocular irritation, corneal damage and loss of vision are possible due to this eyelid malposition.

There are many causes of anterior lamellar disease that lead to cicatricial ectropion. Actinic damage from chronic sun exposure, dermatologic conditions such as rosacea, and even iatrogenic anterior lamellar shortening post blepharoplasty or Mohs reconstruction are all common causes of cicatricial ectropion.

Systemic Diseases

Bilateral cicatricial ectropion can be a result of a variety of systemic diseases such as ichthyosis and psoriatic arthritis. Ichthyosis is an inherited group of dermatoses characterized by dry and scaly skin due to impaired keratinization which can, over time, cause contracture of the lower eyelid leading to ectropion. Psoriatic arthritis is a common chronic inflammatory condition affecting the skin and joints of those with an underlying genetic predisposition. It is characterized by concomitant symptoms of

Supplementary Information The online version contains supplementary material available at https://doi.org/10.1007/978-3-031-63178-8_20.

J. Clark (✉)
University of Louisville, Louisville, KY, USA
e-mail: docclark83@gmail.com

J. Tao (ed.), *Efficient Oculofacial Surgery*, https://doi.org/10.1007/978-3-031-63178-8_20

erythematous, scaly, pruritic plaques most commonly on the extensor surfaces of the knees and elbows along with arthritis of the fingers and lower spine. Ocular manifestations of psoriatic arthritis vary, but the eyelids can be affected by chronic blepharitis and loss of eyelid tissue leading to ectropion. Because of the long-term nature and systemic manifestations of these conditions, symptom recurrence and a potential need for repeated surgery may be necessary.

Dermatologic Conditions

Dermatologic conditions such as ocular rosacea and discoid lupus erythematosus should be considered for anyone presenting with cicatricial ectropion. Discoid lupus erythematosus accounts for most of the chronic cutaneous lupus erythematosus. It is rarely associated with systemic disease, and it typically presents with erythematous, inflammatory scaly plaques affecting areas with exposure to UV light that heal but cause significant scarring and atrophy which can ultimately result in cicatricial ectropion.

Post Blepahroplasty

Post blepharoplasty lower eyelid ectropion is common owing to the pervasiveness of cosmetic lower eyelid or midfacial surgery. Over aggressive resection or poor technique or both can cause the lower eyelid to pull away from the globe.

Infectious Diseases

Periocular infections and associated inflammation may induce cicatricial changes to the skin that can cause ectropion. Surgical repair of ectropion should be delayed until the active infection is resolved and the tissues are quiescent. However, a tension suture tarsorrhaphy (i.e., Frost) may be useful to counteract vectors actively pulling the eyelid away from the globe.

Medications

Antineoplastics, bisphosphonates, and topical antiglaucoma agents have been associated with the development of cicatricial ectropion. Cetuximab, a monoclonal antibody that inhibits cell-signaling pathways used primarily in colorectal cancer treatment, is associated with madarosis and cicatricial ectropion. Cases of cicatricial ectropion with cetuximab have been described as soon as one week after beginning treatment with resolution six week after discontinuation of therapy. Similar ocular reactions have been described with the use of erlotinib, an antineoplastic agent used to treat non-small-cell lung cancer, and 5-flurouracil, a fluorinated pyrimidine used to treat cancers of the breast, colon, and skin. Notably, both topical and systemic 5-Flurouracil have been implicated in the occurrence of cicatricial ectropion. Bisphosphonates is another medication class associated with cicatricial ectropion. They are commonly prescribed to treat osteoporosis, bone metastasis, multiple myeloma and Paget's disease. These drugs have the potential to cause maxillary osteonecrosis ultimately leading to cicatricial ectropion. Lastly, anti-glaucoma agents such as dorzolamide and brimonidine have rarely been associated with ectropion. Of note, compared to other causes of cicatricial ectropion, which typically require surgical correction, most causes of medication-induced cicatricial ectropion resolve with discontinuation of the offending medication.

Trauma

Cicatricial ectropion can occur as a consequence of direct eyelid injury or facial burns. Cicatricial ectropion is a common iatrogenic problem from orbitofacial fracture repair with poor orbitotomy technique.

Other

Radiation to the head and neck poses a significant risk for cicatricial ectropion through skin contraction and distortion, along with muscle atrophy. Treatment should be delayed until radiation therapy has been completed and after adequate revascularization and healing of treated areas.

Clinical Evaluation

Patients may experience epiphora, foreign body sensation, redness, and irritation. Eversion of the lower eyelid can cause lacrimal outflow failure and if chronic, these patients can show complete or partial punctal stenosis. Because the palpebral conjunctiva can be chronically everted, keratinization may ensue. Prolonged ocular exposure can ultimately cause corneal decompensation and in severe cases corneal ulceration or infection. Furthermore, depending on the cause, there may exist neurotrophic disease or follicular keratitis that may warrant separate treatments.

The exam should include assessment of skin shortening. For instance, vertically oriented anterior lamellar striae are a sign of skin tightening. Other signs include limited movement of the lower eyelid with upward gaze and decreased skin recoil upon manual downward lower eyelid distraction. Orbicularis oculi tone can be assessed by having the patient squeeze their eyes closed forcefully. Then, the examiner manually tries to open the eyelids of the patient. The force required to open the eyelids can be graded.

Surgical Management with Full Thickness Skin Graft (FTSG)

Full-thickness skin grafts lengthen the anterior lamella and aid in returning the lower eyelid to a more normal anatomic position. Common donor sites for the skin graft include the upper eyelid, post-auricular, supraclavicular, and upper inner arm areas. It is important to consider the color and thickness of the donor graft and the upper eyelid is generally the best match. In addition to donor site considerations, patient selection is key because a skin graft can leave a conspicuous scar or be associated with color and other mismatch with the surrounding recipient site.

For most anterior lamellar skin grafting procedures, skin grafting is combined with a lateral canthal anchoring procedure such as a lateral tarsal strip. Initially, local anesthesia is injected into the anterior lamella along with the area of the skin graft (Fig. 20.1). A subciliary incision

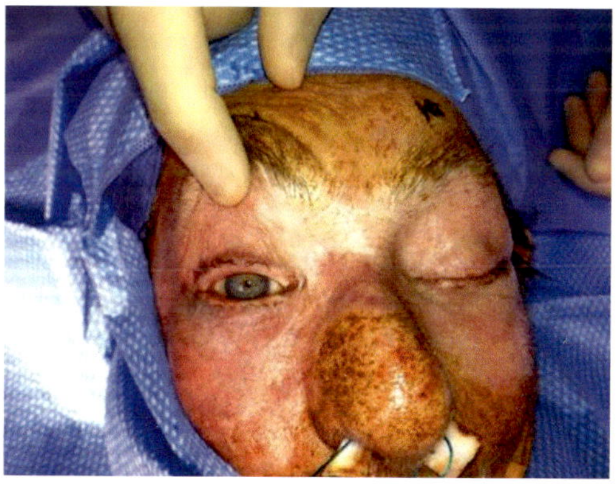

Fig. 20.1 Right lower eyelid cicatricial ectropion with eversion site

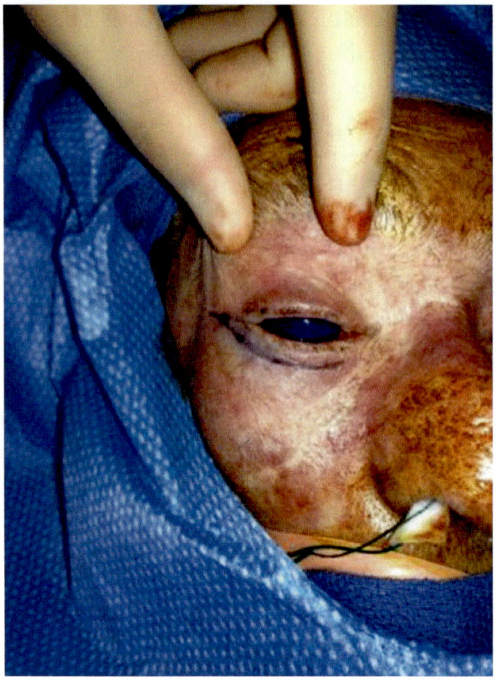

Fig. 20.2 A subciliary incision is planned across the horizontal extent of the lower eyelid. The subciliary incision should extend 5–10 mm past the lateral canthus

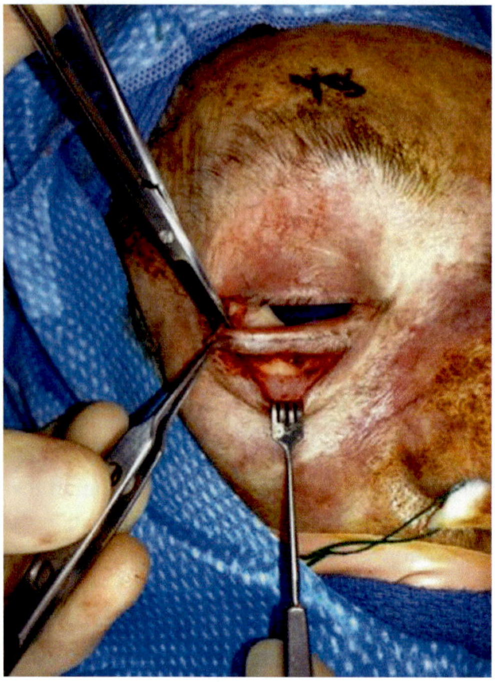

Fig. 20.3 A subciliary incision is fashioned with a scalpel and extended past the canthus. Through this wound cicatricial bands are released. The inferior crus of the lateral canthal tendon is released

is made to release the area of anterior lamellar deficiency. Further dissection is performed to release the lower eyelid completely so that it can be freely mobilized superiorly along with releasing any residual deep cicatricial bands (Figs. 20.2 and 20.3). Complete dissection through middle and deep posterior lamella structures to the level of conjunctiva is often useful to ensure complete release of cicatricial vectors (Figs. 20.3 and 20.4). This more adequately mobilizes the eyelid and prevents ectropion recurrence.

Horizontal tightening is usually performed to treat any laxity as well as anchor the eyelid. A lateral canthotomy is performed with inferior

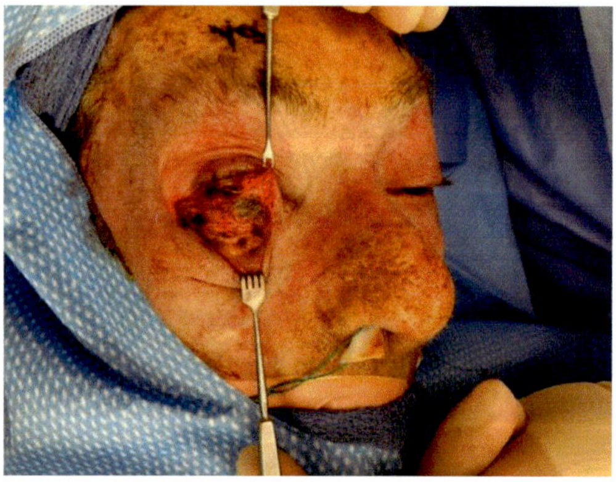

Fig. 20.4 Further dissection is performed through cicatricial bands (often through all eyelid layers except conjunctiva) to freely mobilize the lower eyelid

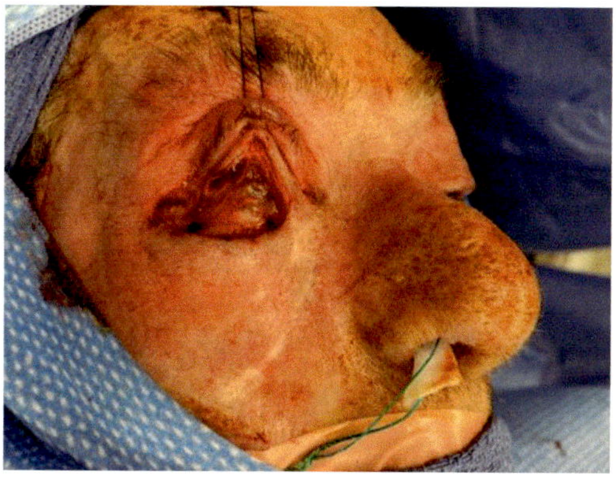

Fig. 20.5 Once all cicatricial bands are released, lateral canthal anchoring is performed with or without formation of a lateral tarsal strip

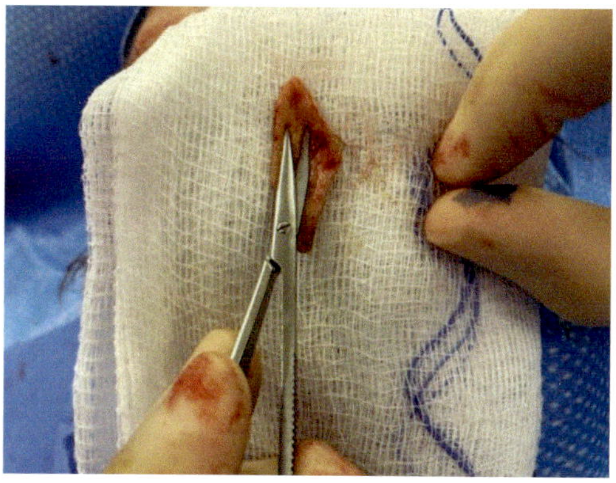

Fig. 20.7 The graft is thinned by trimming subcutaneous fat or muscle with scissors

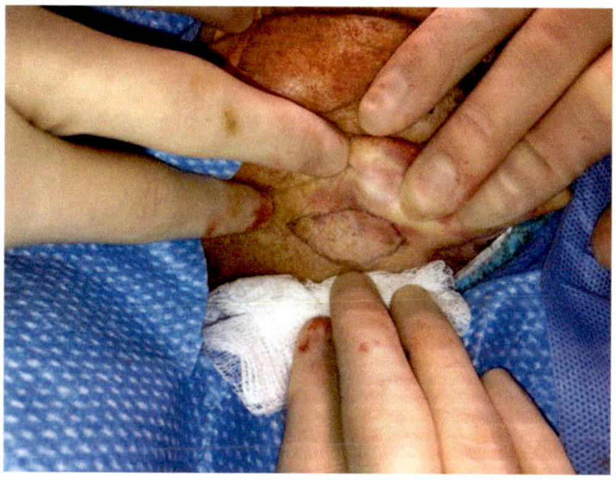

Fig. 20.6 The anterior lamellar defect is measured and an appropriately sized graft is harvested from the donor site (postauricular shown here)

cantholysis and further dissection between the anterior and posterior lamella for approximately 5–10 mm. The released lateral canthal tendon is anchored in the appropriate position along the internal lateral orbital rim at the level of the lateral orbital tubercle (Fig. 20.5). Once all cicatricial bands are released, the eyelid should be easily elevated and rotated to a normal anatomical position flush with eyeball. A Frost suture tarsorrhaphy is placed on upward tension to counter inferior contractile forces from healing as well as gravity. An appropriately sized graft is harvested from the donor site (Fig. 20.6). The ideal donor site is the upper eyelid but if there exists insufficient skin or upper eyelid surgery is otherwise undesirable, other common skin harvest sites are behind the ear (postauricular), along the base of the neck (supraclavicular), in front of the ear (preauricular), or from the inner arm.

The graft is further removed of all subcutaneous fat (or orbicularis oculi muscle if from the upper eyelid) so that only dermis and epidermis remain (Fig. 20.7). The skin graft is placed into position and trimmed to best fit the area of the defect. It is secured with 5-0 or 6-0 plain gut suture. Ideally, the skin should be on slight stretch. A pressure patch is placed over a nonadherent dressing to prevent collection of fluid or dislocation (Video 20-1; Fig. 20.8).

With good technique and proper patient selection, good results can be achieved (Figs. 20.9, 20.10, 20.11 and 20.12). However, patients should be prepared for the potential need for scar modulation or revision described below.

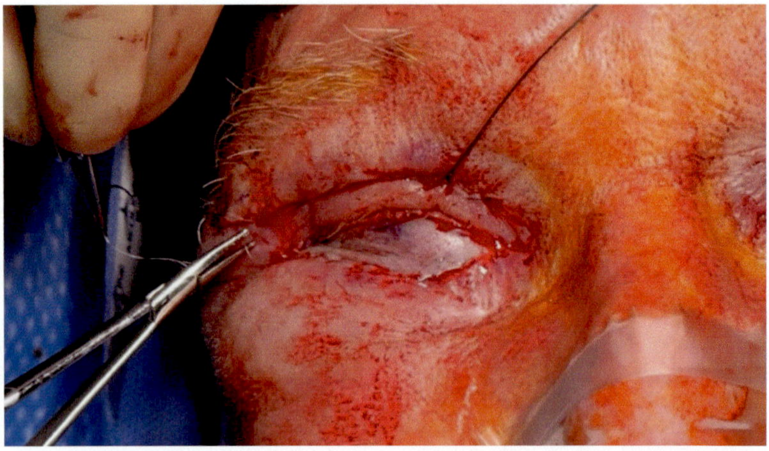

Fig. 20.8 Skin graft placed into position and secured along the perimeter of the defect with a 6-0 plain or 6-0 chromic suture. A 4-0 silk suture is placed to achieve upwards tension for approximately 1 week. After topical antibiotic is applied to the surgical site, a moderate pressure dressing is applied (the authors typically place a nonadherent Telfa® dressing under two folded eyepads, secured with paper tape). Photo credit: Jeremiah Tao

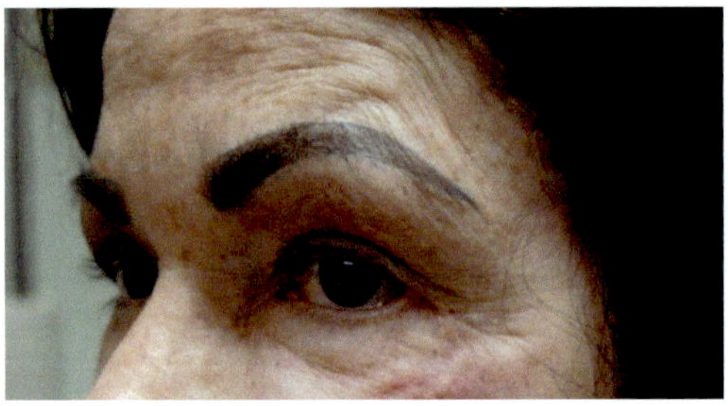

Fig. 20.9 Cicatricial retraction and ectropion after cosmetic blepharoplasty

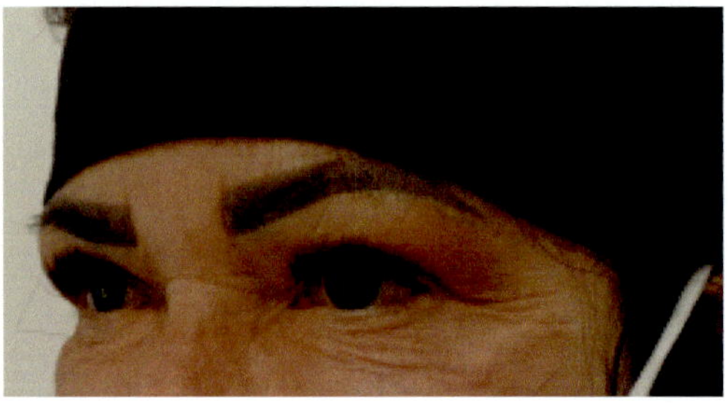

Fig. 20.10 3 years post lower eyelid ectropion repair with skin graft from upper eyelid. Fair complexion and fine rhytids contribute to good aesthetic result and minimally conspicuous scarring. Photo credit: Jeremiah Tao

Other Therapies

Surgical management remains the gold standard for treatment of cicatricial ectropion; however, other nonsurgical treatments have been described and, as aforementioned, include the use of hyaluronic acid, corticosteroid, or 5-fluorouracil injections.

A midface lift (also known as a suborbicularis oculi fat lift (SOOF) lift can obviate a skin graft in some instances. This approach is often pursued in the post cosmetic blepharoplasty setting in which a patient is still seeking an excellent aesthetic outcome. These are performed with or without posterior lamella spacers. Additional canthoplasty or tarsoconjunctival suspension flaps are other adjuncts. These are described in other chapters (Figs. 20.13 and 20.14).

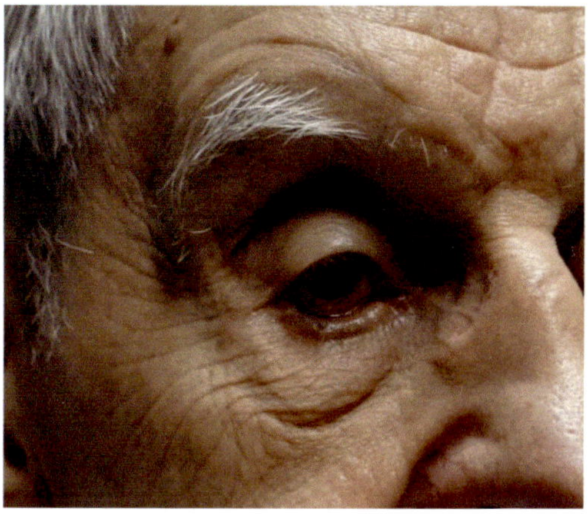

Fig. 20.11 Combined involutional and cicatricial retraction and ectropion. Photo credit: Jeremiah Tao

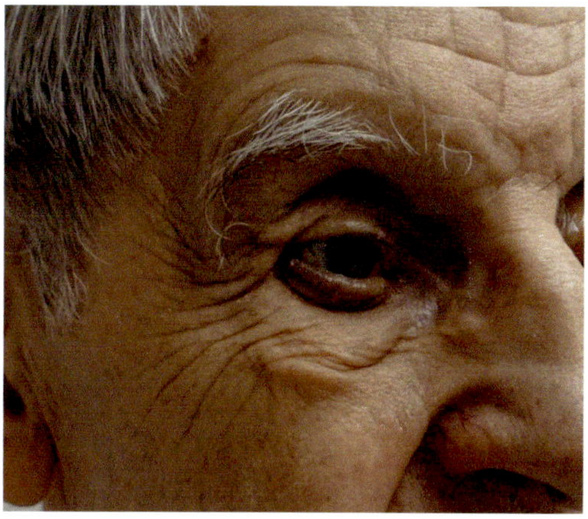

Fig. 20.12 4 months post lower eyelid ectropion repair with skin graft from upper eyelid. Fair complexion and thin skin with inferior edge of graft placed near the palpebromalar groove contribute to good aesthetic result and minimally conspicuous scarring. University of California, Irvine

Complications

Cicatricial ectropion repair with full thickness skin graft typically has a high success rate with minimal graft failure or necrosis. However, it is important to consider some of the complications that can occur with skin grafting.

Graft Failure or Necrosis

A hematoma or seroma can separate the graft from the wound bed. This prevents the graft from receiving vital nutrition from the donor site and increases the risk of graft failure. Appropriate pressure dressing or anchoring sutures can help decrease this risk. Some surgeons also advocate for providing slit incisions to allow egress of fluid and promote adherence and graft-donor opposition. Graft Infection can also occur and may lead to graft failure.

If graft failure is evident, it may require debridement or repeat surgery. However, the authors advocate expectant management and leaving the graft as a biological dressing to cover the wound until the time of revision surgery. In some instances, portions of the graft may take and other areas healed through second intention may result in a stable, adequately positioned eyelid.

Primary Contracture/Secondary Contracture

The full-thickness-skin graft (FTSG) is more likely to have primary contracture after harvesting due to the passive recoil of elastin fibers in the dermis. This will reduce the amount of added anterior lamellar support and makes recurrence more likely or cicatricial retraction a possibility. To avoid this, it is important to harvest a graft that is 1–2 mm larger than the lamellar defect. Split thickness skin grafts (STSG) do not have as much primary contracture because they have a smaller proportion of the dermis.

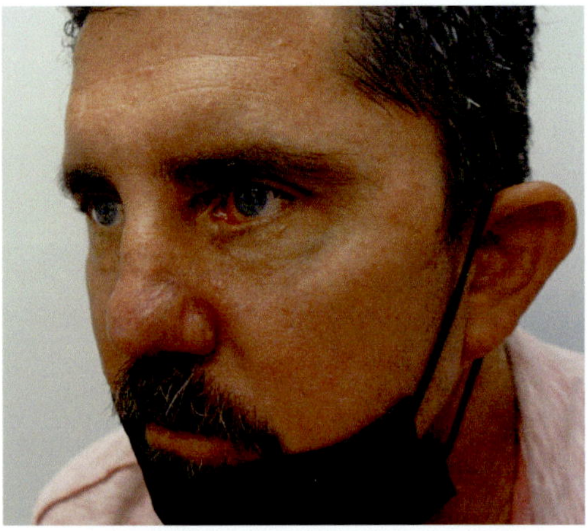

Fig. 20.13 Medial lower eyelid cicatricial retraction and ectropion due to trauma

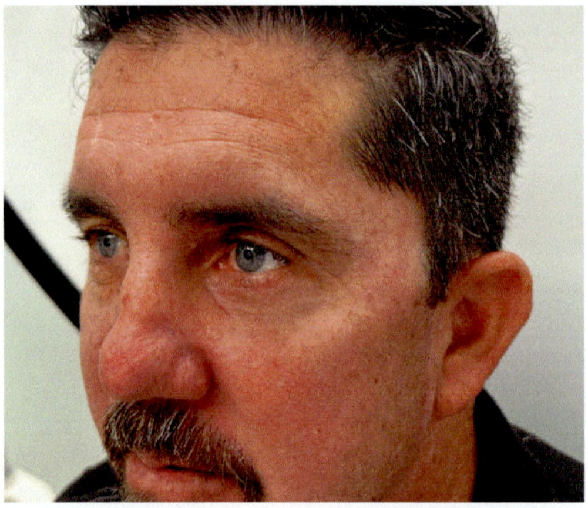

Fig. 20.14 Patient in Fig. 20.13 after eyelid 3 months status post repair with a skin graft harvested from the ipsilateral upper eyelid crease. Photo credit: Jeremiah Tao

Unlike STSG, full thickness grafts are less likely to shrink with time because there is usually a less robust myofibroblast deposition. However, it is possible to see FTSG shrink with time, especially in cases of facial burns or cutaneous chemical injuries.

Scarring

Skin grafts may lead to conspicuous scarring at the graft interface or may result in skin tone or texture mismatch. The use of upper eyelid skin may minimize these risks owing to the more similar and thinner skin. Nevertheless, hypertrophic scarring can be managed medically or surgically. In general, within 6 months, corticosteroid or 5 fluorouracil injections may be useful. Surgical revision may have a role in mature scars.

Donor Site Morbidity

Ipsilateral or contralateral upper eyelid skin is an ideal tissue match for the lateral eyelid defect; however, large grafts may cause anterior lamellar shortage to the upper eyelid. Hence upper eyelid skin harvest should obey resection parameters and principles of blepharoplasty. Additionally, harvesting skin laterally may be more resistant to upper eyelid malposition or lagophthalmos.

The retroauricular site is also a common harvest site. It is usually thin, non-hair-bearing and camouflages a surgical incision well. If a patient wears spectacles, the harvest site should be inferior and away from the resting position of the spectacle temple piece.

Overcorrection

Although rare, it is possible to overcorrect the lower eyelid. Entropion or reverse ptosis can be seen and usually requires raising and debulking the graft to shorten the subciliary anterior lamellae.

Conclusion

Cicatricial ectropion is common. Surgical release of all cicatricial vectors followed with full-thickness skin grafting and horizontal eyelid tightening remains one of the most effective treatments but can leave a conspicuous scar. Patient selection, skin graft harvest site choice and good technique are important variables. In special scenarios, other procedures including midface lift, spacer graft placement, canthoplasty, or eyelid suspension flaps, may be indicated.

Cicatricial Entropion Repair

21

Makayla McCoskey and Nahyoung Grace Lee

Abstract

Cicatricial entropion is in-turning of eyelashes due to scar or another adherence syndrome. Trauma or injury (especially chemical) may induce it, or it may be a result of infection or cicatrizing mucous membrane disease. Surgical repair of cicatricial entropion is offered when the tissues are quiescent and entails everting the eyelid margin to restore proper eyelid position and to protect the ocular surface. This can be achieved through multiple approaches, with severe cases of cicatricial entropion requiring a spacer graft to lengthen the scarred posterior lamella. The underlying cause of eyelid cicatrization can influence surgical decision making and potential systemic nonsurgical treatment. In this chapter, the authors describe evaluation and management of cicatricial entropion.

Supplementary Information The online version contains supplementary material available at https://doi.org/10.1007/978-3-031-63178-8_21.

M. McCoskey
Texas Oculoplastic Consultants, Austin, TX, USA

N. G. Lee (✉)
Harvard Medical School, Boston, MA, USA
e-mail: nahyoung.lee@gmail.com

Keywords

Eyelid entropion · Trichiasis · Conjunctival scar · Pemphigoid · Cicatricial entropion · Mucous membrane graft · Tarsotomy

Introduction

Cicatricial entropion is defined by inversion of the eyelid margin caused by shortening of the posterior lamella, typically due to scarring of the conjunctiva, resulting in tension on the posterior surface of the eyelid and lash inversion toward the ocular surface.

The most common cause of cicatricial ectropion globally is trachoma [1]. Other causes of cicatricial entropion include auto-immune or inflammatory disorders, such as Stevens-Johnson syndrome and ocular cicatricial pemphigoid, other infectious or inflammatory conjunctivitis, drug-induced pseudo-pemphigoid (frequently associated with topical glaucoma medications), as well as a history of eyelid trauma, including thermal burns, chemical burns or prior surgery.

Patients with entropion present with symptoms of ocular irritation and foreign body sensation related to the eyelid malposition and trichiasis. Patients may also present with visual decline in the setting of severe ocular surface irritation or ulceration. On examination, features

J. Tao (ed.), *Efficient Oculofacial Surgery*, https://doi.org/10.1007/978-3-031-63178-8_21

suggestive of cicatricial entropion include resistance to manual traction attempting to restore normal eyelid position, trichiatic eyelash positioning, and scarring or keratinization of the conjunctiva seen on eversion of the eyelid. Other important examination features to note are symblepharon formation, forniceal shortening, possible lagophthalmos, and the status of the corneal surface.

Once a diagnosis of cicatricial entropion is made, it is important to next uncover the underlying diagnosis driving posterior lamella cicatrization. The surgeon should inquire about a history of rheumatologic or autoimmune conditions, prior eyelid trauma, burns, or surgery, history of ocular infections, topical ophthalmic medication use, and whether the patient resides in or has traveled to a trachoma-endemic region. Based on clinical suspicion and history, further testing may be pursued to establish a diagnosis.

Surgical Management

The management of cicatricial entropion requires careful surgical correction of eyelid malposition by lengthening the inadequate, shortened posterior lamella. Additional effects of cicatrization, including fornix shortening and symblepharon formation should also be addressed. It is also important to note that immunomodulation or immunosuppression be considered in cases where there is active inflammation prior to surgery to prevent further inflammation and cicatrization.

The goal of surgical cicatricial entropion management is eversion of the eyelid margin to restore normal positioning and protect the ocular surface. In cases of mild to moderate cicatricial entropion, multiple techniques of performing a tarsotomy or "tarsal fracture" have been described; one such method is described in this chapter [2]. For more severe or extensive cicatricial entropion, surgical attention should be directed toward lengthening the posterior lamella to restore normal eyelid margin position. This can be achieved through the use of either autologous mucous membrane grafts, such as oral labial mucosa, buccal mucosa, hard palate, or banked tissue grafts, such as amniotic membrane [3–5]. The approach to harvesting and placing an oral labial mucous membrane graft for cicatricial entropion repair is also described below.

As a general principal, in cases of chronic, progressive cicatrizing disorders, such as ocular cicatricial pemphigoid and Stevens-Johnson syndrome, it is particularly important to minimize trauma to the conjunctiva and avoid tissue resection; undue trauma to this tissue can stimulate further scar tissue formation and cicatrization, and tissue resection is likely to contribute to further inadequacy of the posterior lamella, putting the patient at risk for lagophthalmos and corneal exposure. It is advisable to have the underlying disorder well-managed, such as with systemic immunomodulatory therapy, to minimize disease activity prior to attempting surgical repair, as the trauma of surgery is a risk factor for progression/reactivation of local disease. However, if it is not possible for the patient to receive systemic immunomodulation, there have also been various conjunctival sparing approaches to entropion repair described in the literature. One such technique is described in detail below [6].

Surgical Techniques

Mucous Membrane Graft

Preparation of Eyelid

The patient is prepped and draped in sterile fashion for surgery. The resting eyelid position is inspected (Fig. 21.1A), and the eyelid is anesthetized with injection of local anesthetic. A traction suture, such as 4-0 silk, is placed through the eyelid margin. The eyelid is then everted to inspect the posterior lamella for the extent and location of cicatricial changes/scar tissue (Fig. 21.1B).

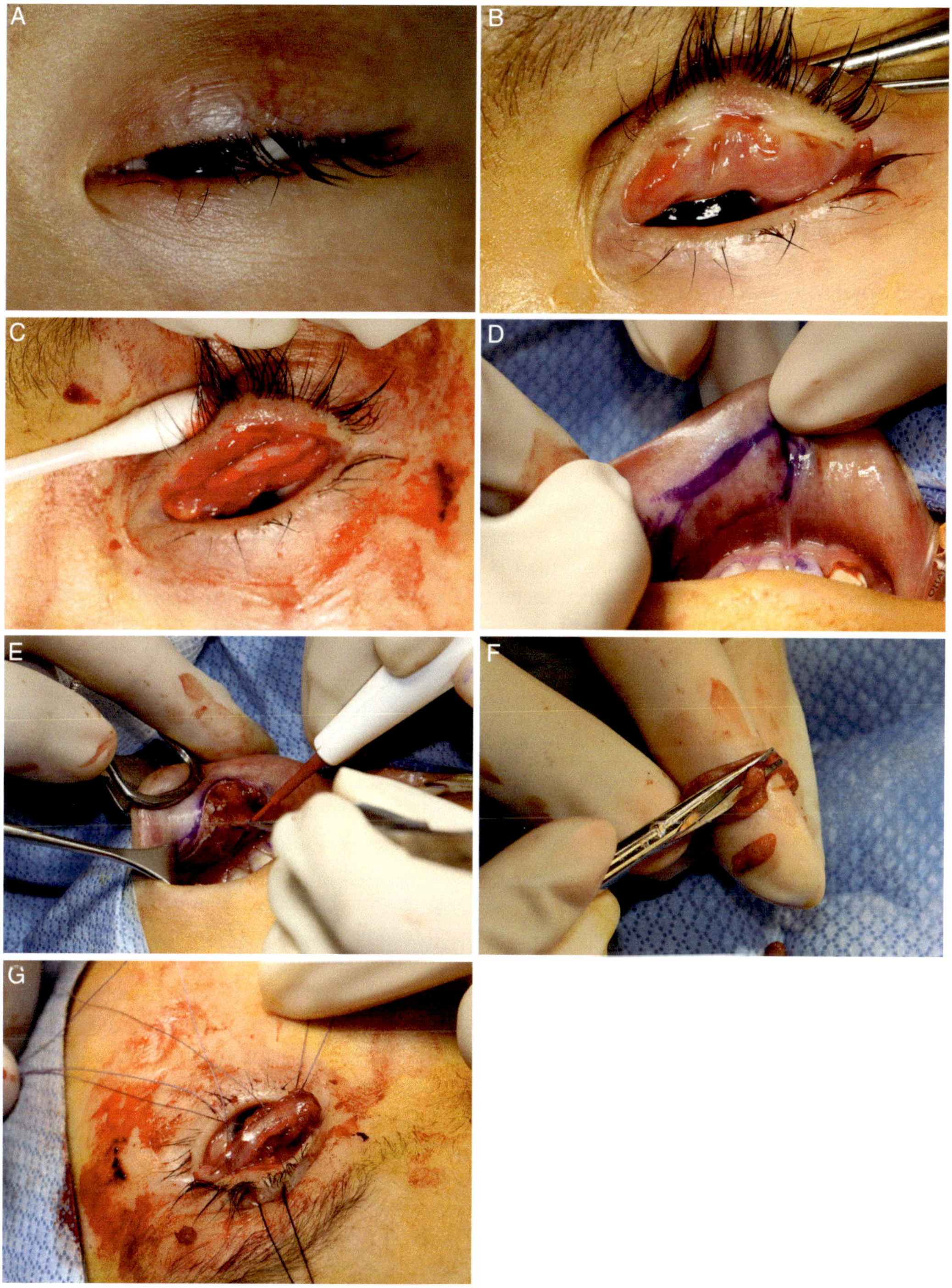

Fig. 21.1 **A** Cicatricial entropion in a 5 year old boy with lash-cornea touch from Stevens Johnsons syndrome. **B** Identification of scarring along the posterior lamella on eversion of the eyelid. **C** Excision of the scarred conjunctiva along the surface of the tarsus. **D** Marking of the oral labial mucous membrane harvest site. **E** Excision of the oral mucous membrane graft. **F** Thinning of the graft with removal of the subcutaneous tissue. **G** Placement of the graft along the upper eyelid tarsus and fornix with forniceal sutures that will be placed transcutaneously and tied externally

An incision is then made with a #15 blade through the conjunctiva and scar tissue 2–3 mm from the eyelid margin and scissors are used to clear scarred conjunctiva off the tarsal surface. This opens a bed for placement of the mucous membrane graft (Fig. 21.1C). This bed should be measured to determine the size of the graft to be harvested.

Oral Labial Mucosal Graft Harvesting

The oral labial mucosa is also prepped for sterility and anesthetized. The donor mucosal site should be inspected and confirmed to be smooth without keratinization or scarring. Then, it is measured and marked, aiming for a size similar or slightly larger in comparison to the recipient posterior lamellar bed (Fig. 21.1D). Electrocautery or a scalpel can be used to incise along the markings and excise the graft tissue (Fig. 21.1E). The mucosal graft is then thinned with scissors, removing subcutaneous fat and any submucosal glands (Fig. 21.1F).

The labial harvest site should be inspected, and good hemostasis should be ensured.

The mucous membrane wound edges are then approximated with continuous running 4-0 or 5-0 chromic gut suture and the patient is encouraged to begin sterilizing mouthwash technique after surgery.

Graft Placement

The labial mucous membrane graft is placed on the posterior surface of the everted eyelid and draped over the previously created posterior lamellar recipient bed (Fig. 21.1G). The graft edge closest to the fornix is secured with a double-armed 5-0 polyglactin suture, passed first through the graft, then into the newly formed fornix, and finally passed out transcutaneous. This is repeated with multiple sutures as necessary along this graft edge. Then, the edge of the graft closest to the eyelid margin is secured to the tarsus with 5-0 polyglactin interrupted sutures, placed in a buried fashion to prevent corneal surface irritation or abrasion.

Antibiotic-steroid ointment is placed in the eye at the end of the procedure.

Margin Tarsotomy

A tarsotomy or tarsal fracture can be performed independently for mild upper eyelid entropion, or in combination with a mucous membrane graft procedure for more severe cases of cicatricial entropion.

While everting the eyelid, a full-thickness incision is made with a #15 blade through the tarsus 2–3 mm from the eyelid margin. Double-armed 5-0 polyglactin sutures are placed through the cut edge of tarsus, with both arms passed transcutaneous near the lash line. These sutures are tied over the skin, and the suture position and tension while tying can be adjusted to titrate the degree of eyelid margin eversion (Fig. 21.2).

External (Conjunctival-Sparing) Approach

In cases where a conjunctival-sparing approach is preferred, such as in ocular cicatricial pemphigoid, an external approach can be employed.

The surgical site is prepped and draped in sterile fashion for surgery, and local anesthetic is injected. An infraciliary (in the lower eyelid) or supraciliary (in the upper eyelid) transcutaneous incision is marked 2 mm from the lash line and then incised with a #15 blade. Westcott scissors are used to expose the anterior surface of the tarsus across the horizontal extent of the eyelid. A 6-0 polyglactin suture is placed in a buried, interrupted fashion from one cut edge of the orbicularis oculi muscle, through the tarsus, to the other cut edge of the orbicularis oculi muscle. Multiple of these sutures should be placed across the horizontal extent of the eyelid with attention paid to placing adequate tension in each suture to achieve good eyelid margin eversion. Once the eyelid margin is felt to be in good position, the cutaneous infraciliary incision can be closed with running, continuous 6-0 plain gut suture.

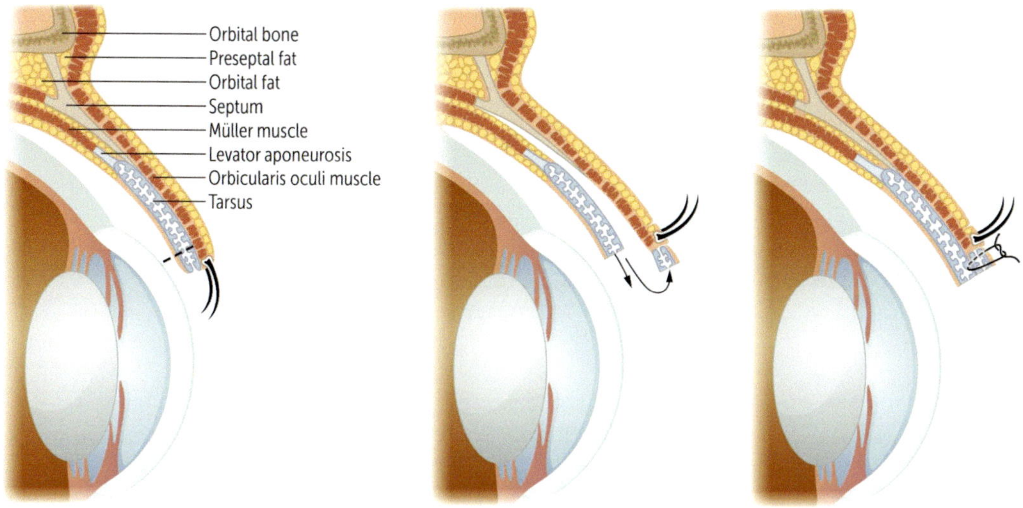

Fig. 21.2 Tarsotomy with posterior lamella super advancement. Illustration by Maureen Lifton

Gray Line Split with Anterior Lamellar Recession with Mucous Membrane Graft

Recessing the anterior lamella is a useful approach when there are broad areas of misdirected lashes. Another benefit of this approach is that, except for at the gray line, it spares the posterior lamella conjunctiva making it a suitable option for cases of chronic progressive cicatricial entropion (Fig. 21.3).

After infiltration with local anesthetic, a scalpel is used to incise the grey line from the lateral canthus to a position lateral to the punctum. Sharp dissection along the submuscular plane on the anterior face of the tarsus is performed using scissors.

With the anterior and posterior lamellae dissociated, the skin, orbicularis muscle, and eyelash follicles are recessed vertically to the anterior, inferior tarsus with interrupted absorbable sutures. It is useful to evert the lash line inferiorly when securing to the anterior, inferior tarsus. By recessing the anterior lamella, dermatochalasis may worsen. A combined or staged blepharoplasty may be useful in some cases.

The bare tarsus is covered with a mucous membrane graft. Oral lower labial mucosa is a typical choice as described previously (Fig. 21.1D–F). The graft is thinned accordingly, and a combination of interrupted and running absorbable sutures are then used to fixate it to the tarsal bed and eyelid margin (Fig. 21.1). The host site may be left bare to heal by second intention or buried 5-0 chromic sutures may help with healing of the donor site. A bolstered temporary suture tarsorrhaphy can then be placed to support the graft in place as it heals for the first postoperative week (Video 21).

Summary

Cicatricial entropion presents a particular clinical and surgical challenge due to the need to address both the eyelid malposition as well as the underlying cause of cicatrization of the posterior lamella. Surgery is aimed at lysing scar tissue and lengthening the posterior lamella to restore appropriate eyelid position. This can be achieved with placement of an autogenous mucous membrane graft, as described herein. However, in cases of progressive inflammatory cicatrizing disease, specifically ocular cicatricial pemphigoid, special consideration must be given to the high risk of disease reactivation with surgical manipulation of the conjunctiva. In these cases, a conjunctival-sparing approach, also described above, may be appropriate [7].

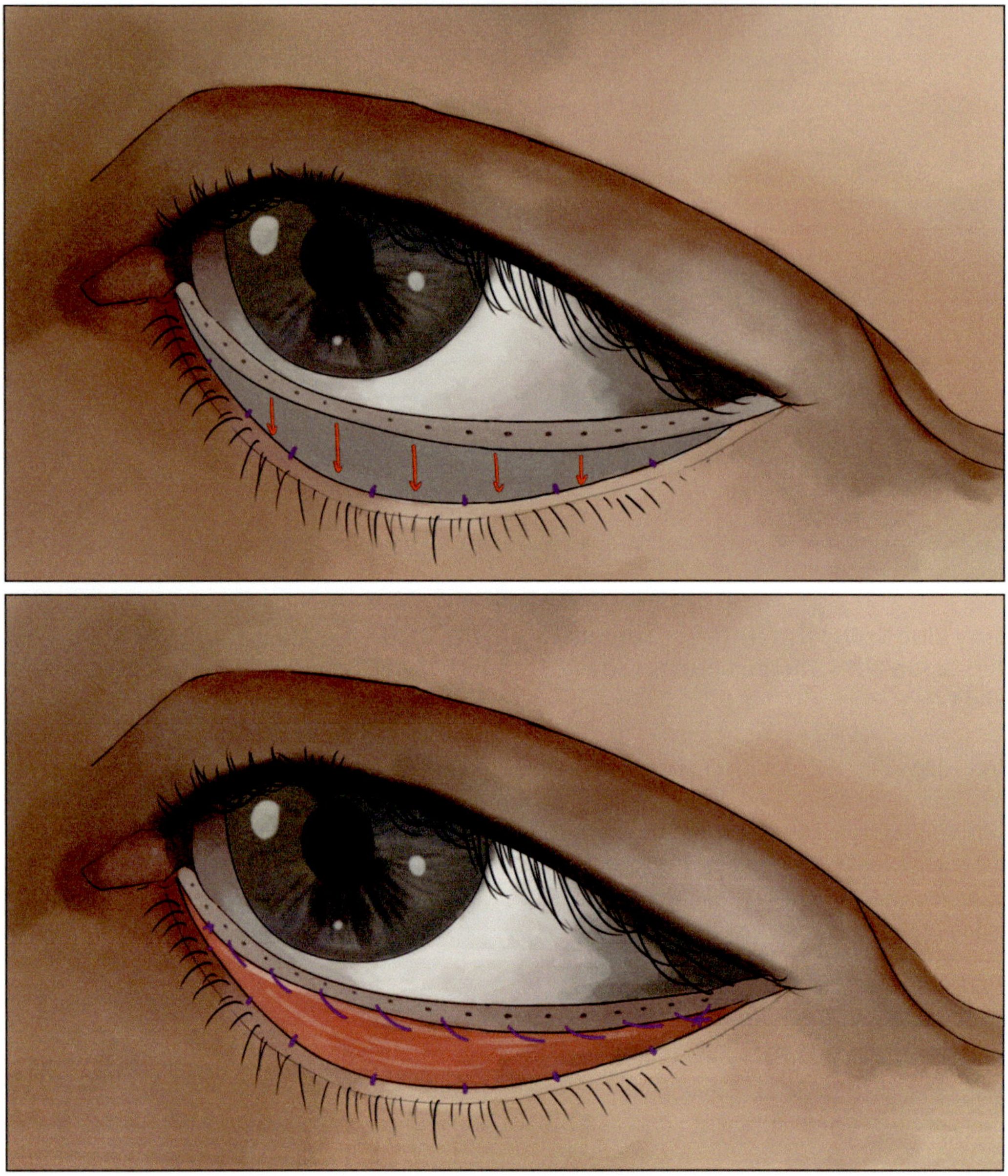

Fig. 21.3 Drawing demonstrating anterior lamellar recession and coverage of margin and superior tarsal defect with a mucous membrane graft

References

1. Rajak SN, Collin JRO, Burton MJ. Trachomatous trichiasis and its management in endemic countries. Surv Ophthalmol. 2012;57(2):105–35. https://doi.org/10.1016/j.survophthal.2011.08.002.
2. Halasa AH, Jarudi N. Tarsotomy for the correction of cicatricial entropion. Ann Ophthalmol. 1974;6(8):837–40.
3. Ti SE, Tow SL, Chee SP. Amniotic membrane transplantation in entropion surgery. Ophthalmology. 2001;108(7):1209–17. https://doi.org/10.1016/s0161-6420(01)00599-1.
4. Leone CR. Mucous membrane grafting for cicatricial entropion. Ophthalmic Surg. 1974;5(2):24–8.
5. Dortzbach RK, Callahan A. Repair of cicatricial entropion of upper eyelids. Arch Ophthalmol. 1971;85(1):82–9. https://doi.org/10.1001/archopht.1971.00990050084013.

6. Choung H, Reshef ER, Tanking T, Freitag SK. A conjunctival-sparing surgical technique for lower eyelid cicatricial entropion repair in ocular cicatricial pemphigoid. Orbit. 2020;39(1):23–30. https://doi.org/10.1080/01676830.2019.1573434.
7. Freitag SK, Grace Lee N, Lefebvre DR, Yoon MK. Ophthalmic plastic surgery (tricks of the trade). Thieme; 2020.
8. Nerad JA. Techniques in ophthalmic plastic surgery. Elsevier; 2010.

Involutional Entropion Repair

22

Kelly H. Yom and Audrey C. Ko

Abstract

Involutional entropion is in-turning of the lower eyelid due to eyelid tissue or ligamentous laxity. Eye irritation or ocular surface damage due to lashes rubbing the ocular surface are indications for repair. Laxity may be present vertically and horizontally in the eyelid, and an overriding of the preseptal orbicularis oculi muscle can be a factor. Different surgical techniques address key pathologic variables in involutional entropion. This chapter details the surgical repair of involutional entropion as well as epiblepharon, a related condition.

Keywords

Involutional lower eyelid entropion · Vertical eyelid laxity · Horizontal eyelid laxity · Epiblepharon

Supplementary Information The online version contains supplementary material available at https://doi.org/10.1007/978-3-031-63178-8_22.

K. H. Yom · A. C. Ko (✉)
Wolfe Eye, Iowa, Iowa City, IA, USA
e-mail: audreykomd@gmail.com

K. H. Yom
e-mail: kelly.hj.yom@gmail.com

K. H. Yom
University of Iowa, Iowa City, IA, USA

Background

Involutional entropion is defined as inward turning of the eyelid margin that can be acquired with age. Seen in up to 2% of the population greater than 60 years old, this condition is often attributed to age-related decreases in collagen tensile strength causing laxity and subsequent malposition of the eyelids [1]. With inward rotation of the eyelid margin, significant and progressive disturbance of the ocular surface may occur (Fig. 22.1). In addition to the disruption of the healthy tear film, the inward directed eyelashes may rub against the cornea, causing irritation, epithelial erosions, ulceration, and, in the most extreme cases, open globes. As such, repair of involutional entropion is crucial to restoring ocular health and quality of life, and though conservative measures such as lubricants, taping, soft bandage contact lenses, and botulinum toxin injections may provide temporary relief, definitive management requires surgical intervention to restore anatomic positioning of the eyelids.

Pathophysiology

There are multiple mechanical forces and anatomical changes that contribute to involutional entropion. Understanding which factors are present drive the surgical approach. Involutional entropion is predominantly seen in the lower

J. Tao (ed.), *Efficient Oculofacial Surgery*, https://doi.org/10.1007/978-3-031-63178-8_22

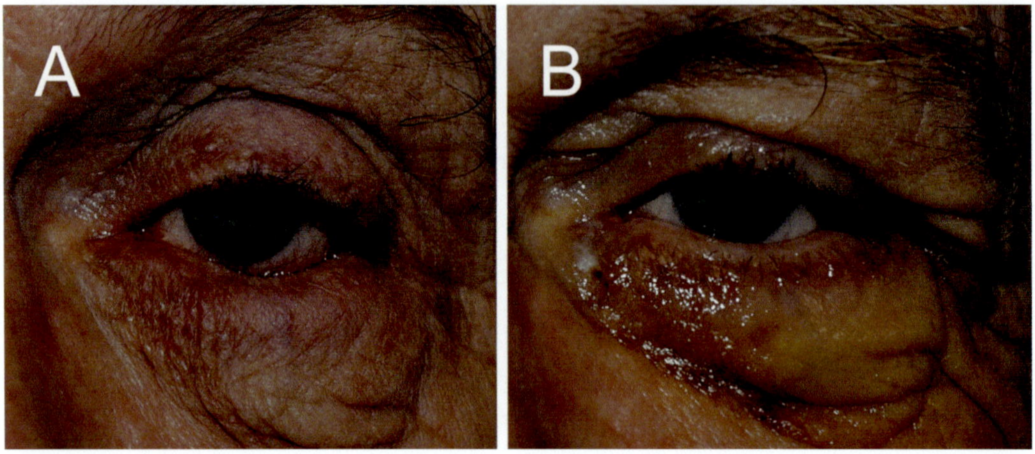

Fig. 22.1 A. Involutional entropion with lash to cornea contact. B After entropion repair

eyelid and can be a result of lower eyelid retractor (a.k.a. capsulopalpebral fascia) dysfunction, horizonal eyelid laxity, overriding of the orbicularis, or any combination of the above [2–4]. A careful exam can determine which of these issues may be contributing to eyelid malposition, as well as rule out spastic or cicatricial causes of entropion.

Eyelid retractor dysfunction is seen when these fibrous bands that normally keep the eyelid margin in place undergo attenuation, dehiscence, or disinsertion from their usual site of insertion at the lower tarsal plate, thus diminishing the vertical pulling force vector preventing inversion of the lower eyelid. While this is usually an idiopathic phenomenon, iatrogenic cases of capsulopalpebral fascia disinsertion have also been reported during routine ophthalmic surgeries [5, 6]. Disinsertion of the retractors can be suspected when the inferior fornix is deeper than normal, the lower eyelid margin is higher than normal, or there is diminished excursion of the lower eyelid on downgaze. If the retractors have become completely detached, this can occasionally be seen at the slit lamp as a white, subconjunctival line several millimeters below the inferior tarsal border.

In addition to retractor disinsertion, horizontal eyelid laxity is also often present in eyelids with involutional entropion. This creates a "floppy" lower eyelid which is more prone to rotating inward. Horizontal eyelid laxity is detected using the distraction test, in which the central eyelid is pulled away from the globe, and if can be distracted more than 6–8 mm, is positive for eyelid laxity. Eyelid laxity can also be detected using the snapback test, in which the eyelid demonstrates slow and incomplete snap back to the globe's surface after being pulled away from the globe anteriorly.

Finally, if the inferior portion of the preseptal orbicularis muscle begins to override the superior portion during eyelid closure, this may also generate sufficient mechanical force to tip the eyelid inward. This is exacerbated if orbital fat has prolapsed into the lower eyelid due to laxity of the orbital septum [7]. Clinically, this can be seen as mounding of the orbicularis oculi, suggestive of an overacting muscle. Epiblepharon is an entity seen more commonly in the pediatric Hispanic or Asian population. In epiblepharon, redundant skin and orbicularis oculi muscle override the eyelid margin and mechanically push lashes against the ocular surface. In many cases of epiblepharon the lash margin may be rotated inwards independent of the redundant anterior lamella.

Surgical Techniques

Correction of involutional entropion should target the underlying factors responsible for the eyelid malposition (i.e., retractor disinsertion, horizontal eyelid laxity, overriding orbicularis). Multiple surgical techniques to repair involutional entropion have been described, with varying degrees of success, recurrence, and complications for each one. Performing procedures that address all vectors of entropion has been shown to result in lower recurrence rates than approaches that address single variables.

Everting Sutures

The simplest and least invasive procedure to address involutional entropion is everting sutures, also known as Quickert sutures [8]. Because this technique may be performed in the office or at bedside, it is useful for patients who cannot tolerate a prolonged or extensive surgery for any reason. Its simplicity make this technique an accessible option for ophthalmologists, and is the least resource intensive in terms of materials and personnel required [9, 10]. However, correction typically only lasts several months and entropion often recurs, as much as 50% of cases within 2 years [11]. Therefore, this technique is often used as a temporizing measure while awaiting optimization for more definitive surgical correction. Recurrence rate is significantly reduced if combined with other surgical procedures, such as the lateral tarsal strip (Fig. 22.2) [12, 13].

1. Two or three sutures are commonly used; either double armed 5–0 polyglactin sutures or double armed 5–0 or 6–0 chromic sutures are ideal.
2. One arm of the suture enters the deep inferior conjunctival fornix. The suture is directed anteriorly and superiorly and will make a full-thickness pass to the external eyelid, passing through the conjunctiva, lower eyelid retractors, orbicularis muscle, and finally skin, exiting just inferior to the lash follicles. The other arm of the suture is placed a few millimeters away and follows a similar path. This functionally tightens the lower eyelid retractors and rotates the eyelid margin away from the globe.

Transverse Full-Thickness Blepharotomy and Everting Sutures

The transverse full-thickness blepharotomy with the everting sutures aims to create a surgical scar between the preseptal and pretarsal orbicularis, to prevent the overriding of the former over

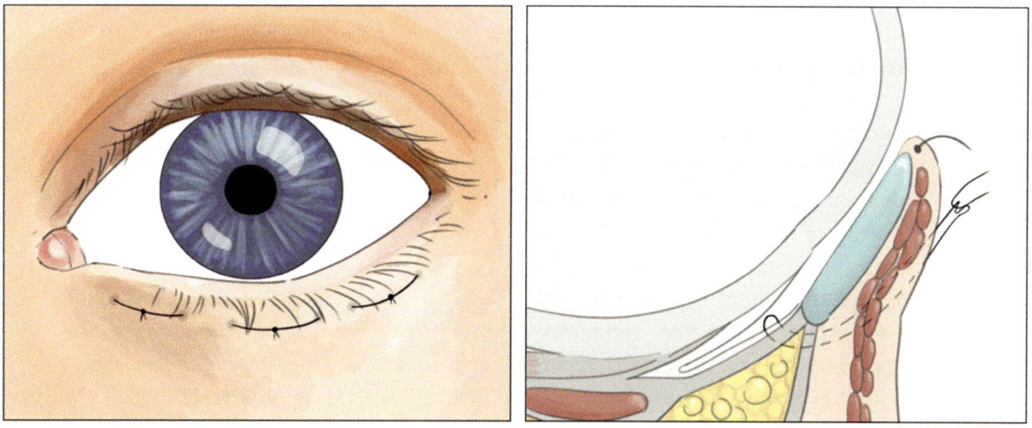

Fig. 22.2 Eyelid everting sutures

the latter; the everting suture facilitates rotation of the eyelid margin outward [14, 15]. While this approach does not address horizontal eyelid laxity, its intention is to create a more durable option for surgical repair of eyelid retractor disinsertion and orbicularis override than everting sutures alone.

1. The skin is marked 4 mm inferior to the lower eyelid margin, running horizontally parallel to the eyelid margin from the punctum to the lateral canthus.
2. A 4–0 silk suture is placed through the lash line of the lower eyelid to provide traction.
3. A full-thickness horizontal incision is made along the marking with a scalpel, and hemostasis is achieved with cautery.
4. If excess skin and orbicularis muscle hypertrophy is present, 1–2 mm of skin and orbicularis muscle can be horizontally excised.
5. A double armed 5–0 or 6–0 polyglactin or chromic gut suture is passed through the conjunctiva and lower eyelid retractors proximal to the incision, then through the orbicularis and skin distally just inferior to the lashes as an everting suture. Both arms of the suture are placed in the same manner to complete a horizontal mattress suture and tied. Up to three everting sutures may be placed.
6. The skin at the blepharotomy incision is closed with running vs interrupted 6–0 sutures; eversion of the eyelid should be apparent at the end of the procedure (Fig. 22.3).

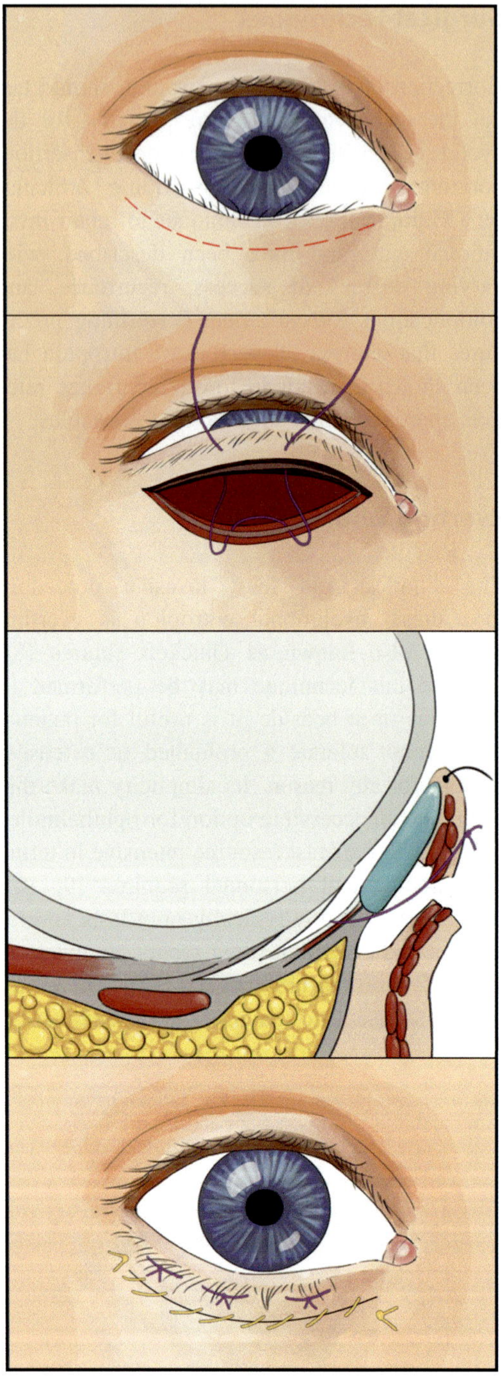

Fig. 22.3 Illustration depicting transverse full-thickness blepharotomy and everting sutures

Retractor Reinsertion

In isolated vertical eyelid retractor disinsertion without significant horizontal eyelid laxity, retractor reinsertion allows for the plication and reattachment of the disinserted lower eyelid retractors to the tarsal plate [16]. This technique facilitates the direct exposure, exploration, and advancement of the retractors, creating a more precise and definitive repair compared to the everting suture procedures above. Retractor reinsertion can be done through either an external transcutaneous or an internal transconjunctival approach [17–20]. Common complications include recurrence of entropion, overcorrection resulting in ectropion, mild eyelid retraction, and pyogenic granuloma formation. Recurrence rates are reduced by combining this procedure with horizontal canthal shortening when indicated [21].

TRANSCONJUNCTIVAL APPROACH

1. A 4–0 silk suture may be placed through the lash line of the lower eyelid to provide traction.
2. A transconjunctival incision is made below the inferior tarsal border with a monopolar cautery. The incision extends from the lateral canthus laterally to the punctum medially and passes through both the conjunctiva and the lower eyelid retractors.
3. The conjunctival flap is elevated, allowing dissection in the plane between the lower eyelid retractors and the lower eyelid fat.
4. Excision of a strip of conjunctiva and lower eyelid retractors measuring approximately 2–3 mm is performed using scissors.
5. The conjunctiva and retractors are reattached to the inferior border of the tarsus with a running 7–0 polyglactin suture, which functionally plicates the lower eyelid retractors and restores anatomical force vectors on the lower eyelid. Eversion of the eyelid should be apparent at the end of the procedure.

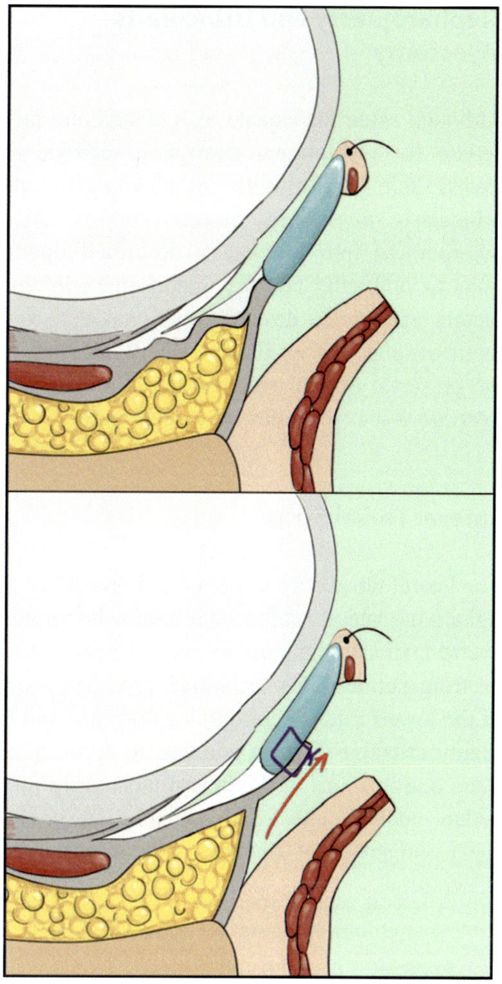

Fig. 22.4 Retractor band tightening through an external subciliary incision

TRANSCUTANEOUS APPROACH (Fig. 22.4).

1. The skin is marked with a surgical pen for a subciliary cutaneous incision inferior to the tarsal plate, running parallel to the eyelid margin along the area of entropion, extending from the punctum medially to the lateral canthus laterally.
2. A 4–0 silk suture may be placed through the lash line of the lower eyelid to provide traction.
3. A subciliary incision is made through the skin along the prior markings with a scalpel or monopolar cautery; hemostasis is achieved with cautery.
4. Division and blunt dissection of the orbicularis muscle is performed, and the orbital septum is opened to reach the level of the lower eyelid retractors. The postoperative fibrous scarring created here through the orbicularis oculi muscle provides a barrier to counteract the overriding of the preseptal orbicularis over the pretarsal orbicularis.
5. The lower eyelid retractors are identified and dissected off the underlying conjunctiva. An interrupted absorbable suture such as 5–0 or 6–0 polyglactin is used to reattach this structure to the anterior inferior tarsal edge. Three sutures are used to plicate the retractors centrally, medially, and laterally. This functionally shortens the retractors and allows for restoration of the force vectors maintaining lower eyelid position.

Blepharoplasty and Orbicularis Myectomy

Although often inadequate as a standalone procedure for involutional entropion, removal of excess skin and muscle (blepharoplasty and orbicularis myectomy, respectively) is often incorporated into previously described operations to optimally address underlying etiologic factors and create desired functional and aesthetic results. By excising a small amount of the preseptal orbicularis, this can eliminate any override that exacerbates the entropion.

Lateral Tarsal Strip

The lateral tarsal strip is a common procedure to tighten the lateral canthus and reduce horizontal eyelid laxity. In combination with placement of everting sutures, this technique provides some of the lowest rates of entropion recurrence and is highly effective [22]. In addition to recurrence, rare complications of the lateral tarsal strip procedure include chemosis, self-limiting granuloma, and persistent trichiasis without entropion.

1. A lateral canthal incision of 1–2 mm is performed with a scalpel or monopolar cautery to create a lateral canthotomy.
2. The inferior crus of the lateral canthal ligament is identified and cut with a monopolar cautery to perform the inferior cantholysis.
3. Scissors are used to dissect between the anterior and posterior lamella of the inferior eyelid for approximately 5 mm so that they are separated.
4. The anterior lamella is excised along the length of the tarsal strip.
5. The superior mucocutaneous junction of the posterior lamella is also excised.
6. The posterior surface of the tarsus is scraped with a scalpel to remove the tarsal conjunctiva, creating a de-epithelialized and isolated strip of tarsus.
7. Trimming of the tarsal strip may be performed with scissors if eyelid laxity persists after pulling the strip superolaterally to the projected site of attachment.
8. A double armed 4–0 braided polyester suture is passed through the tarsal strip and is used to secure the strip to the internal orbital portion of the lateral orbital rim periosteum at the level of the lateral orbital tubercle.
9. The lateral canthus is reapproximated and the lateral canthal angle is reconstructed with a 5–0 versus 6–0 polyglactin or plain suture.
10. The remaining skin incision is closed with interrupted 5–0 versus 6–0 polyglactin sutures. Eversion of the eyelid should be apparent at the end of the procedure.

Canthopexy

In cases of mild involutional entropion, if the lateral canthus is disinserted but reinsertion causes significant tension on the lower eyelid, lateral canthopexy via small incision closed lateral canthoplasty may be used to anchor the lateral canthal tendon through an upper or a lower eyelid incision without the need to expose the entire lateral canthal angle. Compared to the LTS, a canthopexy procedure is faster, uses a smaller incision that heals more quickly, and has reduced risk of webbing or scarring at the lateral canthus.

1. A small horizontal incision is made in the lateral crease line of the upper eyelid. This can also be done concurrently with an upper blepharoplasty incision.
2. Dissection is performed with scissors to the lateral orbital rim.
3. Scissors are then used to release the canthal tendon at the lateral orbital rim. If necessary, the cut edge of the tendon can be trimmed to further shorten the horizontal axis of the eyelid.
4. Both arms of a double armed suture (braided polyester, polydiaxone, or polyglactin) are

passed through the lateral canthal tendon and are anchored to the internal orbital portion of the lateral orbital rim periosteum. This secures the lateral canthus with horizontal shortening, resulting in a greater physiological tone and reduced eyelid laxity.

5. The skin incision is closed with absorbable suture.

Combined horizontal and vertical tightening with anterior lamellar resection (Fig. 22.5) (Video 22.1).

As the three major potential causes of involutional entropion are rarely isolated processes, the authors commonly elect to target all variables at the same surgical setting to more definitively treat entropion. Highly durable results can be achieved with this multimodal approach [22, 23].

1. A subciliary cutaneous incision parallel to the eyelid margin is fashioned from the punctum medially to past the lateral canthus.
2. The anterior lamella is dissected and distracted to expose the lower eyelid retractors. A horizontal full-thickness incision is created following the surgical markings previously created.

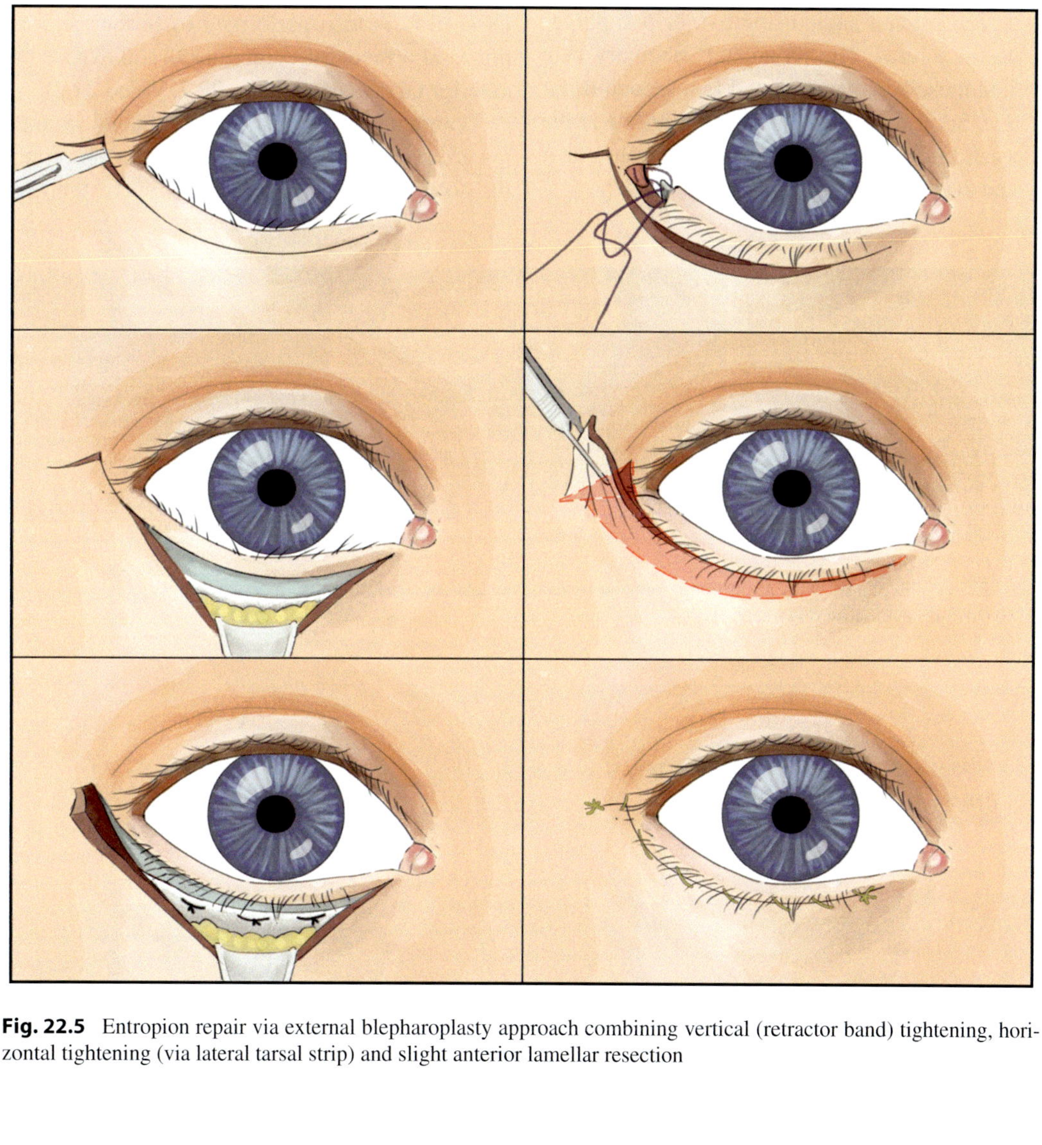

Fig. 22.5 Entropion repair via external blepharoplasty approach combining vertical (retractor band) tightening, horizontal tightening (via lateral tarsal strip) and slight anterior lamellar resection

3. The lower eyelid retractors are tightened by securing the leading edge to the anterior, inferior tarsus using 6–0 polyglactin or chromic gut sutures.
4. The eyelid is tightened horizontally by performing a lateral canthotomy and cantholysis. The lateral eyelid is resected slightly, and the free tarsus is secured to the lateral rim periosteum using 4–0 braided polyester suture or polyglactin sutures, with or without formation of a tarsal strip.
5. Redundant skin and muscle are resected in triangles. The anterior lamella is distracted supertemporal and the skin and muscle past the canthus is resected. The anterior lamella flaps then secured to the periosteum at the lateral canthal angle using 6–0 or 5–0 polyglactin sutures. The redundant subciliary skin and muscle is then resected in a second triangle. Some additional orbicularis muscle at the eyelid margin may be resected to further treat the override.

Epiblepharon Repair

Epiblepharon is a related but separate entity than involutional entropion (Fig. 22.6). It may be a form of mechanical entropion whereby overriding skin and orbicularis oculi muscle push lashes inward. While the anterior lamella override may be a key vector, the lash line is commonly independently rotated against the globe.

The repair begins with an ellipse marked along the length of the eyelid with the first incision one to two millimeters from the eyelash line and the second incision two to five millimeters away from the primary. After local anesthetic injection, an elliptical incision is made, and the anterior lamellar tissue is excised. Dissection is also performed to further remove pretarsal orbicularis oculi muscle and expose the anterior tarsal surface (Fig. 22.7, Video 22.2).

Commonly, the lash line remains rotated inward. Hence, skin and muscle override is not the sole pathologic variable. As such, the lash

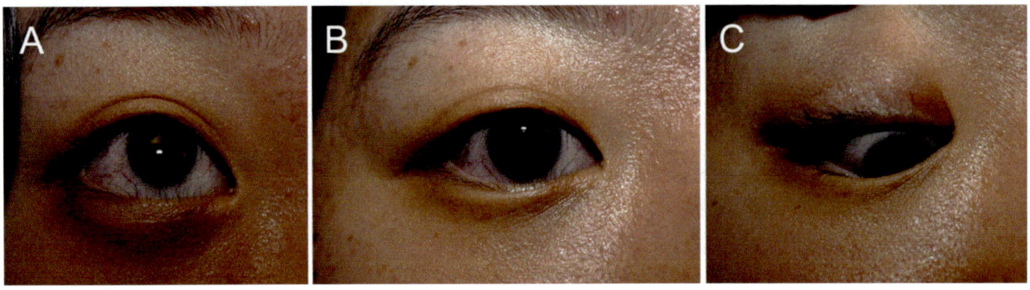

Fig. 22.6 Epiblepharon with an inturned eyelash row (A) and pretarsal skin and muscle redundancy (B), and override especially evident in downgaze (C)

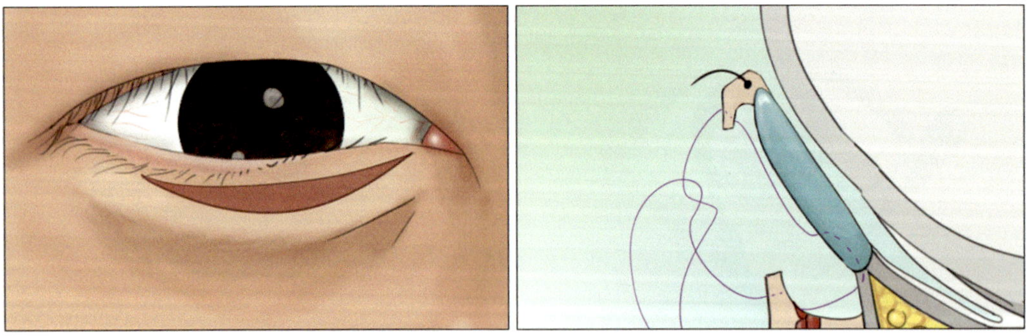

Fig. 22.7 Epiblepharon repair with subciliary elliptical skin and muscle resection then lash rotating sutures

line rotation sutures are necessary. 6–0 polyglactin suture engages the lash line that is anchored to the anterior, inferior tarsus. Typically, 2–5 lash rotation sutures are placed in an interrupted fashion.

This skin is then closed with an absorbable suture in an interrupted fashion. Surgery is typically used in the lower eyelid, but an identical technique may be employed in cases of upper eyelid epiblepharon.

Conclusions

Entropion is one of the most common functional conditions seen in the aging population and may cause eye irritation or ocular surface damage. Three factors contribute to involutional entropion: (1) vertical eyelid laxity (disinsertion or laxity of the lower eyelid retractors), (2) horizontal eyelid laxity, and (3) overriding of the preseptal orbicularis oculi muscle onto the pretarsal orbicularis oculi. Proper surgical repair addresses these variables.

References

1. Damasceno RW, Osaki MH, Dantas PE, Belfort R Jr. Involutional entropion and ectropion of the lower eyelid: prevalence and associated risk factors in the elderly population. Ophthalmic Plast Reconstr Surg. 2011;27(5):317–20.
2. Michels KS, Czyz CN, Cahill KV, et al. Age-matched, case-controlled comparison of clinical indicators for development of entropion and ectropion. J Ophthalmol. 2014;2014: 231487.
3. Jones LT. The anatomy of the lower eyelid*: and its relation to the cause and cure of entropion. Am J Ophthalmol. 1960;49(1):29–36.
4. Neuhaus RW. Anatomical basis of" senile" ectropion. Ophthalmic Plast Reconstr Surg. 1985;1(2):87–9.
5. Hurwitz JJ, Smith D, Corin SM. Association of entropion with cataract surgery. Ophthalmic Plast Reconstr Surg. 1990;6(1):25–7.
6. Putterman AM. Ectropion of the lower eyelid secondary to Müller's muscle-capsulopalpebral fascia detachment. Am J Ophthalmol. 1978;85(6):814–7.
7. Beigi B, Kashkouli MB, Shaw A, Murthy R. Fornix fat prolapse as a sign for involutional entropion. Ophthalmology. 2008;115(9):1608–12.
8. Quickert MH, Rathbun E. Suture repair of entropion. Arch Ophthalmol. 1971;85(3):304–5.
9. Barnes JA, Bunce C, Olver JM. Simple effective surgery for involutional entropion suitable for the general ophthalmologist. Ophthalmology. 2006;113(1):92–6.
10. Wright M, Bell D, Scott C, Leatherbarrow B. Everting suture correction of lower lid involutional entropion. Br J Ophthalmol. 1999;83(9):1060.
11. Jang SY, Choi SR, Jang JW, et al. Long-term surgical outcomes of Quickert sutures for involutional lower eyelid entropion. J Craniomaxillofac Surg. 2014;42(8):1629–31.
12. Scheepers MA, Singh R, Ng J, et al. A randomized controlled trial comparing everting sutures with everting sutures and a lateral tarsal strip for involutional entropion. Ophthalmology. 2010;117(2):352–5.
13. Ho SF, Pherwani A, Elsherbiny SM, Reuser T. Lateral tarsal strip and quickert sutures for lower eyelid entropion. Ophthalmic Plast Reconstr Surg. 2005;21(5):345–8.
14. Wies FA. Surgical treatment of entropion. J Int Coll Surg. 1954;21(6 1):758–760.
15. Bleyen I, Dolman PJ. The Wies procedure for management of trichiasis or cicatricial entropion of either upper or lower eyelids. Br J Ophthalmol. 2009;93(12):1612–5.
16. Jones LT, Reeh MJ, Wobig JL. Senile entropion: a new concept for correction. Am J Ophthalmol. 1972;74(2):327–9.
17. Jones LT. The anatomy of the lower eyelid and its relation to the cause and cure of entropion. Am J Ophthalmol. 1960;49:29–36.
18. Dresner SC, Karesh JW. Transconjunctival entropion repair. Arch Ophthalmol. 1993;111(8):1144–8.
19. Kreis AJ, Shafi F, Madge SN. Transconjunctival entropion repair—the backdoor approach. Orbit. 2013;32(5):271–4.
20. Ben Simon GJ, Molina M, Schwarcz RM, et al. External (subciliary) vs internal (transconjunctival) involutional entropion repair. Am J Ophthalmol. 2005;139(3):482–7.
21. Lee H, Takahashi Y, Ichinose A, Kakizaki H. Comparison of surgical outcomes between simple posterior layer advancement of lower eyelid retractors and combination with a lateral tarsal strip procedure for involutional entropion in a Japanese population. Br J Ophthalmol. 2014;98(11):1579–82.
22. Dulz S, Green S, Mehlan J, et al. A comparison of the lateral tarsal strip with everting sutures and the Quickert procedure for involutional entropion. Acta Ophthalmol. 2019;97(6):e933–6.
23. Collin JR, Rathbun JE. Involutional entropion: a review with evaluation of a procedure. Arch Ophthalmol. 1978;96(6):1058–1064.

Eyelid Surgery Considerations with a Prominent Eye

23

Colin Bacorn and Lily Koo Lin

Abstract

The position of the globe greatly affects the function and appearance of the eyelid and vice versa. This relationship must be considered when operating in the periorbital region. Proptosis should be recognized to avoid an unexpected or suboptimal surgical result. Patients with proptosis or hypoplastic inferior orbital rims often present with lower eyelid retraction and are at increased risk for developing retraction. Upper eyelid retraction may also be present concomitantly with proptosis. Eyelid retraction and proptosis cause patients to be not only dissatisfied with their appearance, but they also may be symptomatic from dry eye and exposure. This chapter outlines prominent eye considerations and techniques to improve the anatomic relationship between the globe and eyelids. The authors also describe upper eyelid retraction repair.

Supplementary Information The online version contains supplementary material available at https://doi.org/10.1007/978-3-031-63178-8_23.

C. Bacorn
The Wilmer Eye Institute, Johns Hopkins University School of Medicine, Baltimore, MD, USA

L. K. Lin (✉)
Ophthalmology and Vision Science, University of California Davis Health, Sacramento, CA, USA
e-mail: lklin@ucdavis.edu

Keywords

Proptosis · Eyelid retraction · Lagophthalmos · Negative vector · Exophthalmos · Thyroid eye disease

Introduction

The close anatomic relationship between the globe and the eyelid carries significant practical implications for changes in position of either structure. An abnormally anterior position of the globe relative to the orbital rim is termed proptosis. The term exophthalmos connotes proptosis due to thyroid eye disease. An abnormally anterior globe position is an important consideration when planning eyelid surgery of any type.

This eyelid-globe relationship may vary normally as a function of age [1, 2], race, or gender [3]. It may be the result of a variety of pathologic processes of the orbit. Eyelid retraction may also contribute to a prominent globe appearance in cases where the globe position is within normal limits.

In Caucasian populations, the palpebral fissure is approximately 10 mm vertically and 33 mm horizontally with the upper and lower eyelids resting in close approximation to the globe along their horizontal extent such that the fornix is a collapsed potential space [4]. Anthropometric measurements vary between

J. Tao (ed.), *Efficient Oculofacial Surgery*, https://doi.org/10.1007/978-3-031-63178-8_23

Table 23.1 Representative normative values of eyelid measurements in middle-aged adults

	Race					
	Caucasian [3, 16]		African [16–18]		East Asian [19, 20]	
	Male	Female	Male	Female	Male	Female
Exophthalmometry (mm)	16.5	15.4	18.2	17.5	15.3	14.4
Vertical Fissure (mm)	9.7	10.1	10.6	10.6	9.7	10.2
Horizontal Fissure (mm)	33.5	32	32.8	32.6	28.6	27.6
Fissure Axis (deg)	4.6	5.2	3.9	5.9	9.6	9.8

published reports; representative normative values are summarized for mid-aged adults in Table 23.1. The upper eyelid rests approximately 2 mm inferior to the superior limbus while the lower eyelid margin rests along the inferior limbus; scleral show (visible superior or inferior sclera in the vertical line transecting the pupil) is abnormal but inferior show is a common feature of the aging or lax eyelid. The size of the globe itself may also vary significantly, such as in cases of buphthalmos or high myopia, and similarly alter this important metric. Abnormalities in any of these factors, in isolation or combination, may result in a prominent appearing globe, as a result surgical techniques to re-establish the normal globe-lid configuration should be tailored to address the relevant factors in each patient.

Globe position relative to the orbital rim is typically quantified with an exophthalmometer which measures the position of the anterior cornea relative to the lateral orbital rim. In cases where the lateral orbital rim is absent or abnormal a similar technique comparing the globe to the inferior and superior orbital rims may be used [5]. Finally, computed tomography (CT) based measurements may be used but there may be systematic differences in measurements obtained by CT and those based on physical techniques which complicate direct comparison.

Commonly associated with the prominent eye is the “negative-vector” eyelid conformation in which the globe protrudes beyond the anterior most projection of the maxilla and inferior orbital rim (Fig. 23.1) [6]. In this position, the eyelid lacks vertical support and as a result is at increased risk of retraction which may exacerbate the prominent appearance of the globe [7]. This anatomic relationship may be present in up to 60% of patients seeking lower blepharoplasty and its recognition in the pre-operative assessment is crucial to prevent poor outcomes [8].

Especially in thyroid eye disease, orbital decompression may be indicated to facilitate or treat retraction or lagophthalmos as eyelid procedures may be futile. (Figs. 23.2 and 23.3) Eyelid procedures are generally performed after decompression and strabismus surgery since these interventions may change eyelid position.

Orbital decompression is detailed in another chapter. Eyelid procedures to manage a prominent eye are described here and as follows.

A straightforward method to correct eye exposure due to lower eyelid retraction in the prominent eye is lateral tarsorrhaphy. By anchoring the lateral lower eyelid margin to the upper eyelid, the lower eyelid is drawn superiorly to rest in a more normal vertical position. The effect can be readily titrated by altering the length of eyelid suspended to tailor the effect to individual patients. Unfortunately, while the technique is safe and simple, it has significant downsides with respect to cosmesis and patient acceptance. The technique necessarily narrows the palpebral fissure and alters the configuration of the lateral canthal angle. It may also cause

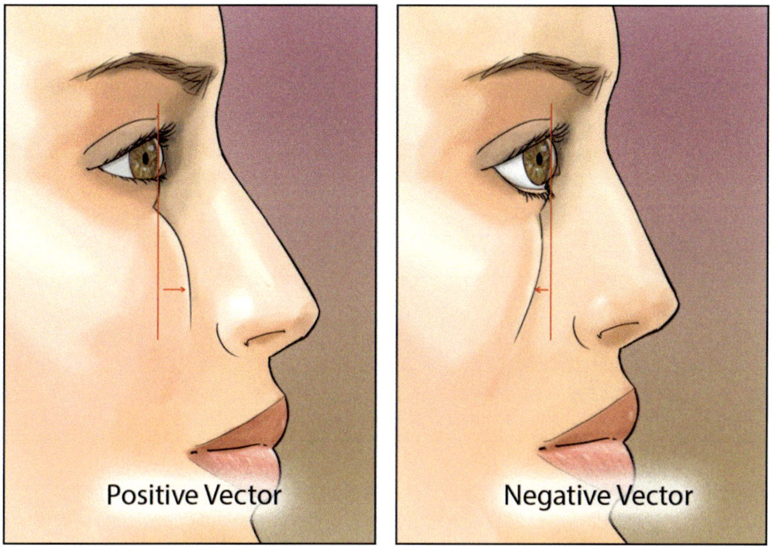

Fig. 23.1 Positive and negative malar vectors. In a positive vector, the globe remains at or behind the plane of the malar eminence. In a negative vector, the globe projects anterior to this plane

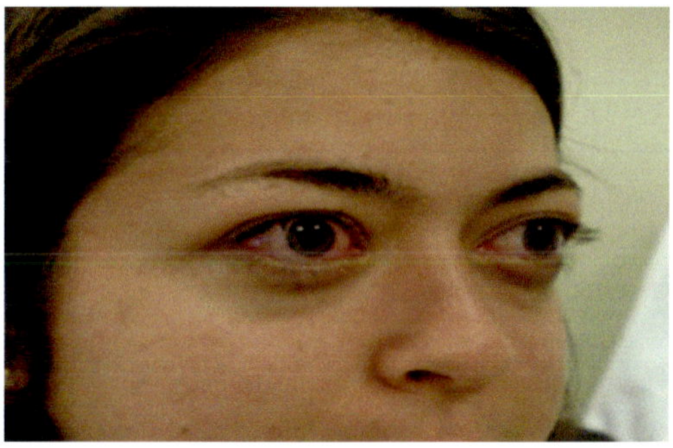

Fig. 23.2 Patient with lower eyelid retraction and proptosis due thyroid eye disease

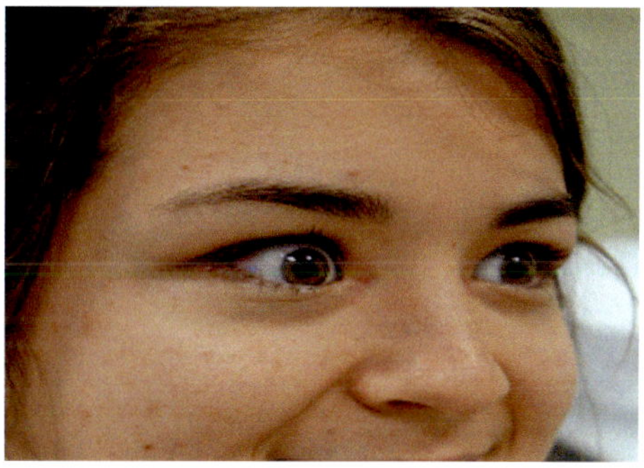

Fig. 23.3 Patient in Fig. 23.2 with improvement in lower eyelid retraction after orbital decompression surgery

the upper lashes to rest in an unnatural fashion. With larger tarsorrhaphies, upper eyelid ptosis may become cosmetically and functionally significant. Due to these downsides, the temporary lateral tarsorrhaphy is best a temporizing measure in cases of exposure keratopathy and used conservatively. The techniques to follow are preferred since they better achieve both functional and aesthetic results.

Non-surgical Enhancement

In patients with mildly prominent eyes with very mild lower eyelid retraction, volumetric enhancement is an option. Injection of fillers, most often composed of hyaluronic acid, may augment volume and elevate the eyelid in a minimally invasive fashion compared

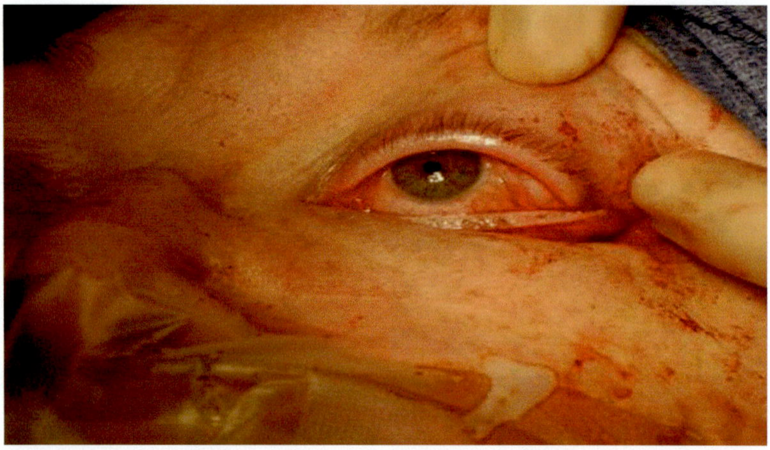

Fig. 23.4 Intraoperative inferior scleral show due to horizontal tightening in the presence of a prominent eye

to open surgery [9–12]. Importantly, these treatments only offer subtle and temporary improvements.

Eyelid Tightening and Canthoplasty

Horizontal eyelid tension is an important consideration that must be assessed concurrently with vertical eyelid height and support. While lax lower eyelids are known to predispose to retraction, it is important to recognize that excess tension may exacerbate a prominent eye. Overly aggressive tarsal strip or horizontal tightening and lateral fixation may cause the eyelid margin to slip beneath the globe and increase inferior scleral show [13] (Fig. 23.4). This effect may be exacerbated in cases when the eyelid is not anchored sufficiently high on the lateral orbital rim. Periosteal anchoring slightly above Whitnall's tubercle or sometimes along the external orbital rim may be required.

Lateral Tarsoconjunctvial Suspension Flap

To obviate the conspicuous nature of intermarginal adhesion tarsorrhaphy, suspension of the lateral lower eyelid to a superior fornix based tarsoconjunctival flap may be preferable. These are detailed in other chapters, but the flap is developed after everting the upper eyelid and the leading edge is sewn to the denuded lateral lower eyelid margin.

Spacer Graft (Video 22.1)

Spacer grafts serve to vertically elongate and, in some cases, mechanically support the eyelid and are of particular use in prominent eyes with concurrent lower eyelid cicatrization from prior surgery or disease (Figs. 23.5 and 23.6) A variety of materials may be used as a spacer graft to help raise the lower eyelid. Preferred autologous options include ear cartilage or hard

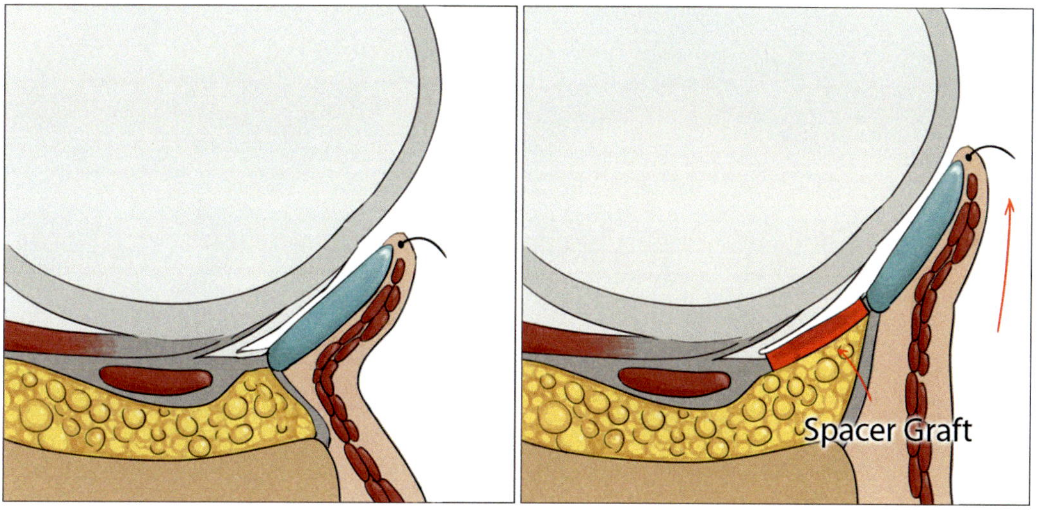

Fig. 23.5 Drawing depicting mechanism of lower eyelid retraction repair with a posterior lamella spacer graft

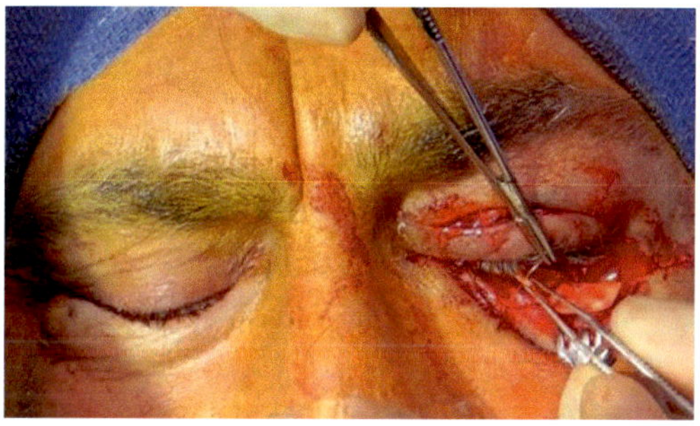

Fig. 23.6 Posterior lamella spacer being sewn into recessed conjunctiva and eyelid retractors

palate. A dermis fat graft may be useful if volume augmentation is desired. Acellular dermal matrix is an off the shelf option that obviates a second surgical site and includes xenografts (e.g., porcine, Enduragen, Stryker Kalamazoo, MI) or allografts (e.g., Alloderm, Lifecell Corp, Branchburg, NJ). Another donor option is human sclera. Spacer grafts may be implanted to the lower eyelid through an anterior or posterior approach and are described in detail in other chapters [14, 15].

Midface Flap

Midface lifting is detailed in other chapters, but it has an important role in the management of lower eyelid retraction in the setting of a prominent eye. Through a subciliary external cutaneous or an internal transconjunctival approach, eyelid and cheek soft tissues are freed from the underlying bone (Fig. 23.7). These tissues are then mobilized in a superolateral direction (Fig. 23.8).

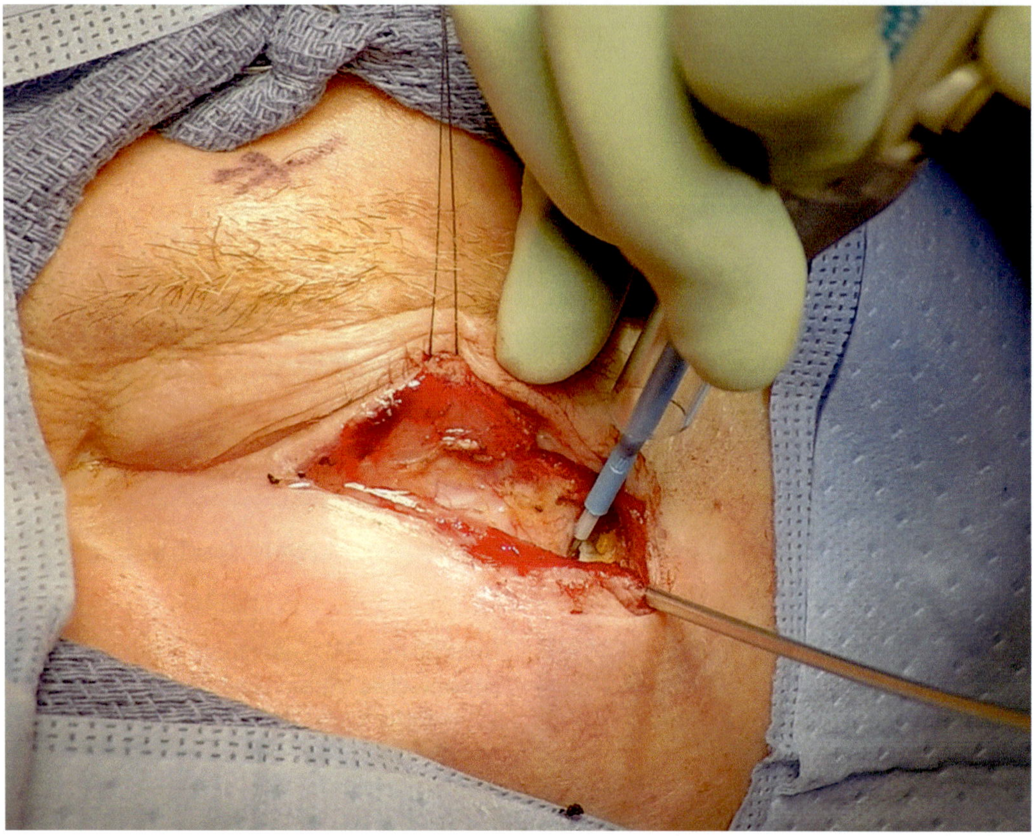

Fig. 23.7 Midface flap being developed through an external blepharoplasty incision

Combined Procedures for Negative Vector Lower Eyelid Retraction (Video 23.3)

In many instances, multiple procedures are combined to treat lower eyelid malposition (Figs. 23.9 and 23.10).

Upper Eyelid Retraction Repair (Video 23.2)

The upper eyelid also may be affected by globe position or, in cases of primary retraction, may contribute to a prominent appearance of the globe. A common scenario is the patient with thyroid eye disease with co-existent proptosis and eyelid retraction.

In levator recession, an eyelid crease incision is created through the skin and dissection is carried through orbicularis and septum to identify the insertion of the levator aponeurosis on the tarsus. The aponeurosis is then disinserted from the superior tarsus with sharp dissection (Figs. 23.11 and 23.12). The levator may be left disinserted or may be linked to the tarsus using a hang-back suture. In some cases, such as recurrence, a spacer graft (donor sclera is common) can be placed between the tarsus and edge of levator to maintain the eyelid in a lower

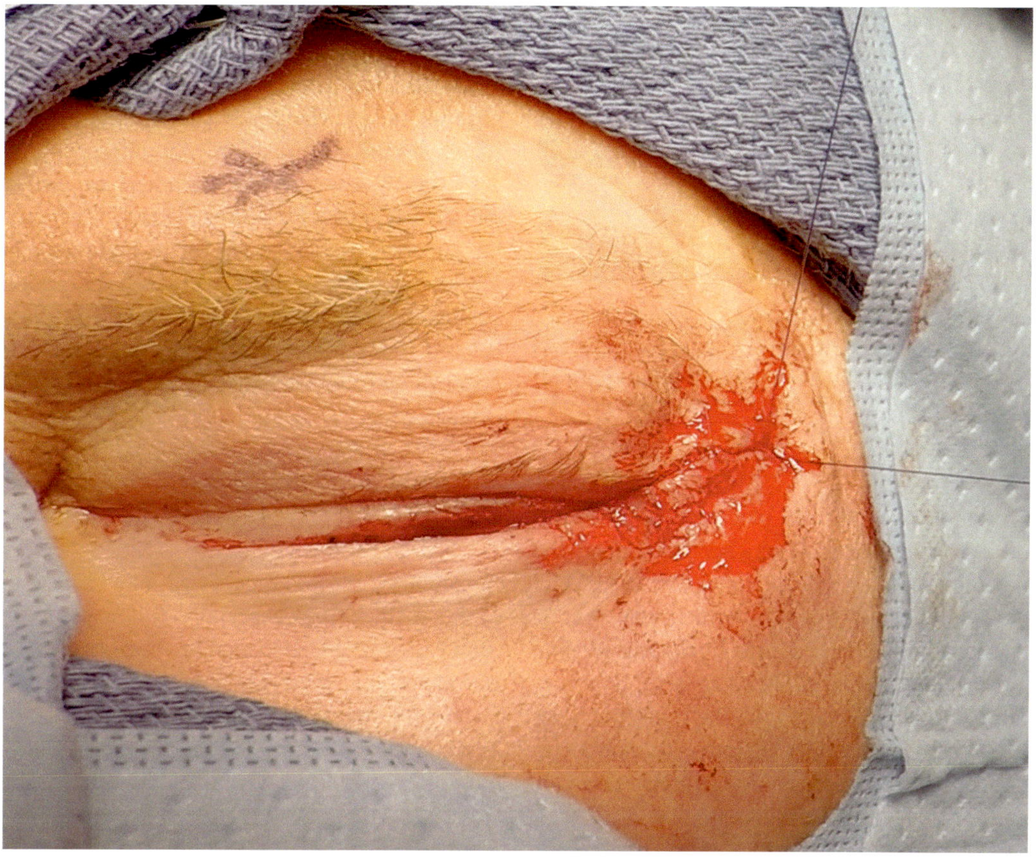

Fig. 23.8 Midface advanced and secured to temporalis fascia

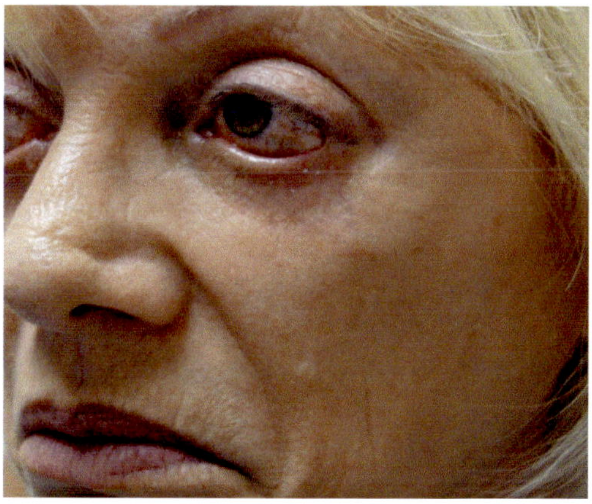

Fig. 23.9 Patient with multivector severe lower eyelid retraction and inferior scleral show

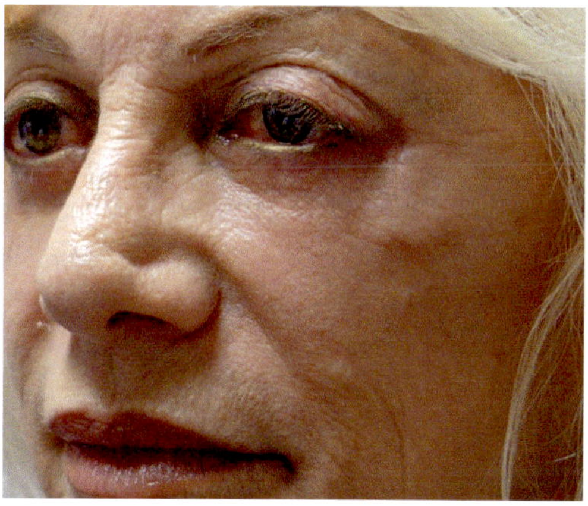

Fig. 23.10 Patient in Fig. 23.9 after lower eyelid retraction repair with combined cheek flap, posterior lamella spacer, canthal anchoring, and a tarsoconjunctival suspension flap

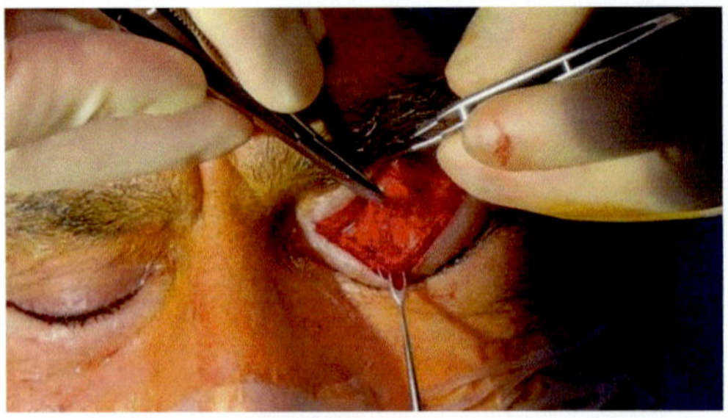

Fig. 23.11 Through an eyelid crease incision, the superior tarsal border is exposed with sharp dissection and the levator is detached and recessed. Dissection proceeds through all layers and down to conjunctiva, that may also be incised, for severe cases

position (Fig. 23.13). En bloc recession of levator and Müller's muscle has been described and may offer additional effect for severe cases. Full thickness blepharotomy in which the skin is incised and all deeper tissues (including septum, levator aponeurosis, Muller's muscle, and conjunctiva) are disinserted from the superior border of the tarsus is another effective technique for the treatment of upper eyelid retraction and may reduce the appearance of a prominent eye. If performed correctly, recession of the levator lowers the MRD1 and improves ocular surface exposure and appearance (Figs. 23.14 and 23.15).

In instances of overcorrection intraoperatively, a non-absorbable 6–0 suture is used to advance the levator onto the conjunctiva or superior tarsus. Hangback sutures may be useful to titrate the position. An interpositional graft (such as auricular cartilage or acellular dermal matrix or donor sclera) between the superior border of the tarsal plate and the recessed levator secured with 6–0 absorbable sutures may be useful. (Video 23.4) If a spacer is used, conjunctiva should not be incised to avoid direct contact between the graft and the ocular surface.

Conclusion

In summary, the prominent eye may exacerbate eyelid malposition, especially following lower eyelid surgery. Understanding eyelid anatomy and identifying these risk factors are important. Successful management of eyelid malposition in the setting of a prominent eye often requires multiple surgical interventions that treat various structures. Upper eyelid retraction repair is commonly seen with proptosis in thyroid eye disease and may be treated with levator recession with or without a spacer graft.

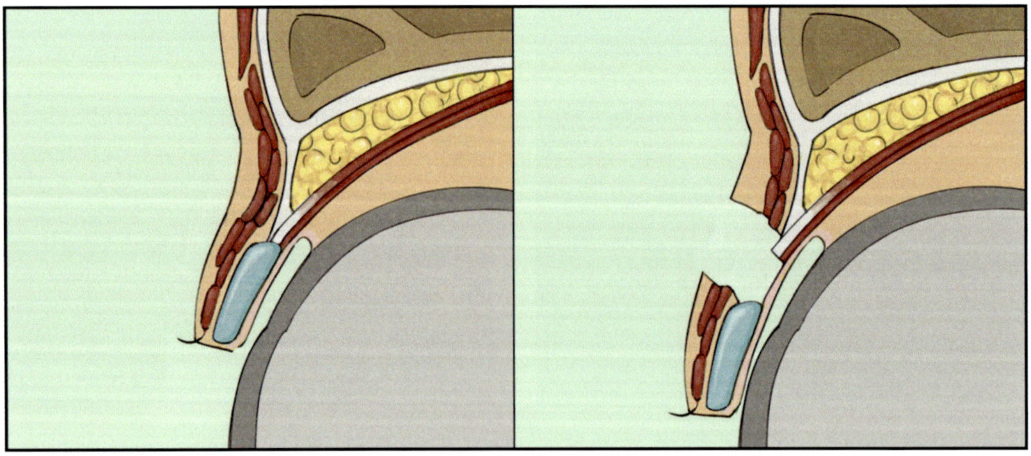

Fig. 23.12 Illustration demonstrating levator recession from a sagittal perspective

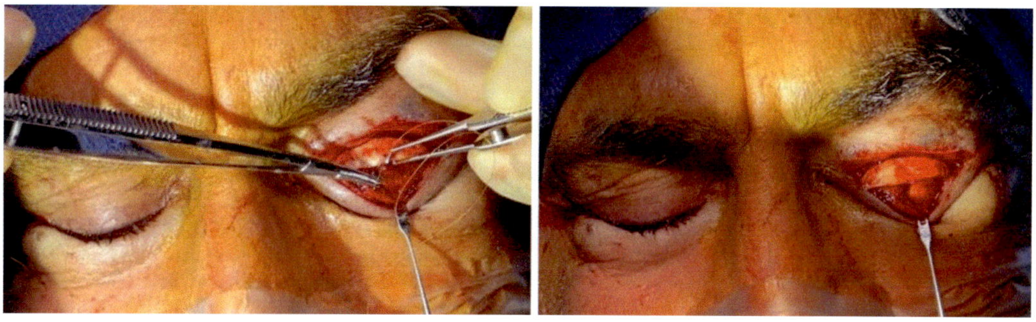

Fig. 23.13 In cases of recurrence or more severe retraction, a spacer graft (donor sclera shown here) is cut into an ellipse and positioned between the upper tarsal border and recessed levator aponeurosis using 6–0 chromic sutures

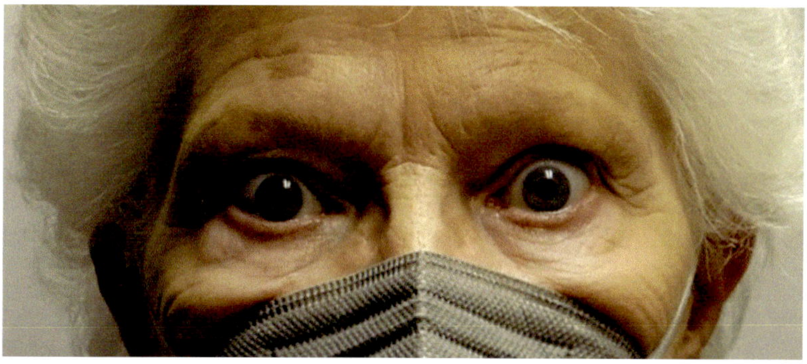

Fig. 23.14 Patient with thyroid eye disease and moderate to severe upper eyelid retraction

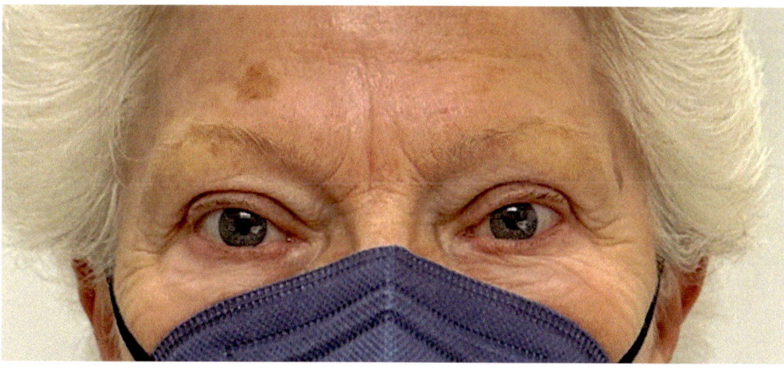

Fig. 23.15 Patient in Fig. 23.10 after bilateral upper eyelid levator recession and good correction of eyelid retraction

References

1. Dijkstal JM, Bothun ED, Harrison AR, Lee MS. Normal exophthalmometry measurements in a United States pediatric population. Ophthal Plast Reconstr Surg. 2012;28:54–6.
2. Ferrario VF, Sforza C, Colombo A, Schmitz JH, Serrao G. Morphometry of the orbital region: a soft-tissue study from adolescence to mid-adulthood. Plast Reconstr Surg. 2001;108:285–292; discussion 293.
3. Migliori ME, Gladstone GJ. Determination of the normal range of exophthalmometric values for black and white adults. Am J Ophthalmol. 1984;98:438–42.

4. Stein JD, Antonyshyn OM. Aesthetic eyelid reconstruction. Clin Plast Surg. 2009;36:379–97.
5. Cole HP, Couvillion JT, Fink AJ, Haik BG, Kastl PR. Exophthalmometry: a comparative study of the Naugle and Hertel instruments. Ophthal Plast Reconstr Surg. 1997;13:189–94.
6. Jelks GW, Jelks EB. Preoperative evaluation of the blepharoplasty patient. Bypassing the pitfalls. Clin Plast Surg. 1993;20:213–223; discussion 224.
7. Rajabi MT, Malmir M, Mahmoudzadeh R, Salabati M, Tabatabaie SZ, Rajabi MB, Hosseini SS. A comparison of lower eyelid retraction in normal individuals with positive versus negative orbital vector. Middle East Afr J Ophthalmol. 2020;27:22–7.
8. Griffin G, Azizzadeh B, Massry GG. New insights into physical findings associated with postblepharoplasty lower eyelid retraction. Aesthet Surg J. 2014;34:995–1004.
9. Xi W, Han S, Feng S, Li K, Brunetti B, Lazzeri D, Tong Y, Zhang Y. The injection for the lower eyelid retraction: a mechanical analysis of the lifting effect of the hyaluronic acid. Aesthetic Plast Surg. 2019;43:1310–7.
10. Hartstein ME. Injectable adjunctive procedures for cosmesis and function. Facial Plast Surg Clin N Am. 2016;24:139–44.
11. Alam M, Kakar R, Dover JS, Harikumar V, Kang BY, Wan HT, Poon E, Jones DH. Rates of vascular occlusion associated with using needles vs cannulas for filler injection. JAMA Dermatol. 2021;157:174–80.
12. Goldberg RA, Soroudi AE, McCann JD. Treatment of prominent eyes with orbital rim onlay implants: four-year experience. Ophthal Plast Reconstr Surg. 2003;19:38–45.
13. Shorr N. Madame Butterfly procedure with hard palate graft: management of postblepharoplasty round eye and scleral show. Facial Plast Surg FPS. 1994;10:90–118.
14. Guthrie AJ, Kadakia P, Rosenberg J. Eyelid malposition repair: a review of the literature and current techniques. Semin Plast Surg. 2019;33:92–102.
15. Kim KH, Baek JS, Lee S, Lee JH, Choi HS, Kim SJ, Jang JW. Causes and surgical outcomes of lower eyelid retraction. Korean J Ophthalmol KJO. 2017;31:290–8.
16. Price KM, Gupta PK, Woodward JA, Stinnett SS, Murchison AP. Eyebrow and eyelid dimensions: an anthropometric analysis of African Americans and Caucasians. Plast Reconstr Surg. 2009;124:615–23.
17. Dunsky IL. Normative data for hertel exophthalmometry in a normal adult black population. Optom Vis Sci Off Publ Am Acad Optom. 1992;69:562–4.
18. Eze BI, Uche JN, Shiweobi JO, Mba CN. Oculopalpebral dimensions of adult Nigerians: report from the Enugu normative ocular anthropometry study. Med Princ Pract Int J Kuwait Univ Health Sci Cent. 2013;22:75–9.
19. Li Q, Zhang X, Li K, Quan Y, Cai X, Xu S, Zhu F, Lu R. Normative anthropometric analysis and aesthetic indication of the ocular region for young Chinese adults. Graefes Arch Clin Exp Ophthalmol Albrecht Von Graefes Arch Klin Exp Ophthalmol. 2016;254:189–97.
20. Cheung JJC, Chang DL, Chan JC, et al. Exophthalmometry values in the Hong Kong Chinese adult population from a population-based study. Medicine (Baltimore). 2019;98: e17993.

Lower Eyelid Retraction—Hard Palate Graft

24

Anne Barmettler and Tiffany Cheng

Abstract

Lower eyelid retraction is common and causes symptoms of ocular irritation and discomfort, as well as issues of cosmesis and facial asymmetry. Moreover, the ocular surface may suffer exposure damage. Prior eyelid surgery, a negative vector facial morphology, and thyroid eye disease are common conditions in which eyelid retraction is present. A spacer graft to the posterior lamella aims to elevate the eyelid margin. Many materials have been used in this context. Hard palate grafts shine due to their similarity to native tarsal tissue with respect to consistency, thickness, stiffness, and the presence of a mucosal surface. In this chapter, the authors describe lower eyelid retraction repair using an autologous hard palate graft.

Keywords

Lower eyelid retraction · Spacer graft · Hard palate graft · Lateral tarsal strip · Lagophthalmos · Thyroid eye disease

Supplementary Information The online version contains supplementary material available at https://doi.org/10.1007/978-3-031-63178-8_24.

A. Barmettler (✉) · T. Cheng
Albert Einstein College of Medicine, New York, NY, USA
e-mail: annebarmettler@gmail.com

Introduction

Lower eyelid retraction can cause symptomatic ocular surface exposure. There exist various etiologies. Commonly, cicatricial vectors occur from prior lower eyelid surgery. A negative vector facial morphology with or without or thyroid eye disease are other common scenarios.

Lower eyelid retraction repair with a hard palate graft is a surgical technique that elevates an inferiorly displaced lower eyelid to restore its normal anatomic height and position. While the use of various spacer grafts has been described in the literature, hard palate grafts stand out for their similarity to tarsal tissue with respect to consistency, thickness, stiffness, and the presence of a mucosal surface. Other spacer grafts commonly used for lower eyelid retraction repair include the following: (1) autologous auricular cartilage, dermis fat, or tarsus, (2) allogenic donor sclera and acellular dermal matrix, (3) xenogenic acellular dermal matrices (e.g., porcine, bovine). Each of these spacer grafts has its own advantages and disadvantages [1–4].

An autologous hard palate graft may minimize cost, especially compared to many biologic tissue device options, while also providing excellent structural support and closely mimicking native tarsal tissue. The technique necessitates familiarity with anatomy of both the lower eyelid and palate.

The procedure begins with a lateral canthotomy and inferior cantholysis to facilitate access

J. Tao (ed.), *Efficient Oculofacial Surgery*, https://doi.org/10.1007/978-3-031-63178-8_24

to the lower eyelid retractors. A traction suture through the lower eyelid margin aids in exposing the posterior lamella, where a horizontal transconjunctival incision is made inferior to the tarsus. Next, an elliptical hard palate graft is harvested and sutured into the newly created incision, inferior to the tarsus. The lateral tarsal strip is fixated to the temporal orbital rim and the canthal angle is then carefully recreated. Lastly, the traction suture is secured to the forehead, as a Frost suture. This technique restores lower eyelid position with excellent cosmesis and durability.

Advantages

- Correction of lower eyelid retraction with a structurally similar tissue
- Excellent cosmesis (the visibility of the hard palate graft contour through the skin is typically less than that of auricular cartilage)
- Amelioration of dry eye symptoms, as less ocular surface is exposed, and the hard palate graft contains mucin-producing minor salivary glands
- No direct cost (compared to acellular dermal matrices)
- Low risk of graft rejection or inflammatory reaction
- Less postoperative graft contracture compared to acellular dermal matrices [5, 6].

Disadvantages

- Increased duration of surgery, exposure to anesthesia, and facility use/fees due to need to harvest donor graft
- Potential prolonged patient recovery time from donor site morbidities

Indications

Lower eyelid retraction can be congenital or acquired, but most often occurs secondary to thyroid eye disease, over-aggressive blepharoplasty, facial nerve paralysis, extraocular muscle surgery or injury, or weakening of the orbicularis oculi [7]. A hard palate graft can be utilized for tectonic support inferior to the tarsus, allowing elevation of the lower eyelid margin. Indications for surgery include severe lower eyelid retraction and/or failure of conservative treatments (i.e. artificial tears, topical ointments) to relieve ocular symptoms. Some alternative non-surgical modalities include hyaluronic acid fillers, steroid injections, and botulinum toxin type A [8]. While these non-surgical modalities provide only a temporary correction, they may be appropriate for poor surgical candidates or those with potentially temporary pathologies (e.g. transient facial palsy).

Hard Contraindications

- Patients with confirmed oral squamous cell carcinoma or other malignancies

Soft Contraindications

- Patients with ocular cicatricial pemphigoid (consider intra- and post-operative steroids)
- Patients with palate abnormalities or prior radiation to the palate
- Patients with coexisting severe or unstable medical conditions
- Patients with liver disease/cirrhosis, bleeding diathesis or coagulopathies.

Considerations

- Aesthetic surgery patients with unrealistic expectations or psychological instability
- Patients who cannot tolerate donor site pain
- Ipsilateral monocular patients may need to avoid patching post-operatively (the Frost suture can be placed more temporally and potentially for a shorter postoperative period).

Preoperative Preparation

- ***Patient Discussion***: As there are several etiologies of lower eyelid retraction, a thorough preoperative history and examination to determine underlying cause and aid in surgical planning. The following components of the pre-operative visit should be obtained:
  - A complete medical and surgical history, including previous surgical attempts at correcting the lower eyelid malposition or fillers to the area
  - Review of systems
  - Family history and social history
  - History of bleeding and use of blood thinners or aspirin-containing products (Patients should be counseled to consult with their prescribing physician to determine when the medications should be discontinued.)
  - Old photographs (To monitor progression of the lower eyelid retraction or to serve as a 'before" picture for comparison with results).
- ***Risks/Benefits/Alternatives and Post-operative Course:*** The risks and benefits of surgery should be discussed, including bleeding, infection, need for additional surgery, as well as:
  - Under- or overcorrection
  - Thickening or visibility of graft contour through the skin
  - Corneal abrasion.

The post-operative course should also be explained, including nausea, headaches, and other side effects from anesthesia, local pain and discomfort at the operative site, avoidance of heavy lifting, contact lens, and make-up application, incision care, and signs of infection (i.e. fever, chills, redness, or discharge from the incision) prompting immediate return.

Examination

Lid position, eyelid laxity, and the presence of scarring or contraction of the anterior, middle, or posterior lamellae should be noted. Lower eyelid retraction can be quantified by measuring the amount of sclera visible between the corneal limbus and the lower eyelid margin in millimeters. Alternatively, the margin reflex distance 2 (MRD2), or the distance between the corneal light reflex to the lower eyelid in primary gaze, can be measured in millimeters (see Fig. 24.1). While any distance greater than 5.5 mm should raise suspicion for lower eyelid retraction, symptoms can still arise in patients with MRD2 less than 5.5 mm. Eyelid laxity can be assessed by the eyelid distraction test, where the distance between the globe and manually distracted lower eyelid is measured, or the snap-back test, where the examiner pulls the lower eyelid away from the globe, lets go, and measures the time to return to original position. A distraction test exceeding 6 mm or delay in snap-back indicates eyelid laxity, which would indicate a need for lateral canthal tendon tightening.

Additional preoperative concerns include malar fat pad positioning and the presence of a negative vector, where a prominent globe or depressed cheeks can lead to poorer outcomes. In these cases, additional treatments, such as orbital decompression or preperiosteal malar fat pad elevation may be helpful.

Determination of spacer graft requirement is often guided by experience but can be as follows [1]:

- The examiner places a finger at the lateral canthus and pushes upward and laterally.

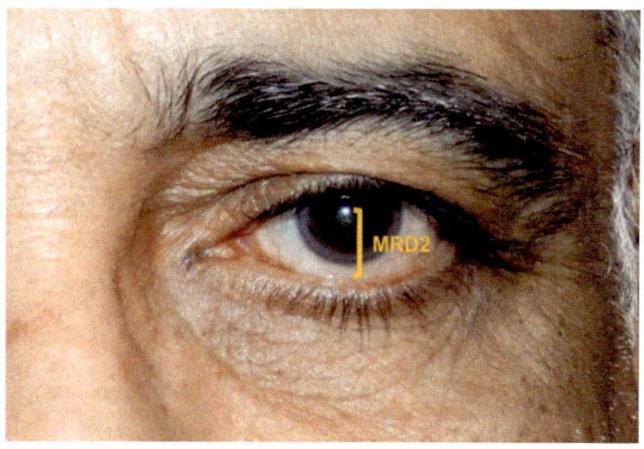

Fig. 24.1 MRD2 of 7 mm in this patient, measured with the patient looking into the light source in primary gaze, indicates severe lower eyelid retraction

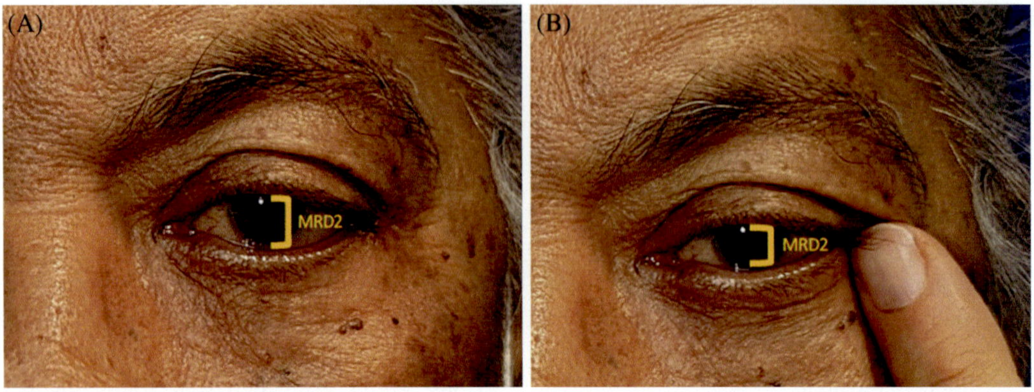

Fig. 24.2 A, B. Examiner demonstrating a method to determine surgical approach. (A) shows a patient with an MRD2 of 6 mm. (B) A finger gently lifts the lateral canthal angle to bring the MRD2 from 6 mm to an acceptable height of 4 mm. This patient most likely will do well with solely a lateral canthal strip

If this maneuver restores the normal position of the lower eyelid, lateral canthal tendon tightening likely will be sufficient (see Fig. 24.2A, B).

- If this maneuver does not restore the position of the lower eyelid margin to above the inferior limbus, a finger is placed at the central lower eyelid margin to lift it superiorly. If this successfully repositions the lower eyelid, a hard palate graft can be considered in conjunction with the lateral canthal tendon tightening.
- If a finger at the lower eyelid margin pushing upwards fails to lift the lower eyelid margin to the superior limbus, additional surgery is likely required, such as a full thickness skin graft or midface elevation.

Symptoms of exposure keratopathy should also be assessed and an anterior slit lamp examination to evaluate the tear film should be conducted. Presence and quantification of lagophthalmos (in millimeters), including corneal show (in millimeters), should be documented. Additionally, frontal and profile photographs of the non-smiling face in primary gaze should be obtained at the pre-operative visit.

Operative Technique (Video 24.1)

(1) ***Lower eyelid retractor release***

First, a lateral canthotomy and inferior cantholysis is done to facilitate access to the lower eyelid retractors and to address any aspect of horizontal laxity. A 4–0 traction suture is placed through the lower eyelid margin at the level of the meibomian glands. The authors prefer a double armed Ticron (Minneapolis, MN, USA) polyester suture on a pre-placed bolster, but silk sutures may be used. The lower eyelid is then everted over a cotton-tip applicator and a conjunctival incision is made approximately 1–2 mm below the inferior border of the tarsus (Fig. 24.3). This incision typically extends from inferior to the punctum to 20 mm laterally. The depth of this incision involves releasing lower eyelid retractors or upon reaching the orbicularis oculi. Hemostasis can be achieved using high temperature cautery.

(2) ***Donor Site Harvesting***

Next, the hard palate graft is harvested from the roof of the mouth. Marking for the donor graft, typically measuring 5 mm wide by 20 mm long,

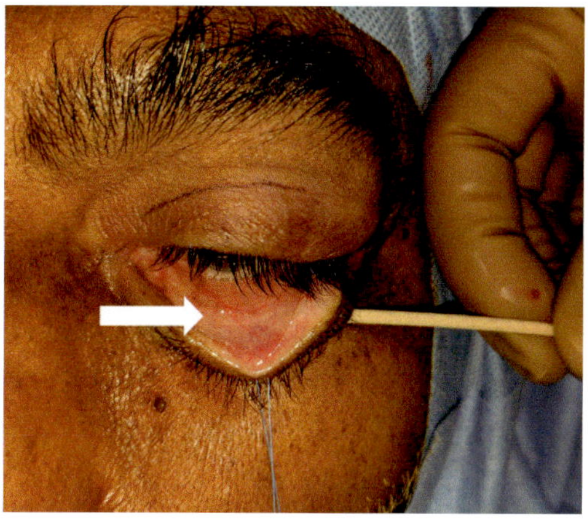

Fig. 24.3 A 4–0 Ticron suture acts as a traction suture through the lower eyelid margin and is pulled inferiorly over a cotton tipped applicator to expose the desired location of the horizontal conjunctival incision inferior to the tarsus (arrow)

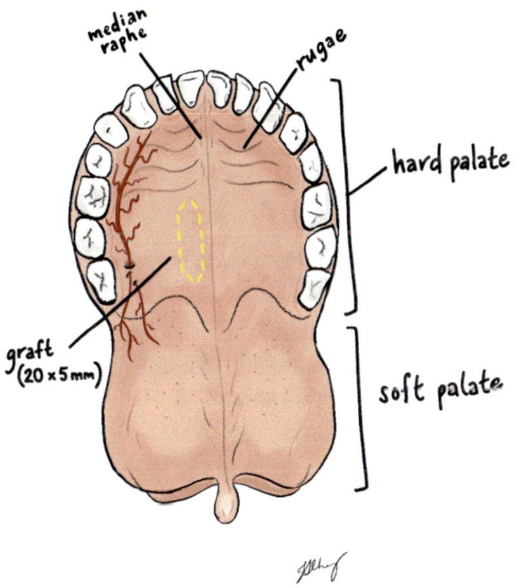

Fig. 24.4 Palate anatomy with desired donor site marked in dotted yellow

can be delineated using cautery. This is usually taken just lateral to the median raphe and behind the rugae (see Fig. 24.4). The dimensions of the graft can be adjusted depending on the patient's need. It is important to avoid the posterior soft palate to prevent palatal fistula. Palpation of the roof will indicate the end of the hard palate and the beginning of soft palate. This incision is carried out from posterior to the mucosal ridge to about 20 mm posteriorly in the shape of an ellipse or elongated hexagon, with a horizontal width of ~5 mm. The graft is then harvested in the submucosal plane, utilizing a 15 blade and Westcott scissors. A size 8 Frazier-tipped suction aids with visualization. Colorado tipped cautery (Stryker, Kalamazoo, Michigan, USA) and thrombogenic materials (Surgicel, Ethicon, Bridgewater, NJ, USA) can be used for hemostasis. The graft can be thinned with scissors to achieve a consistent thickness. Next, the graft can then be placed onto the lower eyelid conjunctival defect and sutured into place using interrupted, buried 6–0 Vicryl sutures (see Fig. 24.5). The authors typically put in eight sutures.

(3) ***Lateral Tarsal Strip***

Attention can then be turned to the lateral canthus, where a lateral tarsal strip is performed. The anterior lamella is dissected from the tarsus with scissors and the tarsus can be shortened to the appropriate length. A double-armed 5–0 non-absorbable suture is then passed posteriorly to anteriorly through the lateral tarsal strip. Each arm is passed through the periosteum of the lateral orbital rim at the level of the lateral orbital tubercle and tied into place using a braided polyester, polyglactin or, polypropylene suture. The lateral canthus is reformed with a circular 6–0 plain gut suture. The skin of the lateral canthus is then closed using a 6–0 plain gut suture.

(4) ***Frost Suture***

Lastly, a Frost suture is used to put the eyelid on stretch. Each arm of the double-armed 4–0 traction is sutured to the area superior to the temporal brow (see Fig. 24.6).

Tips and Pearls

- An oral incision from posterior to anterior helps prevent blood from obscuring the view.
- A graft 1–2 mm larger than the conjunctival defect accounts for graft contraction.

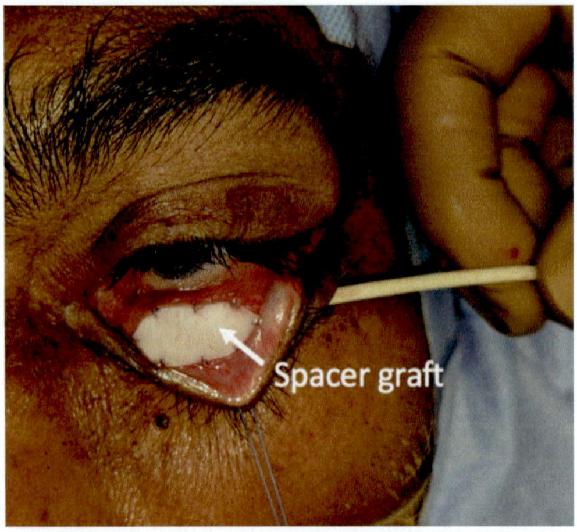

Fig. 24.5 After the horizontal conjunctival incision is made inferior to the tarsus, eight interrupted, buried sutures are used to fixate the spacer graft, which can be hard palate or other materials, such as acellular dermal matrix (shown) or auricular cartilage

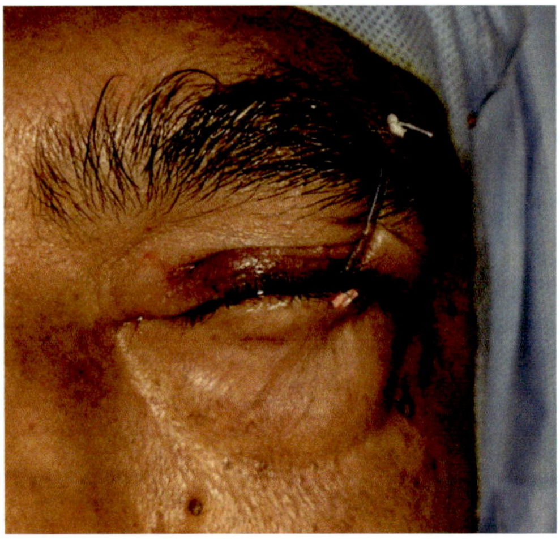

Fig. 24.6 Frost suture

- Avoid extending graft harvesting into the soft palate to avoid risk of fistula. Additionally, the greater palatine vessels are located medial to the second molar and may create significant hemorrhage if inadvertently damaged (see Fig. 24.4).
- When suturing the graft into place, sutures should be cut on the knot and buried to avoid causing ocular irritation.

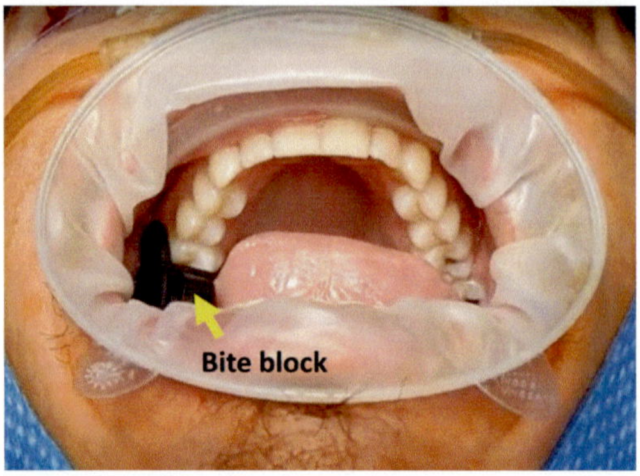

Fig. 24.7 Patient with intra-operative bite block and lip retractor in place with excellent view of the hard palate

- A bite block can improve access. For improved visibility during the surgery, a lip retractor can be used (Ivoclar Vivadent AG, Schaan, Liechtenstein), sweetheart retractor, or tongue depressors can be helpful (see Fig. 24.7).

Complications [9, 10]

- Infection
- Hematoma of eyelid
- Hematoma/prolonged bleeding of palate
- Graft necrosis/dehiscence
- Donor site candidiasis
- Donor site granuloma formation
- Oronasal fistula formation
- Corneal abrasion

Postoperative Care

- The authors place two eye pads over the eye and Frost suture to prevent accidental pulling on the Frost suture during the healing period. The Frost suture is removed in the office four to 10 days later.
- Severe post-operative pain and infections are rare. For prevention of surgical site infection and inflammation, topical antibiotic-steroid ointment (neomycin-polymyxin-dexamethasone) may be used twice daily upon

removal of the eye patch four to ten days postoperatively.

Conclusions

A posterior lamella hard palate spacer graft is an excellent choice for lower eyelid retraction repair. Hard palate is widely considered the gold standard but is associated with some second oral surgical site morbidity.

References

1. Patipa M. The evaluation and management of lower eyelid retraction following cosmetic surgery. Plast Reconstr Surg. 2000;106(2):438–53; discussion 54–9. https://doi.org/10.1097/00006534-200008000-00033.
2. Wearne MJ, Sandy C, Rose GE, Pitts J, Collin JR. Autogenous hard palate mucosa: the ideal lower eyelid spacer? Br J Ophthalmol. 2001;85(10):1183–7. https://doi.org/10.1136/bjo.85.10.1183.
3. Kersten RC, Kulwin DR, Levartovsky S, Tiradellis H, Tse DT. Management of lower-lid retraction with hard-palate mucosa grafting. Arch Ophthalmol. 1990;108(9):1339–43. https://doi.org/10.1001/archopht.1990.01070110155041.
4. Barmettler A, Heo M. A prospective, randomized comparison of lower eyelid retraction repair with autologous auricular cartilage, bovine acellular dermal matrix (Surgimend), and porcine acellular dermal matrix (Enduragen) spacer grafts. Ophthalmic Plast Reconstr Surg. 2018;34(3):266–73. https://doi.org/10.1097/iop.0000000000000946.
5. Park E, Lewis K, Alghoul MS. Comparison of efficacy and complications among various spacer grafts in the treatment of lower eyelid retraction: a systematic review. Aesthetic Surg J. 2017;37(7):743–54. https://doi.org/10.1093/asj/sjx003.
6. Sullivan SA, Dailey RA. Graft contraction: a comparison of acellular dermis versus hard palate mucosa in lower eyelid surgery. Ophthalmic Plast Reconstr Surg. 2003;19(1):14–24. https://doi.org/10.1097/01.Iop.0000040678.19893.F7.
7. Kim KH, Baek JS, Lee S, Lee JH, Choi HS, Kim SJ, et al. Causes and surgical outcomes of lower eyelid retraction. Korean J Ophthalmol. 2017;31(4):290–8. https://doi.org/10.3341/kjo.2016.0059.
8. Grisolia ABD, Couso RC, Matayoshi S, Douglas RS, Briceño CA. Non-surgical treatment for eyelid retraction in thyroid eye disease (TED). Br J Ophthalmol. 2017. https://doi.org/10.1136/bjophthalmol-2017-310695.
9. Kim JW, Kikkawa DO, Lemke BN. Donor site complications of hard palate mucosal grafting. Ophthalmic Plast Reconstr Surg. 1997;13(1):36–9. https://doi.org/10.1097/00002341-199703000-00007.
10. Pang NK, Bartley GB, Bite U, Bradley EA. Hard palate mucosal grafts in oculoplastic surgery: donor site lessons. Am J Ophthalmol. 2004;137(6):1021–5. https://doi.org/10.1016/j.ajo.2003.12.034.

25 Lower Eyelid Retraction Repair with Dermis Fat Graft

Nicole Topilow, Niloofar Radgoudarzi, Catherine Liu, Don Kikkawa, and Bobby S. Korn

Abstract

Lower eyelid retraction can be the result of scar in any eyelid layer. In mild forms, eyelid retraction can be tolerated, but in more severe forms it may cause ocular surface exposure or disfigurement or both. In cases of lower eyelid retraction caused by middle and posterior lamellar deficiencies associated with volume loss, dermis fat grafts are an excellent option for retraction repair. Benefits of autologous dermis fat grafts for lower eyelid retraction repair include good compatibility, abundant donor tissue, and good support for the eyelid. In this chapter, the authors describe considerations and techniques of dermis fat graft lower eyelid retraction repair.

Keywords

Lower eyelid retraction · Lower lid retraction · Dermis fat graft · Autologous

Introduction

The lower eyelid is composed of an anterior lamella (skin and orbicularis muscle), middle lamella (orbital septum), and posterior lamella (tarsus and conjunctiva). When the integrity of any of these three lamellae is disturbed, lower eyelid retraction can occur. For example, anterior lamellar deficiency due to actinic changes, trauma, and surgical removal of lower eyelid skin as in lower eyelid blepharoplasty can cause lower eyelid retraction [1–3]. Poor orbicularis muscle tone due to facial nerve palsy, and scarring of the orbital septum from trauma, lower eyelid blepharoplasty, and orbital surgery can lead to lower eyelid retraction [1–3]. Fibrosis of the capsulopalpebral fascia in thyroid eye disease reduces lower eyelid retractor distensibility and can lead to lower eyelid retraction [1–3]. Regardless of etiology, lower eyelid retraction can result in poor cosmesis, dry eye symptoms, and exposure keratopathy with corneal ulceration and perforation. When aggressive ocular lubrication for mild lower eyelid retraction is insufficient, or in moderate to severe cases of lower eyelid retraction, surgical correction of lid position is necessary.

The clinical examination of the retracted lower eyelid is essential for success. Thus, repair of lower eyelid retraction is directed towards correcting the underlying pathophysiologic changes. In the case of anterior lamellar

N. Topilow · N. Radgoudarzi · C. Liu · D. Kikkawa · B. S. Korn (✉)
Viterbi Family Department of Ophthalmology, Division of Oculofacial Plastic and Reconstructive Surgery, University of California, San Diego, CA, USA
e-mail: bkorn@ucsd.edu

J. Tao (ed.), *Efficient Oculofacial Surgery*, https://doi.org/10.1007/978-3-031-63178-8_25

deficiency, pedicle-based skin flaps or full thickness skin grafting can be employed. To preserve cosmesis, anterior lamellar recruitment can be obtained from lifting of the entire midface. Scarring of the middle lamella can be identified by digital elevation of the lower eyelid. If there is resistance to elevation, middle lamellar scarring is likely present and anterior lamellar supplementation will not be sufficient. Correction of middle lamellar scarring consists of lysis of the cicatrix followed by placement of a suitable spacer graft.

Historically, dermis fat grafts (DFG) have been used for orbital volume augmentation as primary implants at the time of enucleation, in cases of superior sulcus deformity, and in contracted sockets [4]. DFG have also been used with success in cases of lower eyelid retraction caused by middle and posterior lamellar deficiencies associated with volume loss (Fig. 25.4) [3, 5, 6]. One benefit of DFG over more traditional spacer grafts such as hard palate and allografts is that they simultaneously provide volume and posterior lamellar supplementation [3, 7]. The amount of volume provided by the graft can be easily adjusted, and the available harvestable tissue is abundant (ex. hip, abdomen, post-auricular) [3, 6, 7]. Additional benefits of DFG over allografts include the non-immunogenicity of tissue and lack of concern for disease transmission [3, 7]. Compared to hard palate grafts, the donor site healing process is less painful and there is no increased risk of infection from the oronasal flora [3, 8]. Lower eyelid tightening procedures and midface lifting can be simultaneously performed to augment results.

Surgical Technique

See Figs. 25.1, 25.2 and 25.3.

Potential Complications

Potential complications associated with the use of DFG in lower eyelid retraction repair include graft contracture with recurrent lid retraction, keratinization or hair growth on the dermal side, and corneal epithelial defects [3].

Conclusion

Dermis fat grafting is an effective technique for the correction of lower eyelid retraction repair. There is abundant harvestable tissue that is well integrated to the lower eyelid to provide volume and support. There is low harvest site morbidity. Especially in cases of lower eyelid retraction associated with volume loss, dermis fat grafts may have advantages over other customary posterior lamella spacer grafts (Fig. 25.4).

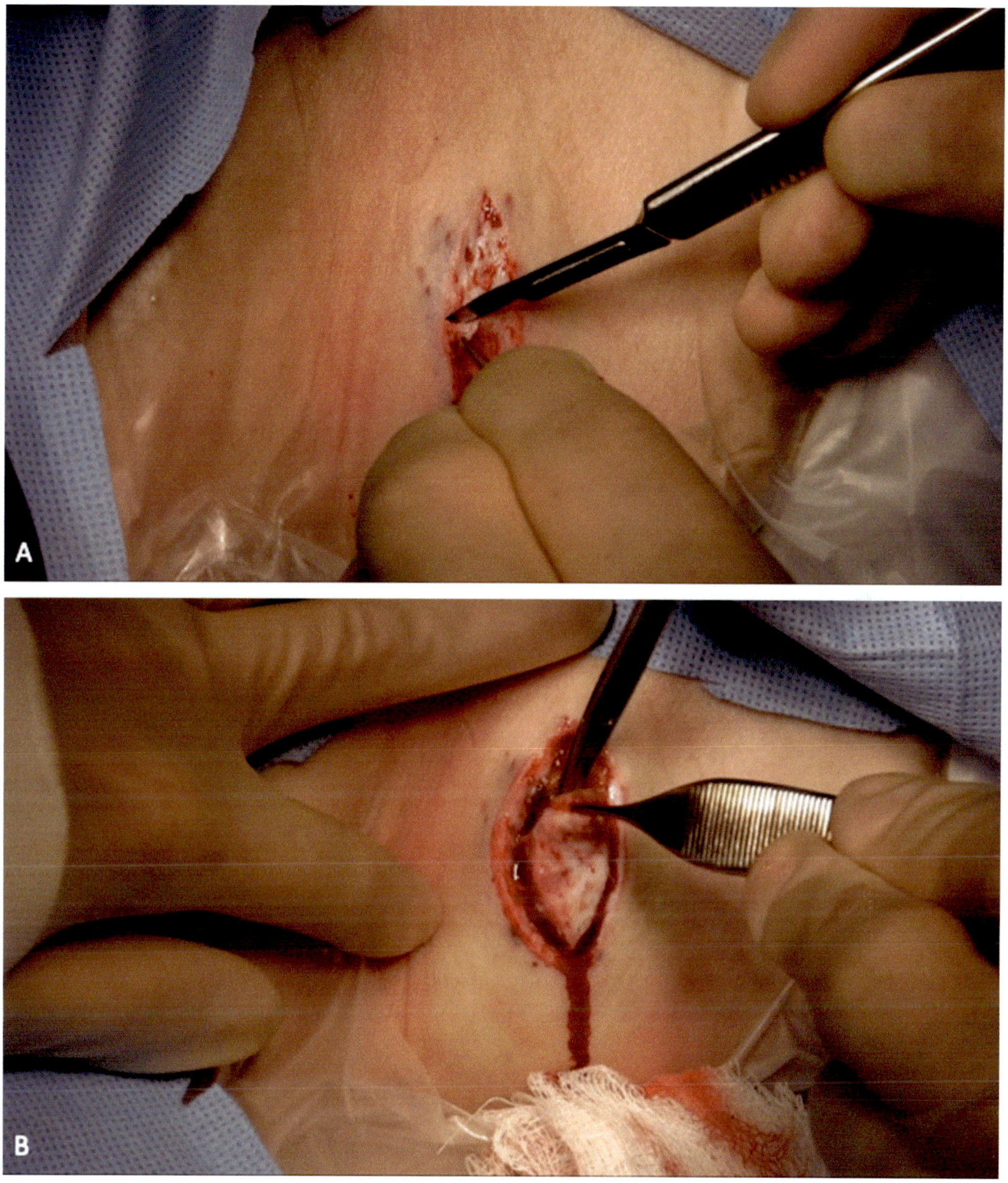

Fig. 25.1 Dermis Fat Graft Harvesting. A: An ellipse measuring approximately 25 × 50 mm is marked on the skin of the hip inferior and posterior to superior iliac crest. The abdomen is another suitable donor site. A #15 blade or diamond burr rotating at 20,000 rpm is used to denude the epithelium down to the level of the deep dermis. Alternatively, the epidermis and adnexal appendages can be removed with direct lamellar excision. B: The graft composed of the deep dermis tissue and underlying fat is harvested using sharp dissection. The wound is closed in deep and superficial layers using absorbable sutures. C: The dermis fat graft can be trimmed according to the area and volume needed for retraction repair. A vertical overcorrection of approximately 1 mm is recommended

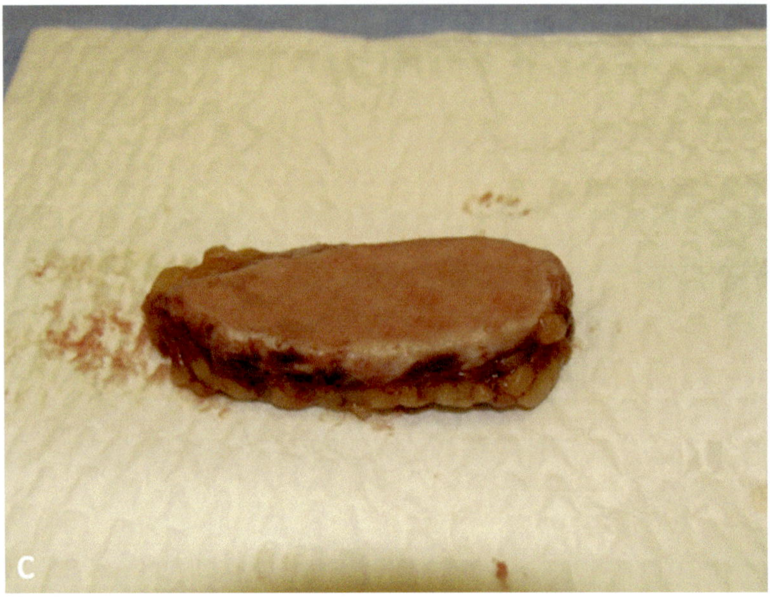

Fig. 25.1 (continued)

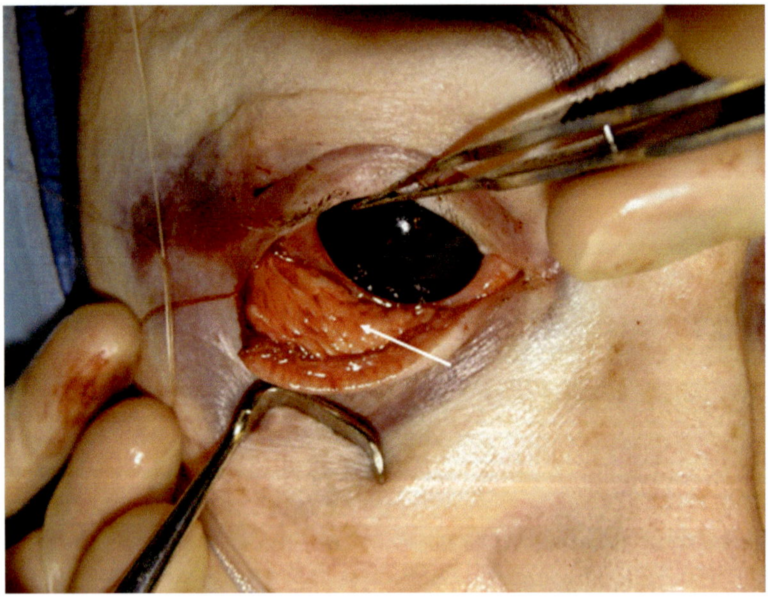

Fig. 25.2 Placement of dermis fat graft. A lateral canthotomy and inferior cantholysis are performed. A transconjunctival incision is made beneath the inferior tarsal border. Scar tissue in the middle lamella is lysed. The graft is placed deep in the inferior fornix with the dermis side facing the ocular surface (white arrow) and the fat side facing anteriorly. The edges of the graft are meticulously affixed to the surrounding conjunctiva with 6–0 rapid absorbing gut suture to allow for post-operative conjunctival epithelial cell migration over the DFG

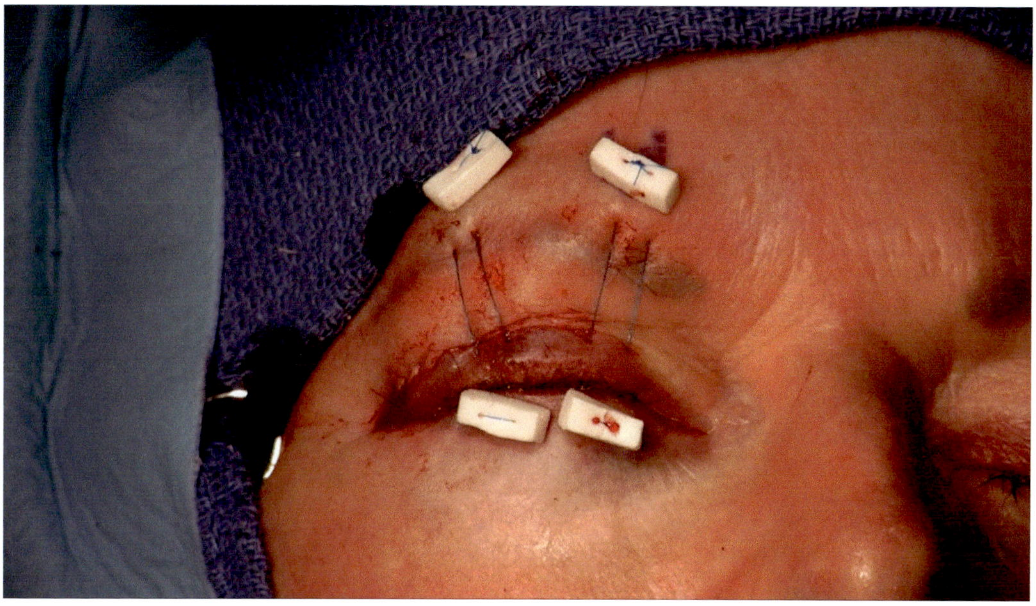

Fig. 25.3 Placement of Frost sutures to maintain the lower eyelid on stretch post-operatively. Two 6–0 polypropylene sutures are passed in a horizontal mattress fashion through the lower eyelid margin, upper eyelid margin, and brow and tied with foam bolsters. To minimize corneal irritation, a large diameter contact lens can be placed. The sutures are removed 1 week after surgery

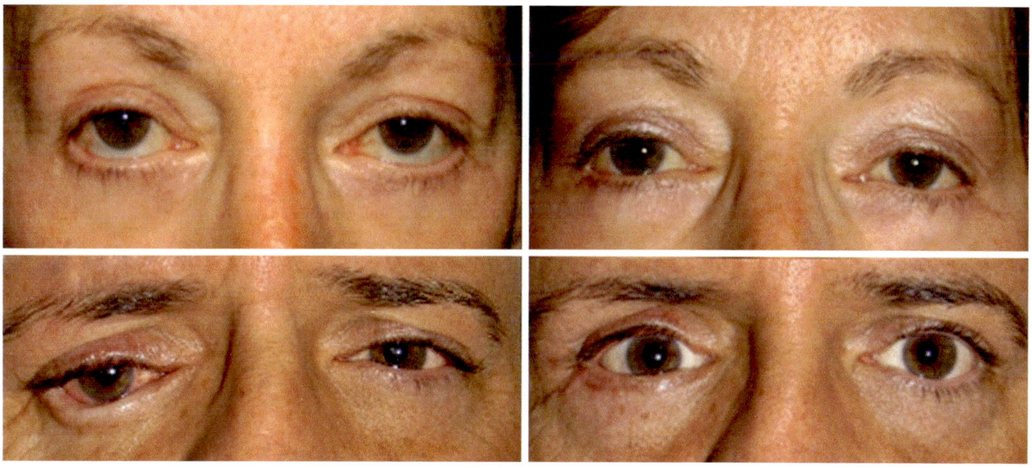

Fig. 25.4 Left: Pre-operative clinical photographs demonstrating bilateral lower eyelid (top) and right lower eyelid retraction (bottom) in two middle aged patients. **Right**: Post-operative clinical photographs demonstrating significant improvement in the lower lid position in both patients following dermis fat grafting

References

1. Kim KH, Baek JS, Lee S, Lee JH, Choi HS, Kim SJ, et al. Causes and surgical outcomes of lower eyelid retraction. Korean J Ophthalmol. 2017;31(4):290–8.
2. Patipa M. The evaluation and management of lower eyelid retraction following cosmetic surgery. Plast Reconstr Surg. 2000;106(2):438–53; discussion 54–9.
3. Korn BS, Kikkawa DO, Cohen SR, Hartstein M, Annunziata CC. Treatment of lower eyelid malposition with dermis fat grafting. Ophthalmology. 2008;115(4):744-51.e2.
4. Smith B, Bosniak S, Nesi F, Lisman R. Dermis-fat orbital implantation: 118 cases. Ophthalmic Surg. 1983;14(11):941–3.
5. Godfrey KJ, Tooley AA, Kazim M. Bipedicle dermis fat graft for orbital volume augmentation and repair of lower eyelid retraction in an anophthalmic socket with prior orbital implant placement. Ophthalmic Plast Reconstr Surg. 2019;35(2):e39–41.
6. Chang HS, Lee D, Taban M, Douglas RS, Goldberg RA. En-glove" lysis of lower eyelid retractors with AlloDerm and dermis-fat grafts in lower eyelid retraction surgery. Ophthalmic Plast Reconstr Surg. 2011;27(2):137–41.
7. Elabjer BK, Miletić D, Bušić M, Tvrdi AB, Bosnar D, Bjeloš M. Dermis-fat graft for correction of recurrent severe upper eyelid retraction in Graves' orbitopathy. Acta Clin Croat. 2018;57(1):173.
8. Park E, Lewis K, Alghoul MS. Comparison of efficacy and complications among various spacer grafts in the treatment of lower eyelid retraction: a systematic review. Aesthet Surg J. 2017;37(7):743–54.

Eyelid Surgery in Facial Paresis

26

Dhruv Sethi, Amy P. Jain and Swapna Vemuri

Abstract

Facial nerve paresis is often associated with eyelid malposition that causes ocular surface exposure. Symptomatic dry eye or vision loss may ensue if the eyelids are not treated effectively. The paretic eyelid may demonstrate loss of upper and lower eyelid tone, ectropion, upper and lower eyelid retraction, lagophthalmos, and an inadequate blink. Inadequate blinking can disrupt the tear pump mechanism and exacerbate epiphora. Concomitant vectors may add to the management. These include a prominent globe, midfacial descent, volume loss, laxity, or cicatricial vectors. Addressing eyelid malposition appropriately demands thorough attention to each vector. Interventions include acute and long-term measures to protect the ocular surface. In this chapter, the authors detail some of the preferred and expedient surgical interventions for paralyzed eyelids.

Supplementary Information The online version contains supplementary material available at https://doi.org/10.1007/978-3-031-63178-8_26.

D. Sethi · S. Vemuri (✉)
Henry Ford Health, Detroit, MI, USA
e-mail: svemuri1@hfhs.org

A. P. Jain
Cedars-Sinai Medical Center,
Los Angeles, CA, USA

Keywords

Facial nerve palsy · Bell palsy · Paretic eyelid · Paralytic eyelid · Paralytic lagophthalmos

Introduction

Facial nerve paresis can result in periocular changes including eyelid malposition that causes exposure keratopathy. In addition to symptoms of dry eye or epiphora vision loss may ensue if the cornea remains unprotected. Medical interventions include eye lubrication, moisture chamber goggles, or taping the eyelid shut. Surgical interventions can be categorized as those that are acute and temporary versus those interventions that provide more durable results.

Acute Management Techniques

1. Medical Management: lubrication, lifestyle, and environmental modifications
2. Minor procedures: temporary serpentine tarsorrhaphy, Botulinum toxin injection, filler.

Ocular surface lubrication can be improved with lubricating eye drops and ointment, a moisture chamber dressing with Tegaderm™ or Saran™ wrap, or taping the eyelids closed. Glad Press N

J. Tao (ed.), *Efficient Oculofacial Surgery*, https://doi.org/10.1007/978-3-031-63178-8_26

Seal™ is a particularly good choice to create a moisture chamber for the eye. While not as adherent as tape, Glad Press N Seal™ sufficiently seals in moisture when placed over and circumferentially around the eye along the sub brow to cheek skin. It may be especially useful at nighttime after placing lubricant ointment into the eye. Bandage soft contact lenses can help retain moisture as well in addition to providing more comfort.

Decreasing free-flowing air from air conditioning, fans, or heaters in addition to a bedside air humidifier help enhance environmental moisture. Warm compresses, omega-3 fatty acids, doxycycline, or autologous serum tears can help improve the quality of the tear film.

Temporary punctal occlusion or permanent punctal cautery helps with tear outflow obstruction to retain more tears on the ocular surface.

If ocular surface lubrication fails, tarsorrhaphy may be necessary. Suture, filler, or neurotoxin tarsorrhaphy can be performed in the office and offer an acute, reversible intervention. They may be ideal in idiopathic facial nerve palsy or other situations in which facial nerve recovery is distinctly possible.

A temporary suture tarsorrhaphy on bolsters or cyanoacrylate glue or Dermabond® glue tarsorrhaphy can be done at the bedside to provide eyelid closure [1, 2]. A serpentine tarsorrhaphy is a useful modification of a bolster temporary tarsorrhaphy that allows for frequent cornea or other ophthalmic checks without needing to replace the tarsorrhaphy. It is usually placed across the full length of the eyelid but a partial tarsorrhaphy can also be placed.

Serpentine Tarsorrhaphy

Technique:

1. The length of tarsorrhaphy required is marked. A bolster spanning the desired tarsorrhaphy length is cut (intravenous tubing works well).
2. Topical anesthetic drops are placed and local anesthetic is administered to the upper and lower eyelid.
3. A 5–0 polypropylene suture on a P3 needle is placed through the end of the bolster (Fig. 26.1A).
4. About 3 mm superior to the eyelid margin and 3–5 mm medial to the lateral canthal angle, the needle is passed through skin of the upper eyelid, then tarsus, and then emerges through the upper eyelid grey line (Fig. 26.1B).
5. The needle enters the lower eyelid grey line and is passed parallel to the eyelid margin and emerging from the grey line more medially (Fig. 26.1C).
6. The suture is zigzagged across the lid from lateral to medial in a serpentine fashion. It emerges through the upper lid skin in the medial one-third, about 3 mm above the lash line. It is ensured that the tarsorrhaphy does not extend more medial to the puncta (Fig. 26.1D).
7. The ends of the sutures are taped to the forehead in a fashion that prevents the suture from slipping through but allows the tape to be removed without disrupting the tarsorrhaphy (Fig. 26.1E).
8. The tarsorrhaphy is unzipped by removing the tape layers and gently opening the eyelids. The tarsorrhaphy can be zipped closed after the ophthalmic exam and the tape is replaced.

Considerations:
The complete visual occlusion or peripheral vision restriction may prevent use in a monocular patient.

Botulinum toxin injected into the levator palpebrae muscle induces transient upper eyelid ptosis to aide in eyelid closure [3, 4]. Soft tissue fillers injected into the upper eyelid or adhesive stick-on weights mechanically lower the upper eyelid [5, 6].

Botulinum Toxin Injection Tarsorrhaphy

Technique:

1. Using a 30 gauge needle, 5 units of botulinum toxin type A (Botox®, Allergan, Irvine CA) are given transcutaneous to the

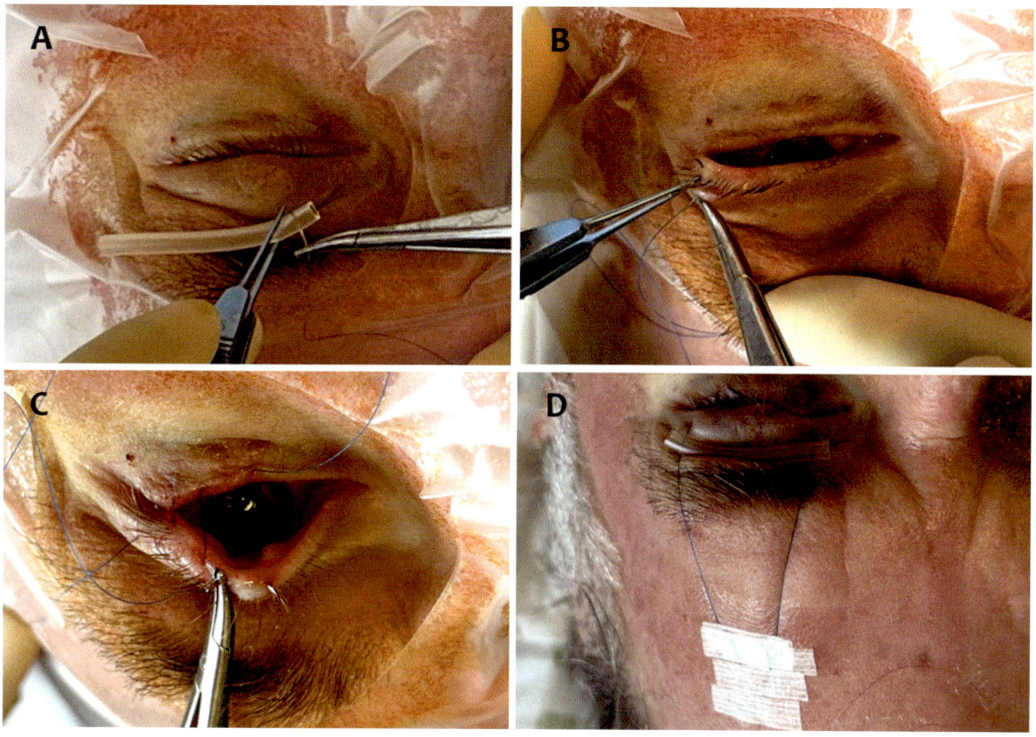

Fig. 26.1 Surgical Steps demonstrating Serpentine Tarsorrhaphy. (A) A 5–0 polypropylene suture on a P3 needle is placed through the bolster. (B) 3 mm superior to the eyelid margin and 3–5 mm medial to the lateral canthal angle, the needle is passed through skin of the upper eyelid, then tarsus, and then emerges through the upper eyelid grey line. (C) The needle is passed into the gray line of the lower eyelid margin and emerging from the grey line more medially. (D) The suture is zigzagged across the lid from lateral to medial in a serpentine fashion. It emerges through the upper lid skin in the medial one-third, about 3 mm above the lash line. (E) The ends of the sutures are taped to the forehead in a fashion that prevents the suture from slipping through but allows the tape to be removed without disrupting the tarsorrhaphy

central upper eyelid beneath the superior orbital rim to achieve temporary (average 3 months) paralytic levator muscle ptosis that closes the palpebral fissure/

Considerations:
Transient superior rectus muscle paresis can result in diplopia as well as reduced Bell reflex.

Filler Injection to the Upper Eyelid

Technique:

1. Using a 30-gauge needle, a hyaluronic acid gel filler (e.g., Restylane®) is injected into the pretarsal or pre aponeurosis area of the central upper eyelid to load the upper eyelid. Small aliquots of the filler are placed at multiple sites in the sub-orbicularis plane. The filler is placed at the area of most severe upper lid retraction or lagophthalmos. The amount of filler placed is titrated based on eyelid position. Approximately 1 cc is required. This induces mechanical ptosis that lowers the upper eyelid margin.

Considerations: Hyaluronidase can be used to dissolve any excessive or unwanted product.

Long-term Management Techniques

1. To improve eyelid closure: permanent tarsorrhaphy, tarsoconjunctival onlay flap

2. To treat horizontal laxity: full-thickness eyelid wedge resection, lateral tarsal strip, medial canthoplasty
3. To correct lower eyelid malposition: medial spindle conjunctivoplasty, full-thickness skin graft, midface lift
4. To correct upper eyelid retraction: levator recession, upper eyelid loading

Several techniques can improve eyelid closure and protect the globe and ocular surface. These can be broadly categorized as ones that improve eyelid closure, address horizontal laxity, or correct eyelid malposition including eyelid retraction and paralytic ectropion. Often, more than one is required.

Eyelid closure techniques help to decrease the palpebral fissure both vertically and horizontally. These can restrict peripheral vision but may be necessary to reduce lagophthalmos and exposure keratopathy.

A lateral or medial permanent eyelid margin tarsorrhaphy effectively helps with improving eyelid closure. The amount of eyelid margin approximation can be adjusted to optimize eyelid closure while limiting peripheral vision restriction [7].

Permanent Tarsorrhaphy

Technique:

1. The upper and lower eyelids are manually pinched to determine the ideal width of tarsorrhaphy. This is marked on the upper and lower eyelid. For a medial tarsorrhaphy, the tarsorrhaphy should be placed lateral to the puncta.
2. A #15 blade is used to make an incision at the eyelid margin along the gray line (Fig. 26.2A). This is done for the length of the tarsorrhaphy along the upper and lower eyelid margins (Fig. 26.2B).
3. Scissors are used to dissect approximately 1–2 mm deep between the anterior and posterior lamella.
4. Scissors or a scalpel are used to denude the mucocutaneous junction of the posterior lamellar lid margin (Fig. 26.2C).
5. Interrupted 5–0 polyglactin horizontal mattress sutures are placed to approximate the posterior lamella of the superior and inferior lid margins (Fig. 26.2D). To achieve this, the needle enters the inferior tarsus medially and exits laterally along the lid margin. It then enters the superior tarsus laterally and exits medially at the margin. This allows the knot to be tied medially and away from the cornea. This fuses the posterior aspect of the upper and lower eyelid margin.
6. The anterior lamella is approximated with a 6–0 nylon horizontal mattress suture tied over bolsters on the upper and lower eyelids (Fig. 26.2E). The sutures are left for 2–3 weeks to allow the eyelid margins to approximate.

Considerations:
Trichiasis and eyelid margin alteration can result if the tarsorrhaphy must be reversed. Additionally, intermarginal adhesion tarsorrhaphy leads to some disfigurement.

To avoid alteration of the eyelid margin, an alternative to the permanent tarsorrhaphy is the tarsal pillar technique or a lateral tarsoconjunctival suspension/onlay flap. Pillars employ tarsoconjunctival flaps from the upper eyelid that are positioned at the medial and lateral limbus and are anchored to the inferior tarsus. A single far lateral tarsoconjunctival onlay flap from the upper eyelid and with the leading edge of the flap attached to the lower eyelid margin may obviate some of the cosmetic concerns pillars visible in the interpalpebral zone 10]. The onlay flap or pillars provide suspender-like support to a paretic eyelid and aide in eyelid closure [8, 9].

Tarsoconjunctival Suspension/Onlay Flap (Fig. 26.3 Video 26.1)

Technique:

1. The upper and lower eyelid are manually pinched together to determine the ideal

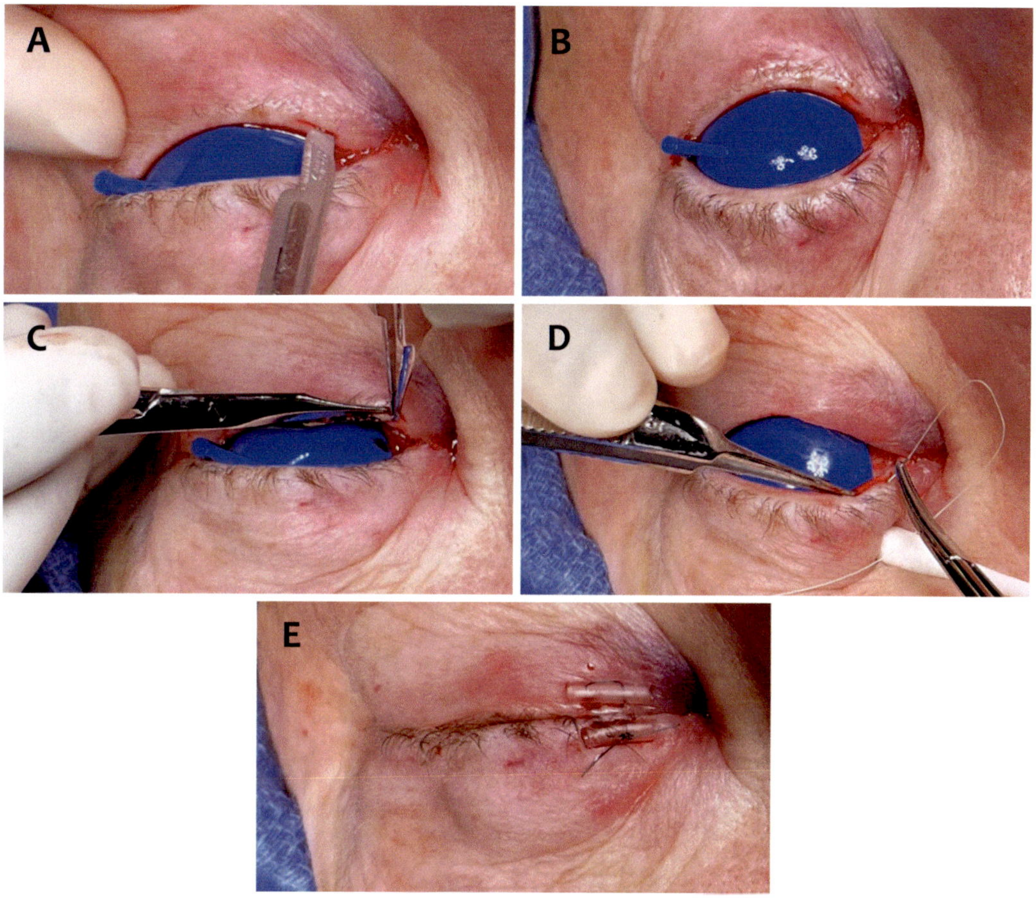

Fig. 26.2 Surgical Steps demonstrating Permanent Tarsorrhaphy. (A) A #15 blade is used to make an incision at the eyelid margin along the gray line. (B) This is done for the length of the tarsorrhaphy along the upper and lower eyelid margins. (C) Scissors are used to denude the mucocutaneous junction of the posterior lamellar lid margin. (D) Interrupted 5–0 polyglactin horizontal mattress sutures are placed to approximate the posterior lamella of the superior and inferior lid margins. (E) The anterior lamella is approximated with a 6–0 Nylon horizontal mattress suture tied over bolsters

amount of eyelid closure. The size of the flap is marked on the skin surface.

2. A 5–0 polyglactin or 4–0 silk suture is placed through the upper eyelid margin to aide in lid eversion over a cotton-tip applicator.
3. Methylene blue is used to mark the tarsoconjunctival flap to be developed ensuring that it is 3–4 mm superior to the eyelid margin.
4. A #15 blade is used to make an incision through tarsus and conjunctiva. Westcott scissors are used to develop the flap. The upper lid traction suture is removed.
5. A #15 blade is used to make an incision along the grey line of the lower eyelid margin to correspond to the length of the flap. The posterior lamella is denuded with scissors or a scalpel.
6. Two to three interrupted 5–0 polyglactin sutures are placed in a horizontal mattress fashion to anchor the tarsoconjunctival flap to the lower eyelid margin.

Paretic lower eyelid malposition also requires addressing eyelid laxity and any need for additional vertical support. Pre-operatively, patient assessment should identify the area of lower lid malposition—medial, lateral, or both. A finger test helps to determine the surgical techniques

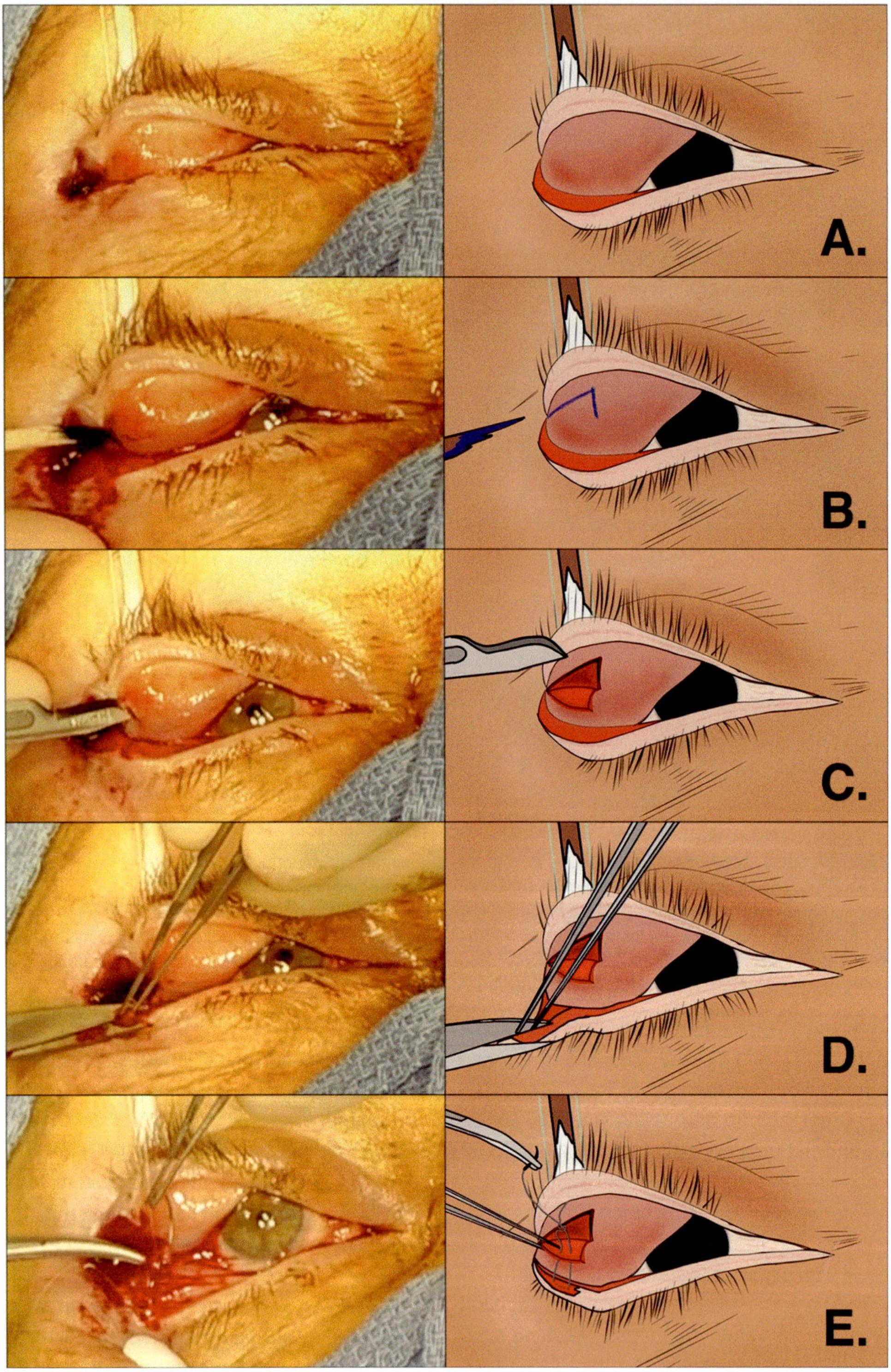

Fig. 26.3 Surgical steps demonstrating a tarsoconjunctival onlay flap

needed to improve eyelid positioning. A finger is placed at the lateral canthus to determine the need for lateral canthal tightening.

With one finger supporting the lateral canthus the central or medial lower eyelid margin may remain out of position and suggest cicatricial or negative vectors need attention. As such, a spacer graft, skin graft, or midfacial lift may be indicated. Importantly these have little utility when the predominant lower eyelid malposition vector is paralytic.

Lower Eyelid Horizontal Tightening

Technique:

1. A #15 blade is used to start a lateral canthotomy.
2. The canthotomy and inferior cantholysis are completed using Westcott scissors.
3. The amount of redundant eyelid is marked and resected.
4. The lateral tarsus is secured with a 4–0 polypropylene, braided polyester, or polyglactin suture. Alternatively, a tarsal strip may be fashioned by dissecting skin anteriorly and conjunctiva posteriorly off the tarsus.
5. The suture secures the lateral tarsus or tarsal strip to the periosteum at the lateral orbital rim.
6. An optional 6–0 polyglactin or plain suture is passed from the lateral upper lid wound edge, through the upper lid grey line. It is then passed through the lower lid grey line and exits through the lateral lower lid wound edge. The suture is tied to recreate the lateral canthal angle.
7. The skin is approximated with absorbable sutures.

In many instances, lower lid horizontal tightening may be combined with a tarsoconjunctival suspension flap to treat both involutional and paralytic vectors (Video 26.2). Horizontal tightening alone, in the setting of paralytic vectors, is generally inadequate.

Medial Canthoplasty

Technique:

1. After punctal dilation, lacrimal probes are passed through the inferior and superior puncta and canaliculi until a hard stop is reached (Fig. 26.4A). These probes are left in position throughout the dissection to protect the canaliculi.
2. A #15 blade is used to make an incision from just anterior to the superior lacrimal punctum, continuing medially around the medial canthal angle and then anterior to the inferior lacrimal punctum. The incision is made along the mucocutaneous junction.
3. Scissors are used to undermine the skin for about 5 mm to reveal the medial canthal tendons and orbicularis oculi muscle (Fig. 26.4B).
4. Three interrupted sutures of 6–0 polyglactin sutures are passed through the orbicularis muscle and inferior crus of the medial canthal tendon to the orbicularis muscle and superior crus of the medial canthal tendon (Fig. 26.4C). Care is taken to avoid engaging canalicular tissue which is guided by the lacrimal probes.
5. The sutures are tied to elevate the medial lower eyelid and turn the lacrimal punctum posteriorly toward the lacrimal lake.
6. Excess skin is excised, and the skin edges are approximated with absorbable suture (Fig. 26.4D).

Considerations: The horizontal palpebral fissure will be shortened. Additionally, there is risk of damage or occlusion of the canaliculi. A modification is to perform a horizontal canaliculotomy and fusion of the anterior cut edge of the upper to lower canaliculus in an attempt to maintain a posterior tear outflow entrance into the canalicular systems (Figs. 26.5, 26.6, 26.7) (Video 26.3). This canaliculoplasty can be performed with or without placement of a temporary silicone lacrimal stent.

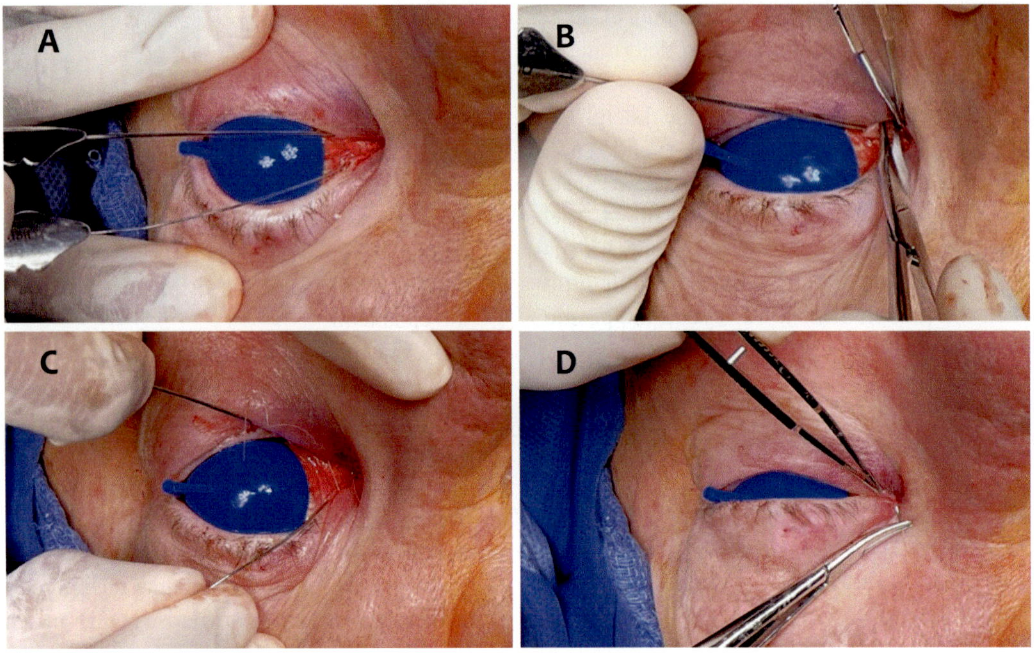

Fig. 26.4 Surgical steps demonstrating medial canthoplasty. (A) After punctal dilation, lacrimal probes are passed through the inferior and superior puncta and canaliculi until a hard stop is reached. (B) A #15 blade is used to make an incision from just anterior to the superior lacrimal punctum, continuing medially around the medial canthal angle and then anterior to the inferior lacrimal punctum. Westcott scissors are used to undermine the skin for about 5 mm to reveal the medial canthal tendons and orbicularis oculi muscle. (C) Three interrupted sutures of 6–0 polyglactin sutures are passed through the orbicularis muscle and inferior crus of the medial canthal tendon to the orbicularis muscle and superior crus of the medial canthal tendon. (D) Excess skin is excised and the skin edges are approximated

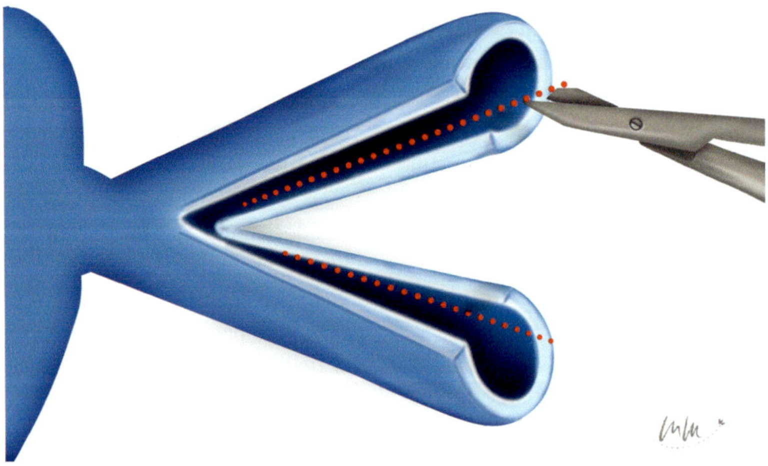

Fig. 26.5 Upper and lower canaliculus opened longitudinally with sharp dissection. *Image courtesy of Dr. Suzana Matayoshi*

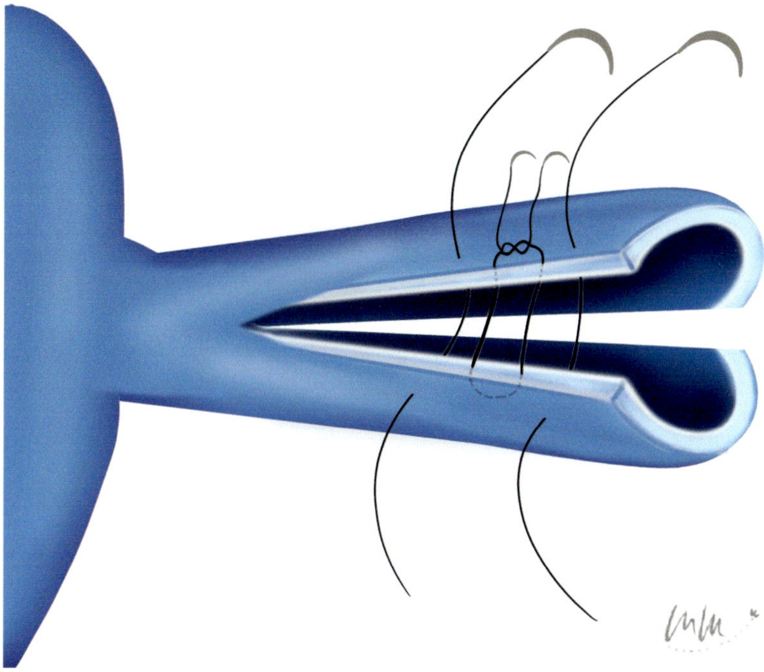

Fig. 26.6 Upper and lower canaliculus fused anteriorly. *Image courtesy of Dr. Suzana Matayoshi*

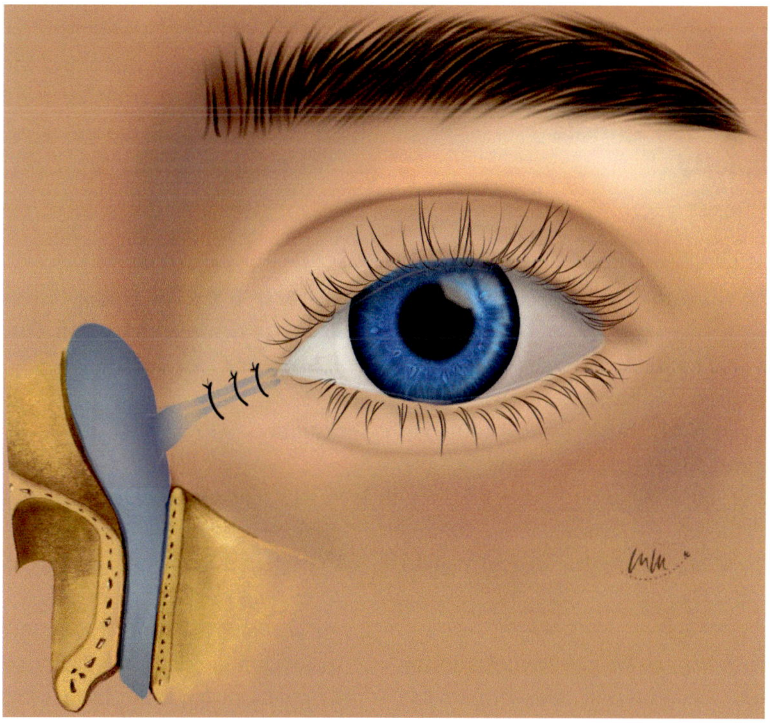

Fig. 26.7 Anterior cut edge of upper and lower canaliculus sewn together. *Image courtesy of Dr. Suzana Matayoshi*

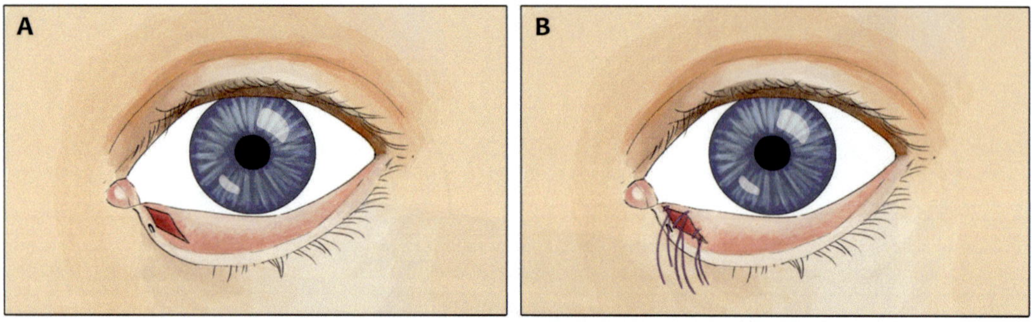

Fig. 26.8 Surgical Steps Demonstrating Medial Spindle Conjunctivoplasty. (A) A diamond shaped medial spindle is marked on the conjunctival surface. A #15 blade is used to incise through conjunctiva-retractor tissue at the markings. (B) Buried interrupted 6–0 polyglactin sutures are placed to approximate the vertical wound edges

If additional paretic lower eyelid malposition (including medial or more diffuse ectropion or retraction) is still present, the following techniques that do not require an additional implant can be adjuncts to horizontal tightening. The techniques further improve lower lid positioning and protection of the ocular surface.

If medial ectropion including punctal ectropion is most prominent, a medial spindle conjunctivoplasty can be done.

Lower Eyelid Medial Spindle Conjunctivoplasty

Technique.

1. The lower eyelid is everted over a cotton-tip applicator.
2. A diamond shaped medial spindle is marked on the conjunctival surface inferior to the lacrimal punctum. A #15 blade is used to incise through conjunctiva-retractor tissue at the markings (Fig. 26.8A).
3. Buried interrupted 6–0 polyglactin sutures are placed to approximate the vertical wound edges (Fig. 26.8B).

Fascial sling or grafts can be placed in the lower eyelid in certain scenarios but add complexity. More importantly, they have limited efficacy and durability for purely paralytic vectors. If there exists skin contracture or midfacial ptosis concomitant to paralytic lid malposition, skin grafting or skin recruitment through midface advancement may be indicated and as described in other chapters (Fig. 26.9).

In a patient with more severely retracted upper eyelid and lagophthalmos or compromised Bell reflex, a gold or platinum weight implant or palpebral spring may be placed to help lower the eyelid and improve closure during blink [11, 12]. Metallic implants, however, add complexity and cost. Moreover, these devices inevitably extrude or cause other complications. In less severe cases of upper eyelid retraction, upper eyelid retractor recession can be considered.

Blepharotomy for Upper Eyelid Retractor Recession (Also Described in Another Chapter)

Technique.

1. A #15 blade is used to make an upper lid skin crease incision. Scissors or a scalpel are used to dissect through skin and orbicularis muscle to the anterior surface of tarsus.
2. At the area of most pronounced retraction, dissection is continued at the superior border of tarsus through the levator muscle aponeurosis and Muller's muscle. The eyelid height is checked, and further dissection is continued at areas of retraction.

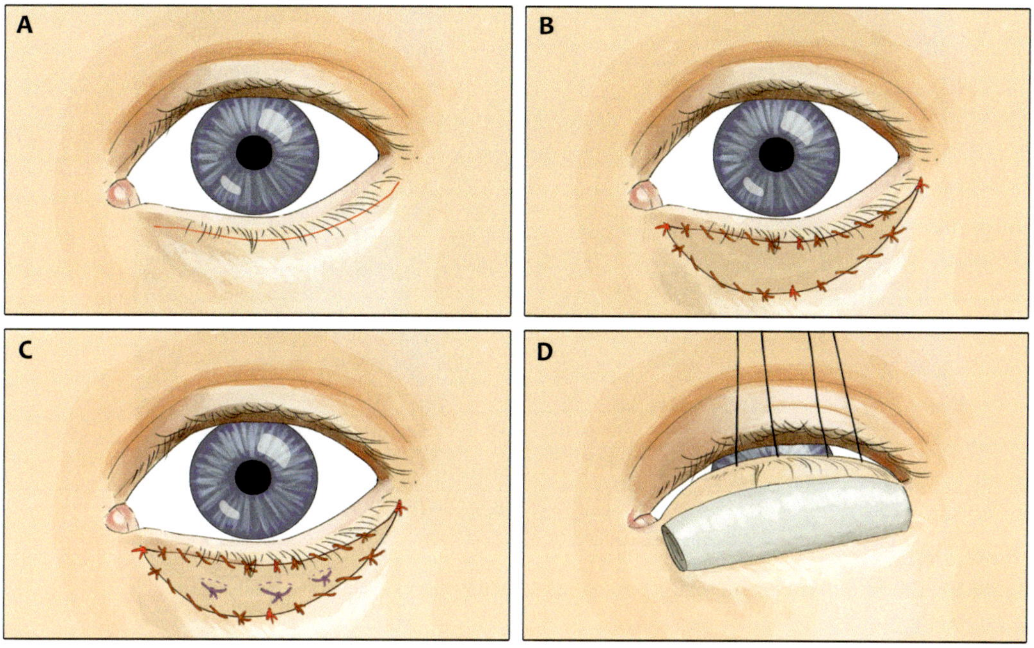

Fig. 26.9 Illustration demostrating skin grafting to the lower eyelid to treat any anterior lamella shortage (has very limited efficacy in paralytic lower eyelid retraction)

3. If additional recession is needed, dissection can continue through conjunctiva. Conjunctiva should be left intact at the eyelid peak. Additional recession can be achieved by cutting the medial and lateral horns of the levator muscle.
4. The skin is closed with a running suture of 6–0 polypropylene or suture of choice.

Conclusions

Eyelid malposition in facial nerve paresis is important to address since the ocular surface protective mechanisms are compromised. Careful pre-operative assessment is necessary to determine the optimal techniques. The choice of procedure also depends on whether a patient requires short-term management or a long-term, permanent solution. Suspension of the lower eyelid with a lateral tarsoconjunctival flap is a highly efficient surgical rehabilitation and has minimal complexity or morbidity (Figs. 26.10 and 26.11). Horizontal tightening lower eyelid procedures are commonly useful adjuncts. Medial eyelid surgery may be indicated, but it is important to consider the lacrimal drainage apparatus. Grafts, slings, upper eyelid levator recession may be useful in special scenarios. Metallic weights and palpebral springs, while part of the armamentarium for eyelid paralysis, add complexity and cost that usually can be avoided using some of the techniques described in this chapter.

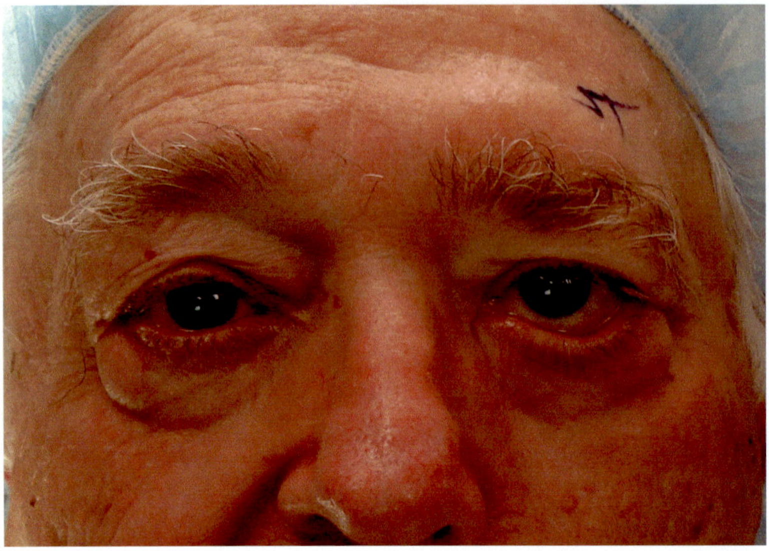

Fig. 26.10 Patient with left lower eyelid ectropion and retraction due to facial nerve paralysis

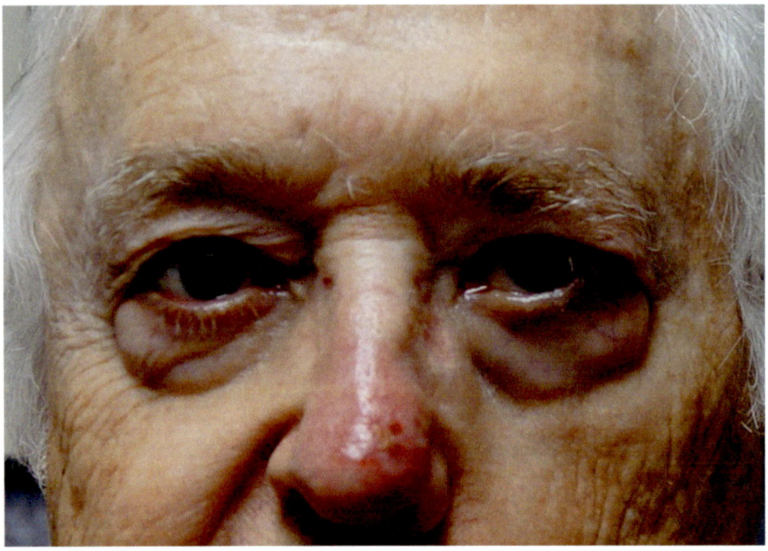

Fig. 26.11 Patient in Fig. 26.10 after a left lateral tarsoconjunctival onlay flap

References

1. Rapoza P, Harrison D, Bussa H, Prestowitz W, Dortzbach R. Temporary sutured tube-tarsorrhaphy: reversible eyelid closure technique. Ophthalmic Surg. 1993;24:328–30.
2. Donnenfeld E, Perry H, Nelson D. Cyanoacrylate temporary tarsorrhaphy in the management of corneal epithelial defects. Ophthalmic Surg. 1991;22:591–3.
3. Adams GG, Kirkness CM, Lee JP. Botulinum toxin A induced protective ptosis. Eye. 1987;603–608.
4. Kirkness CM, Adams GGW, Dilly PN, Lee JP. Botulinum toxin A-induced protective ptosis in corneal disease. Ophthalmology. 1988;95:473–80.
5. Mancini R, Taban M, Lowinger A, Nakra T, Tsirbas A, Douglas RS, Shorr N, Goldberg RA. Use of hyaluronic acid gel in the management of paralytic lagophthalmos: the hyaluronic acid gel "gold weight." Ophthal Plast Reconstr Surg. 2009;25(1):23–6.

6. Robinson C, Tantri A, Shriver E, Oetting T. Temporary eyelid closure appliqué. Arch Ophthalmol. 2006;124(4):546–9.
7. Elner VM, Demirci H, Morton AD, Elner SG, Hassan AS. Transcaruncular medial canthal ligament plication for repair of lower eyelid malposition. Arch Ophthalmol. 2007;125(3):374–9.
8. Tanenbaum M, Gossman MD, Bergin DJ, Friendman HI, Lett D, Haines P, McCord CD Jr. The tarsal pillar technique for narrowing and maintenance of the interpalpebral fissure. Ophthalmic Surg. 1992;23(6):418–25.
9. Steiner GC, Gossman MD, Tanenbaum M. Modified tarsal pillar tarsorrhaphy. Am J Ophthalmol. 1993;116(1):103–4.
10. Tao JP, Vemuri S, Patel AD, et al. Lateral tarsoconjunctival onlay flap lower eyelid suspension in facial nerve paresis. Ophthalmic Plast Reconstr Surg. 2014;30:342–5.
11. Seiff SR, Sullivan JH, Freeman N, Ahn J. Pretarsal fixation of gold weights in facial nerve palsy. Ophthal Plast Reconstr Surg. 1989;5(2):104–9.
12. Levine RE, House WF, Hitselberger WE. Ocular complications of seventh nerve paralysis and management with the palpebral spring. Am J Ophthalmol. 1972;73(2):219–28.

Direct Brow Lift

27

Stephanie H. Noh, Christopher Dermarkarian,
Jenny N. Wang, and Jeremiah P. Tao

Abstract

The direct brow lift or direct brow-pasty is an effective surgery to treat brow ptosis. The direct brow lift offers optimal functional results due to the tissue resection that is in immediate proximity of the eyebrows. The main shortcomings of this procedure are the visible post-operative scar, unnatural brow shape, and potential forehead hypoesthesia, though these risks can be mitigated with appropriate patient selection and good technique. In this chapter, the authors describe direct brow lift surgery including a technique of a medial chevron-shaped supraciliary incision that helps prevent an irregular brow contour.

Keywords

Brow lift · Browplasty · Brow ptosis · Surgical technique

Supplementary Information The online version contains supplementary material available at https://doi.org/10.1007/978-3-031-63178-8_27.

S. H. Noh · C. Dermarkarian · J. N. Wang ·
J. P. Tao (✉)
Division of Oculofacial Plastic and Orbital Surgery, Univeristy of California, Irvine, Irvine, CA, USA
e-mail: jeremiat@hs.uci.edu

Introduction

Upper eyelid and brow position are interdependent. In many patients, upper eyelid dermatochalasis is chiefly due to brow ptosis. Upper eyelid blepharoplasty alone, in this context, may result in suboptimal results. Paradoxically, brow ptosis may worsen owing to eyelid tissue resection inferiorly [1]. In some individuals, frontalis muscle recruitment may abate post blepharoplasty due to the loss of the stimulus of the excess, hooded upper eyelid skin. There exist many techniques to elevate the brow. In general, techniques that include tissue resection may result in more durable and more profound brow elevation [2].

The direct brow lift or direct browplasty is one of the most potent methods of brow elevation [2–5]. In this technique, a supraciliary incision is created to excise skin and subcutaneous tissue, providing direct brow elevation, and treating brow ptosis.

It is important to understand the general anatomy and normal contour of the eyebrow, especially in context of gender variations. A standard male eyebrow rests at the superior orbital rim and the contour is generally flat. A standard female eyebrow rests above the superior orbital rim and is commonly arched temporally [6]. The eyebrow can be considered to have three parts: the head, body, and tail. The eyebrow hairs are oriented upward at the head of

J. Tao (ed.), *Efficient Oculofacial Surgery*, https://doi.org/10.1007/978-3-031-63178-8_27

the brow, horizontal in the body of the brow, and downward in the tail of the brow. Over time, the tissues in the periorbital area begin to sag, leading to brow ptosis. Of note, the frontalis muscle does not extend to the temporal eyebrow; thus, as aging occurs, the patient is more likely to develop a temporal, rather than central, eyebrow droop [6, 7]. Therefore, the goal of any direct brow lift is to excise the skin and subcutaneous tissue necessary to provide appropriate brow elevation and adequate brow contour.

One potential shortcoming of the direct brow lift is a visible supraciliary scar [2, 3, 5]. This negative outcome can be mitigated by proper patient selection and good wound closure technique. Thick brows, usually in male patients, can help hide the incision [4]. In addition, pre-existing horizontal creases and rhytids in the forehead may better camouflage the scar. Another chief risk is hypoesthesia. The supraorbital nerve deep to the brow head can be damaged during incision and if dissection is too deep [3, 5] (Fig. 27.1). Fortunately, hypoesthesia can be avoided with care to resect more superficially at the head of the brow. In most cases, numbness is temporary.

Direct brow lifts offer good control and precision over the amount of lift achieved and in turn, the resulting function and contour. This is particularly helpful in cases that require significant elevation (i.e., severe brow ptosis from unilateral facial palsy). If there is significant temporal eyebrow droop, one may consider performing direct temporal brow lift [8]. Although this may correct temporal hooding of eyebrow skin, it has no effect on the central eyebrow.

In the standard direct brow lift, an ellipse of skin and subcutaneous soft tissue is resected. Since the medial and lateral ends of the ellipse taper, the direct brow lift results in good elevation of the body of the eyebrow with only limited elevation of the head and tail. Given the elliptical nature of the incision, the resulting brow contour seen in a standard direct brow lift often appears overly arched, projecting an unwanted "surprised" or "angry" expression. This result may be less desirable in male patients who naturally tend to have little arch present. The authors utilize a medial chevron-shaped direct supraciliary excision to elevate the head of the brow along with other areas to achieve eyebrows without an irregular, arched contour.

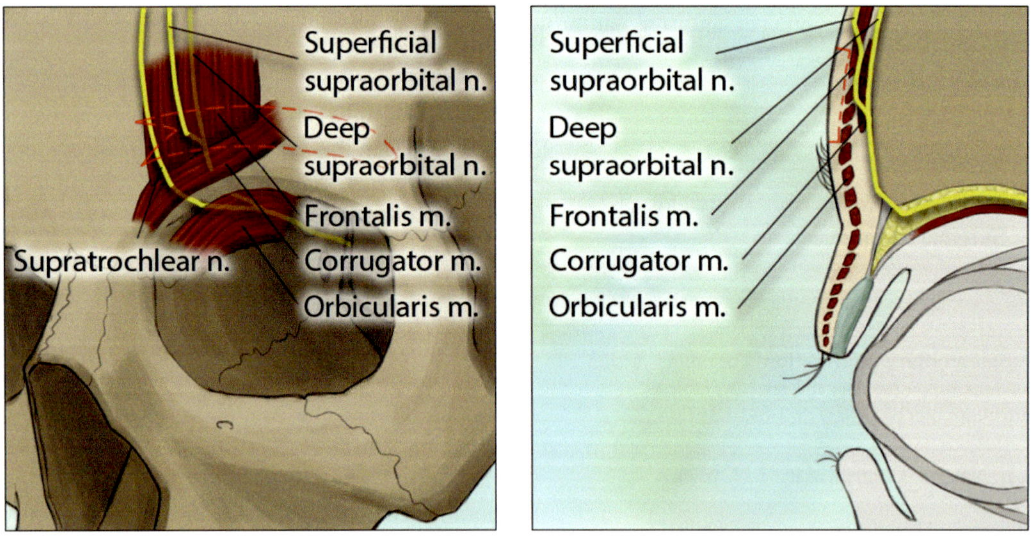

Fig. 27.1 The dashed red line outlines the surgical marking for the medial chevron-shaped incision in relation to important underlying anatomic structures, including the supratrochlear and supraorbital nerves at the brow head. Image courtesy of Michael Han, MD

Surgical Technique (Video 27.1)

The patient is marked pre-operatively to determine the amount of resection (Fig. 27.2A). The eyebrow is held at the desired position at the rim or above the rim and the distance between the actual and ideal brow position is marked. If possible, the resultant wound is designed to coincide with a pre-existing horizontal rhytid. Local anesthesia is then administered. Using a #15 blade, a chevron-shaped incision is created medially and then extended in a tapered fashion to the lateral edge of the brow (Fig. 27.2B). The incision is usually approximately 1 cm in width if possible. After the skin and subcutaneous tissue are excised with scissors, hemostasis is achieved with electrocautery (Fig. 27.2C). Minimal electrocautery is utilized at the medial wound to avoid damage to the supraorbital sensory nerves. Also, the incision and resection are kept slightly more superficial at the head of the eyebrow. Since the supraorbital nerve emerges from the bone at the supraorbital notch, deep dissection or resection are avoided. The deep dermal layer is closed with interrupted, buried 3–0 polyglactin sutures. The subcutaneous tissues are approximated 5–0 polyglactin sutures so that the wound edges are flush and without tension on the skin with subsequent skin sutures. The tissue triangle formed by the chevron incision is distracted superiorly and another resection triangle is demarcated (Fig. 27.2D). The redundant tissue is excised achieving additional lift of the medial brow. To complete the procedure, the skin is closed with a running vertical mattress 5–0 polypropylene suture (Fig. 27.2E). Wound eversion is desired to counteract postoperative contraction that may lead to a depressed scar. The medial resection technique causes some bunching of the central, inter-brow tissues as well as a small Y shaped scar. The bunching relaxes over time and the small scar usually remains inconspicuous.

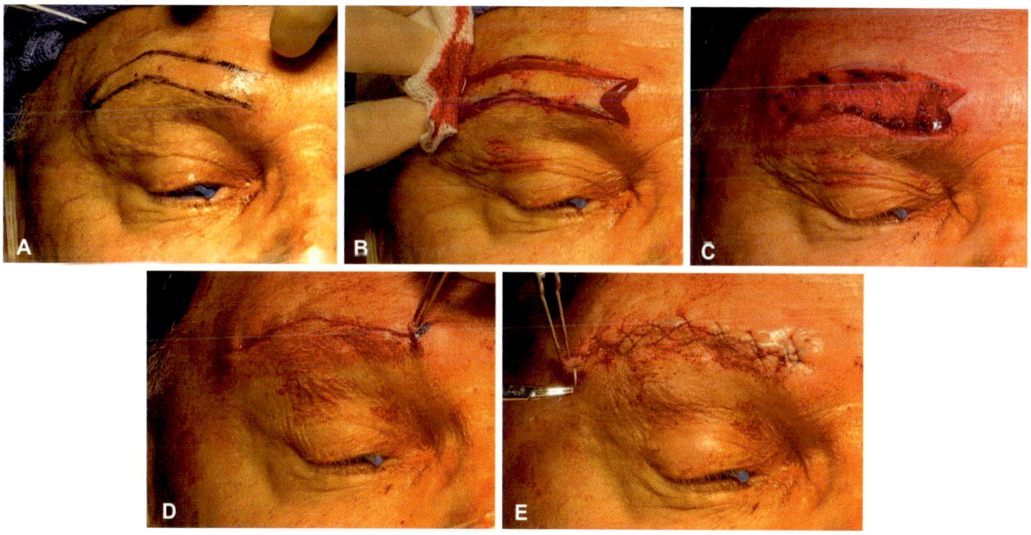

Fig. 27.2 Intraoperative photographs of the direct brow lift utilizing the medial chevron-shaped incision. (A) Preoperative marking. (B&C) The skin and subcutaneous tissue are excised, taking care to avoid deep dissection or resection. (D) After closure of the deep dermal layer and subcutaneous layer, the tissue triangle formed from the chevron incision is retracted superiorly, marked as shown, and then excised. (E) The skin is then closed with a running vertical mattress suture

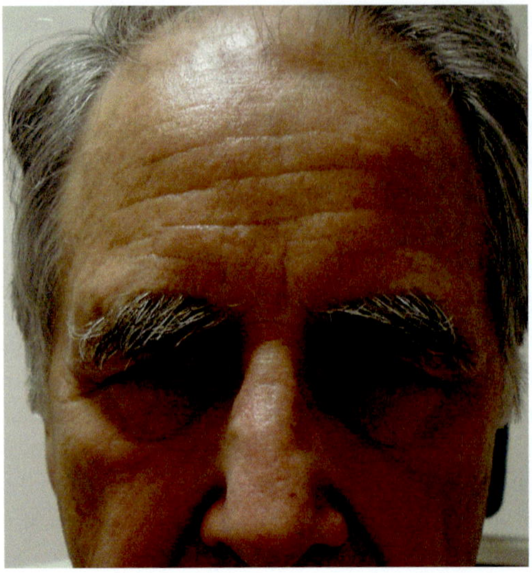

Fig. 27.3 Patient with moderate to severe brow ptosis

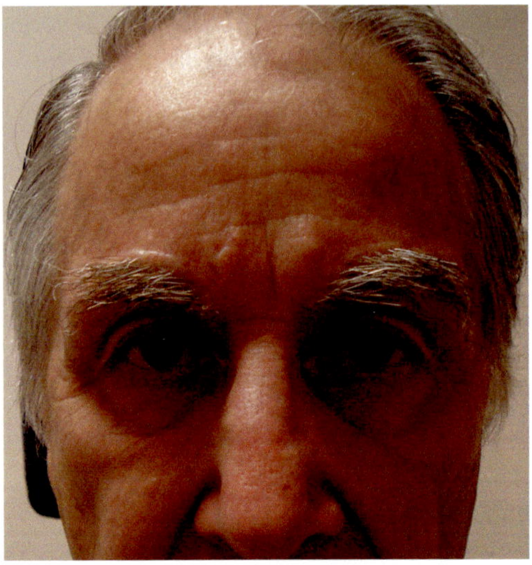

Fig. 27.4 Post-operative photograph of patient in Fig. 27.3 after bilateral direct brow lift

Conclusion

The direct brow lift is a safe, effective, and durable procedure. A modified medial chevron incisional may help preserve the brow's natural contour. The main shortcoming of this procedure is the resulting scar. In general, it offered in functional contexts due to the potential for a visible scar. Proper patient selection is key. In general, older males with thick eyebrows and pre-existing horizontal forehead rhytids are better candidates for this functional procedure. Good surgical technique, with meticulous layered closure and skin wound eversion can achieve favorable cosmetic and functional results as seen in pre and postoperative photographs utilizing the medial chevron incisional technique (Figs. 27.3 and 27.4).

References

1. Lam VB, Czyz CN, Wulc AE. The brow-eyelid continuum: an anatomic perspective. Clin Plast Surg. 2013;40(1):1–19.
2. Karimi N, Kashkouli MB, Sianati H, Khademi B. Techniques of eyebrow lifting: a narrative review. J Ophthalmic Vis Res. 2020;15(2):218–35.
3. Booth AJ, Murray A, Tyers AG. The direct brow lift: efficacy, complications, and patient satisfaction. Br J Ophthalmol. 2004;88(5):688–91.
4. Pascali M, Bocchini I, Avantaggiato A, et al. Direct brow lifting: Specific indications for a simplified approach to eyebrow ptosis. Indian J Plast Surg Off Publ Assoc Plast Surg India. 2016;49(1):66–71.
5. Cho MJ, Carboy JA, Rohrich RJ. Complications in brow lifts: a systemic review of surgical and nonsurgical brow rejuvenations. Plast Reconstr Surg Glob Open. 2018;6(10): e1943.
6. Sedgh J. The aesthetics of the upper face and brow: male and female differences. Facial Plast Surg. 2018;34(2):114–8.
7. Knize DM. An anatomically based study of the mechanism of eyebrow ptosis. Plast Reconstr Surg. 1996;97(7):1321–33.
8. Miller TA, Rudkin G, Honig M, Elahi M, Adams J. Lateral subcutaneous brow lift and interbrow muscle resection: clinical experience and anatomic studies. Plast Reconstr Surg. 2000 Mar;105(3):1120–7; discussion 1128.

Minimally Invasive Direct Lateral Browplasty

28

André Borba

Abstract

The eyebrows have key anatomic relationships with the eyelids. Numerous procedures are available to elevate or stabilize the eyebrows. Most conventional approaches are more invasive, involving extensive skin resection at the hairline or scalp, endoscopic elevation, and temporal and coronal approaches. While these may be indicated for many patients, some patients with mild and lateral brow ptosis may benefit from direct, small incision options. This chapter details a minimally invasive, predictable, and durable technique that removes an ellipse of skin just above the distal third of the eyebrow to elevate the eyebrow tail.

Keywords

Eyebrow · Browplasty · Brow lift · Direct brow lift

Introduction

The position of the eyebrow influences facial expression. The eyebrow also has a close anatomical relationship with the eyelid [1, 2].

Low eyebrows can give the appearance of negative emotions such as loss of vitality, sadness, and tiredness [3]. The lateral aspect of the eyebrow shows significant reductions in height with age [4]. This, along with changes in eyebrow tilt may contribute to lateral eyelid hooding and eyelash ptosis that are manifestations of this aging [5].

The decline in the positioning of the eyelids and eyebrow may be due to changes in all tissue planes from the soft tissues to bone [6, 7]. Loss of underlying supraorbital structures accentuates local excess skin [8].

Many patients have a combination of dermatochalasis, upper eyelid ptosis, and brow ptosis. Importantly, subtle lowering of the brow after blepharoplasty can result in an undesired result [9]. Several studies demonstrate that upper blepharoplasty lowers the brow [9–11]. Beyond mitigating brow lowering effects, direct brow lift procedures may be indicated for aesthetic indications.

A. Borba (✉)
Department of Ophthalmology, Division of Oculoplastic, University of São Paulo, São Paulo, São Paulo, Brazil
e-mail: prof.dr.andreborba@gmail.com

Eneas Aguiar Street, Sao Paulo 25505403000, Brazil

Division of Oculoplastic, University of Sao Paulo Medical School, 255 Eneas Aguiar Street Office 4079, Sao Paulo 05403000, Brazil

J. Tao (ed.), *Efficient Oculofacial Surgery*, https://doi.org/10.1007/978-3-031-63178-8_28

Several procedures are available to prevent eyebrow drooping after upper blepharoplasty. These include internal and external brow-lifting techniques. Open surgical techniques and endoscopic techniques are available. These are necessary in more severe brow ptosis but are generally more invasive. Side effects include scarring, sensitivity alterations, and hairline distortion [8].

Direct elevation of the eyebrow with tissue resection is a traditional and widely used technique. Castañares [12] and has variations. When the entire brow is ptotic, this incision is along the extent of the brow. While effective and powerful in its lift, this leaves an undesirable, visible scar. In general, this technique is reserved for highly functional indications and patients not concerned about appearance or a conspicuous scar. Preexisting horizontal forehead rhytids and thick eyebrows better camouflage these scars, and this procedure is typically reserved for elderly males who are not concerned about a facial scar. These procedures are detailed in the previous chapter.

A modified direct technique is described in this chapter. The procedure is less invasive and involves removing an ellipse of tissue above the lateral eyebrow [13]. Owing to its shorter, less conspicuous scar, it may have broader indications, including aesthetic.

Indications

The procedure is ideal for patients with minimal or no medial brow ptosis and with descending lateral eyebrows due to heredity or aging. In addition, patients with eyebrow problems caused by excess skin, commonly seen in elderly patients with excess loose skin. Lastly, a lateral direct incision may be indicated to raise the eyebrow tail for aesthetic reasons. This is sometimes incorporated in rejuvenation strategies with a goal of a "fox eye" appearance. The advantages of this technique are its simplicity and durability (especially compared to other techniques such as browpexy or endoscopic lifting).

Surgical Technique

Preoperative planning and marking are important. With the patient in the standing position, the skin at the lateral brow is pinched with the thumb and index finger, observing the effect. It is essential to mark the incision with the patient in the upright position to assess gravitational effects on the anatomical positioning. In cases that blepharoplasty will be also be performed, direct browplasty is performed before blepharoplasty and the amount of eyelid skin excision is adjusted accordingly.

The markings should form an an ellipse, the maximum height between 8 and 12 mm from the upper eyebrow hairline. The lower limit should skirt the upper portion of the supercilium, to better camouflage the scar. The medial limit of resection varies. In cases where the patient has an angulation between the body and tail of the eyebrow, the medial limit should be the most acute angle formed between body and tail. In general, this distance varies between 1.0 and 1.8 cm. The lateral limit of the incision must coincide with the end of the eyebrow tail. In some patients, excess lateral skin may form a dog ear deformity, that can be trimmed in small triangles. Figure 28.1 shows an illustration with the step-by-step technique.

After marking the limits of resection (Fig. 28.2A), local anesthesia is administered. The skin incision is made with a scalpel blade, with caution to avoid injury to the hair follicles, removing the epidermis and dermis, (Fig. 28.2B, C). Hemostasis should be minimal and with care to preserve the brow follicles. The wound is closed in layers. The subcutaneous plane is sutured with inverted non-absorbable sutures (Fig. 28.2D, E); Next, the skin is closed with 5–0 0r 6–0 nonabsorbable sutures (Fig. 28.3).

Figures 28.4 and 28.5 demonstrate results of direct eyebrow tail lift with concomitant upper eyelid blepharoplasty, and Fig. 28.6 demonstrates the results of direct eyebrow tail lift alone.

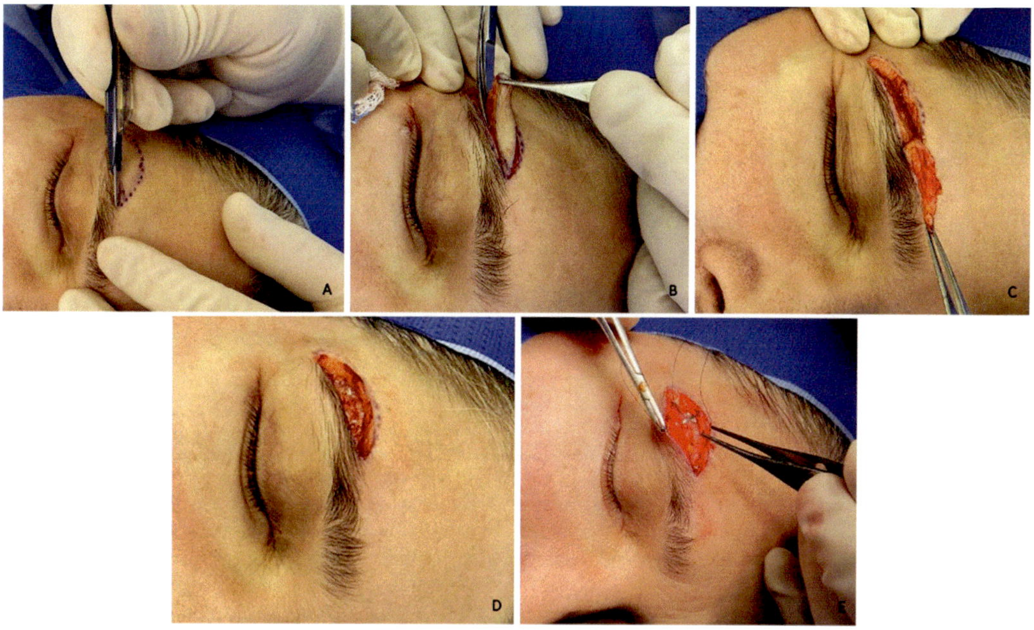

Fig. 28.1 Illustration demonstrating (A) delimitation of the incision, (B) removal of the skin portion with a scalpel, (C) after skin removal, (D and E) subcutaneous suture with 5.0 polyglactin and (F) skin closure with 6–0 nylon

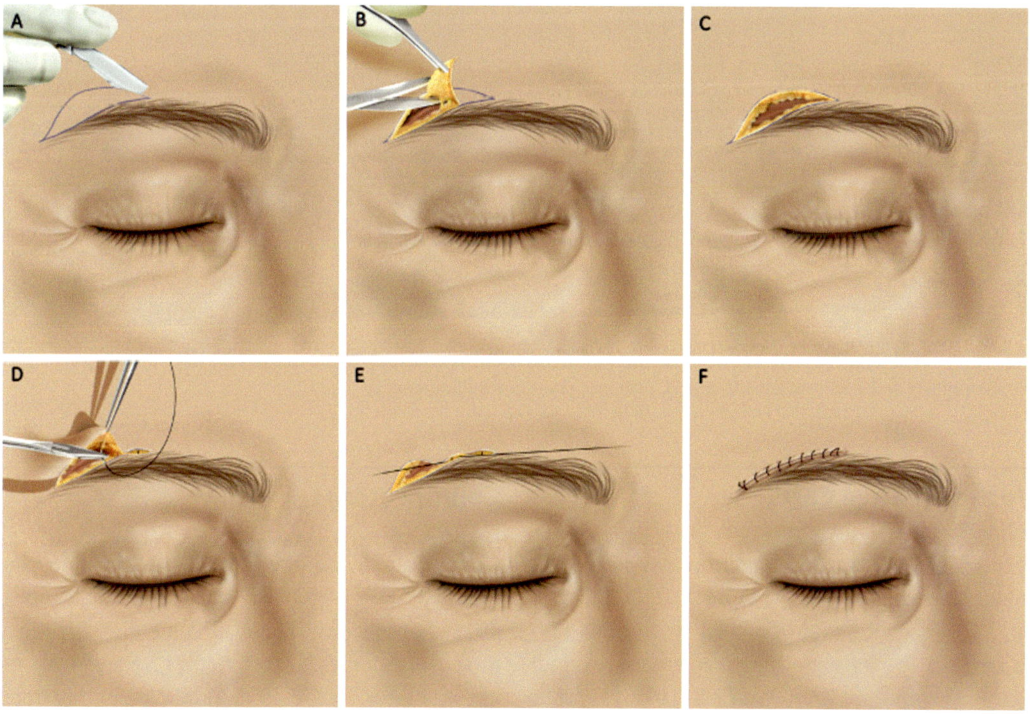

Fig. 28.2 Surgery images showing (A) skin incision, (B and C) removal of skin and subcutaneous tissue, (D) appearance after removal, and (E) suturing of the subcutaneous tissue

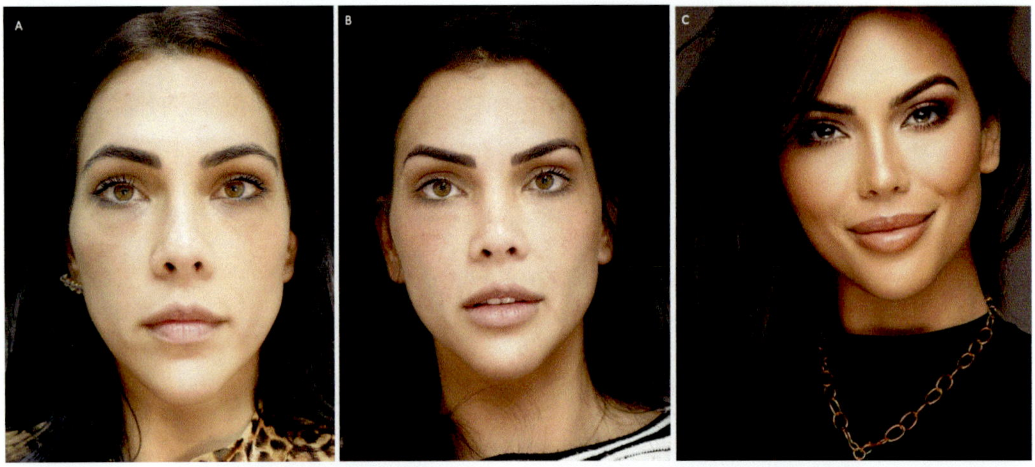

Fig. 28.3 (A) Preoperative photo of a patient with dermatochalasis and lateral brow ptosis and (B) the same patient three months after blepharoplasty and lateral direct brow lift surgery with the technique described. Note that the patient had permanent eyebrow makeup, which further camouflaged the surgical incision wound

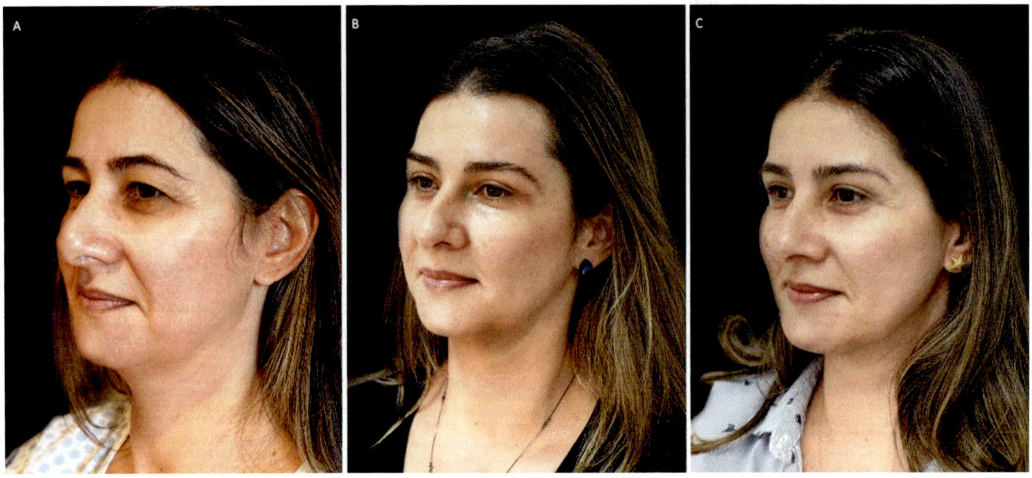

Fig. 28.4 (A) Preoperative photo of a patient with dermatochalasis and eyebrow tail ptosis, (B) 30-days photo after blepharoplasty and eyebrow tail lift, and (C) images six months after surgery

Post-operative Care

Post op care similar to blepharoplasty is recommended, such as cold compresses on the eye site. The patient should be seen within 24–48 h to remove the dressing and inspect the wound. The stitches are removed 8–14 days after surgery.

Complications

Complications of the procedure are rare and minimal compared to the traditional open, direct approaches. There is some risk of injury to sensory nerves, motor nerves, or even vascular structures, but these complications are rare. Other complications include scars and other

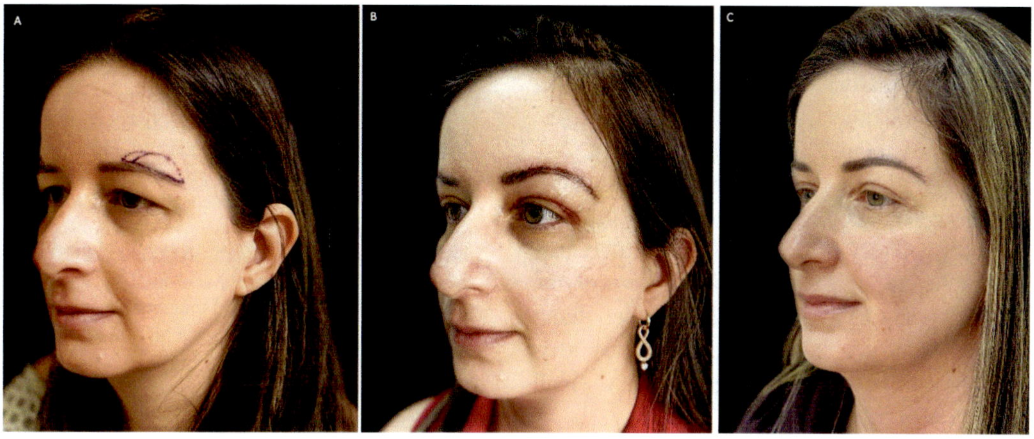

Fig. 28.5 (A) Preoperative photo of a patient with dermatochalasis and lateral brow ptosis with the demarcation of possible incisions, demonstrating the medial extent of one proposed incision, (B) patient 15 days after the more medial extending incision was performed and (C) patient six months after surgery

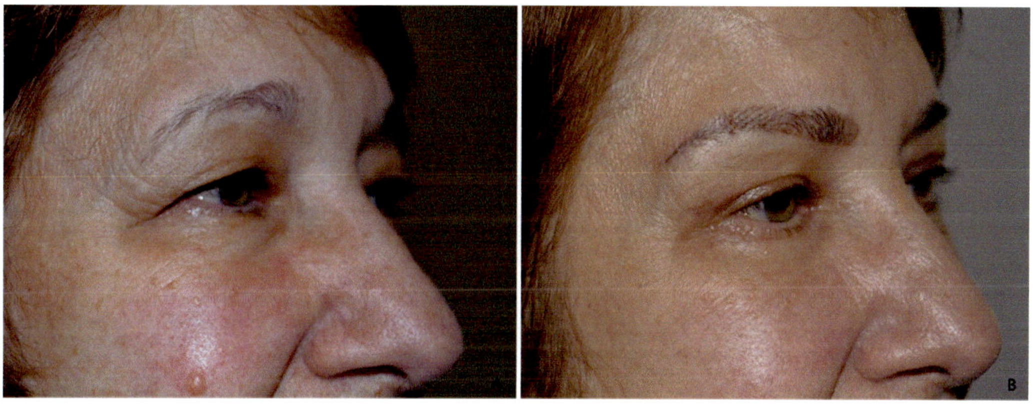

Fig. 28.6 (A) Preoperative of a 33 year old without dermatochalasis who sought only surgical elevation of the brow tail, (B) patient 30 days after surgery

healing defects that can be modified later, CO_2 laser or direct excision of scar may be beneficial for scars that persist and are conspicuous. Some scars may require cover with makeup (Fig. 28.3).

Discussion

The ideal position of the eyebrows varies according to age, gender, and ethnicity [3, 4]. In general, a descending lateral brow may be undesirable [14, 15].

Aesthetically, lateral eyebrow ptosis is considered an early sign of aging [16–18]. It may contribute to lateral upper eyelid hooding as well. A minimal incision direct browplasty may be an excellent choice to correct these issues.

The eyebrow must be carefully examined for ptosis. Direct browplasty should be considered concomitant to upper blepharoplasty in many patients. Excess eyelid skin promotes a compensatory mechanism to keep the eyelid open that involves the use of the frontalis muscle and a reduction in the action of the orbicular. When the excess skin is removed, this compensatory mechanism is lost, and the eyebrow falls.

A short incision direct lateral browplasty may be less invasive than other open brow lifting approaches, owing to its shorter incision. The procedure is straightforward and requires minimal instrumentation or fixation devices, unlike endoscopic or other lifts [19, 20, 26, 29]. The results are reproducible and durable [8, 21].

The technique described here corroborates reports by others showing good results with direct browplasty [23–28]. Slight differences include the elliptical excision above the eyebrow and focus on the brow tail. Like other direct incisions, scarring may be a concern and revision procedures may be necessary in a small percentage of patients [12, 13, 22].

Conclusion

A short incision, lateral direct browplasty efficiently elevates the eyebrow tail in a durable manner and achieves a satisfactory aesthetic outcome with proper patient selection and good technique.

References

1. Ding A. The ideal eyebrow: lessons learnt from the literature. Aesthetic Plast Surg [Internet]. 2021 Apr 25;45(2):536–43. Available from: https://doi.org/10.1007/s00266-020-01920-x
2. Berisha F, Johnston A, McOwan PW. Identifying regions that carry the best information about global facial configurations. J Vis [Internet]. 2010 Sep 28;10(11):27–27. Available from: https://doi.org/10.1167/10.11.27
3. Baker SB, Dayan JH, Crane A, Kim S. The Influence of Brow Shape on the Perception of Facial Form and Brow Aesthetics. Plast Reconstr Surg [Internet]. 2007 Jun;119(7):2240–7. Available from: http://journals.lww.com/00006534-200706000-00039
4. Asaad M, Kelarji AB, Jawhar CS, Banuelos J, Taslakian E, Wahood W, et al. Eyebrow height changes with aging. Plast Reconstr Surg-Glob Open [Internet]. 2019 Sep;1. Available from: http://journals.lww.com/01720096-900000000-97765
5. Delyzer TL, Yazdani A. Characterizing the lateral slope of the aging female eyebrow. Can J Plast Surg [Internet]. 2013 Aug 1;21(3):173–7. Available from: http://journals.sagepub.com/doi/https://doi.org/10.1177/229255031302100302
6. Briceño CA, Zhang-Nunes SX, Massry GG. Minimally invasive options for the brow and upper lid. Facial Plast Surg Clin North Am [Internet]. 2015 May;23(2):153–66. Available from: https://linkinghub.elsevier.com/retrieve/pii/S1064740615000139
7. Paskhover B, Durand D, Kamen E, Gordon NA. Patterns of change in facial skeletal aging. JAMA Facial Plast Surg [Internet]. 2017 Sep;19(5):413–7. Available from: https://doi.org/10.1001/jamafacial.2017.0743
8. Savetsky IL, Matarasso A. Lateral temporal subcutaneous brow lift. Plast Reconstr Surg-Glob Open [Internet]. 2020 Apr;8(4):e2764. Available from: https://doi.org/10.1097/GOX.0000000000002764
9. Hollander MHJ, Contini M, Pott JW, Vissink A, Schepers RH, Jansma J. Functional outcomes of upper eyelid blepharoplasty: a systematic review. J Plast Reconstr Aesthetic Surg [Internet]. 2019 Feb;72(2):294–309. Available from: https://linkinghub.elsevier.com/retrieve/pii/S1748681518304200
10. Prado RB, Silva-Junior DE, Padovani CR, Schellini SA. Assessment of eyebrow position before and after upper eyelid blepharoplasty. Orbit [Internet]. 2012 Aug 9;31(4):222–6. Available from: https://doi.org/10.3109/01676830.2011.648801
11. Lee JM, Lee TE, Lee H, Park M, Baek S. Change in brow position after upper blepharoplasty or levator advancement. J Craniofac Surg [Internet]. 2012 Mar;23(2):434–6. Available from: http://journals.lww.com/00001665-201203000-00023
12. Castañares S. Forehead wrinkles, glabellar frown and ptosis of the eyebrows. Plast Reconstr Surg. 1964;34:406–13.
13. Pelle-Ceravolo M, Angelini M. Transcutaneous brow shaping: a straightforward and precise method to lift and shape the eyebrows. Aesthetic Surg J [Internet]. 2017 Sep 1;37(8):863–75. Available from: https://academic.oup.com/asj/article/37/8/863/3072682
14. Yalçınkaya E, Cingi C, Söken H, Ulusoy S, Muluk NB. Aesthetic analysis of the ideal eyebrow shape and position. Eur Arch Oto-Rhino-Laryngology [Internet]. 2016 Feb 28;273(2):305–10. Available from: https://doi.org/10.1007/s00405-014-3356-0
15. Schreiber J, Singh N, Klatsky S. Beauty lies in the "Eyebrow" of the beholder: a public survey of eyebrow aesthetics. Aesthetic Surg J [Internet]. 2005 Jul;25(4):348–52. Available from: https://doi.org/10.1016/j.asj.2005.05.002
16. Guo H, Hu G, Xu Q, Qin H, Li F, Kang L, et al. [Anthropometric analysis of facial aging in 1200 Han adult people in Dalian]. Zhonghua Zheng Xing Wai Ke Za Zhi [Internet]. 2016 Jan;32(1):29–35. Available from: http://www.ncbi.nlm.nih.gov/pubmed/27197477
17. Yun S, Son D, Yeo H, Kim S, Kim J, Han K, et al. Changes of eyebrow muscle activity with aging. Plast Reconstr Surg [Internet]. 2014 Apr;133(4):455e-463e. Available from: http://journals.lww.com/00006534-201404000-00004
18. Almeida ART de, Sampaio GÂ de A, Queiroz NPL. Hyaluronic acid in the rejuvenation of the upper third of the face: review and update. Part 2: temporal and supraorbital regions. Surg Cosmet Dermatology

[Internet]. 2017;9(2). Available from: https://doi.org/10.5935/scd1984-8773.20179201
19. Bahmani Kashkouli M, Karimi N, Sianati H, Khademi B. Techniques of eyebrow lifting: a narrative review. J Ophthalmic Vis Res [Internet]. 2020 Apr 6; Available from: https://knepublishing.com/index.php/JOVR/article/view/6740
20. Foustanos A, Drimouras G, Panagiotopoulos K. Lateral brow lift: a multi-point suture fixation technique. Arch Plast Surg [Internet]. 2015;42(5):580. Available from: https://doi.org/10.5999/aps.2015.42.5.580
21. Osaki TH, Ferreira CAA, Osaki MH. Improving the results of upper eyelid blepharoplasty: zetaplasty to correct lateral eyebrow sliding. Rev Bras Cir Plástica – Brazilian J Plast Sugery [Internet]. 2016;31(3):398–401. Available from: https://doi.org/10.5935/2177-1235.2016RBCP0065
22. Arneja JS, Larson DL, Gosain AK. Aesthetic and reconstructive brow lift: current techniques, indications, and applications. Ophthalmic Plast Reconstr Surg [Internet]. 2005 Nov;21(6):405–11. Available from: http://journals.lww.com/00002341-200511000-00001
23. Pascali M, Bocchini I, Avantaggiato A, Carinci F, Cervelli V, Orlandi F, et al. Direct brow lifting: specific indications for a simplified approach to eyebrow ptosis. Indian J Plast Surg [Internet]. 2016 Jan 13;49(01):66–71. Available from: https://doi.org/10.4103/0970-0358.182243
24. Homer NA, Zhou S, Watson AH, Nakra T. Nuances of the direct brow lift: oculoplastic surgeons' perspective. Am J Cosmet Surg [Internet]. 2021 Mar 15;38(1):5–10. Available from: https://doi.org/10.1177/0748806820940930
25. Feinendegen DL. The direct brow-lift using the flat incision technique. Aesthetic Plast Surg [Internet]. 2012 Apr 12;36(2):468–71. Available from: https://doi.org/10.1007/s00266-011-9786-9
26. Pascali M, Avantaggiato A, Bocchini I, Carinci F, Cervelli V. Comparison among three different fixation techniques in temporal brow lift surgery. J Craniofac Surg [Internet]. 2015 May;26(3):906–10. Available from: https://journals.lww.com/00001665-201505000-00071
27. Cohen BD, Reiffel AJ, Spinelli HM. Browpexy through the upper lid (BUL): a new technique of lifting the brow with a standard blepharoplasty incision. Aesthetic Surg J [Internet]. 2011 Feb 1;31(2):163–9. Available from: https://academic.oup.com/asj/article/31/2/163/202007
28. Eftekhari K, Peng GL, Landsberger H, Douglas R, Massry GG. The brow fat pad suspension suture: safety profile and clinical observations. Ophthalmic Plast Reconstr Surg [Internet]. 2018 Jan;34(1):7–12. Available from: https://journals.lww.com/00002341-201801000-00002
29. Nahai FR. The varied options in brow lifting. Clin Plast Surg [Internet]. 2013 Jan;40(1):101–4. Available from: https://linkinghub.elsevier.com/retrieve/pii/S0094129812001101

Open Forehead Lift

29

Loreley D. Smith, Y. Stephanie Zhang, Michael M. Han, Jeremiah P. Tao, and Seanna R. Grob

Abstract

Open forehead lift procedures are a traditional and powerful approach to address the aging upper face or brow ptosis. Forehead lifting serves to restore a more youthful appearance, as well as a functionally and aesthetically improved brow position. This chapter describes the anatomy of the forehead and brow, including tissue planes. It includes a review of the pathophysiology of brow ptosis and the preoperative examination of the aging upper face. Lastly, the authors describe the specifics of open forehead lift surgery, as well as potential complications.

Keywords

Open forehead lift · Open brow lift · Mid-forehead brow lift · Pretrichial brow lift · Coronal brow lift

Introduction

The eyebrows are an important landmark of the upper face. They convey emotions and play a crucial role in facial aesthetics. The ideal brow is a standard that differs based on age, cultural preferences, societal norms, current fashion, gender, and personal preferences [1–4]. Brow ptosis, or the descent of the brow, most often occurs due to involutional changes with aging, but other etiologies include trauma, infection, and iatrogenic facial nerve injury must also be evaluated and excluded [3, 5, 6]. The patient with brow ptosis may present with aesthetic concerns or they may have functional consequences of visual field obstruction.

Various surgical procedures exist to successfully address functional and aesthetic brow ptosis ranging from browpexy to direct tissue resection. Open forehead lifting, like other techniques that elevate tissues through resection may provide more profound and durable results. Open forehead lifts can be performed through various incisions including mid-forehead, pretrichial and coronal approaches. Incision selection

Supplementary Information The online version contains supplementary material available at https://doi.org/10.1007/978-3-031-63178-8_29.

L. D. Smith · Y. Stephanie Zhang
Department of Ophthalmology, University of California San Francisco, San Francisco, CA, USA

L. D. Smith
The Pacific Center for Oculofacial and Aesthetic Plastic Surgery, San Francisco, CA, USA

M. M. Han · J. P. Tao (✉) · S. R. Grob
Division of Oculofacial Plastic and Orbital Surgery, University of California, Irvine, CA, USA
e-mail: jeremiat@hs.uci.edu

J. Tao (ed.), *Efficient Oculofacial Surgery*, https://doi.org/10.1007/978-3-031-63178-8_29

is determined after evaluation of the patient and a careful discussion of the patient's goals and expectations. Anatomy of the forehead and brows are key, as is evaluating features of an individual patient.

Surgical Anatomy and Pathophysiology of Brow Ptosis

Anatomy of the Forehead and Brow

The position of the brow varies according to age and gender. In general, the female brow is higher (above the supraorbital rim), thinner, and has a higher point of arc that typically is on the sagittal plane of the lateral limbus or lateral canthus. In contrast, the male brow sits lower (on or below the level of the supraorbital rim), thicker, and travels with a straighter trajectory [1, 2, 5]. The skin of the eyebrow represents a transition zone between the thinner skin of the eyelid and thicker skin of the forehead and scalp. Typically, the brow is divided into three anatomic parts: the head, body, and tail. The eyebrow skin contains cilia directed at different angles that define each aspect of the brow [7].

Tissue Planes in the Upper Face

Several soft tissue layers comprise the upper face and brow which can be separated into two regions, medial to the temporal line and lateral to the temporal line. The temporal line is the anterior attachment of the temporalis muscle and the adjacent fascial structures to the underlying skull [8].

Medial to the temporal line, the soft tissue layers from superficial to deep include the skin, subcutaneous tissue, musculoaponeurotic layer (including the frontalis muscle and galea aponeurotica), loose areolar tissue, and periosteum (Table 29.1) [6, 8, 9]. The galea aponeurotica is a broad band of fibrous tissue that extends from the frontalis muscle across the top of the skull to the occipitalis muscle posteriorly [10, 11]. The galea aponeurotica layer and connected frontalis and occipitalis muscles are equivalent to the superficial musculoaponeurotic system (SMAS) elsewhere in the face [6, 8, 9, 12].

Lateral to the temporal line the layers are more complex. The layers from superficial to deep consist of skin, subcutaneous tissue, the temporoparietal fascia (loose layer of tissue in which the temporal branch of the facial nerve lies), the deep temporalis fascia,

Table 29.1 Tissue layers in the face

General face	Central forehead/scalp (medial to the temporal line)	Temporal forehead (lateral to the temporal line)
• Skin • Subcutaneous fat • Mimetic muscles • SMAS and related layers (temporoparietal fascia, platysma, galea aponeurotica)* • Retaining ligaments • Deeper muscle and fat pads • Periosteum	• Skin • Superficial fascia and connective tissue • Galea aponeurotica/frontalis* • Loose areolar tissue with emissary veins and arteries • Periosteum	• Skin • Superficial fascia and connective tissue • Temporoparietal fascia* • Deep temporalis fascia (superficial and deep subdivisions separated by temporal fat pad) • Temporalis muscle • Periosteum

SMAS = Superficial Musculoaponeurotic System
* Denotes contiguous planes

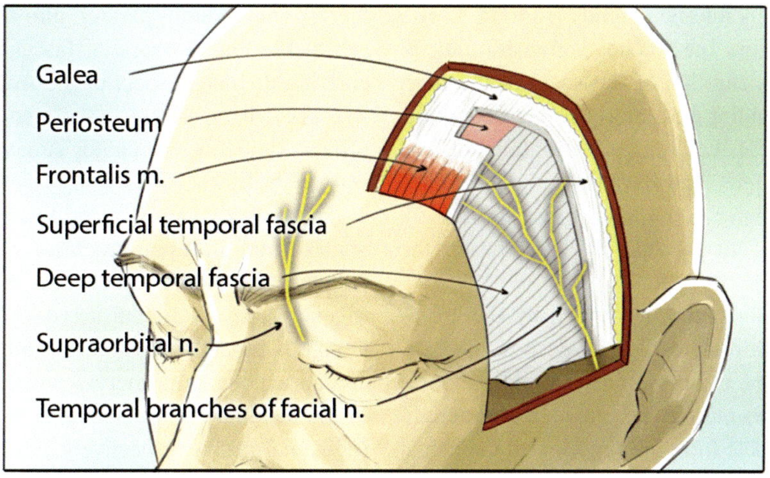

Fig. 29.1 Anatomic landmarks in the upper face

temporalis muscle and periosteum overlying the skull (Table 29.1) [8, 12]. The deep temporalis fascia is an important landmark for dissection planes in the temporal upper face (Fig. 29.1). Dissection should be carried out superficial to the glistening deep temporalis fascia and deep to the temporoparietal fascia to avoid inadvertent injury to the facial nerve [8, 12]. As one dissects toward the zygomatic arch, the temporalis fascia splits around the superficial temporal fat pad producing the superficial and deep layers of the temporalis fascia [8].

As mentioned previously, medial to the temporal line, the galea aponeurotica and connected frontalis and occipitalis muscles is equivalent to the SMAS in this region. Temporally, the temporoparietal fascia is an extension of the SMAS in the lower face. The SMAS is a dense fibrous layer of connective tissue that invests the mimetic muscles and coordinates the various actions of the facial muscles in the lower face. In contrast to the muscles of facial expression in the lower face, the temporalis muscle is a muscle of mastication. It is innervated by cranial nerve V and has a strong attachment to the underlying skull and loose attachment to the overlying soft tissues. This allows for contraction of the muscles of mastication with minimal movement of the overlying soft tissue. This differs from the muscles of facial expression which have strong attachments to the overlying soft tissue. Contraction leads to muscle movement and subsequent facial expression. This also explains the dissection planes during open brow lift procedures. Medial to the temporal line, the frontalis has loose attachments to the underlying tissue. An easy tissue dissection plane is in the loose areolar tissue, otherwise known as the subgaleal or pre periosteal plane. A subperiosteal approach is available but is more difficult to free owing to tighter connective tissue attachments. Temporally, it is important to maintain a plane that is on the deep temporalis fascia, below the temporoparietal fascia, to protect the facial nerve. Intraoperatively, the conjoined tendon is the boundary between the forehead and temple that should be released to connect the temporal and medial dissections.

Forehead Muscles and Innervation

At the eyebrow, the vertical fibers of the frontalis muscle and horizontal fibers of the orbicularis muscles interdigitate. The position of the brow represents a dynamic interplay between elevating and depressing forces [6]. The frontalis is the main elevator or retractor. The depressors, or protractors, include the orbicularis oculi, corrugator supercilii and procerus muscles [12].

The frontalis muscle extends from the brows superiorly across the forehead, transitioning to the galea aponeurotica of the scalp at the hairline, and extending posteriorly to the occipitalis muscle [10, 11]. Laterally, the frontalis ends at the temporal line. The frontalis may be confluent or may have a midline bifurcation [13]. Contraction of the frontalis muscle elevates the brows [10, 11].

The glabellar region is formed by the corrugator supercilii muscles that lie deep to the hair-bearing skin of the brow on each side and the central procerus muscle. The corrugator supercilii muscles originate from the superior orbital rim at the medial end of the brow and terminate at the lateral third of the brow [12, 14]. These muscles have an oblique and transverse head and insert into the dermis of the medial aspect of the eyebrow above the supraorbital rim bilaterally. The transverse head serves to pull the brow medially, while the smaller oblique head runs parallel to the depressor supercilii and serves to depress the medial brow [15–17]. These actions lead to the vertical lines of the glabella, perpendicular to their orientation, commonly known as the "elevens." The procerus muscle is a pyramidal shaped muscle in the midline of the glabella that extends from the superior nasal region to merge with the frontalis and skin between the eyebrows superiorly [7, 18]. Contraction creates horizontal lines in the central glabella and upper nose.

The orbicularis muscle is radially oriented and consists of 3 portions: orbital, preseptal and pretarsal [19]. At the brow, the superior borders of the orbital orbicularis muscle fibers interdigitate with the vertical fibers of the frontalis. There is a dense fibrous attachment of the brow to the superior orbital rim that extends inferiorly to the arcus marginalis of the superior orbit. Along with the corrugator and procerus muscles, the orbicularis oculi muscles serve to close the eye and depress the brow [19].

The frontalis muscle is innervated by the temporal branch (otherwise known as the frontal branch) of the facial nerve (cranial nerve VII) [11]. The facial nerve exits the skull at the stylomastoid foramen. The temporal branch crosses the zygomatic arch, passing into the areolar tissue of the temporoparietal fascia, subsequently entering the deep aspect of the frontalis muscle. Branches of the facial nerve also innervate the orbicularis oculi, corrugator supercilii, and procerus muscles [16, 20, 21].

The sensory supply to the forehead and scalp comes from the supratrochlear and supraorbital branches of the ophthalmic division of the trigeminal nerve (cranial nerve V) [11, 22]. The temple is innervated by the zygomaticotemporal and auriculotemporal nerves which are branches of the maxillary and mandibular branches of the trigeminal nerve, respectively [9, 23]. The scalp is supplied by extensions of these nerves from the forehead, as well as by branches of dorsal rami of cervical spinal nerves and the cervical plexus posteriorly [12]. It is notable that subgaleal divisions of these nerves travel to the vertex of the scalp and are at risk of damage with horizontal incisions that penetrate the galea in this region.

Attachments

The layers of the forehead and brow are anchored to the periosteum at several locations that must be released to achieve an effective forehead and brow lift. The lateral and medial aspects of the forehead meet at the temporal line on each side. This site is otherwise known as the zone of adhesion. Superiorly, the temporal line is formed by the fusion of the temporoparietal fascia, deep temporal fascia and frontoparietal periosteum at the origin of the temporalis muscle [12]. Anteriorly, the deep temporal fascia becomes adherent to the periosteum at the superior temporal lateral orbital rim. The galea aponeurotica also fuses at this point, forming the conjoined tendon. Along the superior orbital rim, the galea aponeurotica and periosteum create the arcus marginalis, anchoring the brow [12]. Releasing the attachments at the superior orbital rim and conjoined tendon down to the lateral canthus during forehead lifts allows for the creation of a contiguous plane of SMAS and related fascia (e.g., temporoparietal fascia, galea aponeurotica).

Danger Zones

During an open forehead lift approach, the temporal branch of the facial nerve is at risk. In the temporal area, the nerve crosses the zygomatic arch and courses superomedially in the deep layers of the temporoparietal fascia [24, 25]. The path of the temporal branch can be estimated by Pitanguy's line, which is a line drawn from 0.5 cm (cm) inferior to the tragus to 1.5 cm above the lateral taper of the ipsilateral brow [12, 26, 27]. The sentinel vein can serve as a helpful landmark intra-operatively as it lies within 2 mm (mm) of the temporal branch of the facial nerve [12, 25, 28–30].

Dissection temporally must be in the plane deep to the temporoparietal fascia and superficial to the deep temporalis fascia overlying the temporalis muscle. Dissection along this plane avoids iatrogenic damage to the overlying facial nerve. In contrast, the facial nerve branches in the lower face run deep to the SMAS, thus dissection is carried out superficial to the SMAS to avoid iatrogenic nerve injury [31].

Care should be taken to avoid injury of the supraorbital and suptratrochlear neurovascular bundles, branches of the ophthalmic division of cranial nerve V that ascend from the superior orbital rim [11, 22]. They provide sensory innervation of the forehead and scalp to the vertex. Damage to these nerves may cause hypoesthesia and paresthesia. The supratrochlear neurovascular bundle exits from the supratrochlear notch located approximately 1.75 cm from the midline on each side. The supratrochlear nerve branches superiorly and medially to provide sensation to the midline glabellar region, medial upper eyelid, portions of the conjunctiva and the upper lateral nose [32–34]. Lateral to the supratrochlear neurovascular bundle, the supraorbital nerve exits the superior orbital rim through the eponymous foramen or notch to innervate the frontoparietal skin and upper eyelid [33–36].

Pathophysiology of Brow Ptosis

Most forms of brow ptosis are acquired and can generally be categorized as age-related, myogenic, traumatic, infectious, spastic, neoplastic, or iatrogenic. Age-related changes are the most common underlying cause of brow ptosis. With age, there is increased skin laxity and progressive elastosis of the connective tissue and frontalis muscle that leads to soft tissue descent. This is first seen at the lateral brow, but eventually can affect the entirety of the brow. The temporal brow often descends first due to loss of temporal volume and the lack of frontalis muscle to assist in elevation. Various environmental factors can affect the onset and progression of brow ptosis, including genetics, sun exposure and radiation. The ptotic brow can be aesthetically displeasing and functionally cause visually significant field obstruction by exacerbating eyelid hooding or by directly obstructing vision, if severe.

Although involutional brow ptosis is the most common, it is important to recognize other etiologies [3, 6]. Paralysis or weakness of the frontalis muscle can cause brow ptosis on one or both sides. This may be due to a congenital defect or facial nerve paralysis from Bell palsy [37], infectious [6, 38], traumatic [25], neoplastic and/or iatrogenic [6] etiology.

In addition, brow ptosis secondary to recent botulinum toxin injection, should be considered [39]. Neurotoxin induced brow droop is generally transient, therefore reassessment after it was worn off (usually 3–6 months) is important prior to considering surgical intervention.

Preoperative History and Evaluation of Brow Ptosis

History

There exist numerous etiologies of brow ptosis and atypical causes must be considered in the correct context. Timing of onset or a waxing and waning course may suggest an etiology due to chemo denervation or a potentially transient Bell palsy. Past medical history of neurological or otologic procedures may suggest an iatrogenic cause. Ocular history should also be obtained with a focus on eyelid procedures that may predispose the patient to a complicated surgery or postoperative ocular surface exposure.

Examination

The forehead, brows and eyes are a central feature of facial beauty. In particular, the forehead and eyebrows relay emotion. Patient s may state that those around them incorrectly perceive them as "tired" or "angry" appearing secondary to involutional changes in the upper face, and they may wish to modify their appearance based on this perception.

Examination of the forehead, brow, eyelids, globe, and cranial nerves should be completed as part of the assessment (Table 29.2). If the patient has received prior chemodenervation to the frontalis and/or glabella, repeat examination should be performed at least 90 days following the injection.

The brows should first be examined in a neutral position without recruitment of the frontalis. The examiner may gently place their fingers on the frontalis above the brows to prevent frontalis contraction. The degree of brow ptosis, any visual obscuration, and location of brow descent temporally and/or centrally should be assessed.

In addition to the evaluation of the position of the brows, the arch and curvature should be assessed. If the eyebrows are tattooed or painted on, the surgeon should carefully assess the true position of the brow, looking for the transition from the thicker brow tissue to the thinner eyelid tissue. Any brow asymmetry should be noted and should prompt a more thorough evaluation for weakness or paralysis of the frontalis muscle. Asymmetric brow ptosis can also present due to asymmetric dermatochalasis and/or blepharoptosis, further emphasizing the importance of examining the patient with a relaxed frontalis [40]. Often it is helpful to compare exam findings with younger pictures of the patient to assess the progression of brow ptosis and to assess for any long-standing asymmetries.

The forehead height should be assessed, along with hair density and presence of a receding hairline. A shorter forehead (hairline to brow distance) can be exaggerated with a pretrichial or mid-forehead approach, whereas a high forehead may be exaggerated by a coronal approach. A patient with thinning or receding hair may have more obvious scars with a pretrichial or coronal approach.

The position of the eyelids should also be evaluated for malposition and lagophthalmos. The eyes should be examined for any ocular surface disease that could worsen following surgical brow and/or eyelid intervention.

The cranial nerve exam should be conducted with a focus on the facial nerve especially if there is concern for facial nerve damage from traumatic, infectious, compressive, inflammatory, or infiltrative etiologies. Adequate time, in general at least 6 months, should be allowed after trauma for any potential nerve recovery before surgical intervention.

In this chapter, we focus on surgical approaches of open forehead lifting. These include the mid-forehead lift, pretrichial brow lift, and coronal brow lift which will be discussed in detail (Table 29.3).

Table 29.2 Physical examination of the face

Brow	Neutral position, asymmetry, arch, density of brow hairs
Forehead	Rhytids, height, curvature, hairline position
Lid	Position, Hering's law, lagophthalmos, incomplete blink
Ocular surface and globe	Signs and symptoms of dry eye or exposure
Cranial nerves	Especially CN VII tone and symmetry

Surgical Approaches for Brow Ptosis Using Open Forehead Lift

Mid-Forehead Lift

The mid-forehead brow lift may be suitable for those with deep forehead rhytids and a receding hairline for whom the coronal approach is not desirable [41–43]. The proximity to the brow increases the mechanical advantage of brow lift compared to endoscopic or coronal approaches, and only moderate undermining is required, decreasing the risk of hematoma or nerve injury [44–46]. In some patients, this incision can also be utilized to lower the frontal hairline [47]. The primary limitation with this technique is incision placement. Even with impeccable closure, some degree of visible scarring is inevitable, and expectations should be discussed at length with the patient. These incisions also may cause hypesthesia caudal to the incision, i.e., to the upper forehead and top of the head.

There are two notable relative contraindications to this approach. The mid-forehead lift is not ideal in patients that lack transverse forehead rhytids as this can lead to a clearly visible scar. This approach should also be used with caution in those with a pre-existing short brow to hairline distance to avoid further reduction of the forehead [41, 45, 48].

Prior to beginning the procedure, the brow position is assessed, and the forehead is marked either with a single, linear mark across the entire forehead (Fig. 29.2), or with a separate mark in the mid-forehead on each side. Separate incisions, placed in different rhytids on each side, can offset a visually obvious, long scar [44, 46, 49]. The amount of tissue to excise can be marked pre-operatively, or the redundant tissue flap can be marked and excised intra-operatively. If marking pre-operatively, care should be taken to place the upper limb of the excision in a forehead crease, as this will be the resultant position of the scar post-operatively. It is imperative that

Table 29.3 Open forehead lift: key points

Procedure	Outcome	Advantages	Disadvantages and other considerations
Mid-forehead	- Elevates brow - Allows for advancement of the hairline (shortening of the forehead)	- Can lift entire brow equally - Can equalize brow asymmetries - Avoids potential arch - Minimal undermining	- Visible scar in forehead rhytids/ can deepen forehead rhytids - Should only be performed in patients with deep forehead rhytids - Avoid in short foreheads as it shortens the hairline to brow distance
Pretrichial	- Elevates brow and forehead - Shortens forehead - Allows for alteration of hairline	- Effective lift of entire forehead and brow - Scars can be hidden in the hairline - Smooths frontalis and glabellar rhytids - Exposure to frontal calvarium	- Large flap dissection with increased risk of hypoesthesia and/or parasthesia - Potential for scarring and/or alopecia
Coronal	- Elevates brow and forehead	- Effective lift of entire forehead and brow - Scars hidden behind hair line - Elevates the hairline / lengthens the forehead - Smooths frontalis and glabellar rhytids	- Largest flap of any open forehead lift approach - Large flap dissection - Higher risk of hypoesthesia and/or parasthesia, especially posterior to the incision

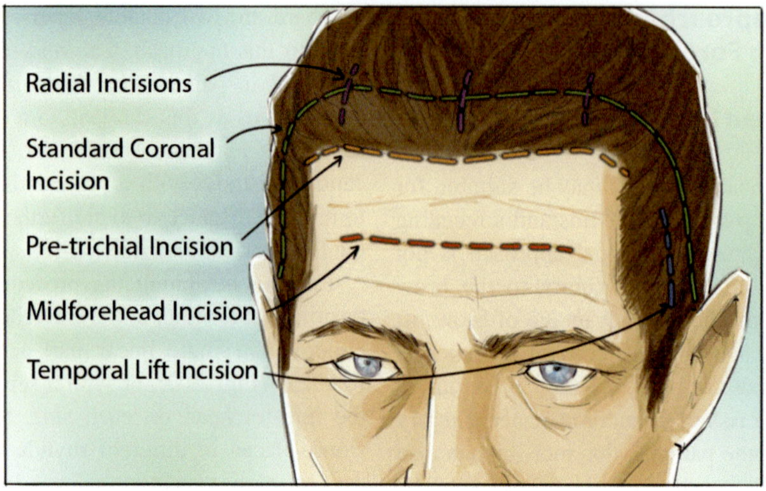

Fig. 29.2 Open forehead lift incisions

the upper edge precisely follows the forehead crease, even if it is slightly irregular. Depending on the surgeon's preference, marking can be performed while the patient is sitting up, or in the supine position in the operating room. The neurovascular bundles medially may also be palpated and marked pre-operatively. Under sedation or general anesthesia, local anesthesia is instilled and the patient is prepped and draped in a routine fashion for surgery.

A # 10 or 15 blade is used to make an incision along markings. If the incision is carried laterally to the conjoined tendon, the incision must not extend past the skin to avoid inadvertent damage to the facial nerve. Blunt dissection is carried down to the subcutaneous layer with Stevens tenotomy or Metzenbaum scissors, avoiding violation of the frontalis muscle. Once the loose, subcutaneous aponeurotic layer overlying the frontalis muscle is reached, this plane is used to dissect inferiorly to the superior orbital rim, visualizing the orbicularis oculi muscle on each side. Dissection is also carried superiorly for approximately 1 cm to facilitate tension-free closure and wound eversion. If the patient also requires frontal hairline advancement, additional undermining may be necessary. Through these incisions, weakening of the corrugator and procerus muscles may be performed by careful blunt dissection or resection [41–43, 46]. The procerus can be weakened in a similar fashion. Care should be taken not to aggressively disrupt the glabellar muscles as this can lead to undesirable spreading of the head of the brows.

Suspension sutures may be placed, although tissue resection alone may achieve lift [44, 46, 49]. The scalp flap is lifted and a 4-0 polydioxanone suture is passed in a horizontal mattress fashion through the orbicularis oculi at the midpoint of the brow (at or near the level of the pupil) to the periosteum at the upper margin of the skin excision. An additional suture can be passed in a similar fashion at the lateral arch point of the brow for additional lift and contour of the temporal brow. This suture is passed in a trajectory directed upward and outward. The sutures can be adjusted and secured once the brows are symmetric and in appropriate position [44, 46, 49].

At this point, attention is turned to excision of the redundant forehead flap. If this was marked pre-operatively, then the redundant tissue is excised as marked. Otherwise, the scalp flap is retracted superiorly. If suspensory sutures have been placed, the brows have already been elevated to the desired height, however, if not, the scalp flap is elevated superiorly until the brows are in the ideal position. The redundant scalp tissue is grasped, and a scalpel is used to make a full-thickness, penetrating incision through the flap to indicate the amount of tissue to be excised. This can be performed in a few places along the flap. The tissue is then excised with facelift scissors or blade.

Once the redundant tissue is removed, wound closure is performed in a layered fashion. The dermis is closed with deep absorbable monofilament (e.g., 5-0 polydioxanone or poliglecaprone 25) sutures or absorbable, braided (e.g., 5–0 polyglactin) sutures. The skin is then closed with non-absorbable, monofilament (e.g., 5–0 polyamide 6 or polypropylene) sutures as running vertical or horizontal mattress suture or a simple running suture. Wound edges should have sufficient eversion to optimize the appearance of the post-operative scar.

Antibiotic ointment is applied, and a compressive dressing is placed for 24–48 h to prevent postoperative hematoma formation. The placement of a drain is not necessary. Skin sutures may be removed after 7–10 days.

Pretrichial Brow Lift (Video 29-1)

The pretrichial brow lift is best suited when moving the hairline further superior or posterior is undesirable [12, 50]. The pretrichial incision provides excellent exposure of the frontal calvarium and periosteum. Relative contraindications to this approach include patients with a history of poor scarring and a receding or low hairline [51]. Some degree of visible scarring is inevitable, and expectations should be outlined. Patients who have bangs or like wearing their hair forward, as opposed to those that pull their hair straight back into a ponytail, are good candidates for this procedure since this helps camouflage scarring.

Marking of the brow can be performed with the patient sitting up or in the supine position in the operating room. The location of the neurovascular bundles medially may be marked pre-operatively. A marker can be used to mark a slightly irregular line along the anterior hairline, posterior to the vellus hairs, following into the peak of temporal recession (Fig. 29.2). The incision can extend downward toward the helix of the ear on each side. Alternatively, the incision can be placed approximately 4–5 mm posterior to the hairline at the point of follicular density change, allowing for better hair regrowth through a beveled incision [52]. The pretrichial brow lift can also be performed with the use of an endoscope. The mark is made in a similar fashion at the anterior hairline, extending to the peak of temporal recession bilaterally. A separate temporal mark for the endoscope can be placed on each side, similar to a temporal brow lift incision (Fig. 29.2). The location of this mark is made by following the trajectory of the lateral canthus to the tail of the brow then temporally to the helix of the ear. On average, this mark is 2–3 cm in length and is placed 1.5–2 cm posterior to the hairline.

Once the markings have been completed, the hair is combed, parted, and tied with hair rubber bands to separate and clear the hair from the field. Local anesthesia is instilled and the patient is prepped and draped in a routine fashion for surgery.

A # 15 or # 10 blade is used to make the incision. Centrally, this can be subcutaneous, subgaleal or subperiosteal [48, 50–54]. The incision can be made perpendicular to the skin or can be beveled. A beveled incision perpendicular to the hair follicles is thought to better promote hair regrowth through the incision, and help camouflage the scar [50–52, 55]. Conservative hemostasis should be employed to avoid injury to the hair follicles. Blunt dissection with Metzenbaum scissors, an elevator or with finger dissection is carried out to a point approximately 2 cm above the superior orbital rims. As the flap is elevated, tension will be felt at the conjoined tendon temporally on each side. If the surgeon extended the incisions temporal to the conjoined tendon, Adson forceps are used to grasp the incision and Metzenbaum scissors are used to bluntly dissect to the level of the glistening deep temporalis fascia. It is imperative to dissect in the proper, deep plane laterally to avoid inadvertent damage to the frontal branch of the facial nerve. The Metzenbaum scissors are then used to bluntly spread in the plane overlying the deep temporalis fascia toward the tail of the brow. The elevator is then inserted and used to expose the deep temporalis fascia broadly toward the lateral canthus. The conjoined tendon is then freed with either an elevator or scissors to connect the temporal and central dissection planes. Following temporal dissection, the tail of the brow should be mobile.

Attention is then turned to the central portion of the flap again. The dissection is carried down to the root of the nose centrally. A retractor can be utilized to assist in dissection around the supraorbital neurovascular bundles. The periosteum along the rim should be released with a combination of blunt and sharp dissection. The glabellar muscles can then be carefully weakened with sharp dissection perpendicular to the muscle fiber plane with or without resection.

With the forehead flap free, the redundant tissue is excised. An assistant may push the tissue superiorly over the incision, demonstrating the amount of tissue overlap. A central cut is made in the redundant flap with a scalpel, marking the amount of tissue to be removed. This can be performed in 3–4 locations across the flap, ensuring proper brow elevation and contour along the way. The flap can be stabilized with skin staples or sutures at these incision sites and brow position can be assessed during this process. If the patient's hairline is to be adjusted, this portion is modified to remove some non-hair-bearing skin and some hair-bearing skin as desired. The tissue to be excised typically measures between 1–2 cm.

After hemostasis is achieved, wound closure should be performed in a layered, meticulous fashion to forestall objectionable scarring. Layered closure of the central forehead flap includes closure of the galea aponeurotica followed by the subcutaneous layer, and finally, the skin. Closure of the galea is performed with absorbable monofilament (e.g., 2-0 or 3-0 polydioxanone) sutures in a buried fashion. The subcutaneous closure is then performed with deep, buried absorbable monofilament (e.g., 4-0 or 5-0 polydioxanone) sutures or absorbable braided (e.g., 4-0 or 5-0 polyglactin) sutures. The deep sutures should ensure the skin edges approximate with minimal tension. The skin is then closed with non-absorbable monofilament (e.g., 5-0 polyamide 6 or polypropylene) sutures. A few interrupted sutures can be passed followed by a running, locking, vertical mattress suture. The skin within the hairline can be closed with skin staples. Wound edges of the pretrichial incision should have sufficient eversion to optimize the appearance of the post-operative scar (Fig. 29.3).

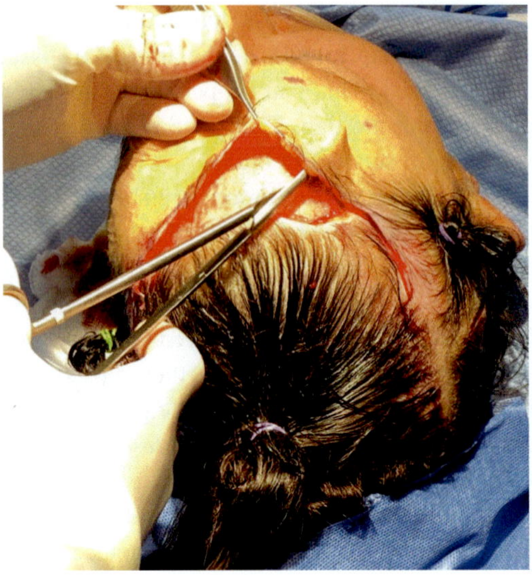

Fig. 29.3 Pretrichial incision and dissection

At this point, the hair is rinsed to remove any accumulated blood. It is then shampooed, rinsed with water, and gently dried. A compressive head dressing is placed for 24–48 h to prevent post-operative hematoma formation. The placement of a drain is not necessary. Skin sutures and staples may be removed after 7–10 days (Fig. 29.4).

Coronal Brow Lift

The open or coronal brow lift is a traditional surgical approach associated with a durable lift [43, 47, 55, 56]. Like the pretrichial approach, the coronal lift provides excellent exposure, allowing the surgeon to address various aspects of upper facial aging. This approach is best suited for patients with a normal to low hairline,

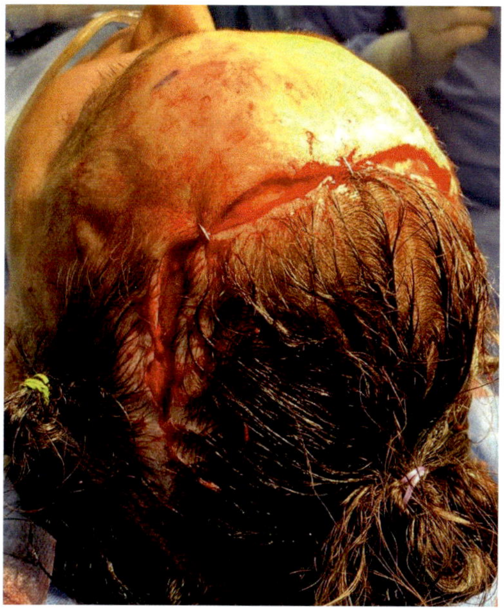

Fig. 29.4 Pretrichial incision following flap resection

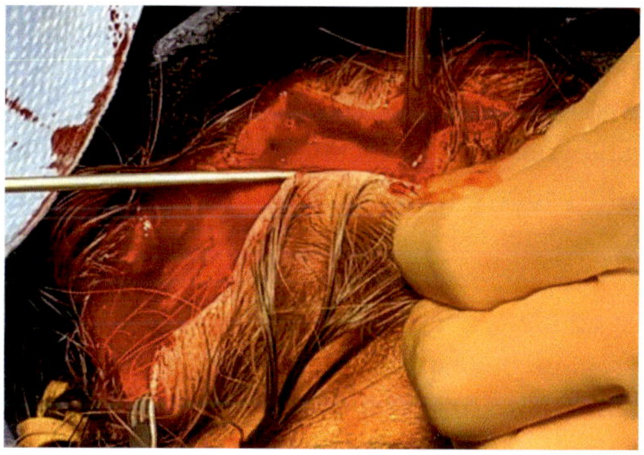

Fig. 29.5 Coronal incision and dissection

and should be avoided in those who are balding, have thin hair, or a high hairline [12, 43, 47, 57–59]. Disadvantages of this procedure include elevation of the frontal hairline, possible hypoesthesia or paresthesia, the potential for hair loss, and an unsightly incision [12, 47, 56–58]. Patients should be adequately counseled pre-operatively (Fig. 29.5).

Straight incisions are easier to manage, however an irregular or corrugated "zig zag" incision may avoid a line that may appear as an unnatural hair parting [55]. The incision should be placed several centimeters posterior to the hairline (approximately 2–8 cm) and extend from a point superior to the tip of the helix of the ear, or posterior to it, to the same point on the opposite side (Fig. 29.2) [43, 57, 58, 60]. Once the marking has been completed the hair is combed, parted, and tied with hair rubber bands to separate and clear the hair from the field. Usually under general anesthesia, local anesthesia is instilled after the skin is marked and the patient is prepped and draped in a routine fashion for surgery.

A # 10 or 15 blade is used to make an incision. The incision may be beveled to promote hair regrowth through the resultant scar, helping camouflage the scar post-operatively. Further steps are identical to the pretrichial approach described above.

Complications of Open Forehead Lift Procedures

Hematoma

During the acute postoperative period, hematoma formation may be encountered. Drains are not typically necessary following open brow lift procedures; however, adequate hemostasis should be assured at the termination of the case. Equally critical is the avoidance of excessive cauterization to avoid other complications, such as hair loss and paresthesia. Slow postoperative bleeding may be controlled with pressure alone. If a hematoma is encountered post-operatively, it should be evacuated immediately to avoid flap necrosis.

Infection

Wound infection is a potential issue during the postoperative period, albeit rare. The scalp, brow, and eyelids are extremely vascular, thus helping to minimize the incidence of infection. If infection is encountered, the patient should be placed on appropriate antibiotic coverage and monitored carefully.

Nerve Injury

A common side effect of brow surgery is hypoesthesia or paresthesia of the forehead and scalp. Peri-incisional, scalp and forehead anesthesia should be discussed with patients preoperatively. Most patients will experience some degree of temporary hypoesthesia from raising the forehead flap [62]. In particular, the coronal brow lift can result in anesthesia of the scalp posterior to the incision due to transection of the deep division of the supraorbital nerve [17]. This typically recovers within weeks but may take many months [56–58, 63].

The supratrochlear and supraorbital neurovascular bundles are also at risk of injury and should be identified to preserve and minimize any forehead hypoesthesia. Although direct injury is uncommon, neuropraxia secondary to tractional forces frequently occurs, but recovers within a few weeks [62]. Rarely, injury to the supraorbital nerves may cause neuralgia [45].

Special care should be taken to avoid injury of the frontal branch of the facial nerve. Dissection in the temporal region should remain in a plane above the glistening deep temporalis fascia. The frontal branch is at risk of damage during any brow procedure, most notably the temporal and coronal approach. It can also be seen with the midforehead lift if the incision is extended deeper than the skin at the lateral aspect on either side [45, 64]. Local edema and tension may cause temporary paresis which should recover [45].

Incision Scar

Scarring of the incision site is a universal side effect of all brow surgery. Appearance of the forehead scar is difficult to predict, but will be more evident, at least initially, in approaches where the incision is not hidden (e.g., midforehead lift). Widening of the scar is the most troublesome outcome. Depending on the patient's skin tone and prior or current exposure to the sun, hyper or hypopigmentation of the scar can occur. The use of silicone gel, and/or skin resurfacing, or injections using triamcinolone and/or 5-fluorouracil can improve the appearance of the post-operative scar [64, 65]. Surgical scar revision or laser resurfacing may be indicated if medical options are unsatisfactory.

Alopecia

Alopecia is a rare complication following open brow lift procedures. Of the approaches discussed, it is understandably the most common following the coronal approach [67]. This complication can be minimized in open approaches by beveling the incision. This avoids damage to dermal appendages and allows for hair growth through and around the forming scar. Minimizing cautery at the scalp edges also avoids damage of the surrounding follicles.

Brow Asymmetry

Most patients will have some degree of preexisting brow asymmetry. This should be noted, photographically documented, and discussed with patients to avoid poor patient satisfaction post-operatively.

Iatrogenic causes of post-operative brow asymmetry may result from asymmetric flap resection or suspension [62]. If over resection or asymmetric suspension does occur, revision surgery with release and re-suspension should be considered.

Lagophthalmos

Lagophthalmos may occur from brow lift, especially if combined with upper eyelid surgery. Temporary lagophthalmos is common in the acute post-operative period. Patients noted to have pre-existing lagophthalmos, xerophthalmia or a poor Bell phenomenon should be counseled preoperatively. Lagophthalmos should be treated with lubricating eye drops and ointment. In some cases, additional surgery may be needed to address post-operative lagophthalmos.

Conclusion

In summary, the open forehead lift is an excellent option to achieve durable brow elevation. These approaches offer aesthetic improvement to the face by the elevating effect, as well as the opportunity to weaken muscles that contribute to undesirable rhytids of the upper face. The long wound and potential for scarring or hypesthesia are drawbacks, but these can be mitigated by thoughtful incision placement and good closure technique.

References

1. Gunter JP, Antrobus SD. Aesthetic analysis of the eyebrows. Plast Reconstr Surg. 1997;99(7):1808–16.
2. Sclafani AP, Jung M. Desired position, shape, and dynamic range of the normal adult eyebrow. Arch Facial Plast Surg. 2010;12(2):123–7.
3. Glass LR, Lira J, Enkhbold E, Dimont E, Scofield S, Sherwood PR, Winn BJ. The lateral brow: position in relation to age, gender, and ethnicity. Ophth Plast Reconstr Surg. 2014;30(4):295–300.
4. Feser DK, Grundl M, Eisenmann-Klein M, Prantl L. Attractiveness of eyebrow position and shape in females depends on the age of the beholder. Aesthetic Plast Surg. 2007;31(2):154–60.
5. Shaw LT, Phelps PO. The basics of brow ptosis. Dis Mon. 2020;66(10): 101038. https://doi.org/10.1016/j.disamonth.2020.101038.
6. De Jong R, Hohman MH. Brow ptosis. [Updated 2022 May 2]. In: StatPearls [Internet]. Treasure Island (FL): StatPearls Publishing; 2022. Available from: https://www.ncbi.nlm.gov/books/NBK560762/. Accessed 25 Sept 2022.
7. Branham G, Holds JB. Brow/Upper Lid anatomy, aging and aesthetic analysis. Facial Plast Surg Clin North Am. 2015;23(2):117–27.
8. Nerad JA. Techniques in ophthalmic plastic surgery—a personal tutorial, 2nd ed. Elsevier, Inc.; 2021.
9. Kashkouli MB, Abdolalizadeh P, Abolfathzadeh N, Sianati H, Sharepour M, Hadi Y. Periorbital facial rejuvenation; applied anatomy and pre-operative assessment. J Curr Ophthalmol. 2017;29(3):154–68.
10. Costin BR, Plesec TP, Sakolsatayadorn N, Rubinstein TJ, McBride JM, Perry JD. Anatomy and histology of the frontalis muscle. Ophthalmic Plast Reconstr Surg. 2015;31(1):66–72.
11. Pessino K, Patel J, Patel BC. Anatomy, head and neck, frontalis muscle. [Updated 2021 Jul 31]. In: StatPearls [Internet]. Treasure Island (FL): StatPearls Publishing; 2022. Available from: https://www.ncbi.nlm.nih.gov/books/NBK557752/. Accessed 25 Sept 2022.
12. Angelos PC, Stallworth CL, Wang TD. Forehead lifting: state of the art. Facial Plast Surg. 2011;27(1):50–7.
13. Abramo AC, Do Amaral TP, Lessio BP, De Lima GA. Anatomy of forehead, glabellar, nasal and orbital muscles, and their correlation with distinctive patterns of skin lines on the upper third of the face: reviewing concepts. Aesth Plast Surg. 2016;40(6):962–71.
14. Isse NG, Elahi MM. The corrugator supercilii muscle revisited. Aesthet Surg J. 2001;21(3):209–15.
15. Janis JE, Ghavami A, Lemmon JA, Leedy JE, Guyuron B. Anatomy of the corrugator supercilii muscle: part I. Corrugator topography. Plast Reconstr Surg. 2007;120(6):1647–53.
16. Yu M, Wang SM. Anatomy, head and neck, eye corrugator muscle. [Updated 2021 Aug 11]. In: StatPearls [Internet]. Treasure Island (FL): StatPearls Publishing; 2022. Available from: https://www.ncbi.nlm.nih.gov/books/NBK542280/. Accessed 25 Sept 2022.
17. Knize DM. Anatomic concepts for brow lift procedures. Plast Reconstr Surg. 2009;124(6):2118–26.
18. Beer JI, Sieber DA, Scheuer JF 3rd, Greco TM. Three-dimensional facial anatomy: structure and function as it relates to injectable neuromodulators and soft tissue fillers. Plast Reconstr Surg Glob Open. 2016. https://doi.org/10.1097/GOX.0000000000001175.
19. Tong J, Lopez MJ, Patel BC. Anatomy, head and neck, eye orbicularis oculi muscle. [Updated 2021 Jul 26]. In: StatPearls [Internet]. Treasure Island (FL): StatPearls Publishing; 2022. Available from: https://www.ncbi.nlm.nih.gov/books/NBK441907/. Accessed 25 Sept 2022.
20. Brown TM, Drake TM, Krishnamurthy K. Anatomy, head and neck, procerus muscle. [Updated 2021 Aug 11]. In: StatPearls [Internet]. Treasure Island (FL): StatPearls Publishing; 2022. Available from: https://www.ncbi.nlm.nih.gov/books/NBK534763/. Accessed 25 Sept 2022.
21. Caminer DM, Newman MI, Boyd JB. Angular nerve: new insights on innervation of the corrugator supercilii and procerus muscles. J Plast Reconstr Aesthet Surg. 2006;59(4):366–72.
22. Green JP, Goldberg RA, Shorr N. Eyebrow ptosis. Int Ophthalmol Clin. 1997;27:97–122.
23. Patel BC. Surgical eyelid and periorbital anatomy. Semin Ophthalmol. 1996;11(2):118–37.
24. Liebman EP, Webster RC, Berger AS, DellaVecchia M. The frontalis nerve in the temporal brow lift. Arch Otolaryngol. 1982;108(4):232–5.
25. Lettieri S. Frontal branch of the facial nerve: galeal temporal relationship. Aesthet Surg J. 2008;28(2):143–6.
26. Pitanguy I, Ramos A. The frontal branch of the facial nerve: the importance of its variations in face lifting. Plast Reconstr Surg. 1966;38(4):352–6.
27. Sanderson KG, Conti A, Colussi M, Connolly C. A simple clinical application for locating the frontotemporal branch of the facial nerve using the

zygomatic arch and the tragus. Aesthet Surg J. 2020;40(5):NP223–7.
28. Trinei FA, Januszkiewicz J, Nahai F. The sentinel vein: an important reference point for surgery in the temporal region. Plast Reconstr Surg. 1998;101(1):27–32.
29. Friedman T, Lurie D, Westreich M. Rembrandt's sentinel vein. Aesth Surg J. 2007;27:105–7.
30. Sabini P, Wayne I, Quatela VC. Anatomical guides to precisely localize the frontal branch of the facial nerve. Arch Facial Plast Surg. 2003;5(2):150–2.
31. Pankratz J, Baer J, Mayer C, Rana V, Stephens R, Segars L, Surek CC. Depth transitions of the frontal branch of the facial nerve: implications in SMAS rhytidectomy. JPRAS Open. 2020;26:101–8.
32. Zito PM, Chauhan PR. Anatomy, head and neck, supratrochlear. [Updated 2021 Jul 31]. In: StatPearls [Internet]. Treasure Island (FL): StatPearls Publishing; 2022. Available from: https://www.ncbi.nlm.nih.gov/books/NBK557549/. Accessed 25 Sept 2022.
33. Domeshek LF, Hunter DA, Santosa K, Couch SM, Ali A, Borschel GH, Zuker RM, Snyder-Warwick AK. Anatomic characteristics of supraorbital and supratrochlear nerves relevant to their use in corneal neurotization. Eye (Lond). 2019;33(3):398–403.
34. Kikuta S, Yalcin B, Iwanaga J, Watanabe K, Kusukawa J, Tubbs RS. The supraorbital and supratrochlear nerves for ipsilateral corneal neurotization: anatomical study. Anat Cell Biol. 2020;53(1):2–7.
35. Knize DM. A study of the supraorbital nerve. Plast Reconstr Surg. 1995;96(3):564–9.
36. Beer GM, Putz R, Mager K, et al. Variations of the frontal exit of the supraorbital nerve: an anatomic study. Plast Reconstr Surg. 1998;102:334–41.
37. Holland NJ, Weiner GM. Recent developments in Bell's palsy. BMJ. 2004;329(7465):553–7.
38. Coulson S, Croxson GR, Adams R, Oey V. Prognostic factors in herpes zoster oticus (Ramsay Hunt syndrome). Otol Neurotol. 2011;32(6):1025–30.
39. Czyz CN, Burns JA, Petrie TP, Watkins JR, Cahill KV, Foster JA. Long-term botulinum toxin treatment of benign essential blepharospasm, hemifacial spasm, and Meige syndrome. Am J Ophthalmol. 2013;156(1):173–7.
40. Lam VB, Czyz CN, Wulc AE. The brow-eyelid continuum: an anatomic perspective. Clin Plast Surg. 2013;40(1):1–19.
41. Brennan HG, Rafaty FM. Midforehead incisions in treatment of the aging face. Arch Otolaryngol. 1982;108(11):732–4.
42. Johnson CM Jr, Waldman SR. Midforehead lift. Arch Otolaryngol. 1983;109(3):155–9.
43. Shorr N, Seiff SR. Cosmetic blepharoplasty: an illustrated surgical guide. Thorofare: Slack Inc.; 1986.
44. Powell B, Younes A, Friedman O. Evaluation of the midforehead brow-lift operation. Arch Facial Plast Surg. 2011;13(5):337–42.
45. Patel BC, Malhotra R. Mid forehead brow lift. [Updated 2022 May 24]. In: StatPearls [Internet]. Treasure Island (FL): StatPearls Publishing. 2022. Available from: https://www.ncbi.nlm.nih.gov/books/NBK535452. Accessed 25 Sept 2022.
46. Cook TA, Brownrigg PJ, Wang TD, Quatela VC. The versatile midforehead browlift. Arch Otolaryngol Head Neck Surg. 1989;115(2):163–8.
47. Karimi N, Kashkouli MB, Sianati H, Khademi B. Techniques of eyebrow lifting: a narrative review. J Ophthalmic Vis Res. 2020;15(2):218–35.
48. McGuire CS, Gladstone HB. Novel pretrichial browlift technique and review of methods and complications. Dermatol Surg. 2009;35(9):1390–405.
49. Dunn BS, Humphrey CD, Kriet JD. Functional browlifting. Facial Plast Surg. 2022. https://doi.org/10.1055/a-1883-0483.
50. Spiegel JH. Scalp advancement and the pretrichial brow lift. Facial Plast Surg. 2018;34(2):145–9.
51. Dunn T, Hohman MH. Pretrichial brow lift. [Updated 2022 May 15]. In: StatPearls [Internet]. Treasure Island (FL): StatPearls Publishing; 2022. Available from: https://www.ncbi.nlm.nih.gov/books/NBK570632/. Accessed 25 Sept 2022.
52. Niamtu J 3rd. The subcutaneous brow- and forehead-lift: a face-lift for the forehead and brow. Dermatol Surg. 2008;34(10):1350–61.
53. Tower RN, Dailey RA. Endoscopic pretrichial brow lift: surgical indications, technique and outcomes. Ophth Plast Reconstr Surg. 2004;20(4):268–73.
54. Pollock H, Pollock TA. Subcutaneous brow lift with precise suture fixation and advancement. Aesthet Surg J. 2007;27(4):388–95.
55. Walrath JD, McCord CD. The open brow lift. Clin Plast Surg. 2013;40(1):117–24.
56. Kerth JD, Toriumi DM. Management of the aging forehead. Arch Otolaryngol Head Neck Surg. 1990;116(10):1137–42.
57. Karabulut AB, Tumerdem B. A comparison between subgaleal and subperiosteal brow lift. Plast Reconstr Surg. 2000;106(7):1652–3.
58. Karabulut AB, Tumerdem B. Forehead lift: a combined approach using subperiosteal and subgaleal dissection planes. Aesth Plast Surg. 2001;25(5):378–81.
59. Dayan SH, Perkins SW, Vartanian AJ, Wiesman IM. The forehead lift: endoscopic versus coronal approaches. Aesth Plast Surg. 2001;25:35–9.
60. Flowers RS. The open approach to forehead and brow lifting. Aesth Surg J. 1998;18(6):463–4.
61. Flowers RS, Ceydeli A. The open coronal approach to forehead rejuvenation. Clin Plastic Surg. 2008;35(3):331–51.
62. Lighthall JG, Wang TD. Complications of forehead lift. Facial Plast Surg Clin North Am. 2013;21(4):619–24.
63. Knize DM. Reassessment of the coronal incision and sub-galeal dissection for forehead plasty. Plast Reconstr Surg. 1998;102(2):478–89.

64. Hohman MH, Bhama PK, Hadlock TA. Epidemiology of iatrogenic facial nerve injury: a decade of experience. Laryngoscope. 2014;124(1):260–5.
65. Shah VV, Aldahan AS, Mlacker S, Alsaidan M, Samarkandy S, Nouri K. 5-fluorouracil in the treatment of keloids and hypertrophic scars: a comprehensive review of the literature. Drematol Ther (Heidelb). 2016;6(2):169–83.
66. Khan MA, Bashir MM, Khan FA. Intralesional triamcinolone alone and in combination with 5-fluorouracil for the treatment of keloid and hypertrophic scars. J Pak Med Assoc. 2014;64(9):1003–7.
67. Cho MJ, Carboy JA, Rohrich RJ. Complications in brow lifts: a systematic review of surgical and nonsurgical brow rejuvenations. Plast Reconstr Surg Glob Open. 2018;6(10): e1943.

Midface-Lift Surgery

30

Roberto M. Limongi and Marisa Novaes de Figueiredo Rassi

Abstract

The lower eyelid and cheeks comprise the midface that is a source of many signs of aging or otherwise unsatisfactory aesthetic facial appearance. A midface lift addresses many variables including loose skin, orbital fat herniation, and prominent inferior rim grooves. A midface lift can be useful in reconstructive contexts as well, especially in cases where lower eyelid support is needed. In this chapter, the authors describe an external midface lift surgery approach.

Keywords

Midface lift · Cheek lift · Lower blepharoplasty · Under eye bags · Dermatochalasis · Tear trough deformity · Under eye hollows

Supplementary Information The online version contains supplementary material available at https://doi.org/10.1007/978-3-031-63178-8_30.

R. M. Limongi (✉) · M. N. de Figueiredo Rassi
Division of Oculoplastic Surgery,
Department of Ophthalmology,
Federal University of Goiás, Goiás, Brazil
e-mail: rmurillousp@hotmail.com

Introduction

The middle third of the face is important in eyelid function and has several aesthetic roles. Surrounded by the lower eyelids and lateral corners superiorly, the malar projection laterally, and the upper lip inferiorly, the middle third is the largest segment by surface area and one of the most relevant to facial expression and aging changes. The maxillary and zygomatic bones are underneath and support the soft tissues of the midface. From an ophthalmological perspective, the lower eyelids are instrumental in distributing eye tears, as well as protecting the cornea and eye in general.

The lower eyelids and cheeks are major contributors to facial aesthetics. In the young face, the soft tissues of the middle third appear smooth and without demarcation. As the face ages, the anatomical separations and underlying structures become more defined. Ligaments become more apparent, the skin becomes more flaccid, fascial planes weaken, malar fat atrophies, and eyelid bags protrude. The eyelid-cheek junction becomes increasingly evident, also defined as the inferolateral palpebromalar sulcus and the medial nasojugal sulcus. Since the middle third is contiguous with the lower eyelid, knowledge of the middle anatomy is instrumental for the oculoplastic surgeon. Advanced age along with familial tendency cause laxity of the eyelid skin, sagging of the

J. Tao (ed.), *Efficient Oculofacial Surgery*, https://doi.org/10.1007/978-3-031-63178-8_30

ligaments and muscles of the lower eyelid and the middle third of the face resulting in sagging eyelids and drooping cheeks. This condition produces skin folds, fat pockets and wrinkles, characteristic signs of facial aging. Importantly, laxity of the tissues around the eye can cause changes in eyelid position or tear distribution function.

Midface lifting can be performed using a muscle flap (Fig. 30.1) or direct suturing of SOOF fat (sub orbicularis oculi fat). The external approach is described in this chapter.

In the muscle flap technique, an external incision is made below the eyelashes on the lower eyelid and extends through a crease at the outer corner of the eye. Through this wound, pockets of fat can be removed or transferred to depressions such as the tear trough. The flaccid orbicularis muscle is tightened laterally, smoothing the creases and folds in the eyelid and the entire middle third of the face. A small amount of redundant skin is resected laterally.

External midface lifts may be more invasive than transconjunctival blepharoplasty, but they offer several benefits. First, they are associated with excellent and durable aesthetic results due to treatment of excess skin as well as underlying fat and release of the orbital retaining ligament (Fig. 30.2). Second, they may prevent eyelid retraction complications since the midface flap provides robust support to the lower eyelid. Especially with minimal resection of skin and orbicularis in the subciliary zone, eyelid malposition is a rare complication. Midface lifts, owing to the support they provide the lower eyelid, are often used in reconstructive contexts as well. In particular, they may be used as part of post blepharoplasty eyelid retraction repair.

Surgical Technique (Video 1)

With the patient under local anesthesia, with or without sedation, a subciliary incision is formed from the position that coincides with the middle of the pupil and extends to 5–10 mm beyond the lateral commissure. The skin is dissected from the underlying orbicularis muscle. The lateral orbicularis muscle is incised and dissected from the septum. A supraperiosteal dissection

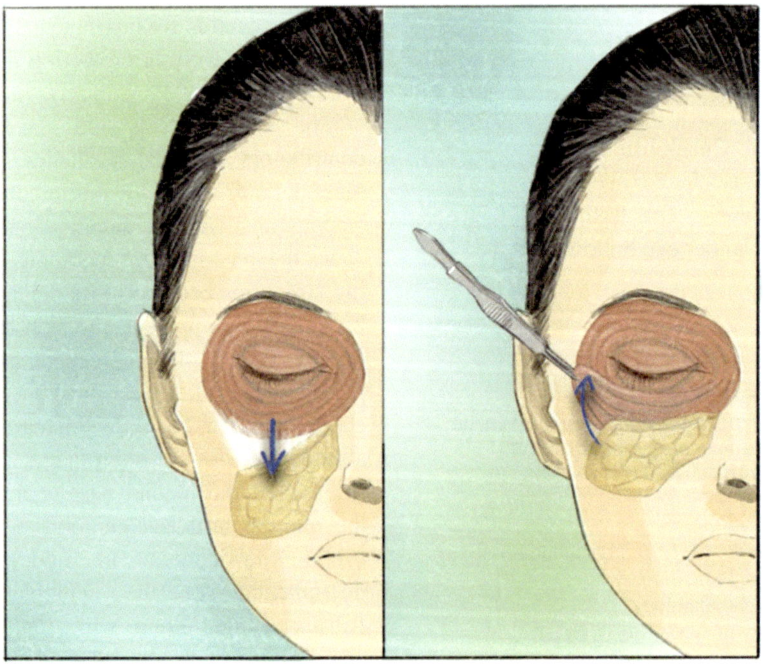

Fig. 30.1 Left—midface drooping, Right—orbicularis/SMAS muscle flap elevating the midface

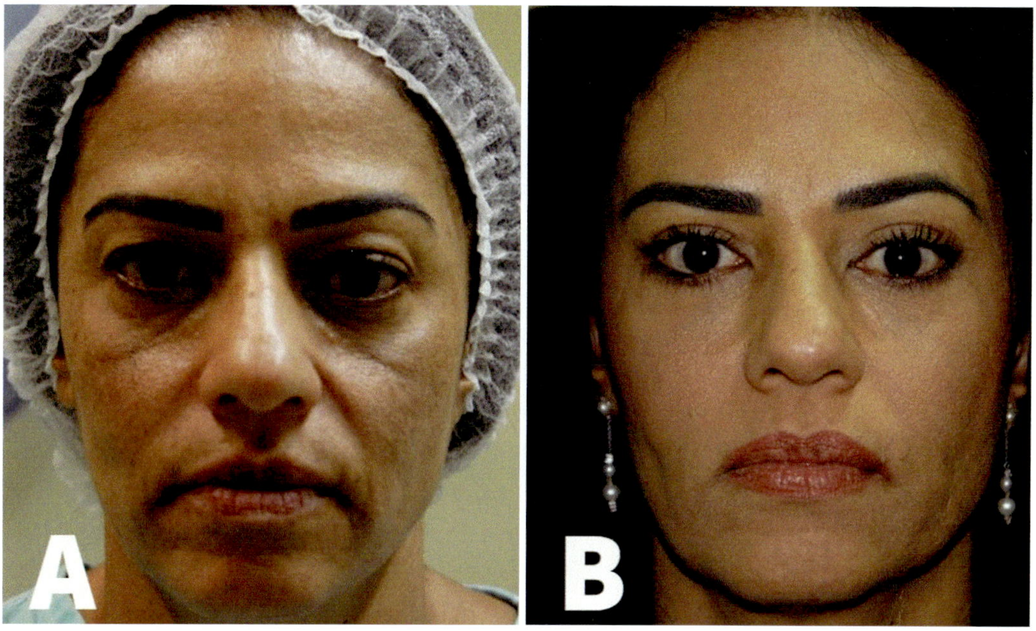

Fig. 30.2 Pre (**A**) and post (**B**) photos of external midface lift

of the inferior orbital rim is performed in the inferior direction of the face. The orbitomalar ligament is detached, and the preseptal and supraperiosteal planes are connected, allowing good mobilization of the midface. Orbital fat herniation (if any) is excised or repositioned into the subperiosteal spaces. A canthopexy or canthoplasty is performed. The latter if significant horizontal laxity is perceived by the lid distraction test. The orbicularis flap is advanced in a superolateral direction, resected slightly, and sutured to the temporal fascia or the periosteum of the lateral border with a 4-0 polypropylene suture. Excess skin laterally is resected conservatively and closed with a 6-0 polypropylene suture (Video 1; Fig. 30.3) Minimal subciliary skin and muscle is resected.

Surgical Complications

Bleeding or bruising is usually minor, self-limiting, and can be managed conservatively. Major postoperative hemorrhages requiring wound exploration are rare. To avoid excessive intraoperative and postoperative bleeding, patients are advised to discontinue preoperative anticoagulant, antiplatelet and nonsteroidal anti-inflammatory drugs and resume them at least 48 h after surgery. Intraoperatively, care is taken to avoid injury to larger blood vessels and cauterize conservatively.

Granuloma, irregularity, and scar formation can occur, especially laterally. Reasons include suture reaction and routine healing, but myocutaneous flap anchorage contributes to this. Redundant muscle flap resection and a continuous suture can minimize contour problems. In some cases of irregularity persisting after many months, an elliptical excision is performed. Entropion or ectropion can occur especially in the lateral lower eyelid. Mechanical entropion can occur if the skin muscle flap overlaps the lateral margin.

As with other lower eyelid blepharoplasty techniques, lower eyelid retraction is a complication. However, the authors believe that retraction is less common due to eyelid and cheek mobilization that resists displacement of the lower eyelids. Other maneuvers that prevent eyelid retraction are conservative skin resection and robust suturing of the skin-muscle flap to

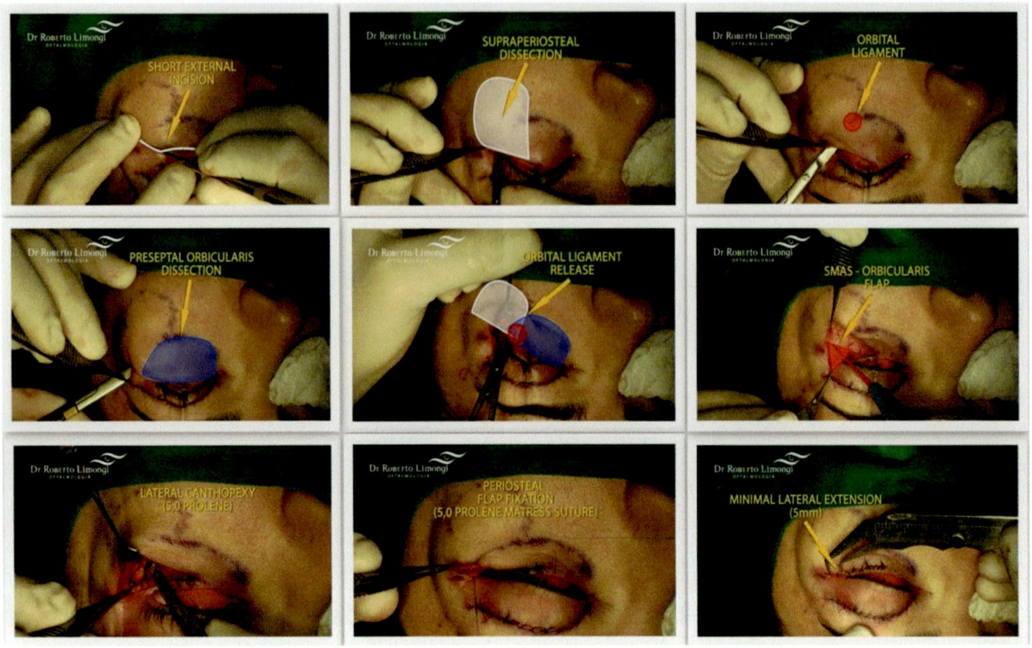

Fig. 30.3 Surgical steps of the external midface lift

the temporal fascia and periosteum of the lateral border. In some patients with pre-existing lower eyelid retraction, a posterior lamella spacer may be indicated concomitant to midface lifting.

Conclusion

Aging in the midface region includes contour irregularities, elevation zones, and areas of depression. The main changes are orbital fat prolapse, soft tissue descent, and deflation, with exposure of the anatomy of the underlying ligaments. These changes can be successfully treated with rejuvenation surgery using good technique and good knowledge of mid-third anatomy. The use of a muscle flap to elevate the middle third of the face can treat these variables and produce good aesthetic results. External midface lifts promote three-dimensional rearrangement of the middle third that fills the tear trough and other depressions while elevating the cheek and eyelid. (Figs. 30.4 and 30.5) Other benefits include increased convexity of the lateral malar area and softening of the nasolabial folds in many cases. Lastly, midface lifts support the lower eyelid and may be useful in both preventing or treating lower eyelid retraction.

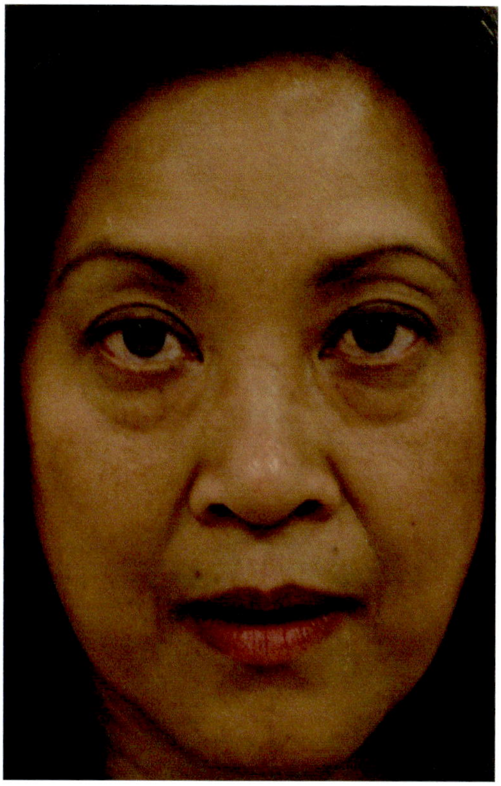

Fig. 30.4 Patient with under eye dark circles with mild fat herniation, and skin redundancy

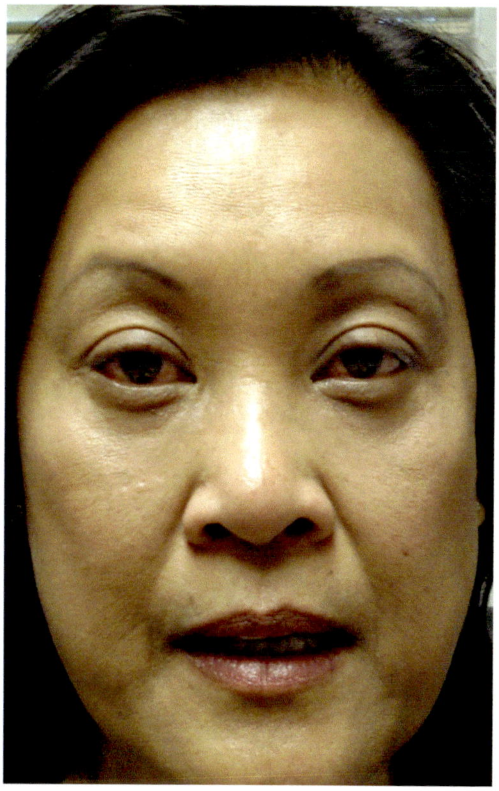

Fig. 30.5 Patient in Fig. 30.4 four weeks after midface lift with excellent correction of lower eyelid and cheek contour. Photo credit: Jeremiah Tao

References

1. Limongi RM. Estética Periocular, vol. 1. In: Livro tema do Congresso Internacional de Oculoplástica em Goiânia. 1st ed. Rio de Janeiro: Cultura Médica; 2018. p. 360.
2. Tao JP, Limongi RM. Short-incision midface-lift in lower blepharoplasty. JAMA Facial Plast Surg. 2016,18(4):313–4. https://doi.org/10.1001/jamafacial.2016.0148. PMID: 27077484.
3. Akaishi P, Limongi RM, Pereira F, Pieroni A. Blefaroplastia. Manual de Condutas Blefaroplastia, vol. 1. 1st ed. Goiânia: Conexão Propaganda e Editora; 2019. p. 108.
4. Strasser EJ. An objective grading system for the evaluation of cosmetic surgical results. Plast Reconstr Surg. 1999;104(7):2282–5.
5. Hester TR Jr, Codner MA, McCord CD, Nahai F, Giannopoulos A. Evolution of technique of the direct transblepharoplasty approach for the correction of lower lid and midfacial aging: maximizing results and minimizing complications in a 5-year experience. Plast Reconstr Surg. 2000;105(1):393–406.
6. Hobar PC, Flood J. Subperiosteal rejuvenation of the midface and periorbital area: a simplified approach. Plast Reconstr Surg. 1999;104(3):842–51.
7. Mendelson BC, Muzaffar AR, Adams WP Jr. Surgical anatomy of the midcheek and malar mounds. Plast Reconstr Surg. 2002;110(3):885–96.
8. Hirabayashi KE, Tao JP. Midface-lift with lateral orbicularis oculi flap excision or imbrication. Dermatol Surg. 2014;40(7):743–7.
9. Viana GAP. Upper and lower lid blepharoplasty. In: Hathiram BT, Khattar VS, Org. Atlas of operative otorhinolaryngology and head and neck surgery, 1st ed, vol 1. New Delhi: Jaypee Brothers Medical Publishers; 2013. pp. 853–66
10. Viana GAP, Magacho B, Cariello A. Anatomia do terço médio da face. In: Limongi R, Matayoshi,

Akaishi P, Pimentel AR, Org. Estética Periocular. 1st ed. Rio de Janeiro: Cultura Médica; 2018, pp. 37–43.
11. Viana GAP. Elevação do terço médio por via transcutânea. In: Osaki TH, Osaki MH, Kikkawa DO, Org. Rejuvenescimento Palpebral e Periorbital. 1st ed. Rio de Janeiro: Elsevier; 2019, pp. 333–40.
12. Freeman MS. Rejuvenation of the midface. Facial Plast Surg. 2018;34:505–23.
13. Mittelman H, Kundaria S, Lam HP. Facelift techniques that restore facial volume. Facial Plast Surg. 2016;32:560–4.
14. Stein R, Holds JB, Wulc AE, Swift A, Hartstein M. Phi, fat and the mathematics of a beautiful midface. Ophtal Plast Reconstr Surg. 2018;34:491–6.
15. Whipple KM, Oh SR, Kikkawa DO, Korn BS. Anatomy of the midface. In: Hartstein M, Wulc A, Holck D, editors. Midfacial rejuvenation. New York, NY: Springer; 2012.
16. Levesque AY, de la Torre JI. Midface anatomy, aging, and aesthetic analysis. Facial Plast Surg Clin North Am. 2015;23(2):129–36.
17. Hwang K, Kim DH, Huan F, Nam YS, Han SH. The anatomy of the palpebral branch of the infraorbital artery relating to midface lift. J Craniofac Surg. 2011;22(4):1489–90.
18. Rea P. Head. In: Essential clinically applied anatomy of the peripheral nervous system in the head and neck. 1st ed. Academic Press; 2016. pp. 21–130.
19. Liu L, Wang H, Wang ZJ. A new approach to lower eyelid-cheek junction rejuvenation. J Cosmet Dermatol. 2019;18(1):45–50.

Deep Plane Facelift and Neck Lift

31

D. J. John Park

Abstract

Facial aging in the lower face is most notable for sagging jowls and laxity at the neck from loss of elasticity in the skin and underlying aponeurotic layer. Facelift and neck lift surgery addresses these changes, restores a more youthful contour and helps rejuvenate the appearance of the face and neck. There is a multitude of variant facelift and neck lift procedures described as well as options for incision planning; and while a thorough discussion of each is beyond the scope of this chapter, a brief overview will be provided to allow an organizational framework on which the reader can expand their knowledge. This chapter details the high superficial musculo-aponeurotoric system (SMAS) pattern deep plane face and neck lift technique.

Keywords

Facelift · Neck lift · Facial aging · SMAS · Deep plane

Supplementary Information The online version contains supplementary material available at https://doi.org/10.1007/978-3-031-63178-8_31.

D. J. John Park (✉)
Plastic Surgery, Newport Beach, CA, USA
e-mail: Johnparkmd@gmail.com

Introduction

With advancing age, tissue elasticity diminishes and loses its ability to maintain elastic tone. This manifests with jowls and marionette lines in the lower face and with plastysmal bands and laxity in the neck. For the subsequent 60 years since the first facelift in 1916 [1], this procedure involved elevation and advancement of subcutaneous flaps, excision of the redundant skin and inset of the flap to tighten the skin without any underlying work on the apoeneurotic layer. The results were not long-lasting and patients often had an overly-done, unnatural appearance. In 1968, Skoog developed a technique to elevate the platysma with the subcutaneous flap as a composite flap, which he published in 1974 [2]. In 1976, Mitz and Peyronie [3] described the superficial musculo-aponeurotoric system (SMAS) , a tissue layer of dense connective tissue and fat just deep to the subcutaneous fat in which the mimetic facial muscles are invested. The expansion of knowledge of the SMAS and its changes with age led to rapid advances in facelifting and the description of many surgical maneuvers to advance the SMAS in a vertical vector.

Understanding the various facelift and neck lift techniques is difficult because of the numerous ways in which this procedure can be done. This is made all the more difficult due to some surgeons making minor changes to a

J. Tao (ed.), *Efficient Oculofacial Surgery*, https://doi.org/10.1007/978-3-031-63178-8_31

well described approach, claiming it as their own procedure, and assigning a unique name for "their" procedure for the sake of marketing and self-promotion. With closer examination, it becomes clear that many similarities exist between these techniques. Therefore, it is most important to understand the principles and concepts as a foundation of knowledge.

In order of technical difficulty, the most common SMAS advancement techniques are as follows: SMAS plication, SMASectomy, low SMAS deep plane facelift, and high SMAS deep plane facelift. What all of these methods share in common is that this aponeurotic layer is advanced superiorly and slightly posteriorly in vector. In SMAS plication, a series of sutures are placed parallel to the nasolabial fold in a manner that imbricates the SMAS and elevates it superoposteriorly. The seam is placed approximately 2 cm posterior to the nasolabial fold in the area where the SMAS is more mobile and less adherent to the sub-SMAS structures. SMASectomy involves excision of the strip of SMAS tissue that would be imbricated in SMAS plication. The primary advantage of this technique is that it is easier to get a smooth suture seam line compared to plication. However, the risk of underlying nerve injury is higher as the sub-SMAS space is exposed. A variant of the SMASectomy procedure involves fashioning an inferolaterally based SMAS flap (instead of excision) and transposing it posteriorly to be secured to the mastoid fascia in order to accentuate the jawline. In a deep plane facelift, the SMAS is elevated as a separate second flap to advance in the desired vector. More extensive dissection in the sub-SMAS plane increases the risk of facial motor nerve injury. In a low SMAS deep plane technique, the incision to lift the SMAS is below the zygomatic arch near the anterior limit of the parotid gland parallel to the nasolabial fold. In a high SMAS deep plane technique, the incision for the SMAS flap is in line with the zygomatic arch and makes a right angle turn just anterior to the tragus and continues inferiorly into the neck. The principal advantage of this high SMAS method is that it is effective in lifting the lateral midface and recruiting lower eyelid skin much like a trans-palpebral approach to mid-facelifts. In addition, the seam line for the SMAS flap is away from the center of the cheek and overlying contour irregularities are much less likely in those with thin skin. However, there is a risk to the frontal branch of the facial nerve, one that is avoided in all the other techniques described above (Fig. 31.1A, B).

Having climbed the surgical learning curve performing each of the above methods, I describe here my preferred approach to face and neck lifting: the high SMAS deep plane facelift.

Surgical Technique

Patients should be of sufficient vitality to undergo surgery, off any anti-coagulant or anti-platelet agents, and with well controlled blood pressure if hypertensive. While some surgeons prefer deep sedation to general anesthesia, I feel that the risk of hypoxic episodes or undersedation are too high with deep sedation. Laryngeal mask airway is contraindicated as the bulk of the laryngeal balloon obscures the natural neck contours (Fig. 31.2).

The endotracheal tube is tied to a 2–0 silk suture which is looped around the central incisor and gauze packed in the mouth to absorb any secretions that may contaminate the field (Fig. 31.3). The whole face and head are prepped in Betadine wash. An under buttock obstetric drain drape is placed under the head to collect irrigation and wash at end of case. The submentum is injected with diluted local anesthetic (0.125% Lidocaine with 1:800,000 epinephrine and 1 mg/cc tranexamic acid). The midline is marked at the mentum and a 3 cm transverse incision made just posterior to the submental crease so as not to create a ptotic (witch's) chin deformity with scar contracture. Subcutaneous flaps are elevated, taking care to leave a cobblestone layer of fat on the flap side while leaving the underlying platysma undisturbed (Fig. 31.4). Liposuction can be done prior

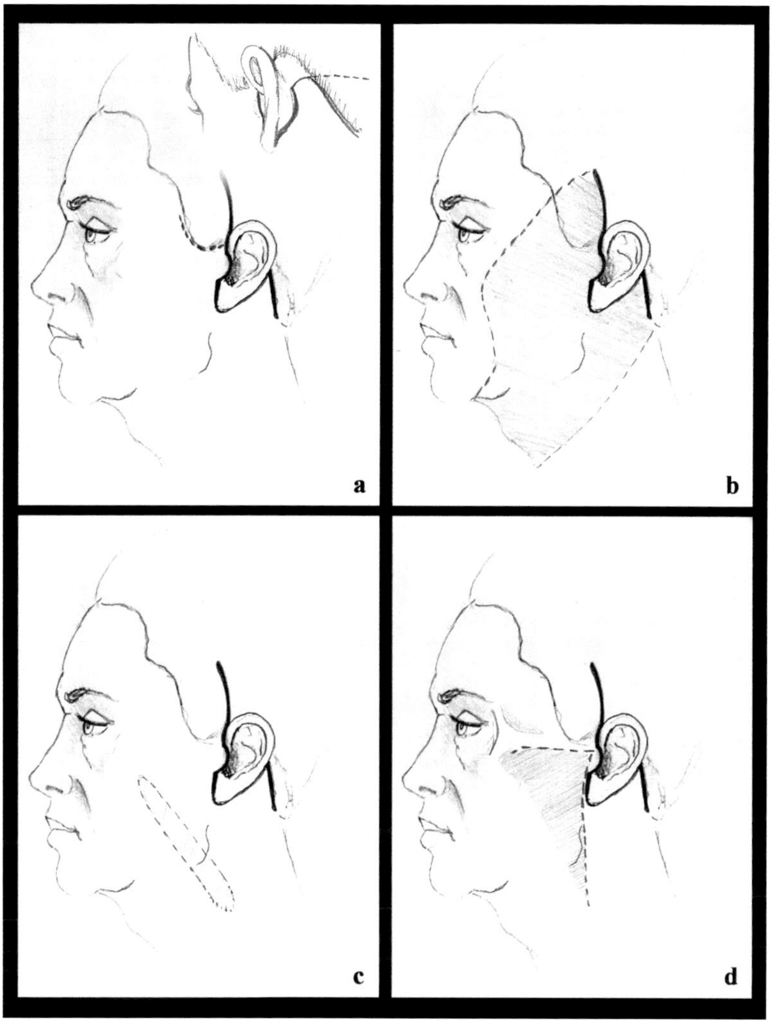

Fig. 31.1 A, B Markings for facelift and neck lift. Markings should be applied with anterior tension on the skin, so scar settles in the desired location. For men, an alternative is to mark the incision along the pre-tragal crease to avoid advancing hair bearing skin to the tragus. For women with a sideburn that terminates higher up, consider making the incision anterior to the sideburn along the hairline to avoid further elevating the sideburn with skin flap advancement. Posterior marking. Classically, the apical point of the posterior flap should be marked at the level of the bifurcation of the antihelix. While this works well for incisions that continue into the occipital scalp, when the incision follows along the posterior hairline, the flap end becomes too narrow and risks flap necrosis

to and/or after flap elevation under direct visualization with a spatulated single port cannula. The platysma is elevated from its medial edge extending laterally and a 3–4 cm back cut made at the level of the hyoid cartilage. The medial edges are brought to the midline and coapted with 3–0 PDS sutures. Tranexamic acid-soaked gauze is packed in the pocket after hemostasis.

The diluted local anesthetic is injected on the first side of the face in the planned area of skin undermining. The incision which was marked pre-operatively is made, starting from the temporal scalp (approximately 3 cm from the helical root). This continues along the anterior border of the ear, around the ear lobule, along the post-auricular sulcus and along the posterior

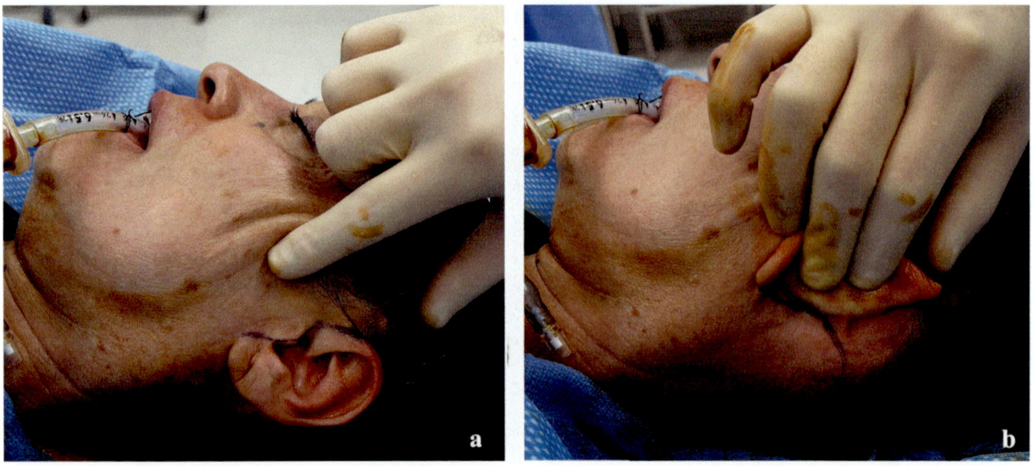

Fig. 31.2 The endotracheal tube is secured to the central incisor with a 2-0 silk suture as shown. An air knot is tied prior to wrapping the suture around tube for better security. The throat is packed with gauze to prevent secretions from contaminating the sterile field

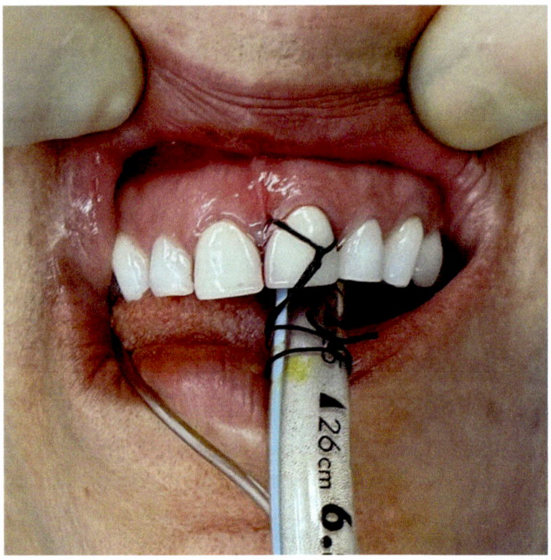

Fig. 31.3 **A** Corset platysmaplasty via submental incision. The incision is marked 5 mm from the submental crease and the flap is elevated anteriorly slightly to ablate the natural submental crease. Notice the medial edge of the right platysma. **B** The medial edges of the two platysmal muscles are advanced medially and coapted together with 3-0 PDS sutures creating a muscular hammock in support of the floor of the mouth. Back cuts need to be made laterally at the level between the hyoid cartilage to allow medialization of the muscle flaps

hairline. In individuals with high sideburns, the incision should follow along the anterior border of the hairline here so as not to further elevate the side burn point. The incision should be post-tragal or more precisely along the tragal ridge. Classically, the incision is pre-tragal for men in order to prevent advancement of hair bearing skin onto the ear. However, I prefer post-tragal incisions for all patients. The follicles can be excised or fulgurated secondarily under local anesthesia. Posteriorly, the incision can follow along the posterior hairline or into the scalp. While the incision is well hidden when extended into the scalp, with more extensive neck laxity, this may result in a step along the posterior hair line with a large area of skin where one would expect hair.

The subcutaneous flap is elevated, taking care to leave a cobblestone layer of fat on the flap side while leaving the underlying SMAS undisturbed. The flap is elevated just past the zygomatic retaining ligament (McGregor's patch) at the malar area, made contiguous with the submental dissection, and past the mental retaining ligament just anterior to the marionette line and jowl (Fig. 31.5). Extreme care should be exercised at the mental ligament as the mandibular branch of the facial nerve is fairly superficial here. Following hemostasis, the flap is tailor tacked with staples and the subcutaneous flap elevated on the contralateral side as described above.

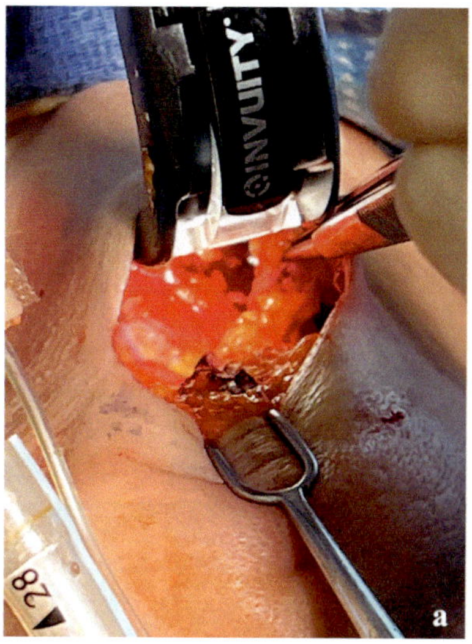

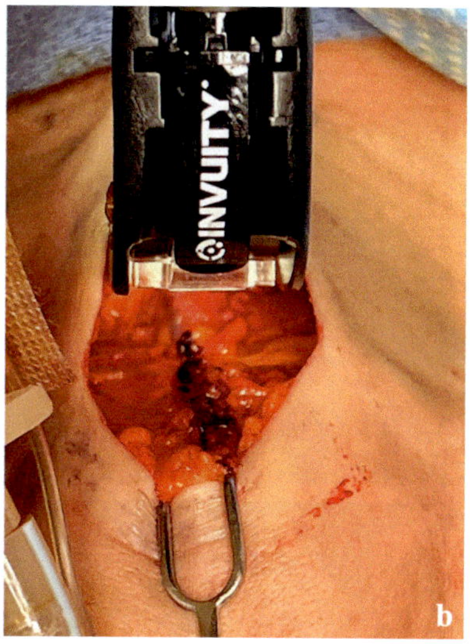

Fig. 31.4 **A** Cutaneous ligaments of the face bind the skin and prevent movement. Dissection should extend past the zygomatic ligament (McGregor's patch), mental ligament, and made contiguous with the submental dissection and approximately two finger breadths from the modiolus. When the zygomatic ligament is not adequately released, dimpling occurs in the lateral submalar area as shown. **B** Skin flap elevation should be carried out with care to allow a uniform thickness and preserving a thin layer of subcutaneous fat while leaving the underlying SMAS undisturbed. **C** Upward traction when making the SMAS incision overlying the zygomatic arch is crucial to prevent facial nerve frontal branch injury. **D** The SMAS flap is elevated to where it is readily mobile. Like the skin flap, the SMAS flap should be released from the zygomatic ligament to get full mobility including the midface. **E** With superior and some posterior tension, a dart incision is made to inset the SMAS flap at the right-angle point. A triangle of SMAS is excised upon superior SMAS advancement. Observe the jowls and midface for effect. **F** Instead of excising a strip of SMAS along the vertical seam and in setting with posterosuperior advancement, an inferiorly based SMAS flap can be fashioned and transposed posteriorly under the jawline and secured to the mastoid fascia to accentuate the jawline

Back on the first side, the high SMAS flap is marked along the zygomatic arch as a transverse line curling slightly downward near its anterior limit at the malar eminence to prevent a Burrow's triangle. The mark continues along the pre-auricular border and down into the neck approximately 4–5 cm below the mandibular angle. The transverse SMAS incision is made with cutting cautery with upward traction on either side of the incision to prevent underlying frontal motor branch injury. The SMAS flap is elevated with cutting cautery and facelift scissors (Fig. 31.5). Care should be taken to ensure that the underlying parotid masseteric fascia is undisturbed, as the facial nerve branches run under this layer (Fig. 31.6). The deep plane dissection is extended until the jowls and neck are freely mobile with manipulation of the flap. The SMAS flap is then advanced superiorly and slightly posteriorly for inset. A dart incision is made to inset the flap at the right-angle point with a buried figure of-eight 3–0 PDS. The redundant SMAS is excised, and the remainder is closed with interrupted 3–0 PDS and a second running layer with 4–0 PDS.

Once repeated for the contralateral side, 10F fluted drains are externalized posteriorly, inset along the submentum, and secured to the scalp with a single surgical staple. The skin is then advanced superiorly and posteriorly. Observe for the desired effect and any unintended irregularities that may need attention. Once set, sequentially cut dart incisions and secure with 4–0 Prolene for the key points of the inset at the ear lobule, root of the helix, superior and inferior limit of the tragus, and at the apical portion of the posterior flap. Optionally, the surgeon can apply aerosolized fibrin (Artiss) prior to inset to

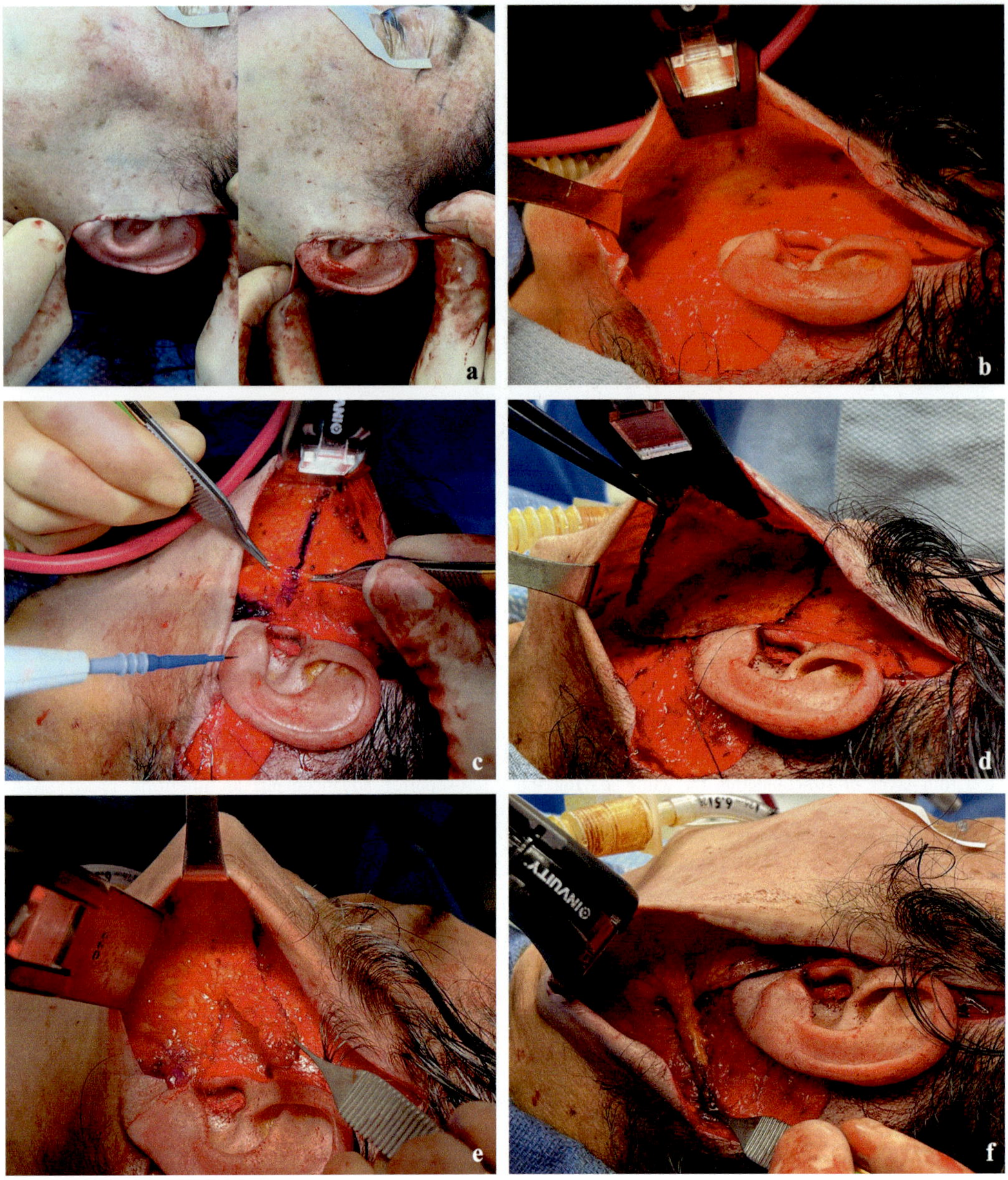

Fig. 31.5 Surgical pearls. **A** Cutaneous retaining ligaments of the face. Anterior platysma ligament (Furnas ligament) is a band of firm adhesion just in front of the ear. Use sharp dissection at this area. Release of the zygomatic retaining ligament (McGregor's patch) is a key maneuver without which, effective facelifting cannot be done. The mental ligament need not be released if platysmaplasty is not done. However, redraping of the skin in this area is needed with platysmaplasty. **B** The great auricular nerve is the most commonly injured nerve with this surgery. The nerve lies on the anterior face of the mid-belly of the sternocleidomastoid muscle, approximately 6–7 cm from the external auditory canal and near the external jugular vein. **C** The facial nerve branches reside deep within the parotid gland, providing a surgical buffer to nerve injury here. The branches continue anteriorly under the parotid-massoteric fascia, a thin semi-translucent layer under which the nerve branches can be seen. Unlike the single frontal and mandibular branches, the midface branches have significant arborization and redundancy, such that nerve injury here often recovers, although dyskinesia may result

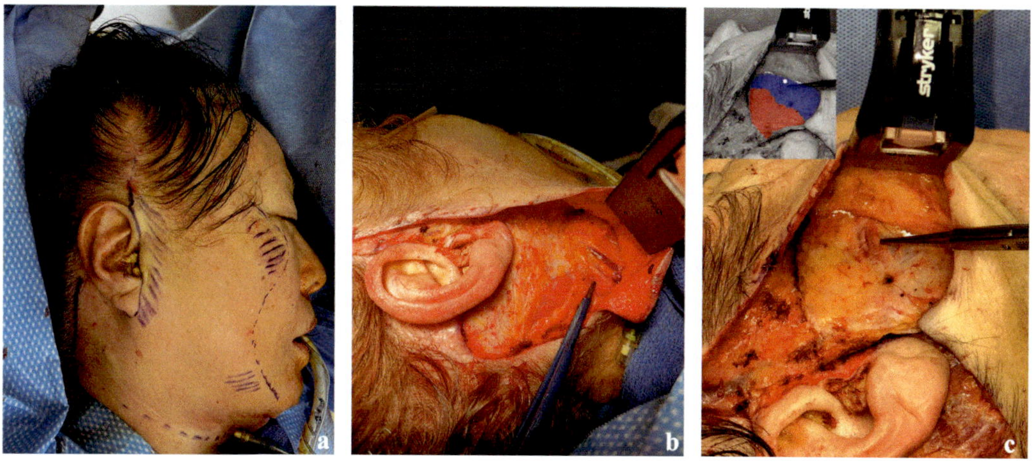

Fig. 31.6 Intraoperative facelift demonstrating a deep plane dissection

facilitate flap adhesion and reduce bleeding risk. The redundant skin is then excised and closed as follows. Anteriorly, 5–0 Monocryl is used as dermal sutures, and the skin is closed with 5–0 Prolene as a simple running closure or with interrupted horizontal mattress sutures if the surgeon prefers and time allows. The scalp here is closed with surgical staples. Posteriorly, the dermis is closed with 4–0 PDS sutures and the skin closed in likewise fashion with 5–0 Prolene except at the post auricular sulcus where 5–0 gut is used. The submentum is closed with 5–0 Monocryl and 5–0 Prolene in two layers.

The face and hair are washed and Xeroform, ABD pad, Kerlex roll, and stretch net knitted (size 6) dressing are applied.

Potential Complications

Complications include bleeding, submental fluid collections or hematomas, great auricular sensory nerve injury, facial motor nerve injury, and flap devitalization and compromise. Bleeding is more likely in individuals with uncontrolled hypertension, haphazard or incomplete cautery hemostasis, and unrecognized relative hypotension under anesthesia. While it may be difficult, hemostasis should be achieved while the blood pressure is as close to pre-operative levels. Secondary submental edema or collections can be avoided with careful hemostasis, elastic compressive band use, and digital massage by the patient. Great auricular nerve injury is the most common nerve injury and presents with numbness at the ear lobe. The nerve runs superiorly along the anterior surface of the sternocleidomastoid muscle and is most at risk during skin flap elevation in this area from approximately 6 cm inferior to the ear lobule extending superiorly. Motor nerve injury was covered above. Arguably the most significant surgical complication may be flap necrosis. As Sir Harold Gillies so aptly stated, “plastic surgery is a constant battle between beauty and blood supply” [4]. Whereas more extensive skin flap elevation, applied tension, or overaggressive monopolar hemostasis on the flap side may yield a more favorable cosmetic improvement, it may compromise the remnant perfusion enough to result in flap devitalization and epithelial necrosis to full thickness flap loss. The surgeon should be vigilant and release sutures and tension early on and/or start hyperbaric oxygen therapy.

Conclusions

Facelift and neck lift are effective surgical options for moderate to severe lower facial and neck aging (Figs. 31.7 and 31.8). While it is important to be familiar with the various

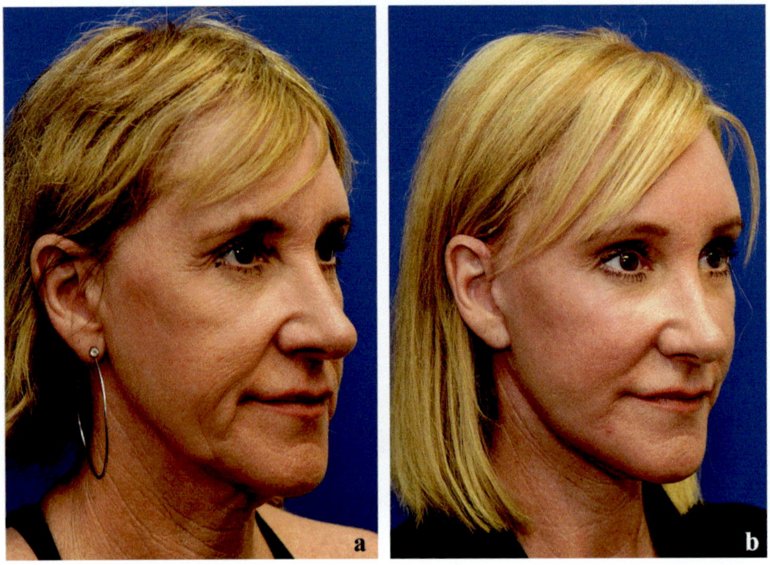

Fig. 31.7 Before and after facelift

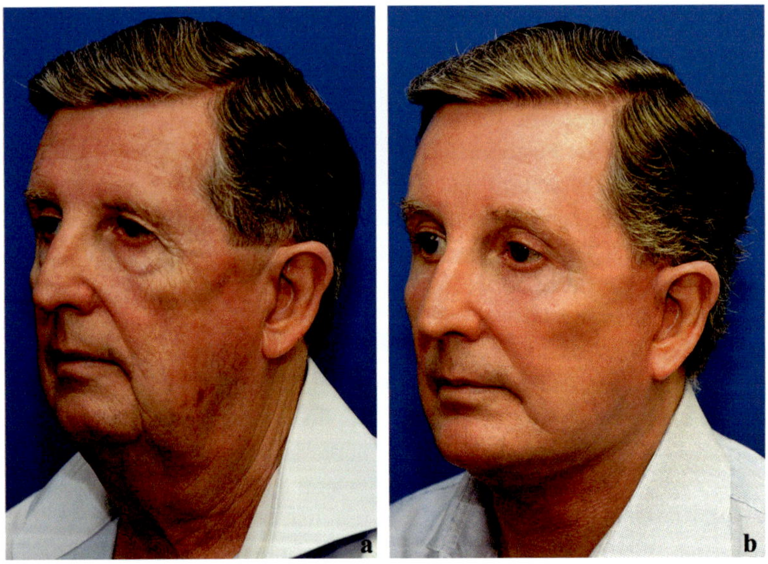

Fig. 31.8 Before and after facelift

techniques including incision options, what matters most is the surgeon utilizing these methods. Put another way, the type of paint or paintbrush used in the painting of a portrait matters far less than the artist who is using those tools. To that end, focus on thoroughly learning the surgical anatomy and the principles of facelift and neck lift procedures, not the types of procedures out there. Climb the learning curve slowly and safely in service to our patients. Start with reconstructive flap elevation in the cheeks and neck to familiarize yourself with the surgical anatomy. Don't swing for the fences and start with a deep plane facelift when plication is much safer, technically easier, and takes less time.

References

1. Locher WG, Feinendegen DL. Aus der Frühzeit der Ästhetischen Chirurgie: Eugen Holländer (1867–1932) und Erich Lexer (1867–1937) als Face-Lift-Pioniere [The early days of aesthetic surgery: facelift pioneers Eugen Holländer (1867–1932) and Erich Lexer (1967–1937)]. Handchir Mikrochir Plast Chir. 2020;52(6):545–51. https://doi.org/10.1055/a-1150-7343.
2. Zimbler MS. Tord skoog: face-lift innovator. Arch Facial Plast Surg. 2001;3(1):63.
3. Mitz V, Peyronie M. The superficial musculo-aponeurotic system (SMAS) in the parotid and cheek area. Plast Reconstr Surg. 1976;58(1):80–8.
4. Gillies H. Direct flaps. In: Gillies H, Millard DR, editors. The Principles and Art of Plastic Surgery. Boston, MA: Little, Brown and Company; 1957. p. 48–54.

Orbitotomy Approaches

32

Lydia Zhong and Robi N. Maamari

Abstract

Due to the dense anatomy of the orbital region, surgical approaches are critical to understand and master. Anatomy, visualization requirements, and sometimes balancing the needs of other disciplines are factors in selecting a particular orbitotomy approach. In this chapter the authors describe several common surgical approaches of the orbit.

Keywords

Orbital surgery · Orbitotomy · Orbital anatomy · Transconjunctival approach · Transcaruncular approach

Introduction

The orbit can be divided into the medial, superior, lateral, and inferior quadrants, as well as the anterior, mid-, and apical orbit in the anteroposterior dimension. Given the density of vital neurovascular structures in and around the orbit including the eye, selection of the surgical approach is a critical decision. The approach to access these orbital spaces is influenced by factors such as patient anatomy, visualization requirements, and balancing the needs of multiple disciplines [1–6]. Common indications for orbital surgery include lesions, trauma, and decompression. This chapter describes the most relevant approaches to the orbit, as well as the indications.

Extraconal Orbital Approaches

The extraconal orbital compartment is the space outside of the musculofascial cone within the orbit. Extraconal approaches to the orbit include transcutaneous approaches, the transconjunctival approach, the transcaruncular approach, and the lateral canthal approach.

A. Transcutaneous Approach

The transcutaneous approach offers a wide range of access to orbital spaces. Three

Supplementary Information The online version contains supplementary material available at https://doi.org/10.1007/978-3-031-63178-8_32.

L. Zhong · R. N. Maamari (✉)
John F. Hardesty, MD, Department of Ophthalmology and Visual Sciences, Washington University School of Medicine, St. Louis, MO, USA
e-mail: maamarir@wustl.edu

J. Tao (ed.), *Efficient Oculofacial Surgery*, https://doi.org/10.1007/978-3-031-63178-8_32

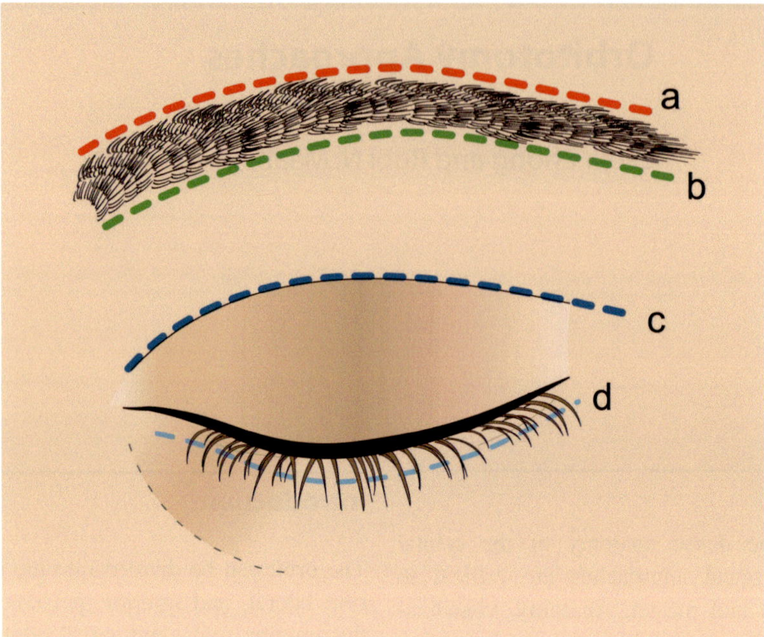

Fig. 32.1 Transcutaneous orbitotomy approaches include (**a**) suprabrow incisions, (**b**) subbrow incisions, (**c**) upper eyelid crease incisions, (**d**) subciliary incisions

transcutaneous approaches that will be discussed are the eyelid crease incision, the subciliary incision, and the supra-brow/sub-brow incision (Fig. 32.1).

1. *Upper Eyelid Crease Incision*

The upper eyelid crease incision provides access to the superior orbital region and can easily be extended laterally within the upper eyelid crease for access to the lateral orbit with a cosmetically desirable result that masks the incision scar. This approach is often used for the removal of supraorbital mass or dermoid cyst, and the orbital lobe of the lacrimal gland can also be readily accessed using this technique. (Fig. 32.2) A lateral orbital decompression can also be performed through this eyelid crease incision.

Surgical Technique

- Preoperatively, the planned upper eyelid incision is marked in the natural eyelid crease which is delineated by asking the patient to open and close their eye.
- A transcutaneous incision is made with a #15 blade and dissection is carried out through the orbicularis muscle to the preseptal level.
- Dissection is carried out in the preseptal plane to the superior and/or lateral orbital rim to the arcus marginalis.
- Using a #15 blade or monopolar cautery, an incision is made at the arcus marginalis to approach the desired orbital region.
- If dissection is to be carried out along the orbital roof, care must be taken to avoid the supraorbital neurovascular bundle containing the supraorbital nerve, artery, and vein. These can be identified preoperatively by palpating and marking the supraorbital notch which contains the neurovascular bundle. Additionally, superomedial dissection must avoid the trochlea of the superior oblique muscle and tendon.
- Next, elevation of the periosteum is performed using an elevator (e.g., Cottle) and dissection is carried out in a subperiosteal

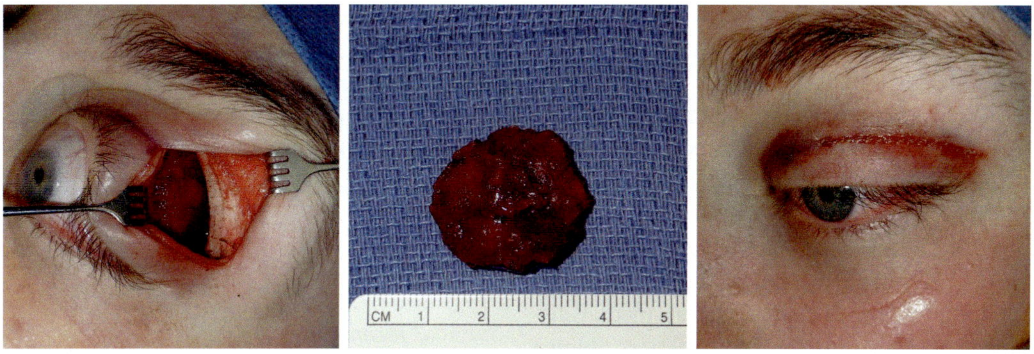

Fig. 32.2 Upper eyelid crease incision. A lateral incision was made to achieve a superolateral orbital approach (left). A Ewing sarcoma lesion was excised (center). The periosteum, orbicularis muscle, and the upper eyelid incision following closure (right)

fashion along the superior and/or lateral orbital wall.

- If dissection is performed along the lateral wall, the zygomaticotemporal and zygomaticofacial neurovascular bundles should be isolated, cauterized, and divided to permit further dissection to the deeper lateral orbital region.
- At the desired orbital depth, the periosteum can be incised and opened to expose the superolateral lacrimal gland or the extraconal region superiorly or laterally. Meticulous dissection must be performed to avoid injury to the levator muscle superiorly and the lateral rectus muscle laterally.
- If surgical intervention involving decompression of the lateral orbital bone is intended, the lateral orbital wall may then be removed superiorly to the level of the superior orbital wall, posteriorly to the level of the dura, and inferiorly to expose the buccal fat. Care must be taken to avoid violation of the dura.
- Once the desired bone decompression, lesion biopsy, or lesion removal is completed, hemostasis must be obtained using bipolar cautery and the periosteum is closed with 5-0 polyglactin suture or left unsutured. While closure of the orbicularis muscle is generally avoided along the medial and central eyelid orbicularis muscle to avoid resulting lagophthalmos, the lateral deep orbicularis muscle can be closed with 5-0 or 6-0 polyglactin suture, and the lateral superficial orbicularis muscle may be closed with 6-0 polyglactin suture. The skin is closed with 6-0 plain gut or polypropylene suture.

2. *Lower Eyelid Subciliary Incision*

The subciliary incision provides access to the preseptal region, infraorbital space, and orbital floor through a well camouflaged incision below the lower eyelid lash line. While this approach conveniently provides direct access to the inferior orbit through an opening in the septum, the transconjunctival approach (described later) has become a more commonly used technique due to the masked conjunctival scar and the reduced risk of postoperative cicatricial ectropion as compared to the subciliary approach.

Surgical Technique

- Preoperatively, a skin marking is made 2 mm inferior to the lower eyelid margin or within an existing lower eyelid skin crease.
- A transcutaneous incision is created using a #15 blade along the subciliary marking.
- The orbicularis oculi muscle is transected to the pretarsal septal level and dissection is carried out inferiorly in a preseptal plane to the inferior orbital rim and arcus marginalis.

- Using a #15 blade or monopolar cautery, an incision is made at the arcus marginalis along the inferior orbital rim.
- Next, elevation of the periosteum is performed using an elevator and dissection is carried out in a subperiosteal fashion along the orbital floor. Care must be taken at the medial infraorbital region as the inferior oblique muscle originates at the maxillary bone in this region. If extensive medial dissection is necessary, the inferior oblique muscle attachment can be released with subperiosteal dissection.
- Care must be taken to avoid injury to the infraorbital neurovascular bundle, which may be identified within the infraorbital canal, separated by a thin layer of bone. In the setting of an orbital fracture repair, care must be taken to identify, decompress, and appropriately separate the infraorbital neurovascular bundle from the intraorbital tissue.
- Following elevation of the periosteum, the periosteum may be incised to access extraconal orbital regions, as needed.
- At closure, the periosteum may be reapproximated with interrupted 5-0 polyglactin suture at the arcus marginalis or may be left unsutured. In general, limited closure of the orbicularis muscle is performed to reduce the risk of postoperative lower eyelid ectropion. The skin is closed with 6-0 plain gut or polypropylene suture.
- To prevent eyelid retraction, a temporary Frost (suspension) suture using 6-0 silk suture is placed through lower eyelid and taped to the forehead and is left in place for several days to further reduce the risk of lower eyelid ectropion.

3. *Suprabrow or Subbrow Incision*

The supra-brow/sub-brow incision provides direct access to the superior orbital rim and orbital roof. This technique is typically utilized to repair extensive fractures of the superior orbital rim and frontal sinus. Additionally, this technique can be utilized in pathology requiring direct visualization, including large bony processes such as an intraosseous orbital rim hemangioma or an orbitofrontal mucocele. This is also a common approach in multi-disciplinary procedures with oculoplastic surgery, ENT, and neurosurgery services for transorbital craniotomy access.

Surgical Technique

- Preoperatively, a suprabrow or subbrow marking is made with attention placed on the supraorbital notch, which demarcates the supraorbital neurovascular bundle.
- A skin incision is made using a #15 blade above or below the brow, following the superior edge of the brow hair (suprabrow) or the contour of the superolateral orbital rim (subbrow).
- Dissection is continued through the orbicularis oculi muscle and the subbrow fat pad to the pre-periosteal plane. Dissection is carried out to the orbital rim.
- The arcus marginalis periosteum is incised and the periosteum can be elevated along the orbital roof and superiorly along the frontal bone or the brow. If the dissection must extend medial to the supraorbital notch, careful dissection can be performed to preserve the supraorbital neurovascular bundle. If the neurovascular bundle travels through a foramen, the foramen can be unroofed using a chisel and mallet, allowing the neurovascular bundle to be removed from the foramen and retracted medially to allow further intraoperative exposure.
- Once adequate exposure is achieved, the orbital rim or orbital roof pathology can be addressed. In cases requiring frontal sinus or anterior cranial access, a bone window can be created at this time.
- Meticulous surgical closure is critical to minimize postoperative scar depression. This is achieved with 4-0 or 5-0 polyglactin sutures to close the orbital rim periosteum. Deep subcutaneous closure is performed with

additional 4-0 or 5-0 polyglactin sutures. Skin closure is performed with 4-0 or 5-0 polypropylene suture in running vertical or horizontal mattress fashion to provide wound eversion and appropriate healing.

B. **Transconjunctival Approach (Video 32.1)**

The transconjunctival approach is often used, particularly to access the inferior orbital spaces with excellent cosmesis. It is the most utilized technique for repair orbital floor fractures or for inferior orbital decompression, also detailed in the respective chapters describing these surgeries.

Once the inferior orbital rim is exposed, posterior dissection is carried out in a similar fashion as described above in the subciliary transcutaneous approach. Either a pre-septal or post-septal approach can be taken, although the pre-septal approach advantageously maintains the septum to prevent orbital fat from protruding and obstructing visualization.

Surgical Technique

- A transconjunctival inferior orbitotomy can be performed without detaching the lateral canthus, however these swinging eyelid maneuvers achieve greater surgical space and expose the planes of subsequent lower eyelid dissection. A lateral canthotomy and inferior cantholysis are achieved with sharp dissection (Figs. 32.3, 32.4 and 32.5).
- A transconjunctival incision is made across the entire length of the lower eyelid 2–4 mm inferior to the tarsus using scissors or a monopolar cautery (Fig. 32.3).
- Dissection is carried out across the lower eyelid from posterior to anterior through the conjunctiva, inferior eyelid retractor band, and orbital septum to the plane between the orbital septum and the orbicularis muscle (Fig. 32.5).
- Dissection is carried out in a septal (either pre or post septal) plane to the level of the inferior orbital rim. An incision is made to the level of the arcus marginalis. The periosteum at the arcus marginalis is incised and the periosteum is elevated to expose the floor (Figs. 32.6 and 32.7).
- Next, the periosteum is elevated and dissection is continued in this subperiosteal plane along the orbital floor. Care must be taken at the medial infraorbital region as the inferior oblique muscle originates at the maxillary bone in this region. If extensive medial dissection is necessary, the inferior oblique muscle attachment at this site can be released with subperiosteal dissection.
- Care must be taken to avoid injury to the infraorbital neurovascular bundle, which may be identified within the infraorbital canal, separated by a thin layer of bone. In the setting of an orbital fracture repair, care must be taken to identify, decompress, and appropriately separate the infraorbital neurovascular bundle from the intraorbital tissue.
- Following elevation of the periosteum, the periosteum may be incised to access extraconal orbital regions, as needed.
- At closure, the periosteum is reapproximated with interrupted 5-0 polyglactin suture at the arcus marginalis or left unstured. The conjunctiva is closed with 7-0 chromic gut suture placed in buried interrupted fashion or loosely in running fashion.
- An optional temporary Frost (suspension) suture using 4-0, 5-0, or 6-0 silk suture is placed through lower eyelid and taped to the forehead and is left in place for 3–5 days to further reduce the risk of lower eyelid entropion and retraction.

C. **Transcaruncular Approach (Video 32.2)**

The transcaruncular approach is a versatile method to access the medial orbit and achieve good visualization to posterior regions approaching the medial orbital apex. This technique can provide access the medial orbital wall with excellent aesthetic results, eliminating the need for cutaneous incisions that may leave scars. This technique is commonly used in medial orbital decompression surgery, medial

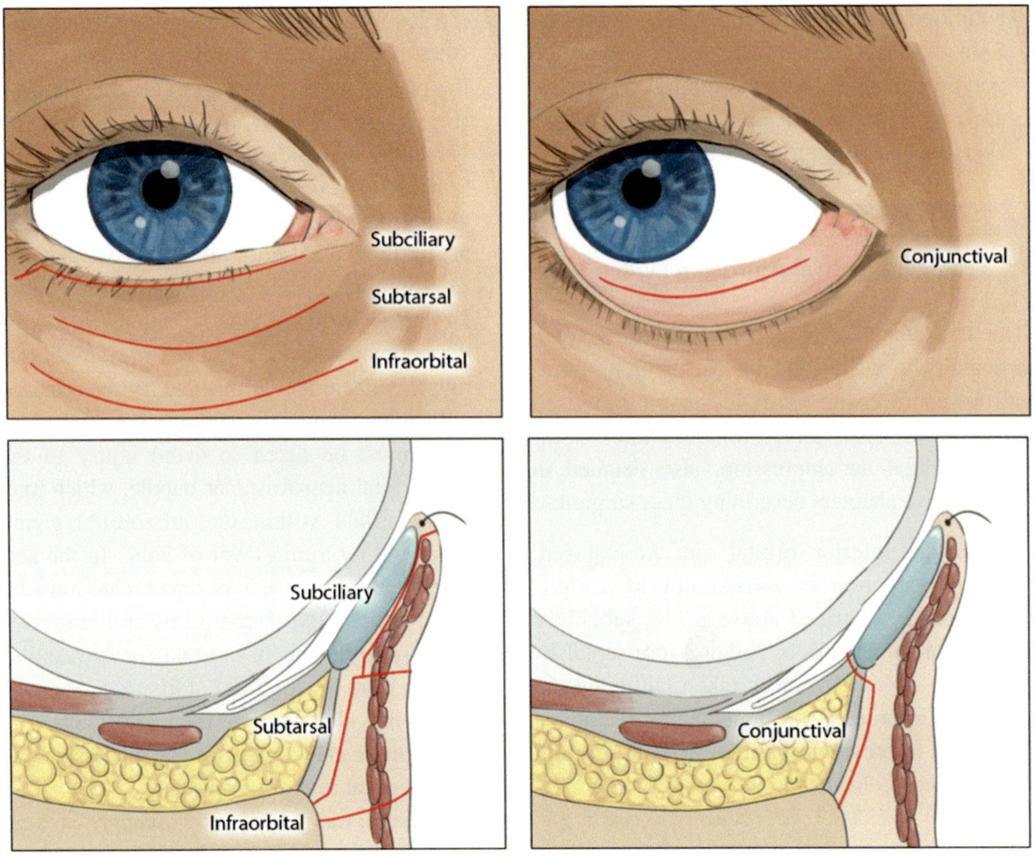

Fig. 32.3 Various inferior orbitotomy incisions (top) and dissection planes (bottom)

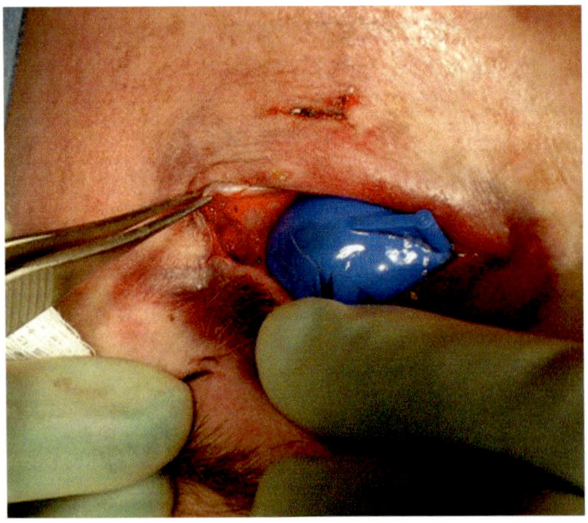

Fig. 32.4 Lateral canthotomy

orbital wall fracture repair, and medial orbital lesion biopsy and/or excision and are also detailed in the respective chapters describing these surgeries.

Surgical Technique

- An eyelid speculum is placed to expose the medial caruncle, plica semilunaris, and conjunctiva.
- Sharp-tipped scissors are used to make a 10–12 mm vertical incision through the epithelial layer between the caruncle and plica semilunaris. Gentle cautery is performed for hemostasis.

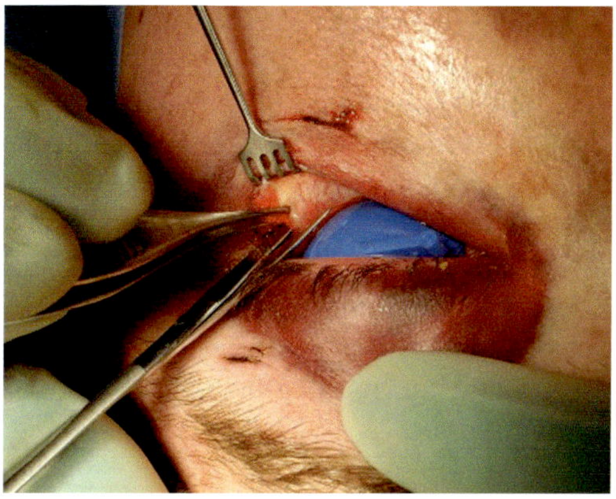

Fig. 32.5 Inferior conjunctival incision

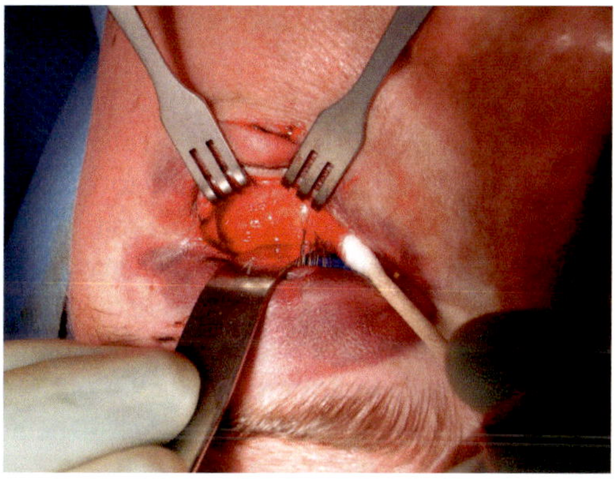

Fig. 32.6 The inferior rim periosteum is exposed by re draping the anterior lamella (skin and orbicularis) anteriorly and pushing fat int to the orbit with malleable such that the rim is approached in the septal plain

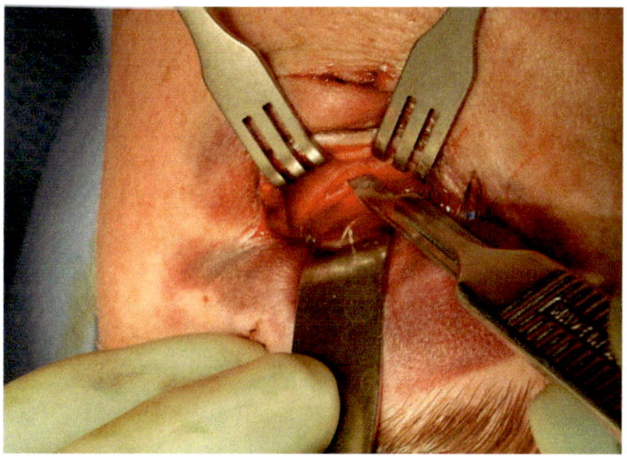

Fig. 32.7 A #15 blade incision cuts septum and periosteum only

- Retraction is performed by an assistant with 4-pronged skin hooks and dissection is carried out in a posteromedial direction in the avascular, fibrous plane of the medial orbital septum to until the periosteum of the medial orbital wall is reached, at a level posterior to the posterior lacrimal crest. Care must be taken to avoid injury the lacrimal sac, as this is located anterior and medial to the dissection plane.
- Ribbon retractors are positioned to allow adequate visualization and the medial orbital periosteum is incised to expose the bones of the medial orbital wall.
- Posterior dissection can be performed in the subperiosteal space to expose the entirety of the medial orbital wall with particular attention to the anterior and posterior ethmoid vessels (Fig. 32.8).
- If orbital tissue must be accessed, the orbital periosteum can be incised at the appropriate location to expose the needed orbital anatomy such as the medial rectus muscle or orbital fat.
- Surgical closure is achieved with closure of the caruncle-semilunaris incision with a deep 7-0 polyglactin suture (optional) and a 7-0 chromic gut suture to close the superficial epithelium. Alternatively, the wound may be left unsutured to heal spontaneously.

D. **Lateral Canthal Approach**

The lateral canthal approach is a common method utilized to access the lateral orbit through a lateral canthotomy and inferior and optional superior cantholysis. As previously mentioned, lateral canthal takedown frequently preceeds fornicieal incisions to increase exposure and achieve proper dissection planes. It is frequently used for lateral orbital decompression and orbital lesion exposure and excision.

E. **Swinging Eyelid Approach**

The swinging eyelid approach utilizes a combined lateral canthal approach and inferior

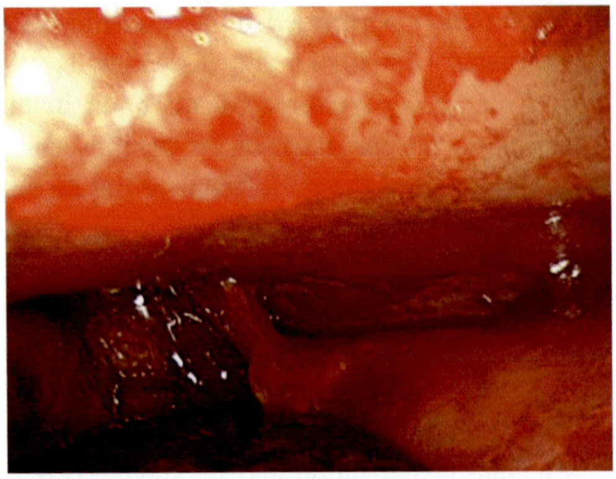

Fig. 32.8 View of the anterior ethmoid artery from a subperiosteal medial orbitotomy

transconjunctival approach to provide extensive access to the inferior orbital rim and orbital floor. In addition, the swinging eyelid approach can be further extended medially to include a joining transcaruncular incision to also access the medial wall (Fig. 32.3).

Intraconal Orbital Approaches

The intraconal orbital component is the space bounded within the muscle cone. Intraconal approaches to the orbit include the perilimbal and fornix conjunctival incision, the vertical eyelid split approach, and combined approaches using the previously described extraconal techniques with further dissection through the intermuscular septum to access the intraconal space.

A. **Perilimbal and Fornix Conjunctival Incision**

Perilimbal and fornix conjunctival incisions offer direct access to the intraconal space through masked conjunctival incisions. These are commonly used to access the medial intraconal space, which can be used to visualize the optic nerve for optic nerve sheath fenestrations and to biopsy or excise medial intraconal lesions.

Surgical Technique

- An eyelid speculum is placed to allow appropriate exposure of the conjunctival medial conjunctival region.
- A medially centered peritomy of the desired size is performed with relaxing incisions. In general, a minimum of a 90° peritomy is needed for adequate exposure, though a 170° peritomy with relaxing incisions allows further exposure.
- The Tenon's fascia is circumferentially released, and the conjunctival flap is reflected.
- The medial rectus muscle is isolated and tagged with a 6-0 polyglactin suture on a double-armed needle and released from its insertion.
- A 5-0 silk traction suture is placed through the medial rectus insertion site. This is used to reflect the globe temporally to provide increased exposure of the medial orbit.
- Dissection is carried out between the globe and medial rectus muscles to expose the medial orbital intraconal space. This allows access to medial intraconal orbital lesions.
- If an optic nerve sheath fenestration is being performed, the ciliary vessels are pushed to the side, and a bare area of the optic nerve is isolated.
- Surgical closure is initiated by re-attachment of the medial rectus muscle at the insertion site using the pre-placed 6-0 double-armed polyglactin suture.
- The conjunctival peritomy is then draped and reattached at the limbus using 7-0 polyglactin suture placed in buried fashion at the superior and inferior corners of the perilimbal region.

B. **Vertical Eyelid Split Approach**

The vertical eyelid split approach allows for superior intraconal exposure compared to the upper eyelid crease incision, which provides more access to the superior extraconal space. This approach is performed by making a vertical full-thickness incision through the eyelid at the junction of the medial one-third and central one-third of the upper lid to access the superior intraconal space (Fig. 32.9).

Surgical Technique

- The junction between the medial and central third of the upper eyelids are vertically marked.
- Sharp scissors are used to make a perpendicular full-thickness marginal eyelid incision carried out to the level of the superior fornix.
- Superiorly, the levator aponeurosis is transected vertically with Westcott scissors.
- Traction sutures using 5-0 silk are placed at the medial and lateral eyelid to allow further visualization.
- An incision is performed through the superior conjunctiva at the superior fornix to the medial canthus. Care must be taken to preserve the levator and Muller muscles.
- Dissection is then performed along the superior medial globe and Tenon's fascia is transected between the medial rectus and superior rectus.
- Care must be taken to identify the medial aspect of the superior rectus muscle, as this is generally the lateral-most aspect of dissection and exposure.
- Medially, dissection is performed to identify the tendon of the superior oblique muscle, which serves as the medial-most aspect of dissection and exposure.
- Deep superior intraconal exploration can be performed posteriorly at this point with care to avoid any vortex veins.
- Following completion of the orbital exploration or orbital mass excision, surgical closure is initiated following meticulous hemostasis with bipolar cautery.
- For surgical closure, the levator aponeurosis is closed with interrupted 6-0 polyglactin sutures placed horizontally.
- The conjunctiva is closed with multiple interrupted buried 7-0 or 8-0 polyglactin sutures.
- At the tarsus, partial-thickness 6-0 polyglactin sutures are placed to reapproximate the tarsus. Orbicularis muscle is closed with 6-0 polyglactin suture in buried fashion.
- The margin is closed with 7-0 chromic suture or 6-0 silk placed at the margin to reapproximate the lash line and gray line.
- The skin is closed with 6-0 plain gut suture and an eye pressure patch is placed overnight.

C. Combined Intraconal Approaches

The upper eyelid crease, transconjunctival, transcaruncular, and lateral canthal approaches can all be utilized as the initial steps to access the intraconal space. Access to the intraconal

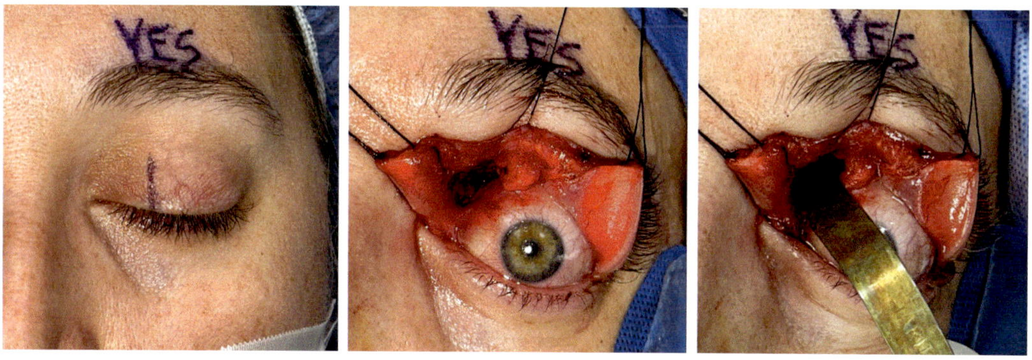

Fig. 32.9 Upper eyelid split intraconal orbitotomy. A vertical incision is marked at the medial third and central third junction of the upper eyelid (left). A full-thickness upper eyelid incision and superior fornix conjunctival incision is made to expose the superior intraconal space (center). A metal ribbon retractor can be inserted to retract the globe inferolateral to increase exposure of the intraconal space (right)

space can be achieved through further dissection through the fascial sheath covering and extending between the rectus muscles via a trans-intermuscular septal approach. For example, in inferolateral intraconal orbital lesion can be accessed through a combined swinging eyelid incision via a lateral canthal and transconjunctival approach with further dissection and exploration through the intermuscular septum between the inferior rectus and lateral rectus muscles to access and remove the intraconal lesion.

Conclusion

Several approaches are available to access the extraconal and intraconal spaces of the orbit. The most appropriate approach depends on anatomy, visualization needs, post-operative cosmesis, and risk to adjacent structures.

References

1. Kersten RC, Kulwin DR. Vertical lid split orbitotomy revisited. Ophthalmic Plast Reconstr Surg. 1999;15(6):425–8. https://doi.org/10.1097/00002341-199911000-00011.
2. Humphrey CD, Kriet JD. Surgical approaches to the orbit. Oper Tech Otolaryngol Head Neck Surg. 2008;19(2):132–9. https://doi.org/10.1016/j.otot.2008.07.002.
3. Rootman J. Orbital surgery: a conceptual approach. 2nd ed. Baltimore: Wolters Kluwer Health-Lippincott Williams & Wilkins; 2014.
4. Weller CL, Tabor MH, Ryan LE, Leyngold IM. Orbital surgery: approaches and techniques. Int Ophthalmol Clin. 2018;58(2):61–84. https://doi.org/10.1097/IIO.0000000000000223.
5. Hu S, Colley P. Surgical orbital anatomy. Semin Plast Surg. 2019;33(02):085–91. https://doi.org/10.1055/s-0039-1685476.
6. Agrawal S, Das D, Modaboyina S, Gupta S, Deora A. Surgical approaches to the orbit—the past and the present. IJOOO. 2021;7(1):5–11. https://doi.org/10.18231/j.ijooo.2021.003.

Lateral Approaches to the Orbit

33

Kalla A. Gervasio and Steven M. Couch

Abstract

Indications for lateral orbitotomy include lateral wall decompression in thyroid eye disease and exploration, biopsy, or removal of lateral orbital lesions in the extraconal or intraconal space or lacrimal gland fossa. Access to the lateral orbit most commonly involves a lateral upper eyelid crease or lateral canthal incision. In this chapter, the authors describe lateral orbitotomy surgical technique.

Keywords

Lateral orbitotomy · Lateral wall orbital decompression · Lateral canthal approach · Bone flap · Bone window

Supplementary Information The online version contains supplementary material available at https://doi.org/10.1007/978-3-031-63178-8_33.

K. A. Gervasio · S. M. Couch (✉)
John F. Hardesty, MD, Department of Ophthalmology and Visual Sciences, Washington University School of Medicine, St. Louis, MO, USA
e-mail: Smcouchmd@gmail.com

Introduction

A lateral approach to the orbit is commonly used for lateral orbital decompression in thyroid eye disease or for removal of lesions located in the lateral extraconal or intraconal orbit, posterior to the globe equator, or affecting the lacrimal gland. Pathology includes benign or malignant tumors, orbital infections such as intraconal or subperiosteal abscesses, and intraorbital foreign bodies. Additional indications include repair of lateral orbital rim or zygomaticomaxillary complex fractures. Depending on the size and posterior extent of the lesion being treated, a lateral orbitotomy with bone removal or fashioning of a bone flap may be utilized (Fig. 33.1). This approach creates extra space and a lateral orbit window to facilitate removal of retrobulbar tumors, such as a cavernous venous malformation that would otherwise be inaccessible or approached blindly from anterior orbitotomy approaches (Fig. 33.2). The most common surgical approaches to the lateral orbit utilize a lateral upper eyelid crease or a lateral canthal incision.

J. Tao (ed.), *Efficient Oculofacial Surgery*, https://doi.org/10.1007/978-3-031-63178-8_33

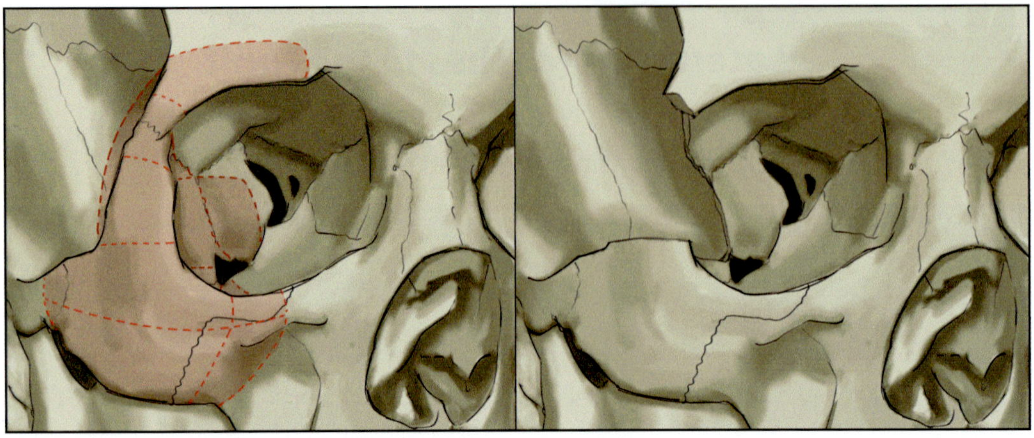

Fig. 33.1 Schematic of bony anatomy of the lateral orbit. The osteotomies may be placed at various locations, depending on surgical exposure needs (left), but traditionally, the inferior cut is at the level of the zygomatic arch and the superior cut is just above the frontozygomatic suture (right)

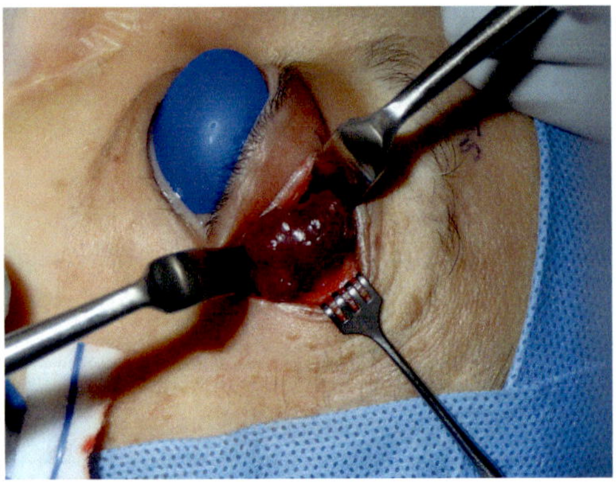

Fig. 33.2 Lateral upper eyelid crease approach with bone flap to intraconal cavernous malformation

Surgical Technique

Lateral Orbitotomy for Decompression, Exploration, Biopsy, or Removal of Lesions

An initial incision is marked using either the lateral upper eyelid crease or an extended lateral canthal incision. If using an upper eyelid crease approach, the incision is made using a #15 blade. If using a lateral canthal approach, an extended canthotomy incision is made using scissors or a #15 blade for approximately 1.5 cm. Next, dissection is performed through the orbicularis muscle. The superior and lateral orbital rim is approached in the septal plane. The periosteum is then incised, exposing the entirety of the lateral rim and lateral orbital wall. The zygomaticotemporal and zygomaticofacial neurovascular bundles are isolated, divided, and cauterized.

In cases involving exploration, biopsy, or removal of lateral orbital lesions, dissection through the periorbita and intermuscular septum is then carried out using a hand over hand technique using malleable or sewall retractors either above or below the lateral rectus muscle. In orbit decompression for thyroid eye disease, bone removal of the lateral orbital wall can then be achieved using either rongeurs, a bone chisel and mallet, a high-speed drill, or an ultrasonic device. Bone decompression includes the greater wing of the sphenoid and may proceed as far as to the level of the dura superiorly and posteriorly and to the buccal fat inferiorly. Alternatively, a thin crest of bone nay be left as a barrier between the orbit and intracranial space. Care must be taken to avoid a cerebrospinal fluid (CSF) leak when removing bone to the level of the dura during this portion of surgery. If a CSF leak occurs, treatment includes tamponade with orbital fat. Fibrin tissue glue may also be useful. Next, the inferior orbital

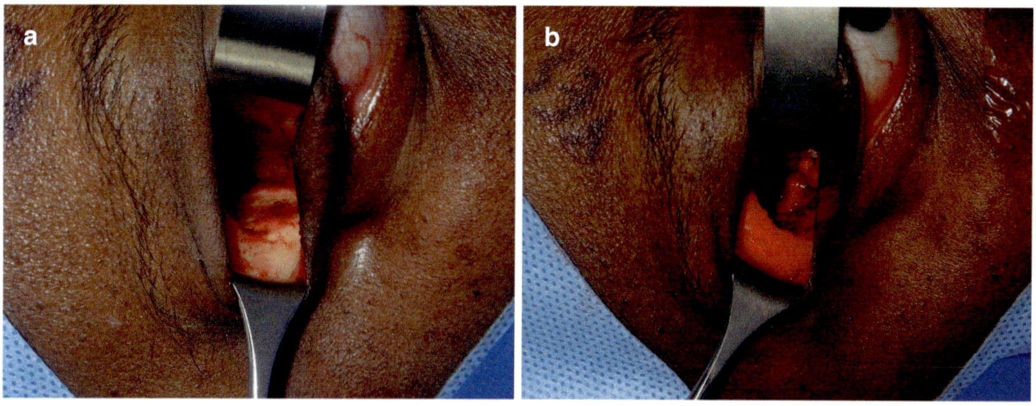

Fig. 33.3 View of lateral orbital wall before (**a**) and after (**b**) bone removal for decompression, note the temporalis muscle underlying the lateral orbital wall

basin is also removed (Fig. 33.3). An approximately 7 mm strut of lateral orbital rim is left intact. Hemostasis is achieved using a combination of cautery, bone wax, and gel foam soaked in thrombin. After adequate bone removal, the orbital periosteum of the lateral orbit is opened with sharp dissection, allowing the contents to protrude into the osteotomy. The periosteum is then closed anteriorly using 5-0 polyglactin suture or it is left un-sutured. If a lateral canthal approach was used, a lateral canthal angle reforming suture is placed using 5-0 polyglactin suture. The extended lateral canthotomy incision is then closed in layers using 6-0 polyglactin suture for the orbicularis muscle and 6-0 plain gut suture for the superficial skin.

Lateral Orbitotomy with Bone Flap (Video 33.1)

The use of a bone flap may be used in cases that require safe access to the posterior orbit, commonly deep intraconal orbital lesions (Figs. 33.6 and 33.7). In some instances of a deep medial orbital tumor, a lateral bone flap may be constructed to prolapse the globe laterally and thereby achieve additional medial orbitotomy space for a safer approach.

A lateral upper eyelid crease (Fig. 33.4) or lateral canthal incision (Fig. 33.5) followed by a preseptal approach to the superior and lateral

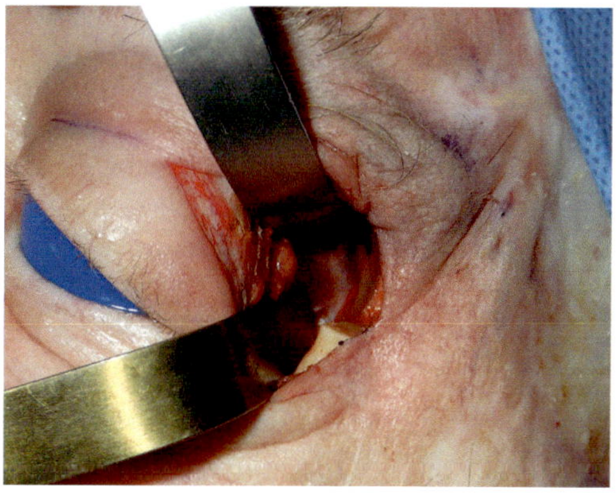

Fig. 33.4 View of orbital apex through lateral upper eyelid crease approach and bone flap to the orbital apex

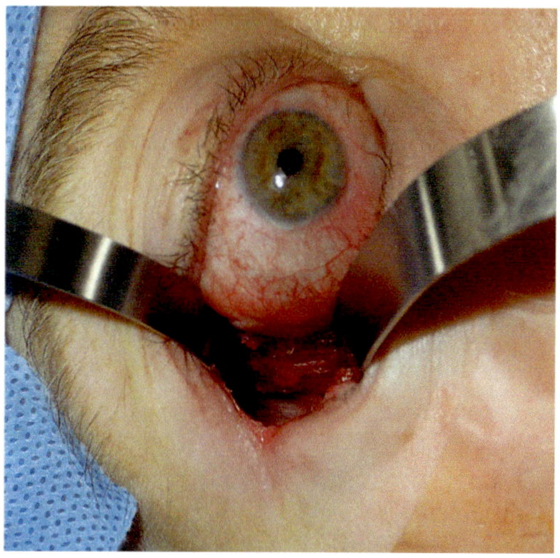

Fig. 33.5 View of lateral orbit through lateral canthal approach

orbital rim can be used as previously described. A periosteal incision is made across the superior, lateral, and inferior rim and the periosteum is reflected temporally into the temporalis fossa. This periosteal incision is carried out medially to expose the lateral orbital wall. The zygomaticotemporal and zygomaticofacial neurovascular bundles are cauterized and divided.

Osteotomies can be fashioned using either an oscillating bone saw, chisel, or piezoelectric knife blade. The procedure is also referred to as a marginotomy. The osteotomies can be made at multiple different areas along the lateral orbit, zygoma and roof of the orbit (Fig. 33.3). Most commonly they are made approximately 8 mm superior to the zygomaticofrontal suture and inferiorly at the junction of the zygomatic body. The bone flap is removed with a large rongeur or similar pliers-type instrument or a bone clamp. Lateral attachments to temporalis are released with electrocautery. A drill or rongeurs can then be used to remove posterior sphenoid bone to create additional space if needed. The lateral orbital periosteum can then be opened using a #11 blade or Westcott scissors. A gentle hand over hand technique may then be used to enter the intraconal soft tissues and facilitate identification and then removal of posterior intraconal lesions (Figs. 33.6 and 33.7). Finally, the bone flap is repositioned. Traditionally, the bone is secured with sutures through predrilled tunnels. Miniplates and screws offer precise and more rigid bone fixation. Periosteum is closed using 5-0 polyglactin sutures or left unstured. Orbicularis muscle is closed using 5-0 or 6-0 oolyglactin suture and the superficial skin is closed with 6-0 plain gut suture. With good technique, the wound is well camouflaged and there is minimal scarring, even early post operatively (Figs. 33.8 and 33.9) [1–4].

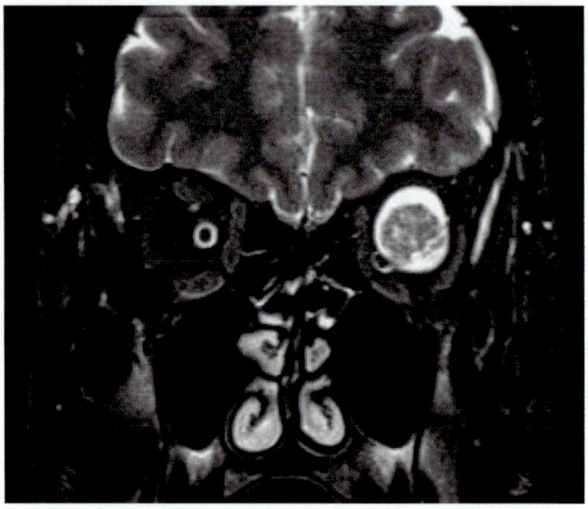

Fig. 33.7 Retrobulbar mass visualized on coronal neuroimaging

Conclusion

The two most common approaches to the lateral orbit include an upper eyelid crease or a lateral canthal approach. Lateral orbitotomy may

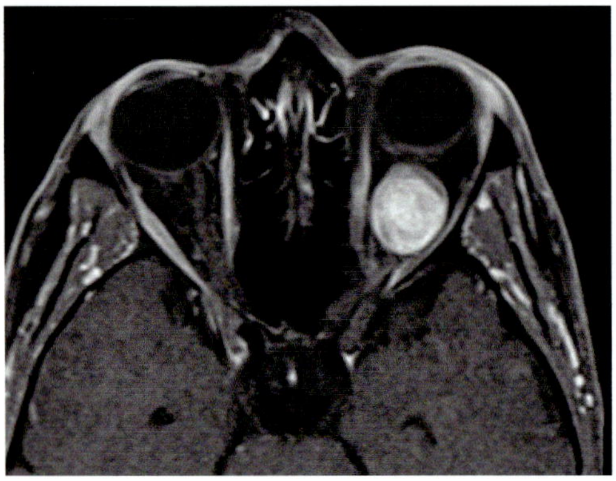

Fig. 33.6 Retrobulbar mass visualized on axial neuroimaging

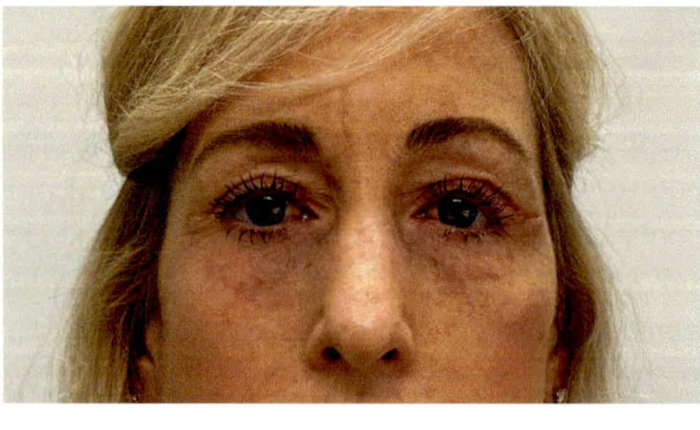

Fig. 33.8 External frontal and oblique view of a patient 1 week status post removal of the intraconal tumor shown in Figs. 33.6 and 33.7 through a lateral bone flap. Minimal scarring, edema, or facial asymmetry are evident

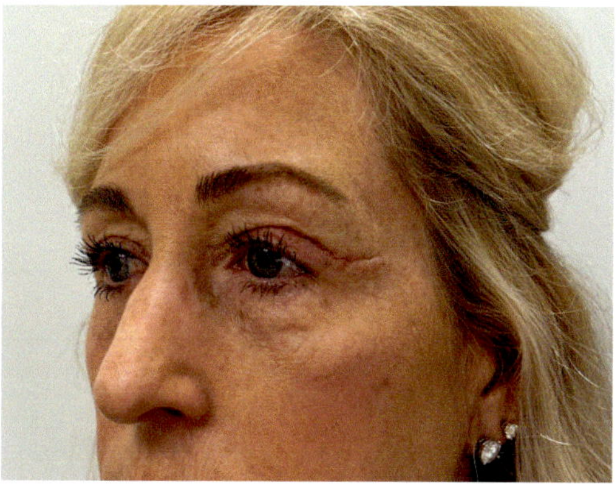

Fig. 33.9 Oblique view of the same patient shown in Figs. 33.6, 33.7 and 33.8 at only 1 week post operative

be used for bony decompression in thyroid eye disease patients or for exploration, biopsy, or removal of lesions in the deep posterior orbit.

References

1. Orbital surgery, Chapter 7, Section 7—Oculofacial Plastic and Orbital Surgery. American Academy of Ophthalmology Basic and Clinical Science Course Book
2. Harris GJ, Logani SC. Eyelid crease incision for lateral orbitotomy. Ophthal Plas Reconstr Surg. 1999;15:9–18.
3. Rootman J. Orbital surgery. Philadelphia: Lippincott Williams & Wilkins; 2013.
4. Rootman DB. Orbital decompression for thyroid eye disease. Surv Ophthalmol. 2018;63(1):86–104.

Orbital Bone Decompression

34

Marc Yonkers

Abstract

Orbital decompression is commonly performed for thyroid eye disease but is also used in other space occupying orbital diseases. Most orbital decompressions are customized with various extent of the orbit floor, medial wall, or the lateral wall removed. In this chapter, the author outlines an orbit decompression protocol that begins with floor and medial wall decompression using direct surgical landmarks. Lateral wall decompression is also described as the third orbital wall decompressed in more severe orbitopathy.

Keywords

Thyroid eye disease · Orbit decompression · Ethmoidectomy · Exophthalmos · Proptosis

Supplementary Information The online version contains supplementary material available at https://doi.org/10.1007/978-3-031-63178-8_34.

M. Yonkers (✉)
Kaiser Permanente, South San Francisco, CA, USA
e-mail: Marc.Yonkers@kp.org

Introduction

Orbital decompression is most indicated for thyroid eye disease (TED), an inflammatory condition of the orbit that has many phenotypes. Hallmarks of the disease are tissue expansion of orbital fat, extraocular muscles, or both. With the rigid bony structure of the orbital walls, orbital tissue expansion often results in proptosis and compression of soft tissue.

Initial treatment goals in TED are to limit inflammation if present. Corticosteroids, immune modulating medication, radiotherapy, or targeted therapy have roles. Surgical decompression may be indicated to create space for enlarged or expanded tissues, namely orbital fat and extraocular muscles. Improving proptosis, reducing orbital pressure and ache, and in rare instances, acutely relieving pressure on the optic nerve are the goals of decompression surgery. In some instances of acute inflammation and congestion of the orbit, orbital decompression may be a useful intervention.

For patients symptomatic from TED, an orbital decompression, is a safe and efficient procedure. Any wall of the orbit may be decompressed, although the roof is generally avoided owing to intracranial risks.

There exist a variety of approaches to orbit bone decompression. A system that begins with orbital floor and medial wall decompression and adds areas of bone removal, including the

J. Tao (ed.), *Efficient Oculofacial Surgery*, https://doi.org/10.1007/978-3-031-63178-8_34

lateral wall when additional decompression is indicated.

Anatomy

The orbital floor is formed by the maxillary bone medially, the zygomatic bone laterally, and the orbital process of the palatine bone posteriorly [1]. It provides vertical support for the orbit and is bordered by the maxillary sinus inferiorly. Medially, the orbital floor is continuous with the medial wall, except for the anterior opening of the nasolacrimal canal. Laterally, the floor is continuous anteriorly with the lateral wall. Posteriorly, the floor and lateral wall are separated by the inferior orbital fissure. Arising from the inferior orbital fissure, the infraorbital groove courses anteriorly and contains the infraorbital nerve, a sensory branch of the maxillary nerve. Identification of the infraorbital groove is an important landmark in an orbital floor decompression as disruption of the nerve can result in numbness from the lower eyelid to the upper lip. The bone of the orbital floor is extremely thin, particularly posterior medially, making it a structural target for decompression surgery.

The medial wall is formed by the frontal process of the maxillary bone, the lacrimal bone, the ethmoid bone, and the sphenoid bone. Like the orbital floor, the medial orbital wall is extremely thin, particularly along the ethmoid bone. The superior aspect of the ethmoid bone contains the anterior and posterior ethmoidal foramen which transmit the anterior and posterior ethmoidal arteries, as well as the anterior and posterior branches of the nasociliary nerve. The ethmoidal foramen passes medially to the lateral aspect of the cribriform plate. The medial wall is bordered by the ethmoidal sinus medially. Superior medially, the medial skull base can have variable descent near the ethmoidal sinus. Therefore, preoperative imaging assessment of this area can help define the extent of a medial wall decompression.

The lateral wall is formed largely by the zygomatic bone and the greater wing of the sphenoid, separated by the zygomaticosphenoid suture, while the upper portion is formed by the frontal bone. Posterior to the zygomaticosphenoid suture, the sphenoid bone expands deep toward the middle cranial fossa to form a trigone, which is the target for a deep lateral decompression [2, 3]. Posterior to the sphenoid bone lies the meninges of the central nervous system, with the outermost layer composed of dura mater.

Preoperative Evaluation with Imaging

A non-contrast computed tomography (CT) of the orbit helps define patient specific anatomy to guide a plan for decompression. Anatomical variations in fat expansion, location and shape of the skull base, and size of the sphenoid are considerations.

Determining fat predominant (Type I, Fig. 34.1) versus muscle predominant (Type II, Fig. 34.2) expansion stratifies diplopia risks [4, 5]. Type I patients have full extraocular motility and usually maintain single binocular vision after orbital decompression of any type. Type II patients, commonly have restricted eye movements on presentation that may worsen over time, with or without intervention. Many type II patients have symptomatic diplopia either in primary or secondary gaze due to tight extraocular muscles and limited ductions. Esotropia and hypotropia are most common, owing to the predilection for medial and inferior rectus involvement. Type II patients should be educated that orbit decompression does not treat strabismus. In fact, hypotropia and esotropia may worsen after floor and medial decompression, respectively. Eye alignment surgery, if necessary, occurs in a subsequent phase. Prism spectacles

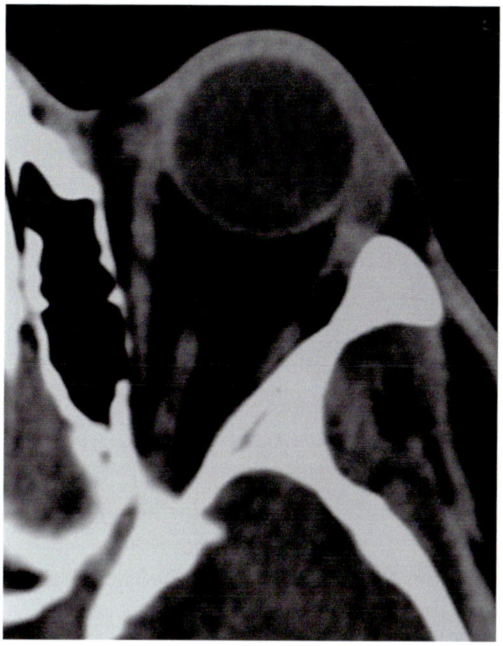

Fig. 34.1 Axial CT demonstrating proptosis due to fat expansion in type I TED

or an eye patch may be useful to alleviate diplopia while awaiting stability for strabismus surgery.

While most patients have significant space between the medial wall and the midline skull base, rare patients may have an inferiorly displaced fovea ethmoidalis and cribriform plate [6, 7]. In these cases, high medial wall decompression should be performed with increased caution.

When considering a lateral wall decompression, the area of bone available for decompression is highly variable [8]. With sufficient sphenoid bone trigone volume, lateral decompression can significantly decompress the orbit. In patients with a small trigone and limited surrounding bone, the effect of a lateral decompression may be limited and add unnecessary risk of cerebrospinal fluid leak, bleeding, and other intracranial complications (Fig. 34.3).

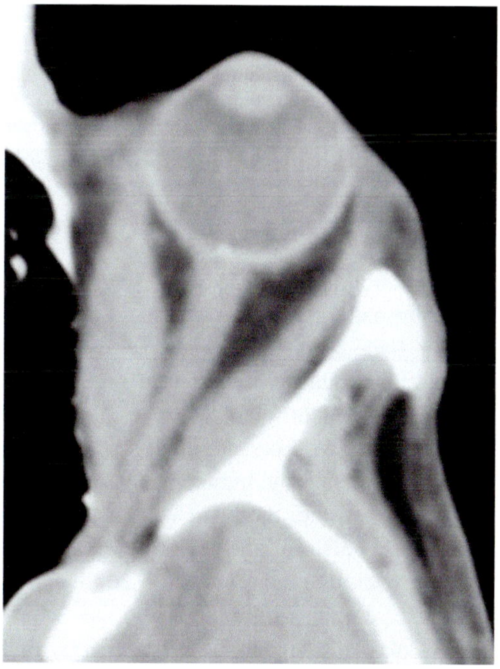

Fig. 34.2 Axial CT demonstrating proptosis due to muscle hypertrophy in type II TED

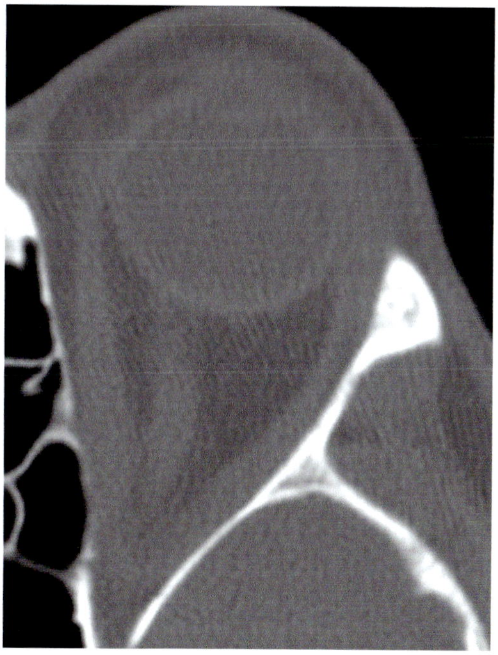

Fig. 34.3 Axial computed tomography scan demonstrating a small sphenoid trigone

Floor and Medial Wall Decompression (Video 34.1)

A combined floor and medial wall decompression is an efficient intervention for many thyroid eye disease patients. Excellent exposure is achieved with minimally invasive incisions. Also, the first areas of decompression include thin bones, making the procedure efficient with minimal instrumentation and short operating times.

Access to the orbital floor is achieved with the swinging eyelid technique [9]. A lateral canthotomy incision and inferior cantholysis are formed followed by a horizontal transconjunctival incision including the conjunctiva and retractor band. The lower lid is then retracted with a Senn or Desmarres retractor to expose the inferior orbital rim. An incision is made on the inferior orbital rim that transects only septum and periosteum to expose the orbital floor. Retraction of the periosteum is then aided by a wide malleable retractor to further expose the floor. Identification of the infraorbital groove and fissure aids in determining the landmarks of the floor (Fig. 34.4). The thin, commonly translucent bone located posterior and medial on the floor is then decompressed with a Kelly forceps and rongeurs. If thicker bone is encountered, an osteotome and mallet may be necessary. Decompressing the medial orbital floor is sufficient for most cases. The roof of the infraorbital groove and the lateral floor are commonly preserved to avoid infraorbital hypoesthesia. However, unroofing of the groove and decompression of the lateral floor may be considered in cases needing greater decompression effect. In these cases, bone is carefully removed from the infraorbital nerve and electrocautery is avoided. Transient V2 hypoesthesia is common, and patients should be reassured that sensation usually recovers within weeks to months. The decompression generally proceeds up to the rim, but the anterior floor may be left intact to prevent hypoglobus in cases needing only modest decompression effect or only need decompression posteriorly (e.g., compressive optic neuropathy).

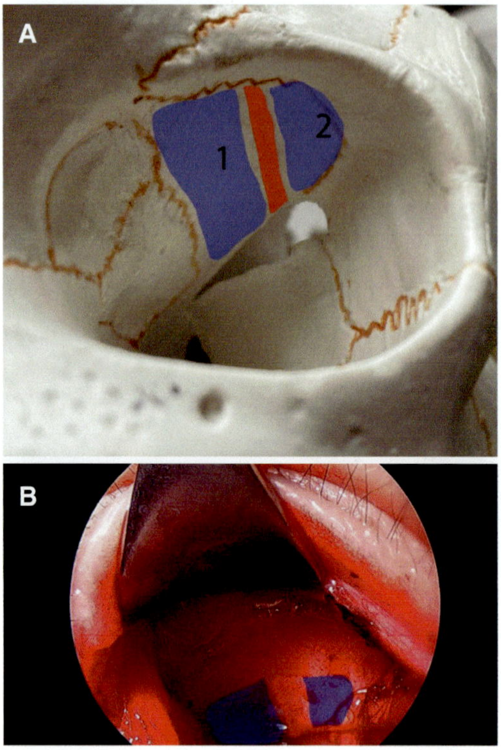

Fig. 34.4 (**A**) Teaching skull view of orbital floor. Areas of decompression outlined in blue including primary target the medial floor (1). Caution around the infraorbital groove (red) is taken to avoid infraorbital hypoesthesia. If necessary, additional floor decompression can be carried to the lateral floor (2) (**B**) Intraoperative surgeon view of the orbital floor

After bone is out fractured and removed a malleable is slightly withdrawn to prolapse the retro-orbital contents into the surgical view. A sickle knife or scissors are used to incise the periorbita and enter the intraconal space. Orbital fat is prolapsed into the bone window and gentle pressure on the globe facilitates seating of the globe back into the orbit. Exposed fat can be gently excised, though prolapse into the decompressed space is adequate for most patients.

The medial wall is accessed through a transcaruncular or transcutaneous incision. The transcaruncular approach is generally preferred for the absence of a cutaneous scar but it may be associated with a slightly narrower surgical view.

After creating a 1 cm vertical incision through the mid caruncle, a skin hook grasps the medial caruncle incision. A malleable ribbon retracts the globe and orbital soft tissues laterally. The periosteum is incised at the level of the posterior lacrimal crest and extended superiorly. The periosteum is then elevated, and the malleable used to further retract the orbital contents.

Subperiosteal dissection should begin superiorly along the thicker orbital roof bone since a more inferior dissection encounters the thin lamina papyracea that collapses easily. Subperiosteal dissection should achieve visualization of the ethmoidal arteries as a landmark denoting the superior border of the decompression (Fig. 34.5). The ethmoid arteries also provide information of the anterior posterior depth within the orbit. The posterior ethmoid artery is typically only 5–6 mm anterior to the optic canal. Like the floor, the thin medial wall is decompressed by out fracturing, then grasping and resecting the bone and sinus tissue, using a Kelly forceps, Kerrison rongeurs, and pituitary (or other front biting) forceps. Once the desired bone and underlying ethmoid air cells are removed to create a medial wall window, the periorbita is incised to prolapse fat into the ethmoid sinus.

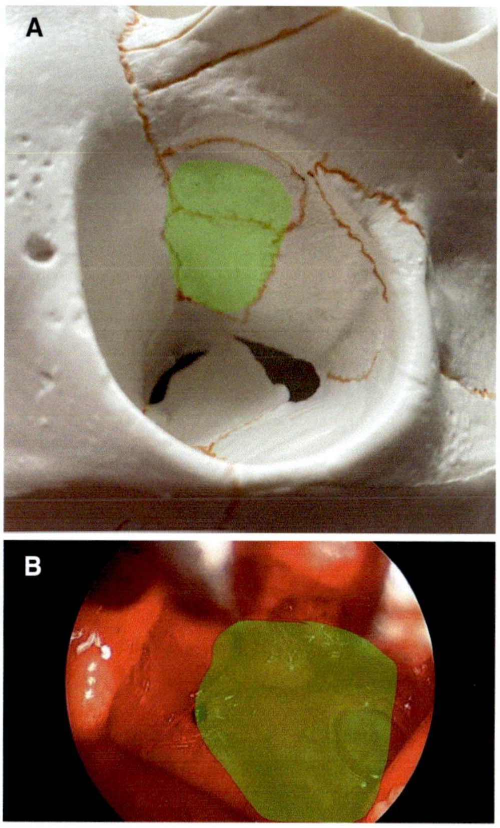

Fig. 34.5 (**A**) Model view of the medial wall. The thin ethmoid and lacrimal bones available for decompression (green). (**B**) Surgeon view of the mediall wall

Separating the thin bone of the floor and medial wall is the denser infraorbital (maxilloethmoidal) strut. For routine mild or moderate decompression, this is left intact, especially anteriorly, to prevent hypoglobus and consecutive strabismus. With more severe proptosis the strut can be removed to further decompress the orbit. In general, the posterior strut is removed first, and anterior aspect removed sequentially, depending on desired proptosis reduction. In cases of optic nerve compression, posterior strut removal facilitates optic nerve recovery.

The caruncle incision can be closed with a buried 6-0 plan gut suture or left to heal by second intention. The lower eyelid transconjunctival incision is also closed with buried 6-0 plain gut suture. In cases with significant lower eyelid retraction, a hang-back technique is useful to recess the lower eyelid retractors and reduce inferior scleral show (Fig. 34.6). The lateral canthus is then repositioned with a 4-0 vicryl suture placed from the lateral tarsus to the lateral orbital rim periosteum. While post-procedure inflammation and edema can be variable, a lateral temporary tarsorrhaphy is an optional step that can help prevent chemosis after the decompression.

On average, a medial orbit floor and medial wall decompression sparing the maxilloethmoidal strut achieves approximately 3–6 mm of proptosis reduction. Lateral floor decompression or strut removal, each add 1–3 mm of additional proptosis reduction effect.

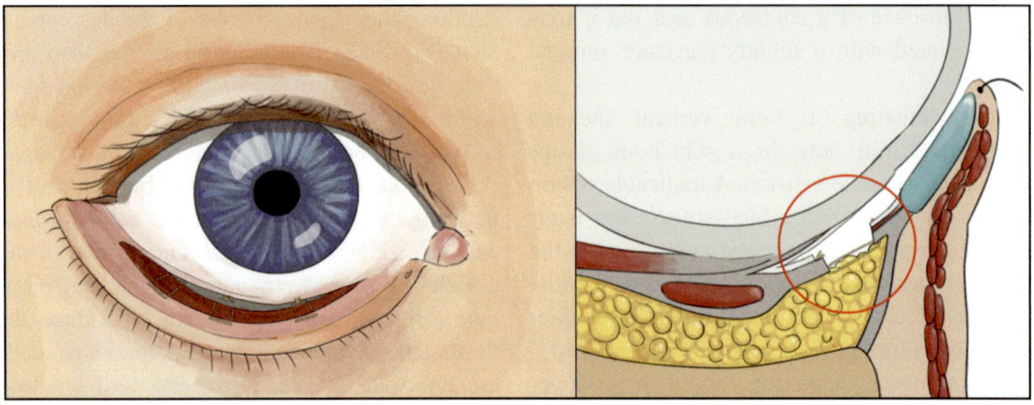

Fig. 34.6 Illustration of hang-back technique used to recess lower eyelid retractors and encourage improvement of inferior scleral show, frontal view on right and sagittal view on left

Lateral Wall Decompression

While a combined decompression of the floor and medial walls is sufficient for most patients with TED, a lateral wall decompression provides additional space. The sphenoid bone lies directly posterior to the globe, which may aid with reduction of axial proptosis.

Decisions on lateral wall decompression are also always tailored to neuro imaging. There exists variability in the size of the sphenoid trigone that largely determines the amount of decompression that can be achieved laterally.

Access to the lateral wall is achieved through an upper eyelid crease incision that can be carried slightly past the canthus. The lateral orbital rim is then exposed and the periosteum is elevated. A malleable retracts the globe medially. The orbital fissures serve as visual landmarks. Preoperative imaging can provide the distance from the lateral orbital rim to the deepest area of the sphenoid bone to apply a high-speed drill for decompression. The area for decompression can expand directly posterior into the trigone, then expand anterolaterally to the zygoma (Fig. 34.7). Deep lateral decompression can expose dura and care should be taken to avoid a cerebrospinal fluid leak. For patients with significant lacrimal gland prolapse, the lacrimal sac fossa can be decompressed with the burr superior and anterior to allow for retro placement of the gland into the orbit. After bony decompression the periorbita can be incised to prolapse orbital fat into the space created. The upper eyelid crease incision is then closed with a running suture.

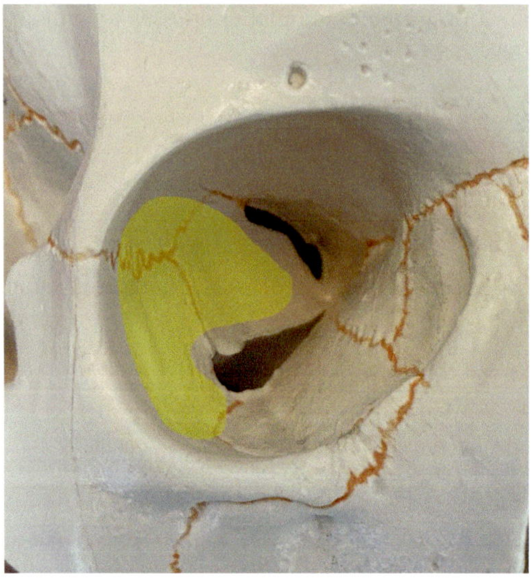

Fig. 34.7 Anterior model view highlighting targeted areas for lateral decompression (yellow)

Complications and Prevention

Overall, orbital decompression is safe and effective for thyroid eye disease patients with proptosis. Complications include asymmetric globe position including residual proptosis, consecutive enophthalmos, or hypoglobus. Appropriate preoperative imaging review, measurements, and discussion of surgical goals will help decrease these risks.

Postoperative edema and exposure can be seen in the weeks after surgery. Chemosis may be present, along with ocular surface exposure. A temporary tarsorrhaphy or a moisture chamber seal and aggressive lubrication are useful. Intraoperative and post procedure steroids may also help with edema and postoperative inflammation.

Infraorbital hypesthesia is a risk of floor decompression. Identification of the infraorbital groove and gentle decompression of the thin orbital bone limits the risk. Mild to moderate hypesthesia will commonly improve in the weeks to months after surgery.

Postoperative bleeding including epistaxis and orbital hemorrhage are limited by adequate intraoperative hemostatic control. Cases displaying signs of intraoperative bleeding may be aided by deep extubation from anesthesia to limit Valsalva and coughing in the immediate post op period. In addition to cautious electrocautery, adjuncts such as gelfoam soaked in thrombin, tranexamic acid (intravenously or mixed in the local anesthesia), or methylcellulose sponges may be useful. For bone bleeding during lateral wall decompression, bone wax can be considered.

Strabismus is inherent to Type II TED, though occurs in less than 4% of Type I patients after decompression [4]. Preoperative counseling on this risk regarding the increased action of extraocular muscles in a decompressed space is helpful. In addition, patients should be counseled that strabismus corrections occur in a subsequent phase of TED rehabilitation.

Cerebrospinal fluid leak is a risk in lateral decompression and can occur very rarely in medial wall decompression. These are often self-limited and self-sealing. Fibrin glue may be useful to help seal the leak intraoperatively. Patients should be monitored closely and in cases of persistent leak, secondary gluing or patching may be indicated.

Conclusion

Orbital decompression is a safe and effective treatment modality for thyroid eye disease (Figs. 34.8, 34.9, 34.10 and 34.11) Owing to the variability of thyroid eye disease phenotypes, decompression is often customized. In this system, we begin with decompression of the medial floor and medial wall with preservation of the maxilloethmoidal strut. The strut is removed, or the lateral floor is also decompressed if a greater effect is desired. Lateral wall decompression is added for more severe cases and depending on

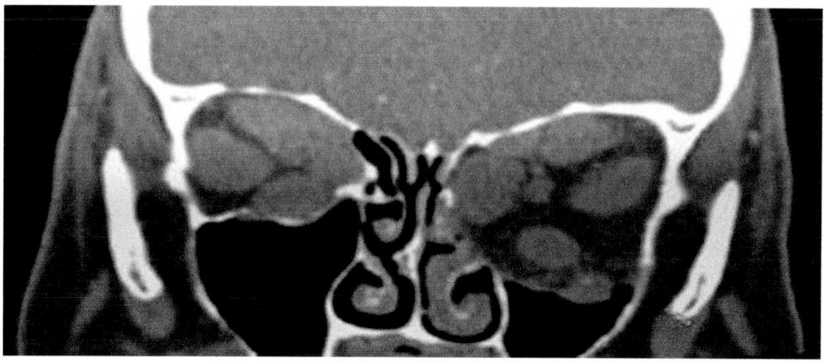

Fig. 34.8 Coronal CT image status post left floor and medial wall decompression. Right orbit is not decompressed to demonstrate appearance pre decompression

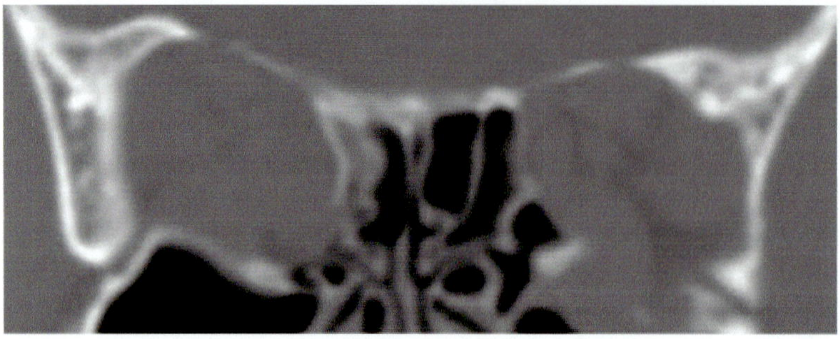

Fig. 34.9 Postoperative CT demonstrating effects of left lateral wall decompression

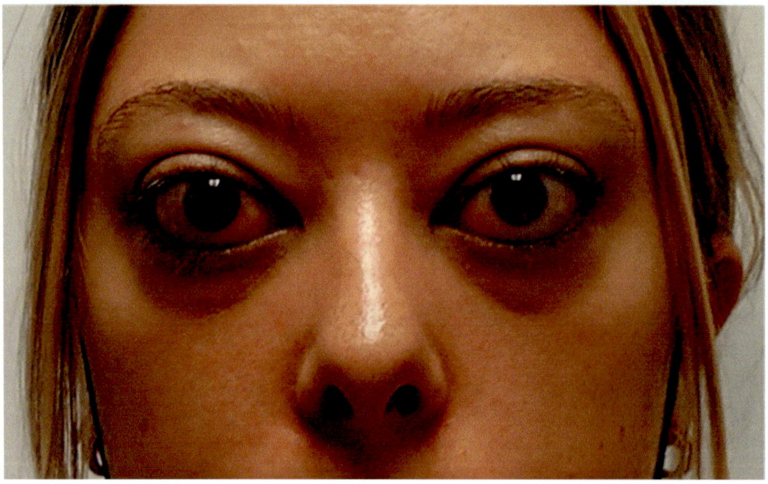

Fig. 34.10 A patient with bilateral exophthalmos due to thyroid eye disease

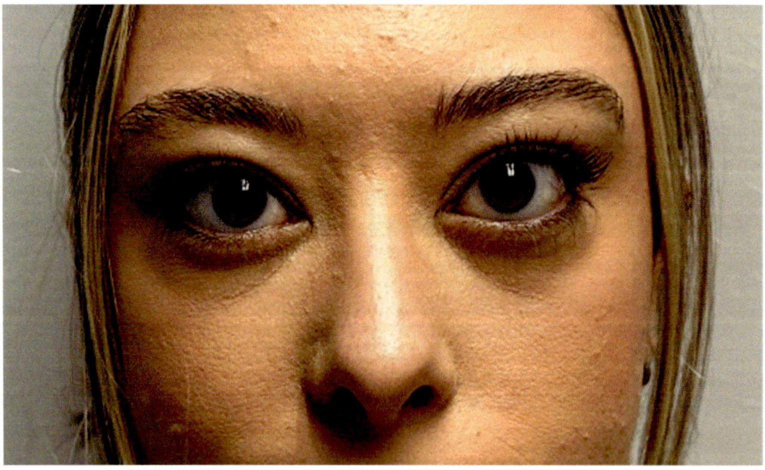

Fig. 34.11 Patient in Fig. 34.9 status post floor and medial wall bone decompression and good reduction of exophthalmos and congestion (whitening of conjunctiva)

imaging findings. This orbital decompression protocol is associated with high surgical efficiency, low risk of cerebrospinal fluid leak, adequate decompression, and minimal surgical scarring.

References

1. Rhoton AL and Natori Y. The orbit and sellar region microsurgical anatomy and operative approaches. Thieme; 1996
2. Goldberg RA, Kim AJ, Kerivan KM. The lacrimal keyhole, orbital door jamb, and basin of the inferior orbital fissure. Three areas of deep bone in the lateral orbit. Arch Ophthalmol. 1998;116(12):1618–24.
3. Beden U, Edizer M, Elmali M, Icten N, Gungor I, Sullu Y, Erkan D. Surgical anatomy of the deep lateral orbital wall. Eur J Ophthalmol. 2007;17(3):281–6.
4. Nunery WR, Nunery CW, Martin RT, Truong TV, Osborn DR. The risk of diplopia following orbital floor and medial wall decompression in subtypes of ophthalmic graves' disease. Ophthalmic Plast Reconstr Surg. 1997;13(3):153–60.
5. Nair AA, Ediriwickrema LS, Dolman PJ, Law G, Harrison AR, Mokhtarzadeh A, Stewart K, Men C, Lucarelli MJ, Van Landingham S, Wingelaar M. Predictive modeling of new-onset postoperative diplopia following orbital decompression for thyroid eye disease. Ophthalmic Plast Reconstr Surg. 2022;38(6):551–7.
6. Kaplanoglu H, Kaplanoglu V, Dilli A, Toprak U, Hekimoğlu B. An analysis of the anatomic variations of the paranasal sinuses and ethmoid roof using computed tomography. Eurasian J Med. 2013;45(2):115–25. https://doi.org/10.5152/eajm.2013.23.
7. Abdullah B, Chew SC, Aziz ME, Shukri NM, Husain S, Joshua SW, Wang Y, Snidvongs K. A new radiological classification for the risk assessment of anterior skull base injury in endoscopic sinus surgery. Sci Rep. 2020;10(1):4600.
8. Lefebvre DR, Yoon MK. CT-based measurements of the sphenoid trigone in different sex and race. Ophthalmic Plast Reconstr Surg. 2015;31(2):155–8. https://doi.org/10.1097/IOP.0000000000000370. PMID: 25658833.
9. McCord CD. Orbital decompression for Graves' disease: exposure through lateral canthal and inferior fornix incision. Ophthalmology. 1981;88(6):533–41.

Orbital Floor Fracture Repair

35

Teresa H. Chen, Maria Belen Camacho,
Christopher R. Dermarkarian, and Jeremiah P. Tao

Abstract

Orbital floor fractures are common after facial trauma. Surgical indications are functional and aesthetic, including but not limited to oculocardiac reflex, diplopia, enophthalmos, and hypoglobus. This chapter details repair of orbital floor fractures using a nylon foil implant.

Keywords

Orbit fracture · Orbit floor · Blowout fracture · Trapdoor fracture · Orbit implant

Introduction

Orbital fractures commonly result from blunt trauma to the midface. They are caused by hydraulic mechanisms, when increased pressure is transmitted from the soft tissues to the orbital walls, and buckling mechanisms, when the deformation of the orbital rim is transmitted to the floor posteriorly [1]. Orbital floor fractures may occur in isolation or concomitant to extra orbital facial fractures and fractures of the other orbital walls, especially the medial wall (Fig. 35.1).

While most orbital fractures do not require urgent surgical intervention, patients with extraocular muscle entrapment and an oculocardiac reflex should undergo surgery within days for quicker recovery and lower risk of permanent restrictive changes [2]. Other indications for surgery include persistent diplopia in primary or downgaze, enophthalmos greater than 2 mm, hypoglobus, a large orbital floor fracture greater than half of the orbital floor, and associated rim or facial fractures causing disfigurement and pathophysiology (Fig. 35.2) [3]. The timing for nonemergent surgical intervention is an area of contention and surgeon preference, but reconstruction is typically performed around 7–21 days, after resolution of posttraumatic edema and before soft tissue scarring [4].

In combined orbit floor and medial wall fractures, disruption of the inferonasal support buttress creates a reconstructive challenge (Fig. 35.3). Access to the orbit can be achieved through different approaches including transconjunctival, transcaruncular, transnasal and transantral endoscopic [5–7]. External subciliary or direct rim incisions have also been described, but are not preferred due to increased risks of cicatricial eyelid changes and visibility

Supplementary Information The online version contains supplementary material available at https://doi.org/10.1007/978-3-031-63178-8_35.

T. H. Chen (✉) · M. B. Camacho · C. R. Dermarkarian · J. P. Tao
Divison of Oculofacial Plastic and Orbital Surgery, University of California, Irvine, CA, USA

J. Tao (ed.), *Efficient Oculofacial Surgery*, https://doi.org/10.1007/978-3-031-63178-8_35

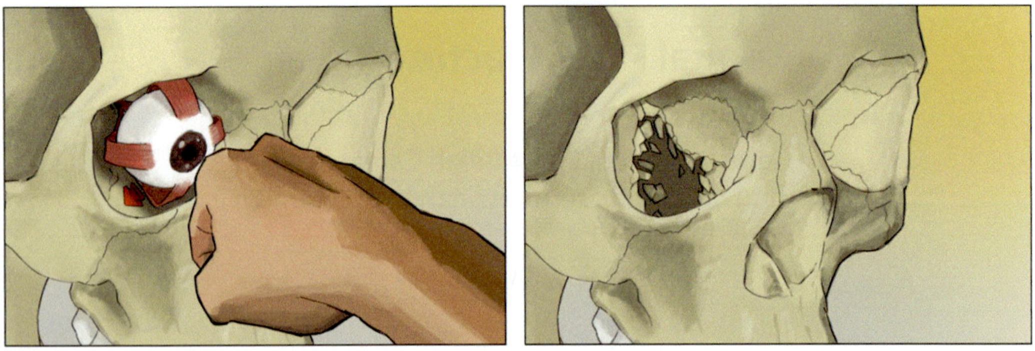

Fig. 35.1 Hydraulic mechanisms for the trauma. Increased pressure is transmitted from the soft tissues to the orbital walls

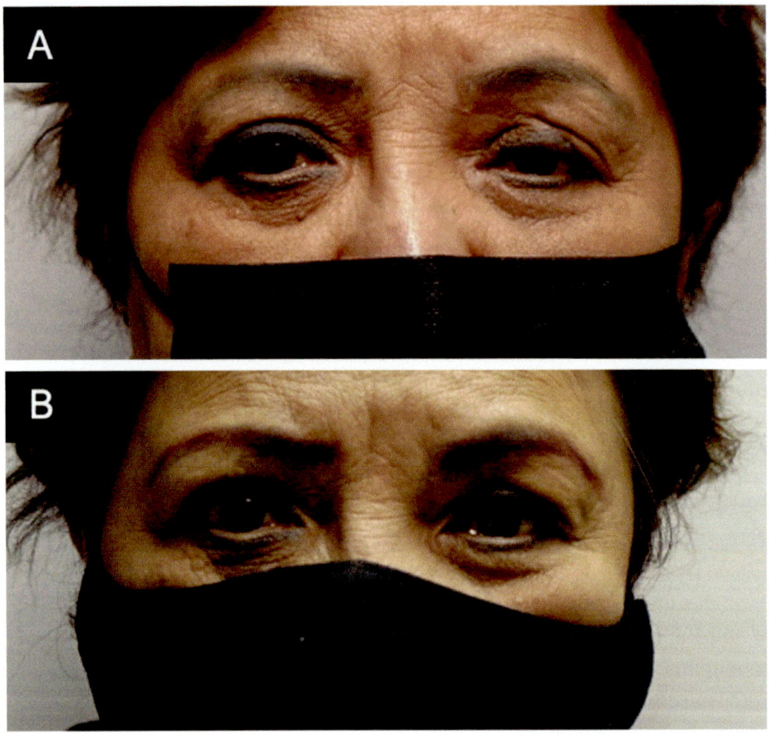

Fig. 35.2 **A** Preoperative clinical photo of patient with left orbital floor fracture causing enophthalmos. **B** Postoperative clinical photo after orbital floor fracture repair with improved globe projection and facial symmetry

of the scar [6]. The repair of combined floor and medial wall fractures are best approached from a combined inferior transconjunctival and medial orbitotomy (caruncular or medial canthal skin incision); this is detailed in another chapter.

A wide variety of implant options exist for orbital wall repair. These include silicone, hydroxyapatite, polytetrafluoroethylene (Teflon), titanium mesh, porous polyethylene, and porous polyethylene with embedded titanium [5, 8–15]. The authors prefer nonporous alloplastic thin implants, such as the nylon foil, because it is both flexible enough to conform to orbital walls yet rigid enough to provide support for the orbital

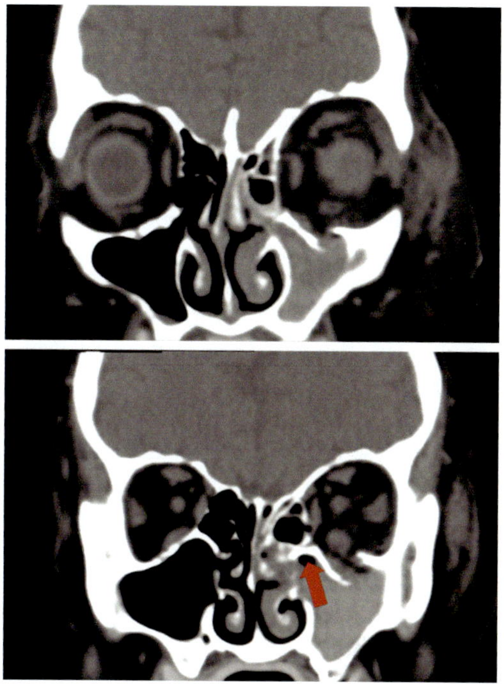

Fig. 35.3 Preoperative coronal CT of moderate sized left orbital floor fracture. The inferomedial strut shows mild displacement (arrow)

soft tissues. The nonporous nature prevents fibrovascular ingrowth and cicatricial changes of the extraocular muscles adjacent to the implant, lowering the risk of post-operative diplopia.

We describe a method of treating orbital floor fractures using 0.35-mm-thick nylon foil implant.

Technique (Video 35.1)

A lateral canthotomy is performed with a #15 blade and continued with straight iris scissors. The inferior ramus of the lateral canthal tendon is severed. The conjunctiva and retractor band are incised between the fornix and inferior aspect of the tarsus (Figs. 35.4 and 35.5). With the eyelid distracted inferiorly, dissection is continued down to the inferior orbital rim in the preseptal plane, where the inferior rim periosteum is incised with a #15 blade and separated from the bone using a periosteal elevator (Fig. 35.6).

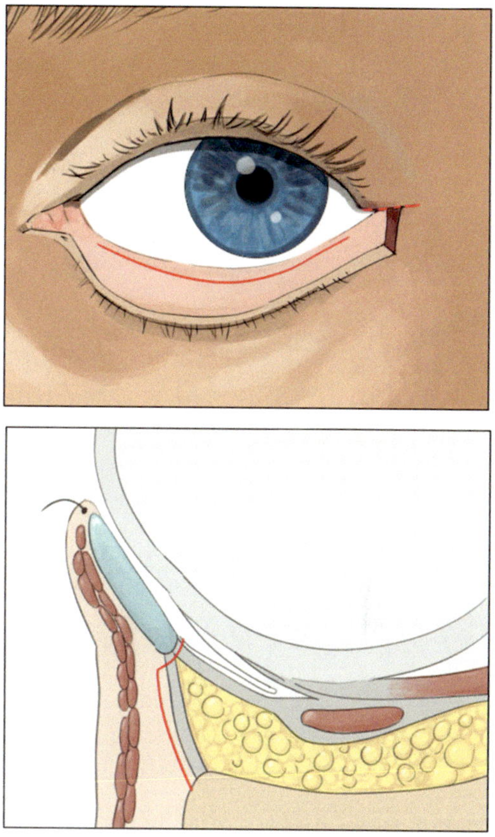

Fig. 35.4 Diagram of swinging eyelid inferior orbitotomy approach. Top shows canthotomy, cantholysis with transconjunctival incision (red). Bottom sagittal drawing depicts the dissection plane from the conjunctival incision to the orbital rim

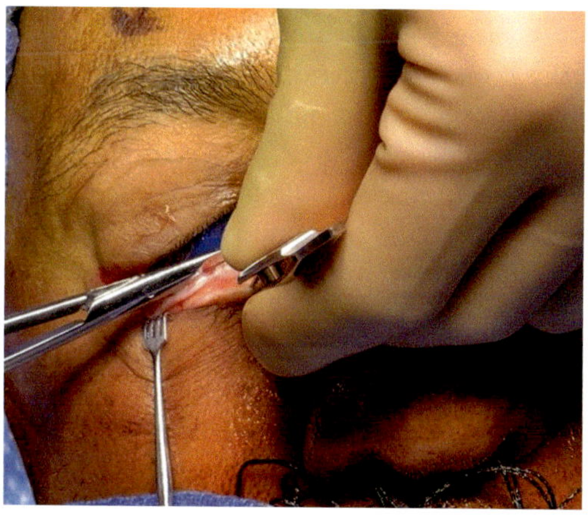

Fig. 35.5 The conjunctiva and retractor band are incised between the fornix and inferior aspect of the tarsus

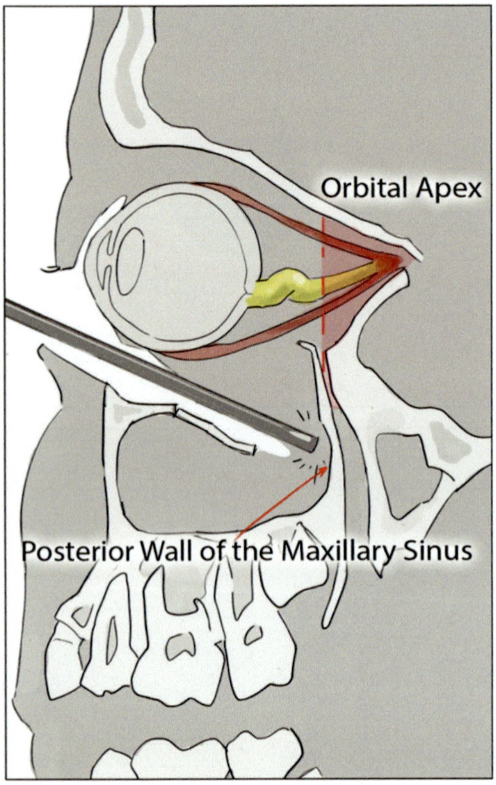

Fig. 35.6 Sagital diagram showing the posterior maxillary sinus as the landmark for the posterior depth of dissection when exposing the posterior ledge of the floor fracture

The orbital floor fracture is exposed, and orbital soft tissues are elevated from the fracture site in a hand-over-hand technique. Care is taken not to injure the infraorbital nerve. The authors often perform an initial slight out fracture especially if there is a concern for orbital soft tissue impingement. Out fractured bones do not necessarily need to be removed, but fragments extending medially toward the maxillary sinus ostium should generally be removed or repositioned to because these fragments may obstruct sinus outflow. The dissection is continued until the entire floor fracture perimeter is visualized. The posterior dissection should not proceed past the pterygopalatine fossa. The authors recommend entering the maxillary sinus through the floor defect and identifying the posterior sinus wall (Fig. 35.7). An imaginary line superior into orbit from the posterior maxillary sinus wall delimits the orbit apex, where dissection should not occur.

If the medial ledge of the floor defect cannot be adequately exposed, a small incision is created at the caruncle and sharp dissection is carried down to the periosteum, which is incised and elevated, thereby elevating the medial canthal tendon and lacrimal sac (Fig. 35.8).

Subperiosteal dissection is continued posteriorly to expose the perimeter of the medial wall fracture and orbital soft tissues are elevated from the fracture. The dissection is directed inferotemporal until continuous with the previous orbital floor dissection.

A 0.35-mm-thick nylon foil implant is cut in an oval pattern that adequately spans the fracture (Fig. 35.9). It is placed from the inferior transconjunctival approach. If medial floor defects need coverage the implant is advanced superomedial in the subperiosteal plane (Fig. 35.10). The implant is positioned to cover the perimeter of the fracture site (Fig. 35.11).

The medial caruncle incision may be left unsutured or is closed using absorbable 6-0 sutures. The inferior palpebral conjunctiva and retractor layer is closed with interrupted 6-0 chromic sutures (Fig. 35.12). The lateral canthus is reapproximated with 4-0 polyglactin suture by attaching free lateral tarsus to the lateral orbital tubercle. The skin is closed with 6-0 chromic sutures. The incisions are then dressed with antibiotic ointment.

Complications

Retrobulbar hemorrhage and subsequent orbital compartment syndrome is fortunately rare, but an important complication. If diagnosed, the surgical wounds should be opened emergently,

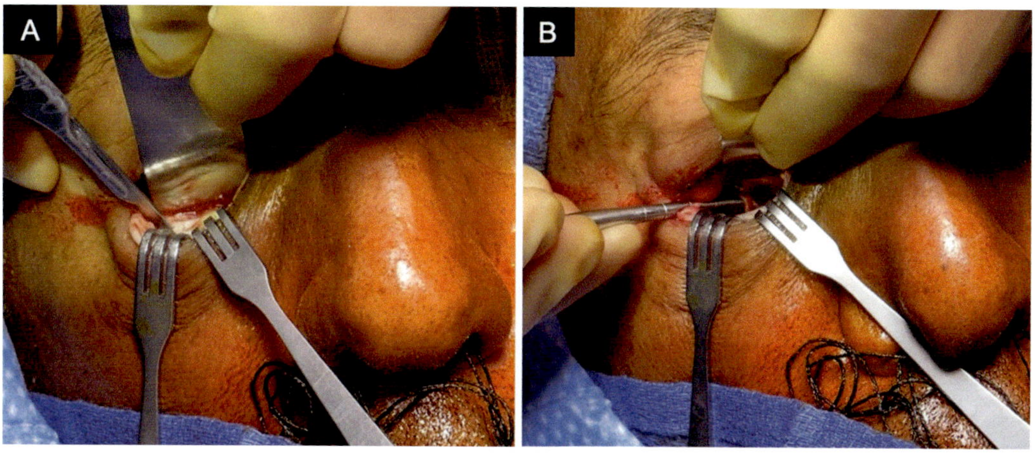

Fig. 35.7 With the eyelid distracted inferiorly, dissection is continued down to the inferior orbital rim in the septal plane, where **A**) the inferior rim periosteum is incised with a #15 blade and **B**) separated from the bone using a periosteal elevator

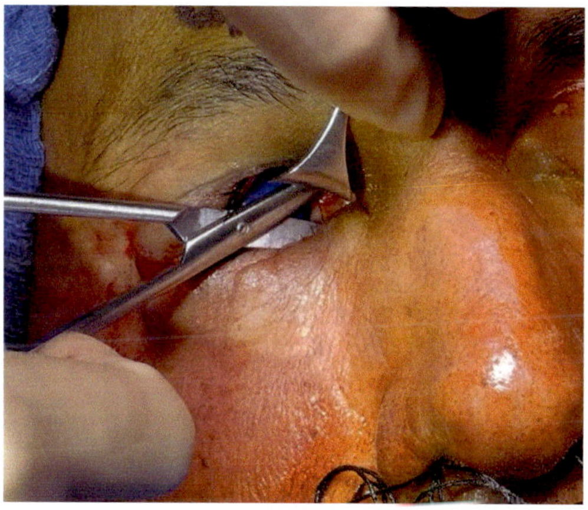

Fig. 35.8 In cases where the medial ledge of the floor cannot be adequately exposed from the inferior orbitotomy, a small incision is created at the caruncle for a medial orbitotomy that aids in orbit wall exposure

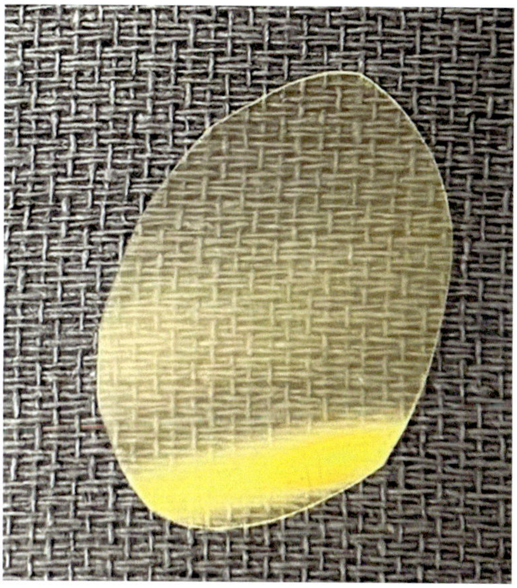

Fig. 35.9 The 0.35-mm-thick nylon implant is cut in an oval pattern

releasing the prior a canthotomy and cantholysis with or without an additional superior cantholysis.

Hypoesthesia is frequent after the injury yet can be exacerbated with orbital floor dissection. Other undesirable results of orbital fracture repair are persistent diplopia, enophthalmos, and eyelid malposition [16–19]. Secondary orbital reconstruction can be considered for cases of prolonged diplopia and enophthalmos. However,

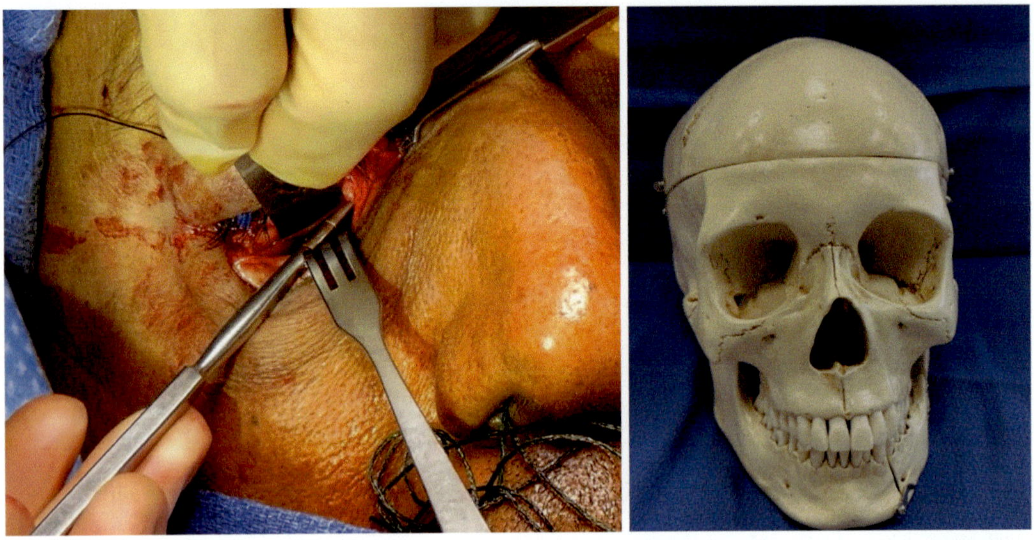

Fig. 35.10 The nylon foil implant is placed in the orbit from the inferior transconjunctival approach. Image right demonstrates nylon foil positioning on the orbital floor in a teaching skull

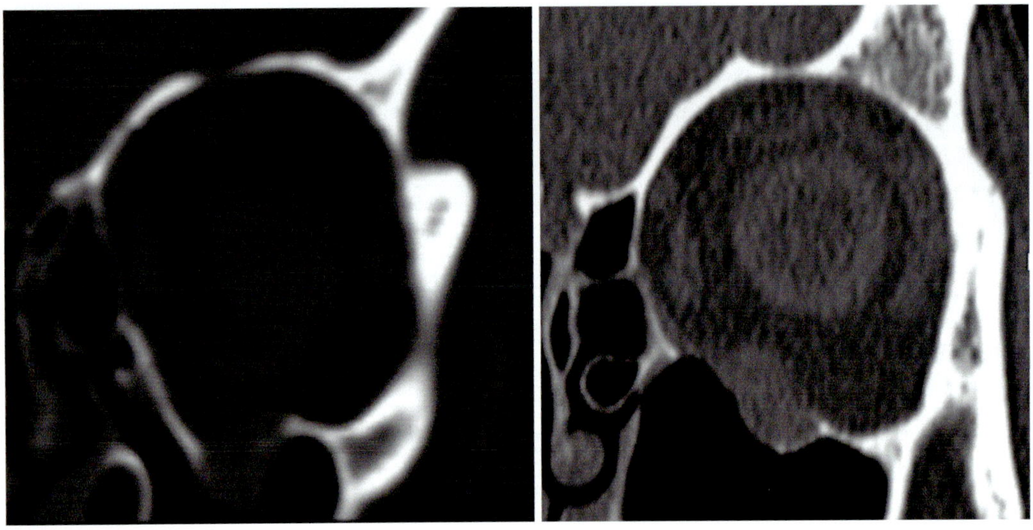

Fig. 35.11 Coronal CT before (left) and after (right) of a successful orbital floor fracture repair with a nylon foil implant

reoperation can be challenging due additional scar and should be considered at many months after the primary operation to allow for recovery. Eyelid malposition, such as lower eyelid retraction, entropion, or ectropion, may occur due to initial trauma or iatrogenic injury during surgery.

Conclusion

Orbital floor fractures occur commonly after trauma to the mid-face. Access the entire floor defect sometimes may benefit from an additional medial orbitotomy approach. With a non-adherent implant well seated in the orbit across

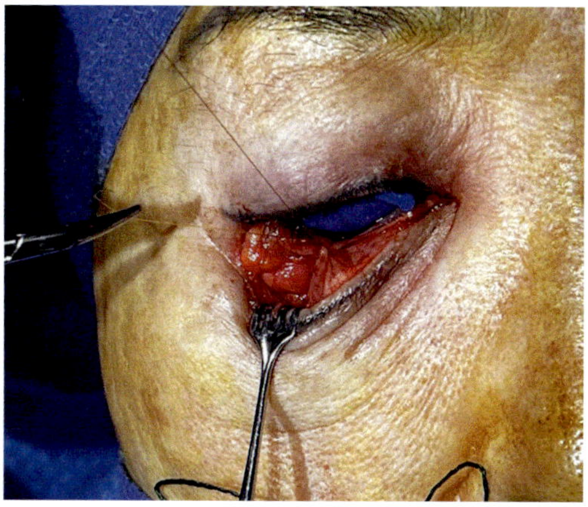

Fig. 35.12 The inferior palpebral conjunctiva and retractor layer is closed with interrupted 6-0 chromic sutures

the fracture site, and with good orbitotomy technique, normal facial appearance, normal eyelid position, and full extraocular motility can be achieved.

References

1. Raflo GT. Blow-in and blow-out fractures of the orbit: clinical correlations and proposed mechanisms. Ophthalmic Surg. 1984;15(2):114–9.
2. Jordan DR, Allen LH, White J, Harvey J, Pashby R, Esmaeli B. Intervention within days for some orbital floor fractures: the white-eyed blowout. Ophthalmic Plast Reconstr Surg. 1998;14(6):379–90. https://doi.org/10.1097/00002341-199811000-00001.
3. Grob S, Yonkers M, Tao J. Orbital fracture repair. Semin Plast Surg. 2017;31(1):31–9. https://doi.org/10.1055/s-0037-1598191.
4. Hawes MJ, Dortzbach RK. Surgery on orbital floor fractures. Influence of time of repair and fracture size. Ophthalmology. 1983;90(9):1066–70. https://doi.org/10.1016/s0161-6420(83)80049-9.
5. Nunery WR, Tao JP, Johl S. Nylon foil "wraparound" repair of combined orbital floor and medial wall fractures. Ophthalmic Plast Reconstr Surg. 2008;24(4):271–5. https://doi.org/10.1097/IOP.0b013e3181788de8.
6. Appling WD, Patrinely JR, Salzer TA. Transconjunctival approach vs subciliary skin-muscle flap approach for orbital fracture repair. Arch Otolaryngol Head Neck Surg. 1993;119(9):1000–7. https://doi.org/10.1001/archotol.1993.01880210090012.
7. Zhou G, Tu Y, Yu B, Wu W. Endoscopic repair of combined orbital floor and medial wall fractures involving the inferomedial strut. Eye (Lond). 2021;35(10):2763–70. https://doi.org/10.1038/s41433-020-01304-0.
8. Schön R, Metzger MC, Zizelmann C, Weyer N, Schmelzeisen R. Individually preformed titanium mesh implants for a true-to-original repair of orbital fractures. Int J Oral Maxillofac Surg. 2006;35(11):990–5. https://doi.org/10.1016/j.ijom.2006.06.018.
9. Choi AH, Barnholtz-Sloan JS, Kim JA. Effect of radiation therapy on survival in surgically resected retroperitoneal sarcoma: a propensity score-adjusted SEER analysis. Ann Oncol. 2012;23(9):2449–57. https://doi.org/10.1093/annonc/mdr616.
10. Su GW, Harris GJ. Combined inferior and medial surgical approaches and overlapping thin implants for orbital floor and medial wall fractures. Ophthalmic Plast Reconstr Surg. 2006;22(6):420–3. https://doi.org/10.1097/01.iop.0000242163.03589.0e.
11. Rubin PA, Bilyk JR, Shore JW. Orbital reconstruction using porous polyethylene sheets. Ophthalmology. 1994;101(10):1697–708. https://doi.org/10.1016/s0161-6420(94)31113-4.
12. Morrison AD, Sanderson RC, Moos KF. The use of silastic as an orbital implant for reconstruction of orbital wall defects: review of 311 cases treated over 20 years. J Oral Maxillofac Surg. 1995;53(4):412–7. https://doi.org/10.1016/0278-2391(95)90714-9.
13. Custer PL, Lind A, Trinkaus KM. Complications of supramid orbital implants. Ophthalmic Plast Reconstr Surg. 2003;19(1):62–7. https://doi.org/10.1097/00002341-200301000-00008.
14. Aronowitz JA, Freeman BS, Spira M. Long-term stability of Teflon orbital implants. Plast Reconstr Surg. 1986;78(2):166–73. https://doi.org/10.1097/00006534-198608000-00003.
15. Polley JW, Ringler SL. The use of Teflon in orbital floor reconstruction following blunt facial trauma: a 20-year experience. Plast Reconstr Surg 1987;79(1):39–43.
16. Biesman BS, Hornblass A, Lisman R, Kazlas M. Diplopia after surgical repair of orbital floor fractures. Ophthalmic Plast Reconstr Surg. 1996;12(1):9–16. https://doi.org/10.1097/00002341-199603000-00002. discussion 17.
17. Hoşal BM, Beatty RL. Diplopia and enophthalmos after surgical repair of blowout fracture. Orbit. 2002;21(1):27–33. https://doi.org/10.1076/orbi.21.1.27.2598.
18. Taher AA. Diplopia caused by orbital floor blowout fracture. Oral Surg Oral Med Oral Pathol. 1993;75(4):433–5. https://doi.org/10.1016/0030-4220(93)90165-z.
19. Jaquiéry C, Aeppli C, Cornelius P, Palmowsky A, Kunz C, Hammer B. Reconstruction of orbital wall defects: critical review of 72 patients. Int J Oral Maxillofac Surg. 2007;36(3):193–9. https://doi.org/10.1016/j.ijom.2006.11.002.

Medial Orbital Wall and Combined Medial Orbital Wall and Floor Fracture Repair

36

Ji Kwan Park, Nicholas R. Levergood, Avi Maun, and Hui Bae Harold Lee

Abstract

Combined medial wall and floor fractures, especially those that involve the maxilloethmoidal strut pose reconstructive challenges. Restoration of the natural support and contour inferomedially is essential to prevent enophthalmos, hypoglobus, or diplopia. Although different orbital implants are available, nonporous implants are preferred since they are associated with good results, low complications and low cost. In this chapter, the authors describe a nylon foil wraparound technique for combined orbital floor and medial wall fractures.

Keywords

Medial orbital wall fracture · Combined medial orbital wall and floor fractures · Wraparound technique · Orbital fracture · Blowout fracture · Maxilloethmoidal strut

Medial Orbital Wall Fractures

The medial orbital wall is formed by the frontal process of the maxilla, ethmoid bone, lacrimal bone, and sphenoid bone. The lamina papyracea of the ethmoid bone, measuring 0.2–0.4 mm in thickness, comprises the majority of the medial orbital wall [1]. The medial orbital wall is the second to the floor as the most common site in orbital wall fractures. Medial wall fractures can be isolated or associated with fractures of the orbital floor or zygomatic complex [2]. Assessment should include damage to the surrounding medial canthal tendon, medial rectus, superior oblique muscles, and lacrimal system [2]. The presence of orbital emphysema may indicate a small non-displaced medial wall fracture. Indications for surgery include medial rectus muscle entrapment, diplopia, and enophthalmos [3]. Typically, the surgery is performed

Supplementary Information The online version contains supplementary material available at https://doi.org/10.1007/978-3-031-63178-8_36.

J. K. Park · H. B. H. Lee (✉)
Oculofacial Plastic and Orbital Surgery, Carmel, IN 46280, USA
e-mail: huibae@gmail.com

J. K. Park
e-mail: jpark9@iuhealth.org

J. K. Park · H. B. H. Lee
Ascension St. Vincent Hospital, Indianapolis, IN 46260, USA

J. K. Park · N. R. Levergood · H. B. H. Lee
Department of Ophthalmology, Indiana University School of Medicine, Indianapolis, IN 46202, USA
e-mail: nlevergo@iu.edu

A. Maun
Brebeuf Jesuit Preparatory School, Indianapolis, IN 46268, USA

J. Tao (ed.), *Efficient Oculofacial Surgery*, https://doi.org/10.1007/978-3-031-63178-8_36

in 1–3 weeks following the injury and after the periorbital edema resolves [4, 5].

Two common surgical options to access the medial orbital wall fractures are the transcaruncular approach and the medial canthal cutaneous incision. The classic cutaneous Lynch incision is associated with a large scar and web formation [6]. A small cutaneous incision anterior to the medial canthal tendon may provide sufficiently wide intraoperative view across fractures of all sizes while minimizing external scar and webbing risks. The transcaruncular approach provides excellent cosmesis owing to the absence of a facial cutaneous incision. It affords adequate surgical exposure in many medial orbital wall fractures.

The surgical technique of medial orbital wall fracture repair using a transcaruncular approach is as follows [7–9].

1. The upper and lower eyelids are retracted using an eyelid speculum.
2. An incision is made using scissors at the mid caruncle through the conjunctiva and underlying Tenons.
3. Blunt dissection using curved Stevens or Wescott scissors is then performed in a plane between the Horner's muscle and medial orbital septum down to the posterior lacrimal crest. Gentle dissection with tips of the scissors over the posterior lacrimal crest in an anteroposterior direction may help identify the posterior side of the posterior lacrimal crest. A malleable retractor is used distract orbital contents laterally, while a Desmarres retractor or 4 pronged skin hook pull the medial caruncle incision toward the midline to expose the medial surgical cavity.
4. The periosteum is exposed and incised with a monopolar cautery. The periosteum is elevated. Subperiosteal dissection is best started superiorly on the thicker frontal bone since it is usually intact and is less prone than the inferior medial wall to collapse.
5. The anterior ethmoidal artery should be visualized to serve as a landmark of anterior–posterior depth of 2–2.5 cm from the lacrimal crest. If the artery obviates adequate exposure of the medial wall defect or subsequent implant seating or both, it may be severed with monopolar cautery.
6. A hand-over-hand technique is used to gradually restore herniated tissue to the orbit. A malleable retractor is placed into the fracture site to pull tissues back into the orbit then a second malleable retractor, suction tip, or elevator is inserted in a slightly deeper into the fracture site before completely withdrawing the first retractor. This technique is done until all herniated tissue from the sinuses has been repositioned into the orbit with a clear view of the fracture ledges. In some instances, especially in fractures that are beyond four weeks, mild further out fracturing of the broken bone with or without partial ethmoidectomy may be useful to expose the perimeter of the fracture.
7. The posterior ethmoidal artery is kept intact to mark the posterior extent of the dissection and avoid damage to the critical structures of the orbital apex, including the optic nerve. Aggressive dissection is avoided posterior to this artery; it is only 5–8 mm anterior to the optic canal.
8. The authors prefer a 0.35 mm thick SupraFOIL® nylon foil implant (S. Jackson Inc, Alexandria, VA) implant trimmed in an ovoid pattern to span across the medial orbital wall defect. The implant is introduced to the orbit. The implant can be introduced through a wound smaller than the width of the implant by folding the implant.
9. The i implant is then positioned in the subperiosteal plane covering the following key ledges: (1) the upper aspect of the medial wall fracture to prevent displacement into the ethmoid sinus. (2) The inferior ledge at the remaining posterior inferomedial strut. Care is given to keep the anterior border of the implant away from the posterior lacrimal crest by avoiding large implants or anterior placement of the implant. Additional anchoring screws or glue is not necessary. Ideally, the posterior aspect of

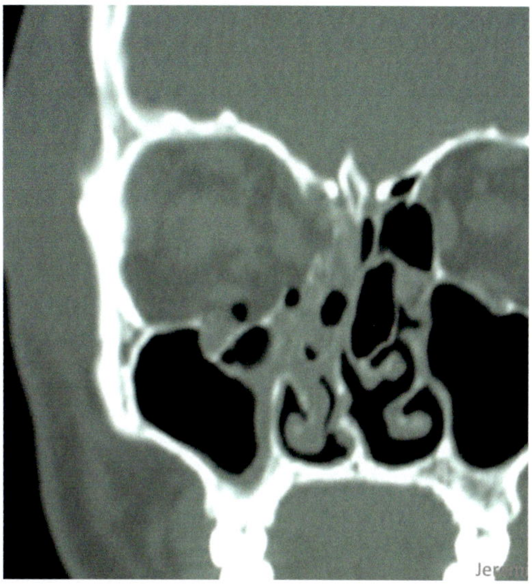

Fig. 36.1 Coronal CT image demonstrating a combined right orbital floor and medial wall fracture

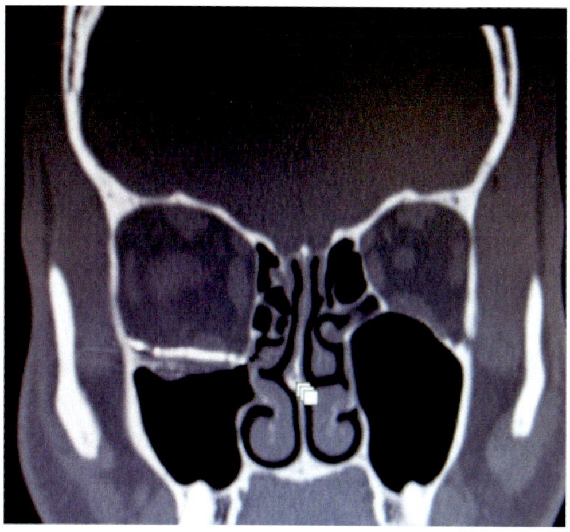

Fig. 36.2 Unnatural orbital contour after attempt at repair of a combined floor and medial wall fracture with a single implant introduced inferiorly. Note the box shape of the orbit with the implant herniating into the ethmoid sinus and no inferomedial orbital structural support

the implant should be visualized seated on the posterior perimeter of the fracture. However, owing to the dangers of dissection at the orbit apex and proximity of the optic nerve, visualization of the implant across the anterior, superior, and inferior perimeter may be sufficient.

10. At the end of the procedure, the caruncle and conjunctiva are closed with interrupted 6-0 chromic or 8-0 Vicryl sutures in a buried fashion or the wound is left unsutured.
11. In addition to routine postoperative instructions and wound care, patients are instructed to refrain from nose blowing for a minimum of 6 weeks after surgery. Eye muscle range-of-motion exercises (consisting of moving eyes in all fields of extreme gaze 5–10 times per day) are recommended in an attempt to maintain maximal extraocular muscle function.

Combined Medial Orbital Wall and Floor Fractures

Combined medial orbital wall and floor fractures present technical challenges and risk enophthalmos and persistent diplopia when not repaired adequately [10] (Fig. 36.1). Many surgeons attempt to address these fractures with a single inferior orbital implant. Unfortunately, since there is no medial support, this strategy is associated with incorrect implant position (often into the ethmoid sinus) with an unsatisfactory orbit contour that unsurprisingly is associated with globe dystopia or eye motility impairments or both (Fig. 36.2).

The inferomedial (a.k.a. maxilloethmoidal) orbital strut is a key structural component to recapture [10]. As such, single plate implant that spans the defects of the floor and medial wall from the medial orbital roof to the lateral edge of the orbital floor is ideal [11]. Alternatively, two overlapping nylon foil implants can be employed [12]. However, the use of multiple thin implants (e.g., nylon foil or porous polyethylene) may increase the risk of implant migration, imprecise coverage of a fractured inferomedial strut [12, 13]. Other mechanisms to maintain structural support include rim fixated devices. A straight titanium plate screwed at the rim and extending posteriorly can be used as support or vault for an overlying plate orbital wall implant. Alternatively, channeled plate implants with titanium plates extensions that can be secure to the rim with screws may have occasional roles.

A highly efficient method to recapture inferior medial orbital support is the wraparound technique. An inexpensive nylon foil implant well seated across both medial and floor fractures defects can recapture a natural orbital wall contour (Fig. 36.3). The wraparound has been associated with minimal resultant enophthalmos, globe dystopia, migration, or restrictive extraocular myopathy [10, 14–17].

Postoperative radiological imaging is superfluous with this and other direct visualization surgical techniques. The use of screws or tissue glue, especially along the orbital walls is discouraged as additional adhesions can impair extraocular muscle function [10].

The surgical steps in the repair of combined medial orbital wall and floor fracture using the nylon foil wraparound technique (SupraFOIL® implant, S. Jackson Inc, Alexandria, VA) are as follows [10, 14, 15] (Video 36.1):

1. A lateral canthotomy is performed with a #15 blade and straight iris scissors. The inferior ramus of the lateral canthal tendon is then cut to complete the inferior cantholysis.
2. The lower palpebral conjunctiva and lower eyelid retractors are incised between the fornix and the inferior aspect of the tarsus. With the eyelid distracted inferiorly with blunt Senn retractors, blunt dissection is continued down to the inferior orbital rim in the septal plane moving the orbicularis muscle anteriorly and orbital fat and orbital septum posteriorly with malleable retractors.
3. The periosteum at the orbital rim is then incised with a blade or monopolar cautery, and a subperiosteal dissection plane is achieved using a Cottle periosteal elevator.
4. The orbital floor fracture is exposed using a hand-over-hand technique as described

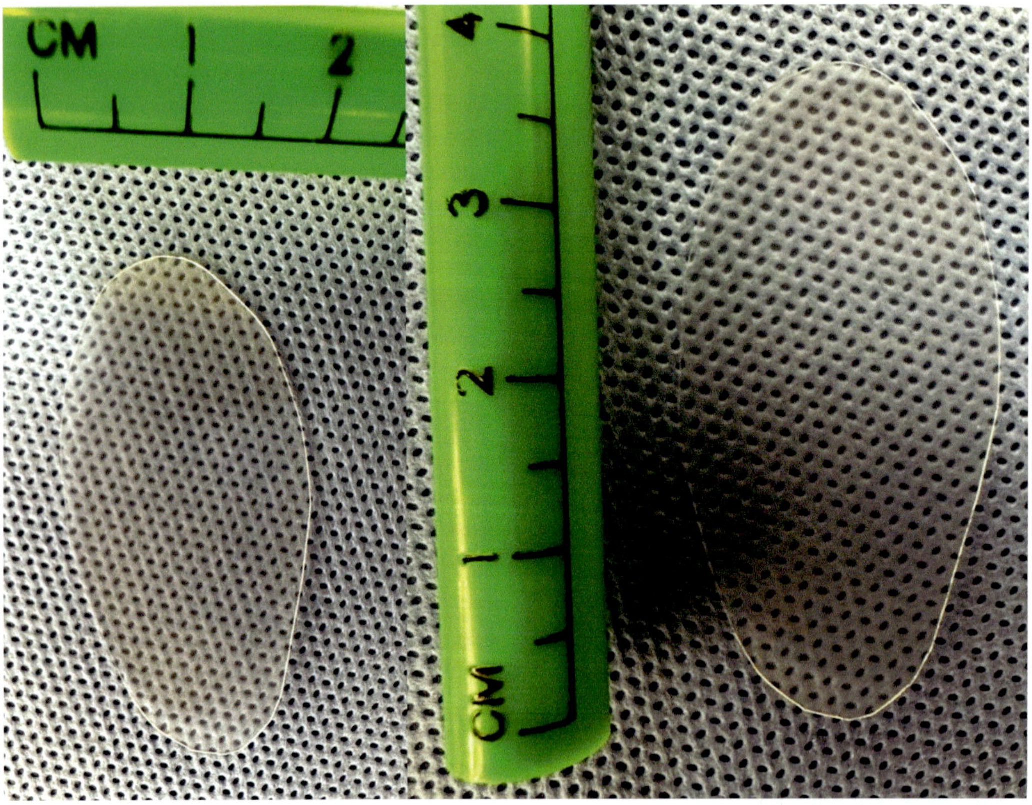

Fig. 36.3 Custom-shaped SupraFOIL® smooth nylon foil implant used in combined medial orbital wall and floor fracture repairs

previously. The dissection remains in the subperiosteal plane until the entire floor fracture perimeter is visualized laterally and posteriorly.

5. The medial wall is exposed through a medial orbitotomy incision (medial canthal cutaneous incision fashioned just anterior to the medial canthal tendon or a transcaruncular incision).
6. Sharp dissection is then carried to the periosteum at the posterior lacrimal crest, with monopolar cautery and the periosteum elevated with Cottle periosteal elevators to elevate the medial canthal tendon and the lacrimal sac. Caution is taken to avoid injury to the nasolacrimal outflow system. Damage to the inferior oblique is avoided to prevent postoperative vertical or torsional diplopia [18].
7. The perimeter of the medial wall fracture is exposed in a hand-over-hand technique. The orbital soft tissues are extracted from the fracture site. The medial dissection is made continuous with the previous orbital floor approach inferomedially and posteriorly.
8. The anterior ethmoidal artery is commonly ligated with monopolar cautery to allow proper implant seating at or above the level of the frontoethmoidal suture. The posterior ethmoidal artery is kept intact to mark the posterior extent of the dissection and avoid damage to the critical structures of the orbital apex including the optic nerve.
9. Following the elevation of all herniated orbital tissues from the fracture sites and identification of bare stable superior, posterior and lateral ledges of the bone under the intact periorbita, a 0.35-mm or 0.4 mm thick SupraFOIL® nylon foil implant is trimmed in an ovoid pattern to span across all fractures as a single unit (Fig. 36.2).
10. The implant is introduced to the orbit from the inferior transconjunctival approach and advanced superomedially in the subperiosteal plane. A temporary silk suture placed at the superior edge of the implant can be used as a lariat that is pulled with a hemostat introduced through the medial orbitotomy incision. The implant is then positioned at the following key ledges: (1) the upper aspect of the medial wall fracture (to prevent displacement in the ethmoid sinus; this typically corresponds to levels above the frontoethmoidal suture line in large medial wall fractures), (2) the posterior ledge of medial and floor fractures at the remaining posterior inferomedial strut; and (3) the lateral aspect of the floor defect (Figs. 36.4 and 36.5).
11. The orbital soft tissue is then to be verified free from impingement by the implant edges through direct visualization of the intact periorbita above the implant and bare bone underneath throughout the defects. A properly positioned implant at the key ledges is confirmed to be firmly seated to avoid any migration or displacement (Figs. 36.6 and 36.7).
12. If a medial canthus cutaneous incision was used, it is closed with a 5-0 polyglactin suture that engages the periorbital overlying the medial canthal tendon on a deep pass to ensure a snug, posterior and medial medial

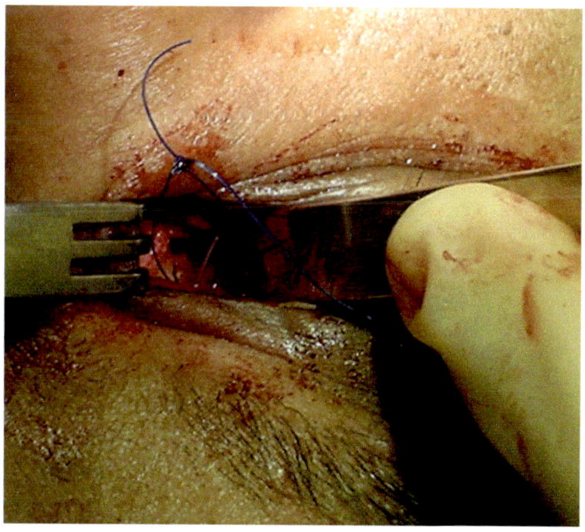

Fig. 36.4 Nylon foil implant seated across a combined floor and medial wall defect with the anterio medial aspect of the implant visualized through the medial orbitotomy incision

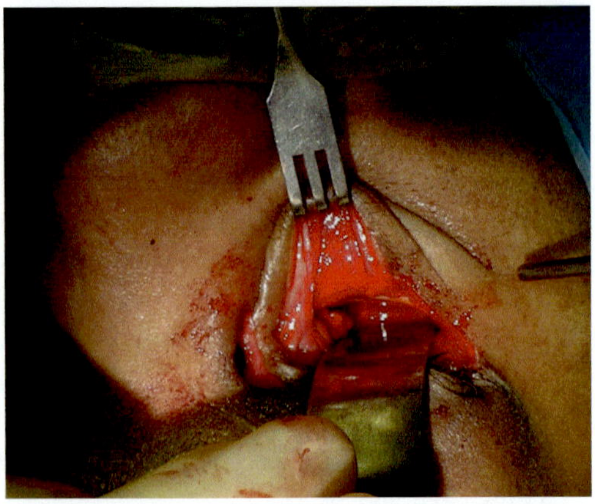

Fig. 36.5 Nylon foil wraparound implant. Inferior aspect of the well seated implant visible through the inferior orbitotomy wound

eyelid commisure. The skin is then closed with 6-0 mild chromic or 5-0 fast-absorbing gut sutures. If a caruncle incision was used, it may be left unsutured or is closed with a single 6-0 chromic suture.

13. The inferior palpebral conjunctiva is then closed without advancing the lower eyelid retractors using two or three interrupted 6-0 chromic sutures.
14. The free inferior lateral tarsus is reattached to the intact upper limb of the lateral canthal tendon as well as the lateral rim periosteum with 4-0 polyglactin suture. The skin is closed with 5-0 or 6-0 absorbing gut suture.
15. In addition to routine postoperative instructions and wound care, patients are instructed to refrain from nose blowing for a minimum of 6 weeks after surgery. Eye muscle range-of-motion exercises (consisting of moving eyes in all fields of extreme gaze 5–10 times per day) are routinely recommended in an attempt to maintain extraocular motility.

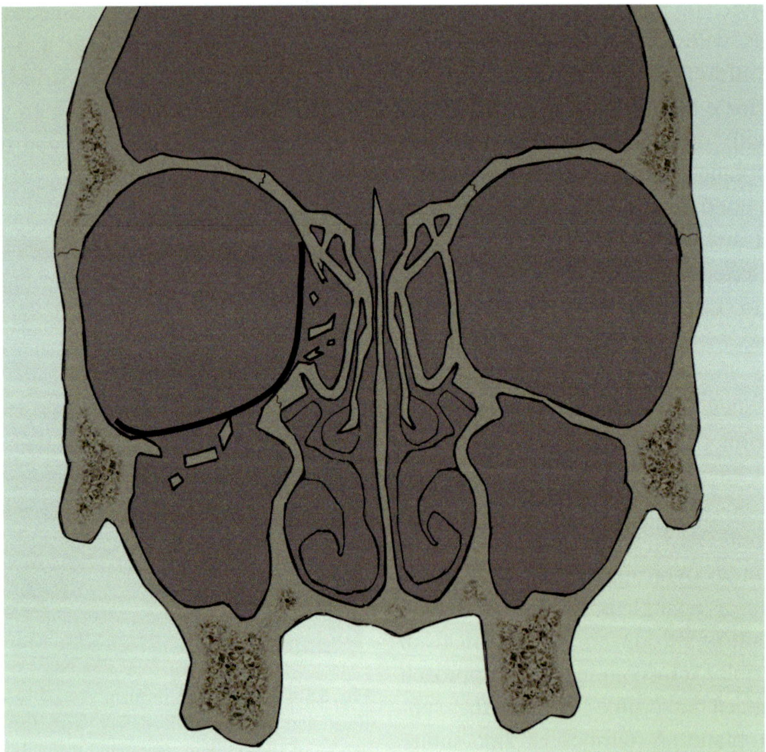

Fig. 36.6 Schematic diagram of a "wraparound" implant that provides complete coverage of all fractures and re-establishment of orbital wall shape and curvature

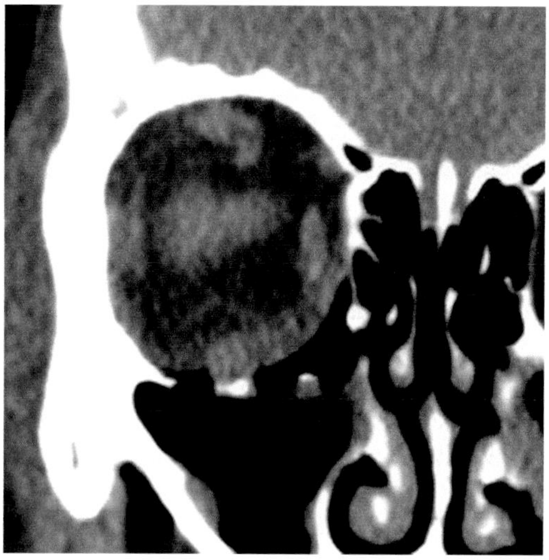

Fig. 36.7 Postoperative coronal CT demonstrating a nylon foil wraparound implant recapturing the normal orbital contours

Additional Surgical Tips

Visualization of the full extent of the orbital fracture margin with complete release and repositioning of the herniated orbital tissue is critical [11]. The combined approach described exposes and reduces orbital contents with an intact periorbita at the anterior, lateral, superior, and posterior extents of the medial orbital wall and floor fractures. Aggressive intraorbital dissection with a transection rather than reduction of herniated orbital tissues may result in hypoglobus, enophthalmos, and diplopia. When wide subperiosteal exposure and intraoperative visualization are achieved, postoperative neuroimaging is superfluous. The wide exposure also assists in the positioning of the implant at the subperiosteal plane along the stable ledges of the bone, which may negate the need for intraoperative forced ductions. A strong superior, posterior and lateral support for the implant is necessary to prevent complications [11]. Correct sizing of the implant is also important to avoid damage to the orbital tissues or muscle entrapment. Proper sizing of the implant also avoids protrusion into the sinuses, orbital rim, or the nasolacrimal crest, or causes pressures around critical structures such as the optic nerve, infraorbital nerve, inferior oblique muscle origin, medial canthal tendon, and the lacrimal sac [10, 19]. Lastly, if the medial orbital wall and the orbital floor are associated with larger facial fractures such as naso-orbitoethmoid complex, zygomaticomaxillary complex, or Le Forte fractures involving the medial and lateral buttress, then these facial fractures should be addressed to allow complete anatomic reduction of the medial orbital wall and floor.

Types of Orbital Implants

While a multitude of orbital implants available [4, 5, 20]. Each implant material poses a certain complication risk regarding various parameters such as the surface (porous versus nonporous), biocompatibility, and ease of use [14, 15]. Decisions on implant selection are commonly influenced by surgeon experience and implant availability [15].

Titanium mesh implants may provide adequate strength while being malleable to cover large defects. Some surgeons utilize these implants customized using preoperative stereolithography constructed to replicate the natural contour of the medial and orbital floor [18]. However, the tissue ingrowth and cicatrization between the gratings may contribute to restrictive strabismus causing orbital adherence syndrome, and removal is extremely difficult [3, 21, 22]. The orbital adherence syndrome from these implants also results in postoperative diplopia and enophthalmos [21].

Porous polyethylene (PPE) implants can be prefabricated to cover defects in the combined orbital medial wall and floor fractures. However, the rigidity and porous features may be undesirable. PPE-imbedded titanium implants manufactured in a pre-shaped design are also available but are associated with high cost. Three versions of these implants include: porous on both sides (MTM), nonporous (barrier) on both sides, or combination (MTB) with a barrier surface placed on the orbital side, preventing soft tissue adherence [18]. The titanium-reinforced

PPE implants allow fixation into the bone that rarely may be beneficial [22]. The nonporous barrier may limit tissue ingrowth, unlike in bare titanium implants. As state previously, these implants are costly and may not add meaningful, if any, benefit [20].

The SupraFOIL® nylon foil implant (S. Jackson Inc., Alexandria, VA) is a nonporous implant that may obviate orbital adherence syndrome and postoperative enophthalmos even in large orbital fractures. Its nonadherent, pliable features allow support for orbital tissues in a natural contour while minimizing soft tissue adherence that may limit eye motility [10, 14–16].

Hemorrhage into a nylon foil implant scar capsule, orbital infection, and enophthalmos have been reported, postoperative implant complications are rare. Several large series report excellent results with normal globe projection, full extraocular motility, and no diplopia [10, 14, 20, 23]. Importantly, the intracapsular hemorrhages reported were with the use of nylon implants much thicker than 0.4 mm [14, 24]. Thin (0.35 or 0.4 mm) nylon foil may have a lower incidence of these bleeding complications yet provide sufficient support for the orbit, even complete loss of inferomedial strut support [10, 14–17].

Resorbable sheets such as poly-l/d-lactide, polyglactin, and polydioxanone are pliable and may be contoured around the defect. However, the long-term stability and support of these implants are uncertain [13]. Other alloplastic implants used in the repair of the medial wall and orbital floor fractures include polyamide, Teflon, Silastic sheets, Marlex mesh, hydroxyapatite, and methylmethacrylate. Patient-specific implants made using 3D printers provide no additional benefit in postoperative orbital volume reduction but are associated with extremely high cost and extended production time [25].

Allogenic materials include irradiated bone, lyophilized dura, lyophilized cartilage, fascia lata, and bovine bone. Autologous materials include bone, cartilage, fascia lata, and periosteum [10, 26–32]. Although most autograft materials are biocompatible donor site morbidity, increased operative time and cost, difficulty in adjusting shapes, and resorption over time are disadvantages [22]. Moreover, these biologic options may adhere to the extra ocular muscles or their surrounding fascial components that may restrict eye motility.

Complications

Complications of orbital fracture repair include blindness, diplopia, mydriasis, and implant-related issues such as infection, extrusion, and cicatricial eyelid changes. Other complications include fistula formation, implant migration, extraocular entrapment, globe elevation, retrobulbar hemorrhage, cyst formation, and dacryocystitis [24, 33–40]. Although transient diplopia due to edema is common and typically resolves within weeks, persistent diplopia may be related to implant positioning, muscle damage from the trauma, fibrosis, or nerve paresis [22]. Delayed surgery and older age may be risk factors for postoperative diplopia [41]. Enophthalmos may occur despite appropriate implant positions due to orbital fat atrophy and damage to the intraorbital fascial septae [42]. Postoperative eyelid malposition after orbital fracture surgeries include lower eyelid retraction, lower eyelid flattening, ectropion, entropion, medial and lateral canthal dystopias [43, 44]. Care and proper surgical planes should be utilized in the manipulation of the eyelid and orbital tissues. Many postoperative complications evolve or improve over time [4, 5, 10].

Summary

Combined medial orbital wall and floor fractures are challenging. A nylon foil wraparound technique may minimize morbidity with maximal surgical efficiency and minimal cost. Good surgical exposure from a combined medial and inferior and medial orbitotomy with direct visualization of implant coverage of the orbital bony defects achieves excellent results. Enophthalmos and diplopia are rare complications.

References

1. Foster JA, Carter KD, Durairaj VD, Kavanagh MC, Korn BS, Nelson CC, et al. Chapter 1. Orbital Anatomy. In: Basic and Clinical Science Course. San Francisco: California: American Academy of Ophthalmology; 2017. p. 8–10. (Orbit, Eyelids, and Lacrimal System; vol. 7).
2. Liss J, Stefko ST, Chung WL. Orbital surgery: state of the art. Oral Maxillofac Surg Clin. 2010;22(1):59–71.
3. Thiagarajah C, Kersten RC. Medial wall fracture: an update. Craniomaxillofac Trauma Reconstr. 2009;2(3–4):135–9.
4. Jain MK, Alexander M. The need of postoperative radiographs in maxillofacial fractures—a prospective multicentric study. Br J Oral Maxillofac Surg. 2009;47(7):525–9.
5. Carpenter D, Shammas R, Honeybrook A, Brown CS, Chapurin N, Woodard CR. The role of postoperative imaging after orbital floor fracture repair. Craniomaxillofac Trauma Reconstr. 2018;11(2):96–101.
6. Campbell AA, Grob SR, Yoon MK. Novel surgical approaches to the orbit. Middle East Afr J Ophthalmol. 2015;22(4):435.
7. Balch KC. The transcaruncular approach to the medial orbit and ethmoid sinus. A cosmetically superior option to the cutaneous (Lynch) incision. Facial Plast Surg Clin North Am. 1998;6:71–7.
8. Nguyen DC, Shahzad F, Snyder-Warwick A, Patel KB, Woo AS. Transcaruncular approach for treatment of medial wall and large orbital blowout fractures. Craniomaxillofac Trauma Reconstr. 2016;9(1):046–54.
9. Lai PC, Liao SL, Jou JR, Hou PK. Transcaruncular approach for the management of frontoethmoid mucoceles. Br J Ophthalmol. 2003;87(6):699–703.
10. Nunery WR, Tao JP, Johl S. Nylon foil "wraparound" repair of combined orbital floor and medial wall fractures. Ophthalmic Plast Reconstr Surg. 2008;24(4):271–5.
11. Cho RI, Davies BW. Combined orbital floor and medial wall fractures involving the inferomedial strut: repair technique and case series using preshaped porous polyethylene/titanium implants. Craniomaxillofac Trauma Reconstr. 2013;6(3):161–9.
12. Su GW, Harris GJ. Combined inferior and medial surgical approaches and overlapping thin implants for orbital floor and medial wall fractures. Ophthalmic Plast Reconstr Surg. 2006;22(6):420–3.
13. Choi JC, Fleming JC, Aitken PA, Shore JW. Porous polyethylene channel implants: a modified porous polyethylene sheet implant designed for repairs of large and complex orbital wall fractures. Ophthalmic Plast Reconstr Surg. 1999;15(1):56–66.
14. Park DJ, Garibaldi DC, Iliff NT, Grant MP, Merbs SL. Smooth nylon foil (SupraFOIL) orbital implants in orbital fractures: a case series of 181 patients. Ophthalmic Plast Reconstr Surg. 2008;24(4):266–70.
15. Campbell BC, Shipchandler TZ, Ting JY, Vernon D, Torabi RS, Miller M, Lee HH. Wraparound nylon foil implant for isolated orbital floor fractures. Am J Otolaryngol. 2022;43(1): 103229.
16. Grob S, Yonkers M, Tao J. Orbital fracture repair. Semin Plastic Surg. 2017;31(01):31–9.
17. Prendes MA, Gudgel B, Kassa EB, Todd AM, Fu R, Abou-Jaoude M, Timoney PJ, Shipchandler TZ, Nunery WR, Lee HH. Intracapsular hemorrhage rates in non-fixated nylon sheet orbital implants for orbital fracture management. Am J Otolaryngol. 2019;40(4):509–11.
18. Scolozzi P, Momjian A, Heuberger J, Andersen E, Broome M, Terzic A, Jaques B. Accuracy and predictability in use of AO three-dimensionally preformed titanium mesh plates for posttraumatic orbital reconstruction: a pilot study. J Craniofac Surg. 2009;20(4):1108–13.
19. Jordan D, Mawn L. Chapter 12: Blowout fractures of the orbit. In: Black EH, Nesi FA, Calvano CJ, Gladstone GJ, Levine MR, editors. Smith and Nesi's ophthalmic plastic and reconstructive surgery. 3rd ed. New York: Springer; 2012. p. 243–63.
20. Ng SG, Madill SA, Inkster CF, Maloof AJ, Leatherbarrow B. Medpor porous polyethylene implants in orbital blowout fracture repair. Eye. 2001;15(5):578–82.
21. Lee HB, Nunery WR. Orbital adherence syndrome secondary to titanium implant material. Ophthalmic Plast Reconstr Surg. 2009;25(1):33–6.
22. Boyette JR, Pemberton JD, Bonilla-Velez J. Management of orbital fractures: challenges and solutions. Clin Ophthalmol. 2015;9:2127.
23. Shah HA, Shipchandler T, Vernon D, Baumanis M, Chan D, Nunery WR, Lee HB. Extra-ocular movement restriction and diplopia following orbital fracture repair. Am J Otolaryngol. 2018;39(1):34–6.
24. Custer PL, Lind A, Trinkaus KM. Complications of supramid orbital implants. Ophthalmic Plast Reconstr Surg. 2003;19(1):62–7.
25. Maher DI, Hall AJ, Gwini S, Artsi EB. Patient-specific implants for orbital fractures: a systematic review. Ophthalmic Plast Reconstr Surg. 2022;38(5):417–24.
26. Smith B, Putterman AM. Fixation of orbital floor implants: description of a simple technique. Arch Ophthalmol. 1970;83(5):598.
27. Chang SH, Custer PL, Mohadjer Y, Scott E. Use of Lorenz titanium implants in orbital fracture repair. Ophthalmic Plast Reconstr Surg. 2009;25(2):119–22.
28. Taban M, Nakra T, Mancini R, Douglas RS, Goldberg RA. Orbital wall fracture repair using Seprafilm. Ophthalmic Plast Reconstr Surg. 2009;25(3):211–4.
29. Büchel P, Rahal A, Seto I, Iizuka T. Reconstruction of orbital floor fracture with polyglactin 910/polydioxanon patch (ethisorb): a retrospective study. J Oral Maxillofac Surg. 2005;63(5):646–50.
30. Baumann A, Burggasser G, Gauss N, Ewers R. Orbital floor reconstruction with an alloplastic resorbable polydioxanone sheet. Int J Oral Maxillofac Surg. 2002;31(4):367–73.

31. Loftfield K, Jordan DR, Fowler J, Anderson RL. Orbital cyst formation associated with Gelfilm use. Ophthalmic Plast Reconstr Surg. 1987;3(3):187–91.
32. Mok D, Lessard L, Cordoba C, Harris PG, Nikolis A. A review of materials currently used in orbital floor reconstruction. Canadian Journal of Plastic Surgery. 2004;12(3):134–40.
33. Liu D. Blindness after blow-out fracture repair. Ophthalmic Plast Reconstr Surg. 1994;10(3):206–10.
34. Girotto JA, Gamble WB, Robertson B, Redett R, Muehlberger T, Mayer M, Zinreich J, Iliff N, Miller N, Manson PN. Blindness after reduction of facial fractures. Plast Reconstr Surg. 1998;102(6):1821–34.
35. Bodker FS, Cytryn AS, Putterman AM, Marschall MA. Postoperative mydriasis after repair of orbital floor fracture. Am J Ophthalmol. 1993;115(3):372–5.
36. Okinaka Y, Hara J, Takahashi M. Orbital blowout fracture with persistent mobility deficit due to fibrosis of the inferior rectus muscle and perimuscular tissue. Annals of Otology, Rhinology & Laryngology. 1999;108(12):1174–6.
37. Jordan DR, Onge PS, Anderson RL, Patrinely JR, Nerad JA. Complications associated with alloplastic implants used in orbital fracture repair. Ophthalmology. 1992;99(10):1600–8.
38. Folkestad L, Westin T. Long-term sequelae after surgery for orbital floor fractures. Otolaryngol Head Neck Surg. 1999;120(6):914–21.
39. Morrison AD, Sanderson RC, Moos KF. The use of silastic as an orbital implant for reconstruction of orbital wall defects: review of 311 cases treated over 20 years. J Oral Maxillofac Surg. 1995;53(4):412–7.
40. Polley JW, Ringler SL. The use of Teflon in orbital floor reconstruction following blunt facial trauma: a 20-year experience. Plast Reconstr Surg. 1987;79(1):39–43.
41. Hossal BM, Beatty RL. Diplopia and enophthalmos after surgical repair of blowout fracture. Orbit. 2002;21(1):27–33.
42. Cole P, Kaufman Y, Hollier L. Principles of facial trauma: orbital fracture management. Journal of Craniofacial Surgery. 2009;20(1):101–4.
43. Kesselring AG, Promes P, Strabbing EM, van der Wal KG, Koudstaal MJ. Lower eyelid malposition following orbital fracture surgery: a retrospective analysis based on 198 surgeries. Craniomaxillofac Trauma Reconstr. 2016;9(2):109–12.
44. Xing Y, Guo Y, Ding X, Li J, Lin M. Eyelid malposition after orbital fracture surgery. Ann Eye Sci. 2020;5:38–38.

Zygomaticomaxillary Complex Fracture Repair

37

Kimberly K. Nguyen, Davin C. Ashraf, Natalie A. Krane, Shravani Mikkilineni, and John D. Ng

Abstract

The zygoma is a thick quadrangular bone that articulates with the frontal, sphenoid, temporal, and maxillary bones and is commonly injured due to its prominence and location. Depending on the extent and location of the injuries, fractures of the zygomaticomaxillary complex can present with various signs and symptoms, resulting in functional and cosmetic complications. The primary goals of surgical intervention are to restore facial symmetry and projection as well as orbital volume and globe position. Importantly, the fracture sites should be widely exposed to obtain adequate reduction while minimizing conspicuous facial scarring. In this chapter, the authors' describe a lateral canthal, transconjunctival, combined with gingivobuccal incisions surgical approach for the repair of zygomaticomaxillary complex fractures.

Keywords

Zygomaticomaxillary complex fracture · Tripod fracture · Orbital fracture · Zygomatic arch · Facial fracture

Introduction

The zygoma is a thick quadrangular bone that articulates with the frontal, sphenoid, temporal, and maxillary bones to create the frontozygomatic, zygomaticosphenoid, zygomaticotemporal, and zygomaticomaxillary sutures, respectively [1–3]. It contributes to the inferior and lateral orbital walls and provides protection for the orbit. It also contributes to the facial contour, namely the malar eminence [4]. Due to its anterolateral projection, it dissipates forces along the cranial base to provide stability and strength to the midface [1]. Given its prominence and location, it is one of the most injured facial bones, comprising approximately 40–57% of facial fractures [1, 2].

Zygomaticomaxillary complex (ZMC) fractures are typically closed, displaced, and

Supplementary Information The online version contains supplementary material available at https://doi.org/10.1007/978-3-031-63178-8_37.

K. K. Nguyen · D. C. Ashraf · J. D. Ng (✉)
Casey Eye Institute Oculofacial Plastic, Orbital and Reconstructive Surgery Division, Oregon Health and Science University, Portland, OR, USA
e-mail: ngj@ohsu.edu

N. A. Krane
ENT/Otolaryngology Facial Plastic Surgery, Oregon Health and Science University, Portland, OR, USA

S. Mikkilineni
Consultants in Ophthalmic and Facial Plastic Surgery, PC, Detroit, MI, USA

J. Tao (ed.), *Efficient Oculofacial Surgery*, https://doi.org/10.1007/978-3-031-63178-8_37

noncomminuted. ZMC fractures often result in midface depression and malar asymmetry, depending on the mechanism of trauma [5]. A "tripod fracture" involves disruption at the inferior and lateral orbital rims, zygomaticomaxillary buttress, and zygomatic arch, compared to a "tetrapod fracture" that involves fracture of all four suture lines [3, 5].

Diagnosis and Clinical Evaluation

ZMC fractures may present with various signs and symptoms depending on the extent and location of the injuries. It is important to obtain a thorough history of the mechanism of injury and obtain an accurate physical examination, evaluating for facial asymmetry or deformity, globe position, and midface stability [1]. Orbital floor fractures may present with diplopia, ocular motility deficits, changes in globe position (e.g. enophthalmos), oculocardiac reflex, infraorbital paresthesia, or muscle entrapment [2, 6]. Displacement of the zygoma posteriorly or inferiorly can increase or decrease the orbital cavity volume, respectively [2]. Depression of the zygomatic arch can be concealed by significant soft tissue swelling but may be detected by the clinical finding of trismus due to collision of the coronoid process or temporalis muscle with the depressed arch [2]. The lateral canthal tendon can also be displaced leading to rounding of the lateral canthus [2]. Other nonspecific signs and symptoms related to trauma include periorbital hematoma or ecchymosis, pain, edema, palpable step-offs, subconjunctival hemorrhage, and epistaxis [2, 6]. Though clinical examination is important, the gold standard for determining the extent of bone injury and displacement is radiographic evaluation.

Imaging and Determining Extent of Fractures

Facial computed tomography (CT) is the most pertinent imaging modality to assess the extent of the fractures (Fig. 37.1) [1]. The axial view is used to assess the zygomatic projection by comparing the anteroposterior and angular dimensions to the unaffected side at the level of the clivus. The coronal view is used to evaluate the zygomatic height while the zygomatic width can be adequately assessed with both the axial and coronal views. Three-dimensional (3D) reconstruction allows for evaluation of the angular

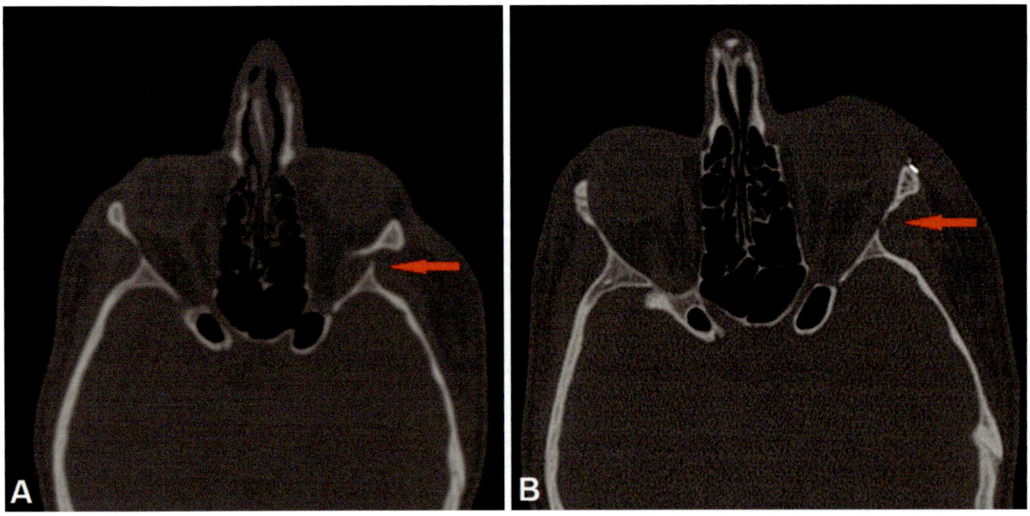

Fig. 37.1 (**A**) Preoperative axial non-contrast computed tomography (CT) scan demonstrated severe displacement of the lateral orbital wall at the zygomaticosphenoid (ZS) suture with resultant impingement of the lateral rectus. (**B**) Postoperative axial non-contrast CT scan demonstrating appropriate reduction of the ZS suture

displacement of the zygoma in the medial and lateral dimension [4].

Translating a 3D fracture into a two-dimensional (2D) imaging modality can be difficult. Additional tools such as computer-aided design/computer-aided manufacturing (CAD/CAM) have allowed for the digital reconstruction of distorted anatomy due to traumatic injury. This allows a 3D reconstructed image to formulate a virtual surgical plan and custom fixation guides [1, 5].

Less commonly used imaging modalities include plain radiographs and ultrasonography [2]. These are essentially obsolete today since CT is nearly ubiquitous at emergency centers.

Surgical Planning

Conservative management can be considered when there is minimal bone displacement and no or minimal symptoms, and especially when there exist medical contraindications to surgery [5]. The primary goals of surgical management are to restore facial symmetry and projection and to restore the orbital volume and globe position [1]. Surgical success depends on the use of optimal approaches and good technique to adequately expose and reduce these fractures [4, 7].

ZMC fractures can be repaired via closed reduction alone or open reduction with internal fixation. Closed reduction alone may be appropriate in cases of isolated, dislocated fractures of the zygomatic arch [6]. However, it can be difficult to assess for adequate reduction of fractures and often results in poor cosmesis [3]. For patients requiring open reduction, access points depend upon which buttresses need repair.

The Gillies' approach is a temporal approach which allows for access to the zygomatic arch. This technique preserves cosmesis as it does not leave facial scars; however, it does not allow for access to the orbit which can result in incomplete reduction. In contrast, the bicoronal scalp approach provides exposure to the lateral orbit and zygoma, but it has limited access to the inferior and medial orbit. It results in a large scalp incision scar with scalp hypoesthesia and the risk of damage to the temporal branch of the facial nerve.

The lateral and inferior buttresses can be accessed via a swinging eyelid approach with a lateral canthotomy and transconjunctival incision. An eyelid crease incision may be utilized to reach the zygomatic arch and frontozygomatic suture if additional exposure is required, with excellent cosmesis. The inferior orbital rim, orbital floor, and frontozygomatic area can also be accessed via a subciliary incision of the entire lower eyelid; however, this provides limited access to the lateral orbital rim and increases the risk of cicatricial ectropion. Lastly, to access the lower maxillary buttress, an intraoral or gingival approach can be utilized [6, 8]. In most cases, a combination of approaches is often required. The authors prefer a lateral canthus, inferior fornix approach combined with a gingival sulcus incision.

Surgical Equipment

The most used instruments include a scalpel, tenotomy scissors, surgeon-preferred forceps, needle drivers, Kocher clamps, suction, and the appropriate sutures. A head lamp is desirable for increased illumination within the orbitotomy surgical cavities or intra-oral incisions that are otherwise not well illuminated. The initial cutaneous incision is typically made with a scalpel and the transconjunctival incision is made with tenotomy or iris scissors. Blunt dissection is carried out with scissors and various retractors are used to obtain adequate exposures. Common retractors include Desmarres or Senn retractors, malleable or orbital ribbon retractors, or double skin hooks. A periosteal elevator is used to access the subperiosteal space. In some cases, a Langenbeck elevator, Carrol Gerard Screws or a bone hook engaged behind the junction of the lateral orbital rim and anterior arch can be used for reduction. After reduction is performed, titanium plates and screws secure the extra orbital facial bones. Nylon foil may be implanted spanning the perimeter of the intra-orbital wall fractures. Intraoperative stereotactic navigational imaging is a new option that may be useful for those not familiar or comfortable with the anatomy visualization afforded during surgery or pre-operative facial imaging [3, 6–9].

Surgical Approach (Video 37.1)

The authors' preferred approach is via a lateral canthal and transconjunctival incision with the addition of an upper gingival incision. To access the lateral orbit, a lateral canthotomy is fashioned and dissection is continued to the periosteum of the lateral orbital rim. To further mobilize the incision, an inferior and superior canthotomy is performed by incising the superficial lateral canthal tendon and inferior and superior limbs of the deep lateral canthal tendon. The inferior orbital rim can be exposed via a tranconjunctival approach with an incision 2–3 mm inferior to the tarsus, extending just lateral to the punctum and connecting to the lateral canthal incision. Dissection to the orbital rim is most efficiently done in a preseptal approach. This avoids orbital fat prolapse into the surgical field of the inferior rim. The arcus marginalis can be reached after the transconjunctival/retractor incision by then retracting the eyelid anteriorly with a Desmarres retractor and using a malleable retractor and Fraser suction tip or cotton-tip applicator to bluntly separate the orbital tissues from the arcus marginalis. No scissor spreading action or sharp dissection is needed to reach the rim. This technique involves a single, small lateral canthus, external incision that obviates disfiguring scars and reduces the incidence of iatrogenic cicatricial malposition. This approach provides a large operative field of exposure from the medial inferior orbital rim continuously to the lateral orbital rim above the zygomaticofrontal suture line [1, 10]. The periosteum at the rim can then be incised with a scalpel or monopolar cautery.

A gingivobuccal incision is used to expose the zygomaticomaxillary buttress or to expand a subperiosteal dissection to access the anterolateral maxillary bone surface (Fig. 37.2) [10]. The intraoral approach involves a horizontal upper sulcus incision from the lateral incisor to the first molar with subsequent elevation of the mucoperiosteal flap. Care is taken to avoid disturbing the infraorbital nerve while allowing for visualization, reduction, and fixation of the lower zygomaticomaxillary buttress [9]. Blunt dissection with a surgical sponge between soft tissue and the periosteal elevator is useful to keep to forestall infraorbital nerve injury as well as keep the surgical plane dry.

Although rarely needed, a hemicoronal incision with a supratemporalis approach can be used, mainly if the zygomatic arch itself requires plating for stability. An incision is made anterior to the tragus that extends from the earlobe to the crus of the helix, then is curved posteriorly and superiorly toward the temporal region posterior to the hairline, creating an approximately 8 cm length incision. The temporal portion of the incision is shaped like a hockey stick and is made 45° to the zygomatic arch. Dissection is continued deep to the superficial temporalis fascia to avoid facial nerve injury and the flap is reflected anterior to the ear along the plane of the subgaleal fascia. The incision is deepened to expose the temporalis muscle and a plane is dissected superficial to the temporalis muscle and at the same depth, dissection is continued until the medial surface of the zygomatic arch is exposed. It is important to avoid over-dissection or total degloving as this can make resuspension more difficult [7].

While retracting the surrounding soft tissue, the periosteum can be incised with a scalpel or electrocautery, and a periosteal elevator can be used to access the subperiosteal space [3, 7]. The zygomatic complex is the first structure to the reduced, which can be achieved with

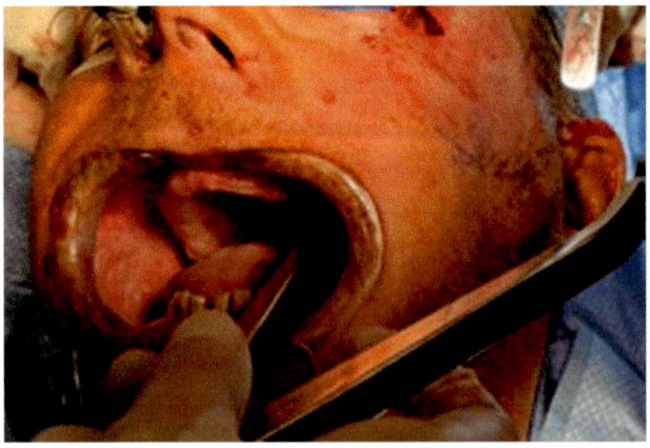

Fig. 37.2 Intraoperative photograph demonstrating reduction of the zygomatic arch using a Rowe zygomatic elevator via a transoral (Keen) approach

a 1 cm curve bone hook placed posterior to the body of the zygoma along the zygomatic arch as it attaches to the lateral orbital rim. This allows for manipulation of the bone in multiple planes of movement. Since the bone is very strong, it reduces the risk of further bone weakening which can occur with use of Kocher clamps or manipulation devices such as the Carrol Gerard screw (Fig. 37.3). If additional reduction is necessary for the zygomaticomaxillary buttress and posterior surface of the zygoma, an elevator can be inserted through the gingivobuccal incision to reduce the zygoma; digital manipulation from below can also be used to hold the repositioned bone in place for fixation [3]. After reduction of the zygomaticomaxillary complex, the next fixation is typically the frontozygomatic buttress, the infraorbital rim, and if a gingival approach was needed, the zygomaticomaxillary buttress [9].

There are different techniques to confirm adequate complete reduction. Prior to the availability of newer technologies, intraoperative positioning relied on temporary fixation of the zygoma with gross inspection of its position [1]. This technique is most effective for evaluating fracture reduction at the sphenozygomatic suture, the most important reference suture for reduction of ZMC fractures [1, 10]. The lateral orbital wall alignment along this suture line viewed from the internal lateral orbit dissection best determines the proper angulation of the zygoma. The lateral orbital wall should essentially follow a straight line from the lateral orbital rim to the sphenoid bone. This complements the proper horizontal, anterior–posterior, and vertical projections of the orbital entrance. If the lateral orbital wall is not in a straight line, the zygoma will be either internally or externally rotated. Internal rotation will result in an over-projected zygomatic arch with temple fullness and a medialized malar prominence. External rotation will result in a concave zygomatic arch with temple depression and a lateralized malar prominence. Intraoperative navigation, if available, may allow immediate assessment of the orientation of the displaced segment but is generally not necessary (Fig. 37.4A–H) [3, 11].

An important consideration for bony fixation with plates is utilizing smaller, separate plates versus large continuous plates (Fig. 37.5A, B). Typically, separate plates across major fractures lines are preferred as it is difficult to conform the curvature of a large, continuous plate to bone. A large plate may be considered in the setting of comminuted fragments along one aspect of the orbital rim.

In rare instances, grafts may be indicated. The material must be biocompatible and amenable to skeletal fixation. Autogenous grafts are commonly used due to their biocompatibility but are limited by donor site morbidity [1, 11]. Calvarial bone is often utilized due to its natural contour and accessibility without the need for an additional incision. It is also resistant to resorption. Cancellous bone grafts are also used due to their ability to revascularize faster compared to cortical bone; however, cancellous bone grafts are weaker than cortical bone. Other autogenous grafting sites include the mandible, iliac crest, and wall of the maxillary sinus [1]. In contrast, alloplastic materials are frequently used due to their ability to spare donor site morbidity and decreased operative time. An example of a non-porous alloplastic graft is titanium mesh, which is a malleable and biocompatible material. Its main advantages include coverage of large areas, use alone or in conjunction with bone grafts, and low infection rates. However, it can be difficult to insert due to its sharp edges and difficult to remove due to fibrovascular ingrowth.

A variety of implants are available to reconstruct the orbital walls. The authors prefer nylon foil because it is relatively inert, is resistant to adherence, conforms orbital wall curvatures, and is inexpensive (Fig. 37.6). Other more costly and possibly more adherent alloplastic options include porous polyethylene or porous polyethylene coated titanium. The authors avoid bare titanium mesh as the fenestrations can facilitate many points of fibrovascular scarring which may cause restrictive strabismus and if later implant removal is indicated the explantation is much more difficult [1, 3, 11].

Internal orbital implants usually do not require fixation and are held in place by the

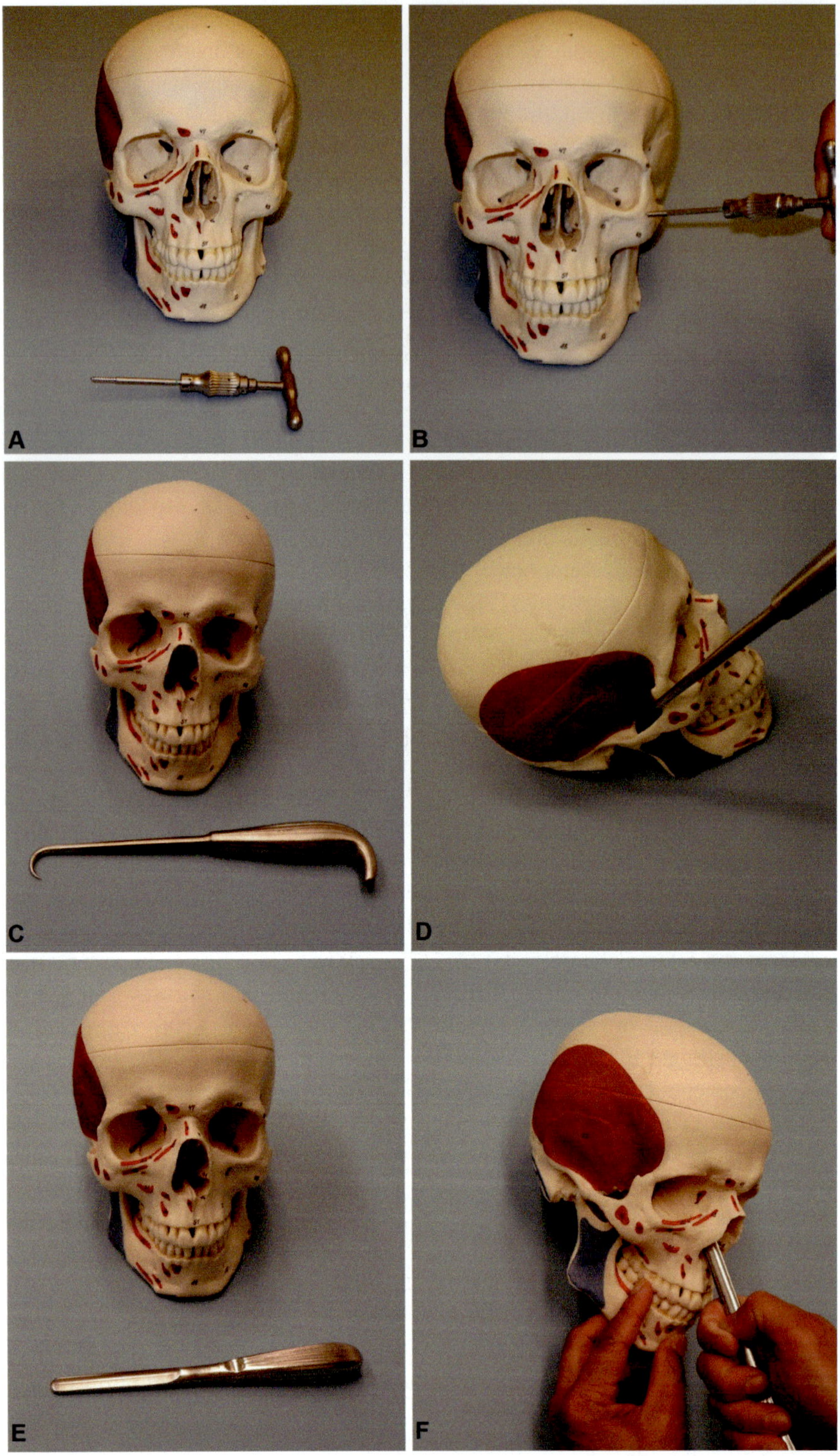

Fig. 37.3 (**A**) Carrol Gerard screw. (**B**) A Carrol Gerard screw may be used for reduction by engaging the malar prominence. (**C**) Bone hook. (**D**) A bone hook may be used behind the junction of the lateral orbital rim and anterior arch for reduction. (**E**) Boies nasal fracture elevator. (**F**) A Boies nasal fracture elevator may be used to reduce the zygoma from an internal approach

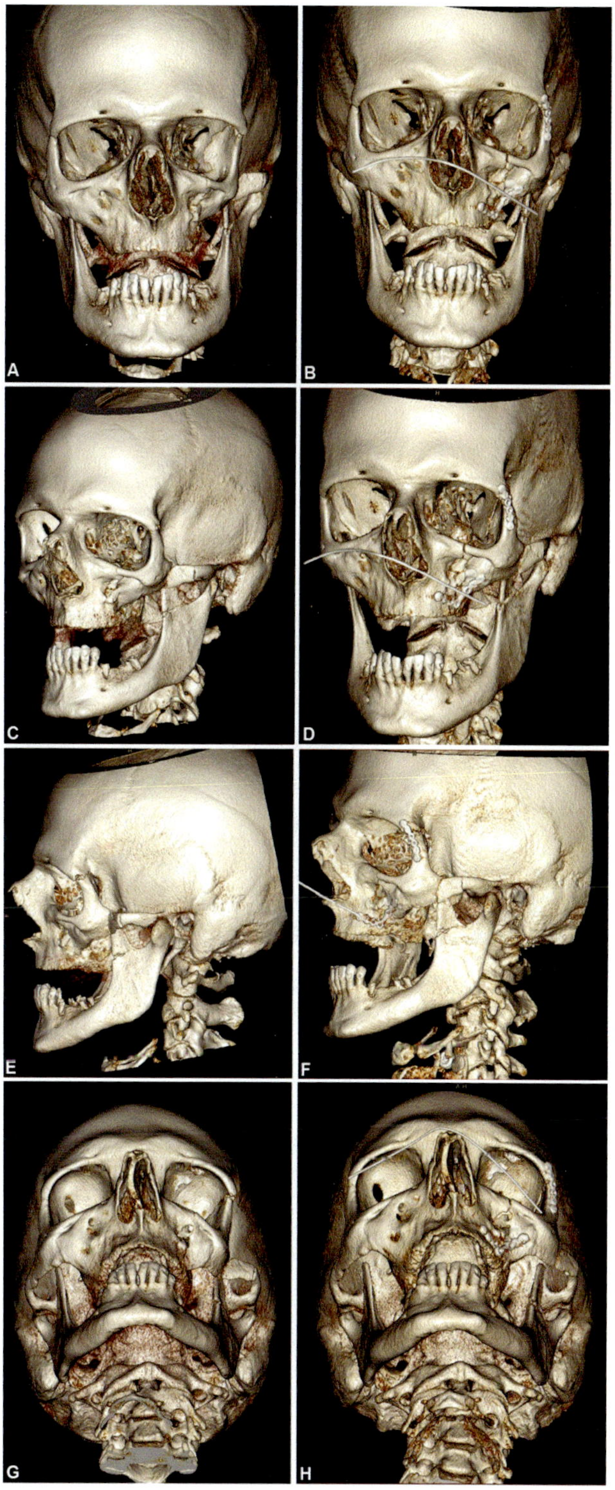

Fig. 37.4 (**A**) Preoperative frontal three-dimensional (3D) CT reconstruction demonstrating severe displacement of the zygomatic arch with narrowing of the facial width and displacement of the lateral orbital rim at the zygomaticofrontal (ZF) suture. (**B**) Postoperative frontal 3D CT reconstruction demonstrating appropriate reduction of the ZF suture and the improved position of the zygomatic arch. (**C**) Preoperative oblique 3D CT reconstruction demonstrating fractures of the zygomatic arch, inferior orbital rim, ZF suture, and ZS suture. (**D**) Postoperative oblique 3D CT reconstruction demonstrating adequate reduction of the ZS suture, ZF suture, infraorbital rim, lateral buttress and zygomatic arch. (**E**) Preoperative sagittal 3D CT reconstruction demonstrating severe displacement of the zygomatic arch and the lateral orbital rim at the ZF suture. (**F**) Postoperative sagittal 3D CT reconstruction demonstrating adequate reduction of the ZF suture, lateral buttress, and zygomatic arch. (**G**) Preoperative Waters' view 3D CT reconstruction demonstrating malar projection asymmetry and narrowing of the facial width. (**H**) Postoperative Waters' view 3D CT reconstruction demonstrating adequate reduction and improved position of the zygomatic arch

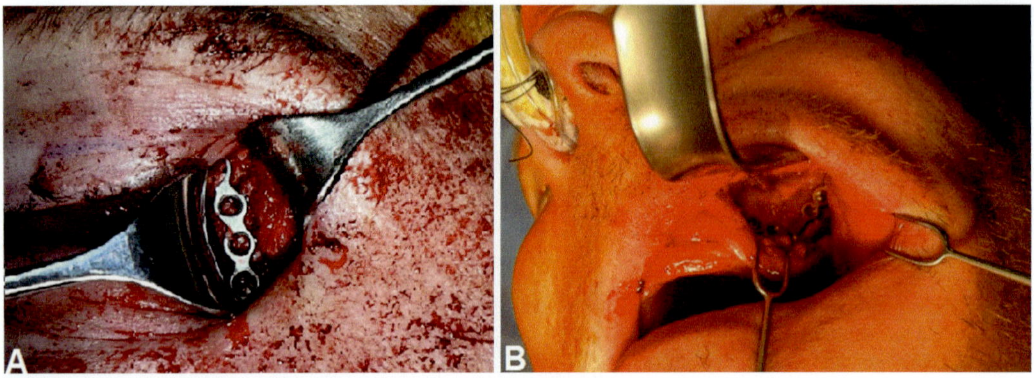

Fig. 37.5 A bent 0.8 mm L-strut plate was fixated along the (**A**) reduced zygomaticofrontal suture and the (**B**) lateral buttress spanning the reduced fracture line

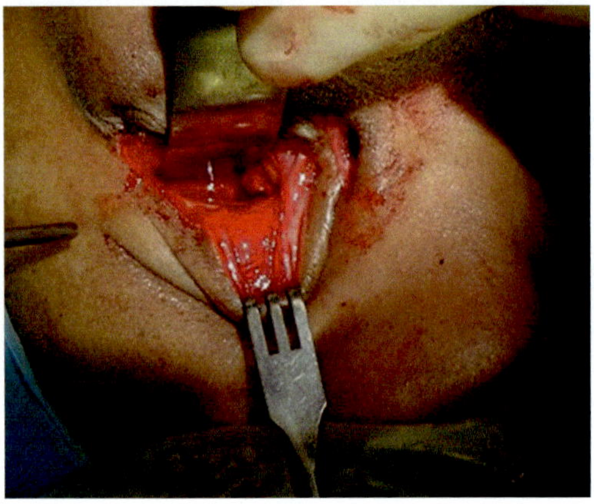

Fig. 37.6 A porous polyethylene (Medpor) implant was used to reconstruct the fractured orbital floor after the infraorbital contents were reduced

surrounding tissue creating a tamponade effect [1, 3, 11]. The conventional repair of the extra orbital bones involves 3-point fixation, involving the zygomaticomaxillary buttress, infraorbital rim, and zygomaticofrontal suture (Fig. 37.7A–C) [4, 10]. Fixation of the frontozygomatic sutures and inferior orbital rim typically involves resorbable 2.0 mm mini-plate systems or titanium mini-plates [3].

After adequate bone fixation, it is important to properly close the wounds. The conjunctiva, without the septum, is closed with 6-0 absorbable sutures. It is important to take minimal suture bites to close the conjunctiva to avoid eyelid retraction [3]. The lateral canthal angle is reformed and resuspended with a 5-0 or 4-0

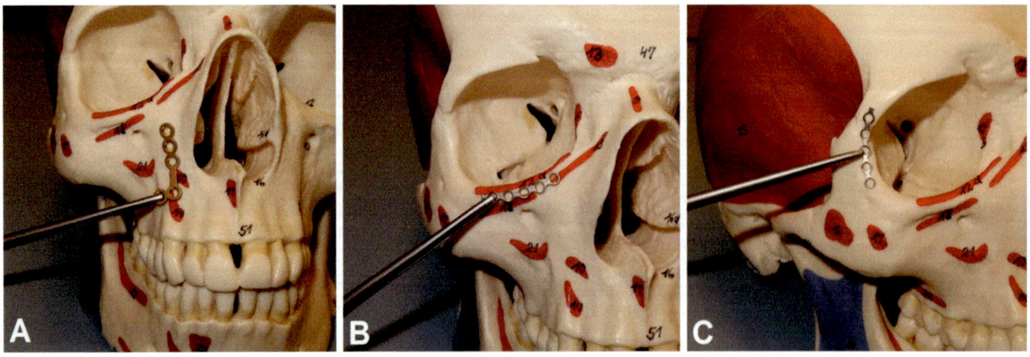

Fig. 37.7 3-point fixation of the (**A**) zygomaticomaxillary buttress, (**B**) infraorbital rim, and (**C**) zygomaticofrontal suture

absorbable suture such as polygalactin to attach the eyelid to the periosteum in a posterior and superior position to prevent ectropion. The height of attachment is usually about 1–2 mm higher than that of the medial canthus. If a gingival incision was made, it can be closed with a 5-0 absorbable suture. Lastly, skin is closed with a 6-0 absorbable suture [3].

Post-operative Evaluation

Post-operatively, it is important to assess for improvement of symptoms including diplopia, extraocular muscle restriction, trismus, and malocclusion. Persistence of symptoms, along with a thorough clinical evaluation of facial symmetry and globe position, can help determine the need for additional surgical intervention. Photo documentation of all facial views is utilized to evaluate for asymmetries or malposition. The zygomatic width, eyelid position, and globe position can be evaluated with the frontal view. The lateral and oblique views can be used to assess malar projection; however, the worm's eye view allows for evaluation of symmetry through direct comparison to the nonoperative side. The worm's eye view can also be utilized for evaluation of globe position (i.e., enophthalmos) relative to the position of the unaffected globe (Fig. 37.8).

Complications

Surgical site morbidity depends on the type of injury and surgical approach. The most common complications include enophthalmos and poor cosmesis related to facial widening or inadequate malar projection, due to inadequate reduction or more commonly improper angulation of the zygoma [1]. Expansion of the orbital volume can be related to improper reduction of the inferior orbital rim and frontozygomatic suture leading to lateral rotation of the anterior maxillary buttress [4]. Cicatricial ectropion or inferior scleral show develop in 5–42% of patients with subciliary and subtarsal lower eyelid incisions which the authors avoid using for these reasons. In contrast, entropion develops in 0–20% of those with a transconjunctival incision. This is usually due to improper closure with either incorporation of the septum or retractors. Overly aggressive dissection of a transconjunctival approach may result in posterior scarring and cicatricial entropion as well [6]. Subciliary, subtarsal, and transconjunctival periorbital approaches can also result in hypertrophic scars, lagophthalmos, and nasolacrimal injury if carried too medially. Intraoral approach can result in paresthesia of the infraorbital nerve and damage to tooth roots if screws are improperly placed [9]. Risks associated with scalp coronal incisions include hematoma, nerve

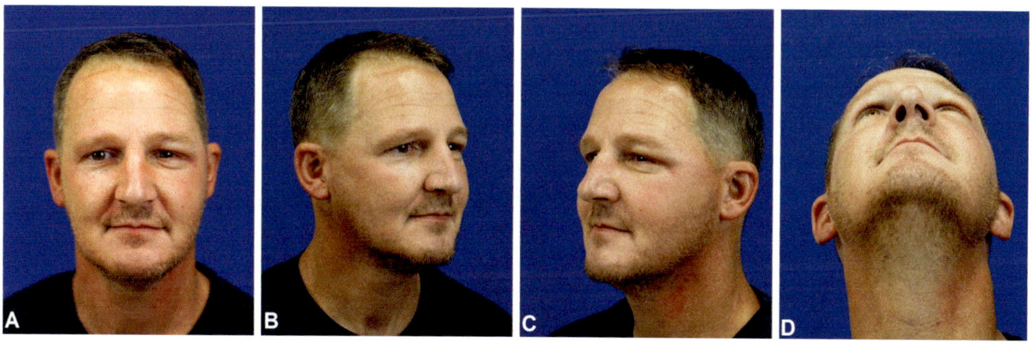

Fig. 37.8 External photographs of the (**A**) frontal, (**B**) right oblique, (**C**) left oblique, and (**D**) worm's eye views demonstrating symmetrical malar prominences, appropriate eyelid position, and well-positioned globes after ZMC fracture repair

injury, alopecia, paresthesia, depression of temporal fossa, and paralysis of the facial nerve [7]. Traumatic injuries can lead to significant challenges and undesirable outcomes in the setting of ZMC fracture repairs and may lead to additional surgical intervention to address these complications.

Conclusions

The optimal repair of ZMC fractures starts with a thorough clinical and radiographic preoperative evaluation. A variety approaches to ZMC fractures have been described but lateral canthal, inferior fornix orbitotomy combined with gingival sulcus wounds may be ideal for the excellent exposure and minimal scarring and eyelid malposition.

References

1. Aman HM, Alenezi A, Ducic Y, Reddy LV. Secondary reconstruction of the zygomaticomaxillary complex. Semin Plast Surg. 2020;34(4):254–9. https://doi.org/10.1055/s-0040-1721761. Epub 2020 Dec 24. PMID: 33380910; PMCID: PMC7759427.
2. Peleg O, Ianculovici C, Shuster A, Mijiritsky E, Oz I, Kleinman S. Three-dimensional intraoperative computed tomography imaging for zygomatic fracture repair. J Korean Assoc Oral Maxillofac Surg. 2021;47(5):382–7. https://doi.org/10.5125/jkaoms.2021.47.5.382. PMID: 34713813; PMCID: PMC8564091.
3. Lee PK, Lee JH, Choi YS, et al. Single transconjunctival incision and two-point fixation for the treatment of noncomminuted zygomatic complex fracture. J Korean Med Sci. 2006;21(06):1080–5.
4. Nasr WF, ElSheikh E, El-Anwar MW, Sweed AH, Bessar A, Ezzeldin N. Two- versus three-point internal fixation of displaced zygomaticomaxillary complex fractures. Craniomaxillofac Trauma Reconstr. 2018;11(4):256–64. https://doi.org/10.1055/s-0037-1604199. Epub 2017 Jul 27. PMID: 30574268; PMCID: PMC6224286.
5. Pau CY, Barrera JE, Kwon J, Most SP. Three-dimensional analysis of zygomatic-maxillary complex fracture patterns. Craniomaxillofac Trauma Reconstr. 2010;3(3):167–76. https://doi.org/10.1055/s-0030-1263082.PMID:22110833;PMCID:PMC3052681.
6. Schneider M, Besmens IS, Luo Y, Giovanoli P, Lindenblatt N. Surgical management of isolated orbital floor and zygomaticomaxillary complex fractures with focus on surgical approaches and complications. J Plast Surg Hand Surg. 2020;54(4):200–6. https://doi.org/10.1080/2000656X.2020.1746664. Epub 2020 Jun 4. PMID: 32493085.
7. Xing Z, Ren R, Xia X, Yang L. Supra-temporalis approach for treating zygomaticomaxillary complex fracture. J Craniofac Surg. 2021;32(3):1087–9. https://doi.org/10.1097/SCS.0000000000007463.
8. Ji SY, Kim SS, Kim MH, Yang WS. Surgical methods of zygomaticomaxillary complex fracture. Arch Craniofac Surg. 2016;17(4):206–10. https://doi.org/10.7181/acfs.2016.17.4.206.
9. Carvalho AC, Pereira CC, Queiroz TP, Magro-Filho O. Intraoral approach to zygomatic fracture: modified technique for infraorbital rim fixation. J Craniofac Surg. 2012;23(02):537–8.
10. Miyazaki H, Okuda K, Ueno K, Wada Y, Kumegawa S, Uemura K, Sakata Y, Asamura S. Swinging eyelid approach to zygomaticomaxillary complex fracture. J Craniofac Surg. 2019;30(7):e655–8. https://doi.org/10.1097/SCS.0000000000005731. PMID: 31574788.
11. van Hout WMMT, de Kort WWB, Ten Harkel TC, Van Cann EM, Rosenberg AJWP. Zygomaticomaxillary complex fracture repair with intraoperative CBCT imaging. A prospective cohort study. J Craniomaxillofac Surg. 2022;50(1):54–60. https://doi.org/10.1016/j.jcms.2021.09.009. Epub 2021 Sep 24. PMID: 34600816.

Medial Canthus Approach to the Naso-orbital Complex

38

Benjamin K. Ghiam, Lalita Gupta, Peter J. Timoney, and Mark A. Prendes

Abstract

The naso-orbital complex and medial orbit may need to be exposed for trauma or other pathology. Direct medial canthus incisions are traditionally avoided by non-oculofacial plastic surgeons, owing to unfamiliarity with the anatomy and concern for a conspicuous facial scar. With good technique and preservation of the underlying tendinous and lacrimal structures, direct medial canthus incisional approaches offer excellent access to the naso-orbito-ethmoid complex without canthal dystopia or a problematic scar. In this chapter, the authors detail medial orbitotomy approaches for trauma and other indications.

Keywords

Medial orbitotomy · Medial canthus incision · Transcutaneous orbitotomy · Naso-orbital ethmoid fracture · Medial orbit fracture

Supplementary Information The online version contains supplementary material available at https://doi.org/10.1007/978-3-031-63178-8_38.

B. K. Ghiam · L. Gupta · P. J. Timoney (✉) · M. A. Prendes
University of Kentucky, Lexington, KY, USA
e-mail: pjtimo2@uky.edu

Introduction

Surgical exposure of the medial orbit and naso-orbital complex is important in many clinical applications including naso-orbital fracture repair, medial orbital abscess drainage, and medial wall decompression of the orbit, among others. The central midface contains various structures, including the lacrimal system, trochlea and superior oblique tendon, cribriform plate, and ethmoidal arteries. In this chapter, the authors detail direct medial canthal approaches to efficiently and safely access a wide range of medial orbit or central midface pathology.

Transcutaneous Lynch Incision and Modifications

In 1921, Lynch described a facial cutaneous surgical approach for the treatment of frontal sinusitis. This procedure is a 3 + cm curvilinear incision that begins from the medial aspect of the eyebrow and extends inferiorly towards the medial canthus, carried up to the periosteum. Lynch described removal of the entire common sinus orbital wall to open and curette the frontal-ethmoid-sphenoid complex, this included removal of the nasal process of the superior maxilla, the lateral edge of the nasal bones, the lacrimal bone, and the lamina papryacea of the ethmoid bone [1].

J. Tao (ed.), *Efficient Oculofacial Surgery*, https://doi.org/10.1007/978-3-031-63178-8_38

This large incision provides good exposure of the medial orbit and naso-orbital complex but may result in a conspicuous scar and webbing. As such, a Z-plasty modification that interrupts the linearity of the scar may accommodate later scar contracture [2, 3]. In addition to the scar, detachment of the medial canthal tendon, without reattachment, may cause telecanthus. Although these modifications to the Lynch incision can decrease web formation, postoperative scarring often remains a concern. Additionally, in each of these approaches, supratrochlear nerve damage and resultant numbness of the medial forehead may ensue owing to the wide dissection plane.

Transcutaneous Medial Canthal Tendon Approach

A transcutaneous medial canthal tendon approach may obviate some of the concerns with a larger and more anterior Lynch incision [4–7]. An array of procedures can be performed through this approach, including naso-orbito-ethmoid fracture repair, medial wall fracture repair, subperiosteal abscess drainage, tumor removal, or medial wall decompression. This approach is useful in patients with a prominent nasal base as well as those with pre-existing vertical creasing at the medial canthus.

A 1.5–2.0 cm vertical incision is placed medial to the medial canthal angle and immediately overlying the medial canthal tendon. After exposing the origin of the anterior medial canthal tendon and elevating the underlying periosteum, the incision provides exposure to the medial orbital wall extending from the nasal dorsum to the orbital apex. The incision that is immediately adjacent to the tendon affords return of the tendon to its anatomic attachment site. This incision is similar to a traditional transcutaneous external dacryocystorhinostomy incision [2]. Importantly, since the medial canthal tendon elevated, it must be resecured medially at the conclusion (described later in this chapter).

Vertical web formation remains a concern if the wound contracts and involves the adjacent eyelids or periorbital skin. A small Z or W configuration to this medial canthal tendon incision may prevent web formation by redirecting tension lines.

Transcutaneous Medial Canthal Tendon Approach Technique

Surgical Technique

A 1.5- to 2.0-cm incision is made immediately anterior, superficial, and in the same plane as the anterior ramus of the medial canthal tendon, shaving the anterior-most fibers of the anterior ramus in many cases (Figs. 38.1 and 38.2). The blade should be kept perpendicular to the nasal bone and should not be angled posteriorly, which may sever the anterior limb of the medial canthal tendon from the attached periosteum or may damage the underlying lacrimal sac.

Sharp dissection is carried down to and through the periosteum just anterior to the anterior lacrimal crest (Fig. 38.3), with concurrent release of orbicularis oculi fibers superiorly, below the trochlea. The anterior ramus of the medial canthal tendon, along with attached periosteum, is then elevated with blunt subperiosteal dissection (Figs. 38.4 and 38.5). Care is taken to preserve the lacrimal outflow structures that

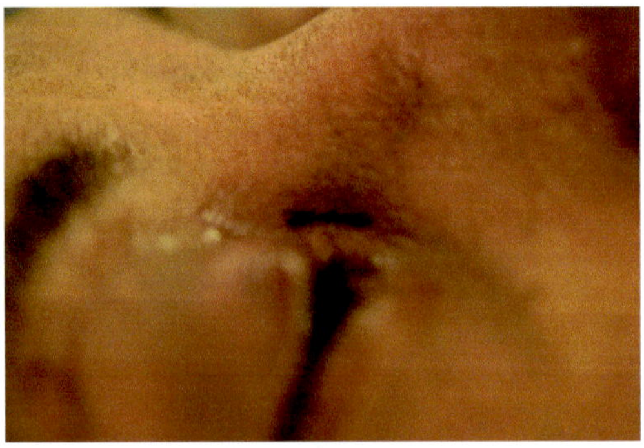

Fig. 38.1 Medial cutaneous incision planned just anterior to medial canthal tendon

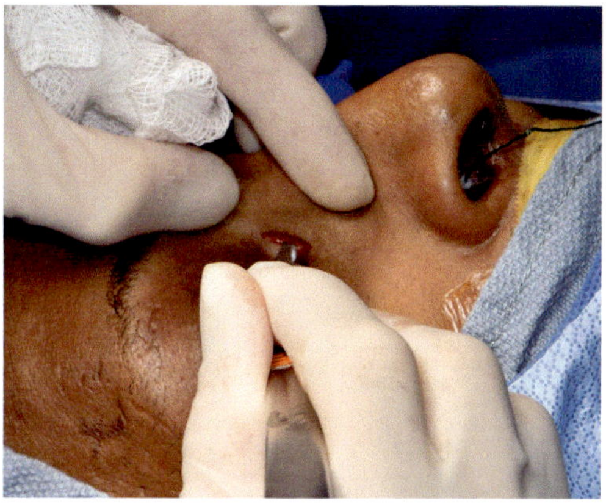

Fig. 38.2 Medial canthal incision fashioned with a #15 blade

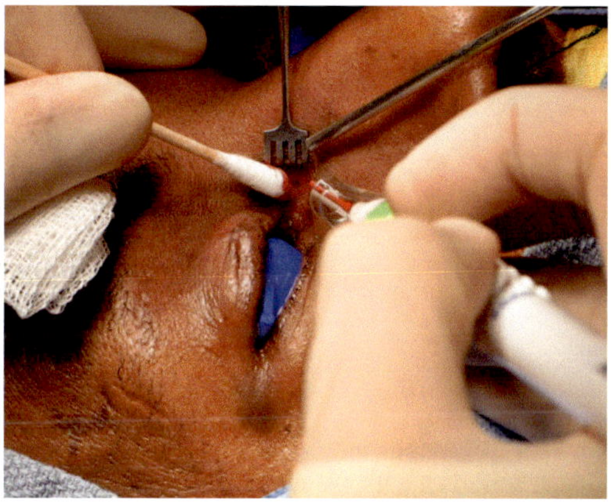

Fig. 38.3 Sharp dissection through orbicularis oculi muscle

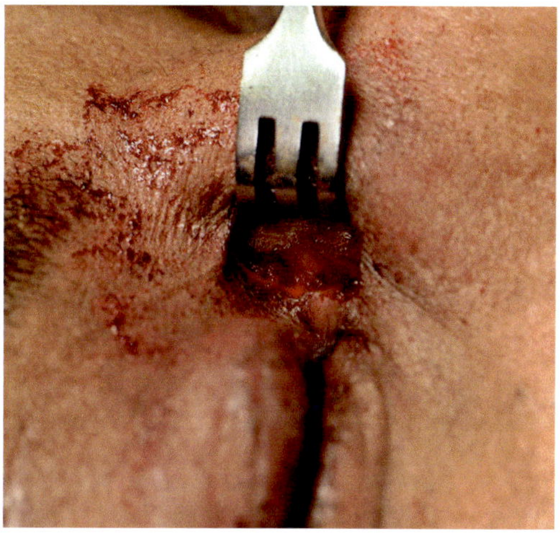

Fig. 38.4 Dissection down to periosteum

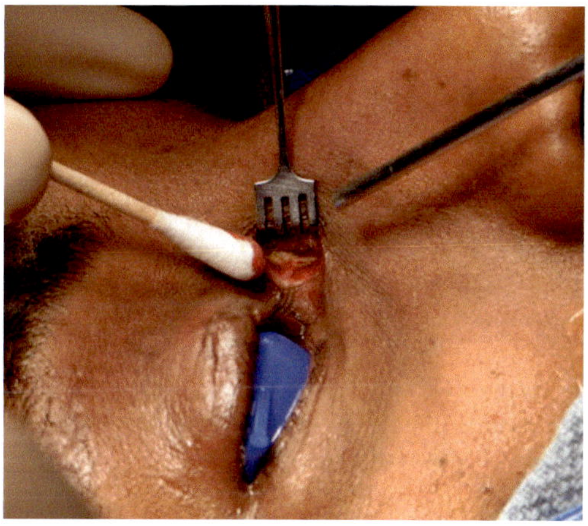

Fig. 38.5 Periosteum opened with sharp dissection

are elevated laterally. The periorbita along with the attached posterior ramus of the medial canthal tendon is then elevated, which completely and easily exposes the entire medial wall of the orbit, extending from the inferomedial orbital strut to the trochlea.

The ethmoidal arteries serve as landmarks to the level of the superior extent of the fovea ethmoidalis, that in turn marks the skull base in this area. The subperiosteal plane can be dissected anteriorly to the nasal dorsum to address open reduction of nasal fractures (Figs. 38.6, 38.7 and Video 38-1).

To prevent medial canthal webbing during closure, the medial canthal tendon, along with periosteum, is re-approximated with a 4-0 or 5-0 polyglactin suture that, on a deep central pass, engages the medial periorbita just deep to the medial canthal tendon (Figs. 38.8, 38.9 and Video 38-2). Alternatively, a small Z or W configuration in lieu of a linear incision may decrease the incidence of vertical web formation. No additional permanent internal sutures are necessary to adequately replace and secure the medial canthal tendon anatomy, provided the tendon has not been released from the

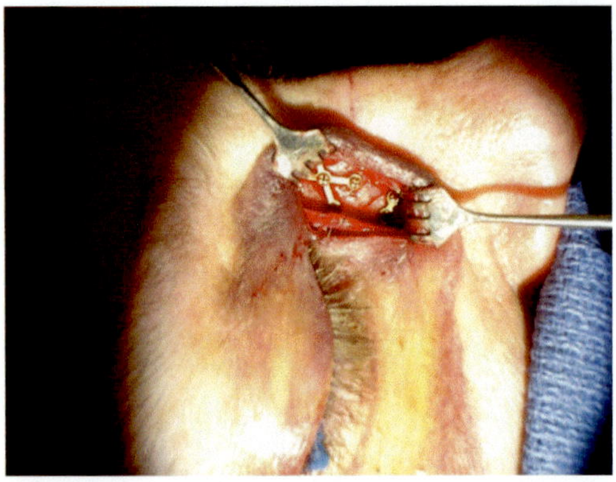

Fig. 38.6 Naso-orbital fractures reduced and plated using a small medial canthus orbitotomy incision

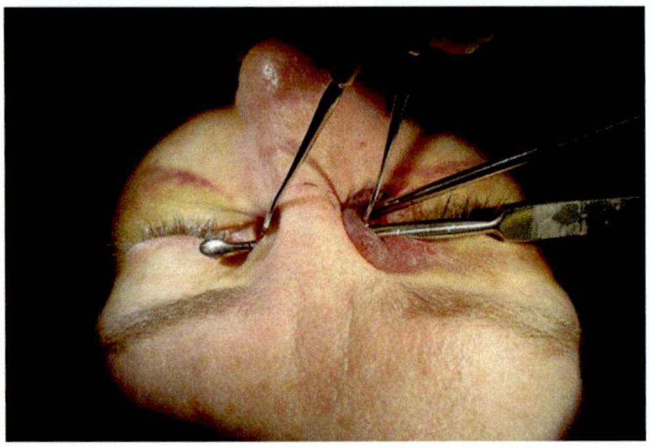

Fig. 38.7 With bilateral medial canthus incisions, the entire central midface can be degloved to repair extensive naso-orbito-ethmoid complex fractures

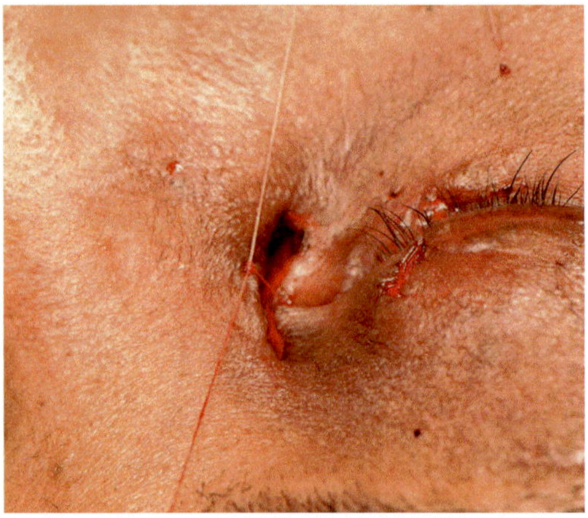

Fig. 38.8 Polyglactin (4-0 or 5-0) grasping skin on the medial and lateral aspect of the incision with a deep ass capturing the anterior medial periorbita

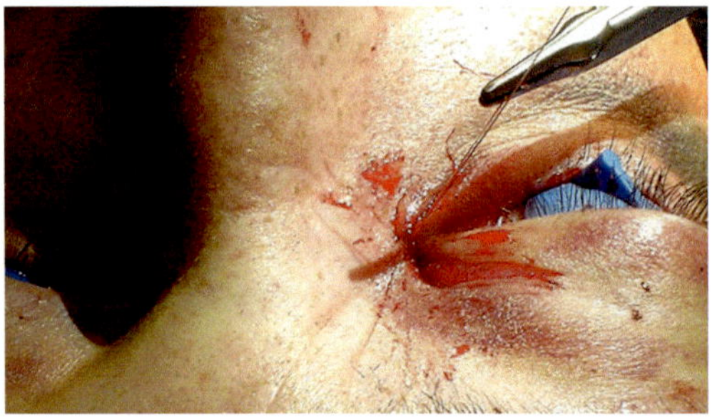

Fig. 38.9 Tightening the closure suture with a deep pass through periorbita pulls the medial canthal tendon medially to resist telecanthus

periosteum during the dissection. An external indentation of the skin into the medial canthal tendon should be observed to ensure the prevention of an epicanthal fold. The skin closure is accomplished with a 5-0 or 6-0 gut suture (Figs. 38.8 and 38.9).

Transcaruncular Incision

Surgical Technique (Video 38-3)

The semilunar fold should be identified and avoided. With Stevens' scissors, a 12 mm vertical incision is created through the lateral one third of the caruncle. The condensed fibrous layer just deep to the caruncle is incised in the direction of the posterior lacrimal crest. A narrow malleable retractor is then used distract orbital soft tissues laterally. The malleable is advanced posteromedial to the posterior lacrimal crest. With the malleable retractor the posterior lacrimal crest, Stevens' scissors are spread to expose the periosteum. The dissection plane is along the medial aspect of the medial orbital septum between the orbital septum and Horner's muscle.

The periorbita along the posterior lacrimal crest is incised with electrocautery. With a periosteal elevator, the dissection is continued posteriorly in a subperiosteal plane. The subperiosteal dissection should start superiorly overlying the thicker frontal bone. An inferior starting point is less optimal because the thin underlying lamina paprycea bone commonly fractures. The subperiosteal pocket can be extended inferiorly with a cantilever technique, torquing the malleable with the elevator. This exposes the lacrimal fossa and medial orbit (Fig. 38.10).

The anterior and posterior ethmoidal arteries should identified to provide landmarks (both superior-inferior positioning as well as anterior–posterior depth) (Fig. 38.11). The arteries sometimes obstruct access to the wall, namely implant placement for a medial wall fracture. In these instances, the arteries may be severed with electrocautery. Of note, this access and cautery of the ethmoidal artery is useful in rare cases of recalcitrant epistaxis. With the medial orbital content distracted laterally after wide subperiosteal dissection, this approach allows wide exposure of the medial wall up to the orbital apex. At the conclusion of the case, the caruncle is closed with interrupted 6-0 vicryl or gut sutures or left to heal by second intention.

In cases requiring access to the inferior and medial orbital walls, the transcaruncular approach may be combined with an inferior conjunctival fornix approach. This approach begins with a lateral canthotomy and inferior fornix incision (swinging eyelid). The inferior fornix incision is then extended medially and superiorly through the caruncle. The transcaruncular dissection is performed as previously described. After the inferior oblique muscle is cut with scissors at its origin, it is then later sutured back to the periosteum at its origin [8–12].

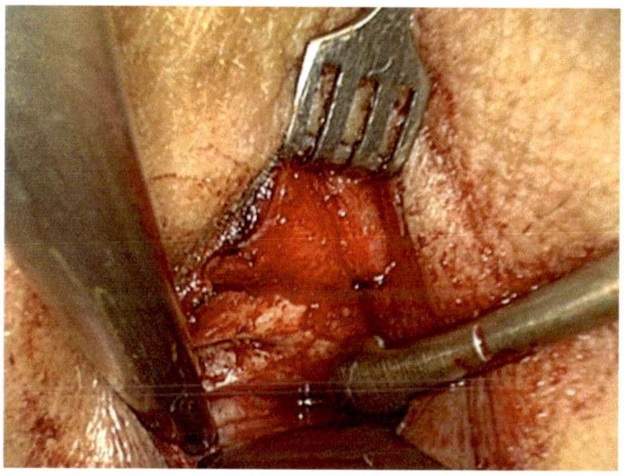

Fig. 38.10 Lacrimal sac fossa and medial wall exposed with periosteal elevation

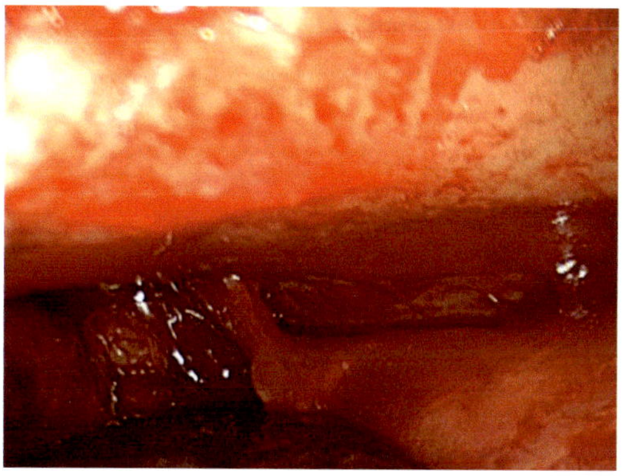

Fig. 38.11 Anterior ethmoid identified as a key anatomical landmark

Coronal Incision

A coronal approach to the orbit, introduced by Tessier (1969) for orbital decompressions, is a more invasive approach [13]. This approach involves an ear-to-ear incision made through the scalp, 1 cm behind the hairline. A flap at the level of the periosteum is reflected down to the supraorbital rim, and periorbita is further dissected laterally and medially. This technique is more often performed for combined neurosurgical procedures [13–16].

Benefits to this approach include wide access to the superior bony orbit, and decent exposure to both the lateral and medial walls. The coronal incision may be useful when there is a concern for conspicuous facial scars with periorbital skin incisions. In facial trauma, frontal bone, frontal sinus, and orbit roof fractures may be best treated through a coronal incision. Other procedures that can be performed with this incision include forehead lifts, correction of glabellar rhytids, and browplasty not to mention craniotomy and other neurosurgical or craniofacial surgeries [13–17]. Today, coronal incisions are largely abandoned in favor of less invasive direct incisions for orbit decompression for thyroid eye disease or orbit fracture repair.

Conclusion

Surgical access to the medial orbit can be transcutaneous or transconjunctival (transcaruncular). Cutaneous incisions afford the opportunity to additionally access extra-orbital facial bones. The transcaruncular approach does not expose the extra orbital central midface but leaves no cutaneous scar and is an excellent medial orbitotomy approach. Medial canthal skin incisions should be constructed and repaired with knowledge and attention to anatomy including the lacrimal drainage apparatus, and the medial canthal tendon .

References

1. Lynch RC. The technique of a radical frontal sinus operation which has given me the best results. Laryngoscope. 1921;31:1–5.
2. Esclamado RM, Cummings CW. Z-plasty modification of the Lynch incision. Laryngoscope. 1989;99:986–7.
3. Burm JS, Oh SJ. Direct local approach through a W-shaped incision in moderate or severe blowout fractures of the medial orbital wall. Plast Reconstr Surg. 2001;107:920–8.
4. Timoney PJ, Sokol JA, Hauck MJ, Lee HB, Nunery WR. Transcutaneous medial canthal tendon incision to the medial orbit. Ophthal Plast Reconstr Surg. 2012;28(2):140–4. https://doi.org/10.1097/IOP.0b013e318248e62c. PMID: 22410662.
5. Nunery WR, Tao JP. Medial canthal open nasal fracture repair. Ophthal Plast Reconstr Surg. 2008;24:276–9.
6. Nunery WR, Tao JP, Johl S. Nylon foil "wraparound" repair of combined orbital floor and medial wall fractures. Ophthal Plast Reconstr Surg. 2008;24:271–5.
7. Nunery WR, Nunery CW, Martin RT, et al. The risk of diplopia following orbital floor and medial wall decompression in subtypes of ophthalmic Graves' disease. Ophthal Plast Reconstr Surg. 1997;13:153–60.
8. Garcia GH, Goldberg RA, Shorr N. The transcaruncular approach in repair of orbital fractures: a retrospective study. J Craniomaxillofac Trauma. 1998;4:7–12.
9. Shorr N, Baylis HI, Goldberg RA, Perry JD. Transcaruncular approach to the medial orbit and orbital apex. Ophthalmology. 2000;107(8):1459–63. https://doi.org/10.1016/s0161-6420(00)00241-4. PMID: 10919889.
10. Balch KC, Goldberg RA, Green JP, Shorr N. The transcaruncular approach to the medial orbit and ethmoid sinus. A cosmetically superior option to the cutaneous (Lynch) incision. Facial Plast Surg Clin North Am. 1998;6:71–7.
11. Fante RG, Elner VM. Transcaruncular approach to medial canthal tendon plication for lower eyelid laxity. Ophthal Plast Reconstr Surg. 2001;17:16–27.
12. Moe KS. The precaruncular approach to the medial orbit. Arch Facial Plast Surg. 2003;5(6):483–7. https://doi.org/10.1001/archfaci.5.6.483. PMID: 14623685.
13. Krastinova D, Rodallec A. Basedowian orbitopathy [in French]. Ann Chir Plast Esthet. 1985;30:351–8.
14. Härting F, Koornneef L, Peeters HJF, Gillisen JPA. Fourteen years of orbital decompression in Graves' disease. A review of technique, results and complications. Orbit. 1986;5:123–9.
15. Kalmann R, Mourits MP, van der Pol JP, Koornneef L. Coronal approach for rehabilitative orbital decompression in Graves' ophthalmopathy. Br J Ophthalmol. 1997;81:41–5.
16. Baldeschi L. Orbital decompressions. In: Wiersinga WM, Karger KG, editors. A Multidisciplinary approach to Graves' Orbitopathy. Basel Switzerland, 2007a.
17. Saks ND, Burnstine MA, Putterman AM. Glabellar rhytids in thyroid-associated orbitopathy. Ophthal Plast Reconstr Surg. 2001;17:91–5.

Evisceration

39

Cameron B. Nabavi

Abstract

Evisceration is commonly performed for a blind, nonsalvageable eye. Endophthalmitis with no vision potential is the classic indication. Other indications include phthisis bulbi or some instances of a blind painful eye. Importantly, a suspected intraocular malignancy (e.g. melanoma or retinoblastoma) is a contraindication owing to the probability of leaving tumor behind. Many believe evisceration is associated with optimal prosthesis motility. Other advantages are that it is technically less difficult and is quicker to perform than other types of eye removal. This chapter details preoperative features and surgical techniques of evisceration.

Keywords

Blind painful eye · Phthisis · Evisceration · Enucleation · Implant · Orbit · Socket surgery

Supplementary Information The online version contains supplementary material available at https://doi.org/10.1007/978-3-031-63178-8_39.

C. B. Nabavi (✉)
Ohio State University, 262 Neil Ave. Ste 430, Columbus, OH 43201, USA
e-mail: nabavieye@gmail.com

Indications for Evisceration

Endophthalmitis with no vision potential is the classic evisceration indication. Many surgeons advocate enucleation for a blind painful eye, owing to severing of all attachments and removal of the eyeball intact. However, evisceration may be appropriate in certain situations such as pain due to a blind hypertensive eye. Evisceration should not be performed if there exists any concern for intraocular malignancy. If the posterior segment of the eye cannot be viewed imaging (B-Scan, CT scan or MRI) to confirm no intraocular tumor should be considered. Eye removal surgery as prophylaxis for sympathetic ophthalmia after globe trauma is sometimes performed, but evisceration may be especially undesirable owing to the high probability of incomplete removal of exposed uvea that contains the purported antigen. Evisceration may be undesirable for moderate or severe phthisis bulbi since the sclera may be too contracted to receive a sufficiently sized orbital implant.

Benefits of Evisceration Surgery

Evisceration is useful for several reasons. Preservation of extraocular muscle attachments to intact sclera may be associated with better prosthesis motility [1]. Technically, evisceration

J. Tao (ed.), *Efficient Oculofacial Surgery*, https://doi.org/10.1007/978-3-031-63178-8_39

is more expedient, and unlike enucleation that almost always requires general anesthesia, it can sometimes be performed with intravenous sedation with a retrobulbar block.

Patient Preoperative Consultation and Discussion

Patients should be informed of the risks include bleeding, infection, socket discharge, cosmetic deformity, migration of implant, extrusion of implant, socket contraction, reduced socket motility, ptosis and ectropion [2]. The benefits include improved cosmesis, reduced pain and improved self-esteem and confidence in social situations in those with significant phthisis. Alternatives include observation, medical treatment with atropine and prednisolone drops, or enucleation surgery. While alloplastic implants are generally preferred in the primary eye removal setting to replace volume, dermis fat grafting can be considered.

Surgical Technique

Evisceration with Intraconal Implant Behind Posterior Sclera

Typically, an evisceration can be performed under general anesthesia or intravenous sedation with a retrobulbar and peribulbar nerve block.

The procedure begins with a 360 degree peritomy (Fig. 39.1). A stab incision 2.5mm posterior to the limbus is placed to gain access to the suprachoroidal space (Fig. 39.2). A 360-degree sclerokeratectomy is completed 2.5mm posterior to the limbus (Fig. 39.3).

An evisceration spoon (or periosteal elevator) is used to remove the intraocular contents (Fig. 39.4). (A periosteal elevator may be used in lieu of an evisceration spoon.) The contents should be examined grossly for any obvious tumor and then sent for permanent pathological examination. Hemostasis of the vortex veins and optic nerve is then achieved. Examination and removal of ocular implants such as a scleral buckle or glaucoma devices should be performed at this time (Fig. 39.5). A stab incision temporal to the optic nerve is then placed to gain

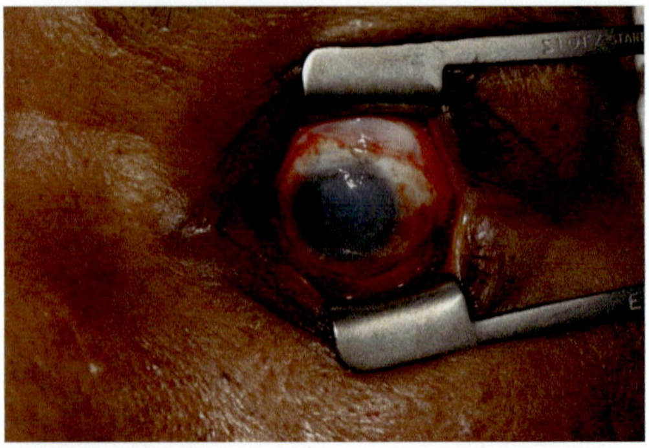

Fig. 39.1 Conjunctiva is dissected off the sclera circumferentially posterior to the limbus

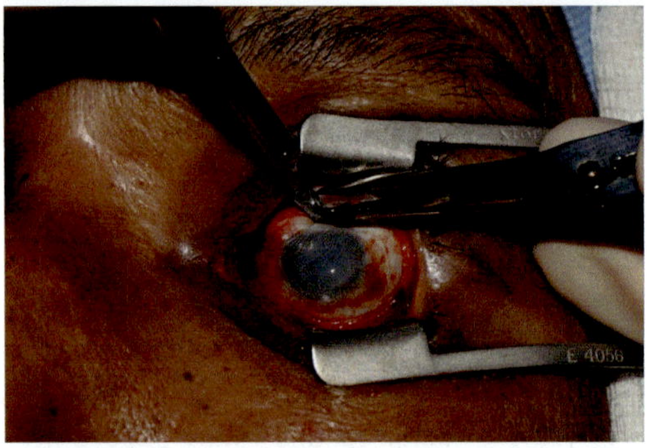

Fig. 39.2 Post limbal stab incision is created to initiate the sclerkeratectomy

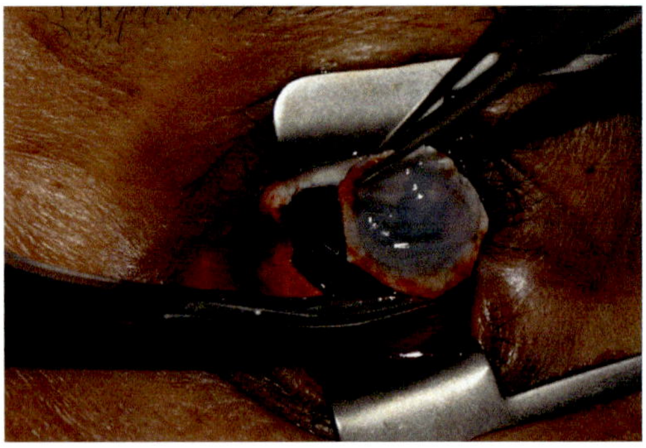

Fig. 39.3 360 degree sclerokeratectomy performed with scissors

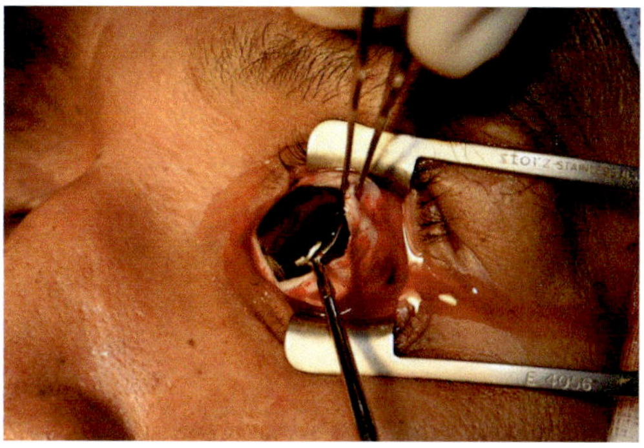

Fig. 39.4 Intraocular contents separated from sclera with an evisceration spoon

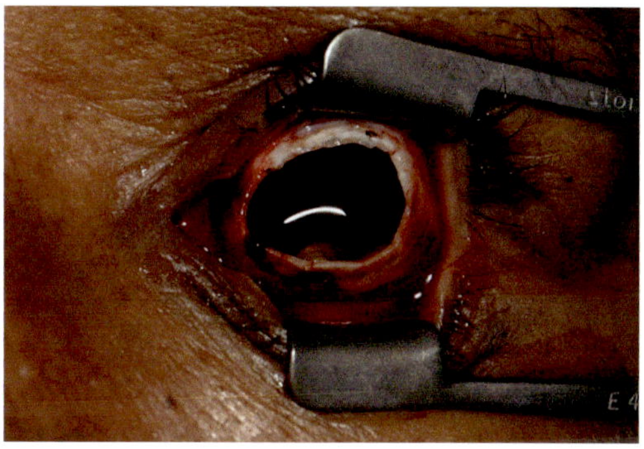

Fig. 39.5 Intrascleral contents removed

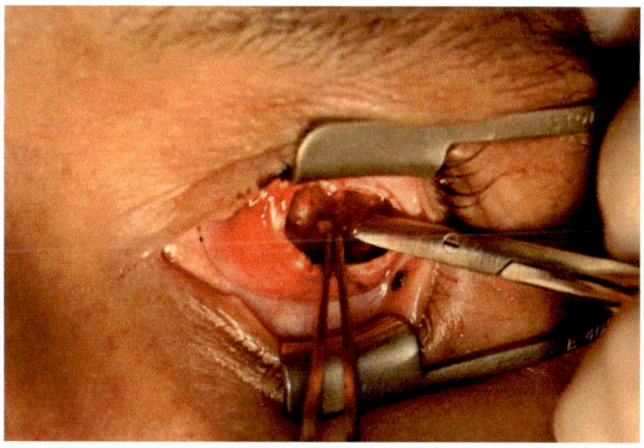

Fig. 39.6 A stab incision is placed temporal to the optic nerve and the optic nerve is transected, allowing anterior mobilization of the posterior sclera

access to the intraconal space where scissors are placed to transect the optic nerve and mobilize the posterior sclera anteriorly [3, 4] (Fig. 39.6).

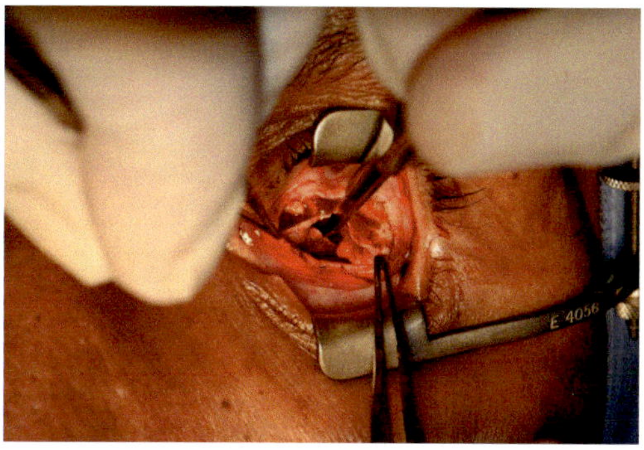

Fig. 39.7 The posterior scleral incision is extended in the 12 to 6 o'clock meridian toward the anterior sclera

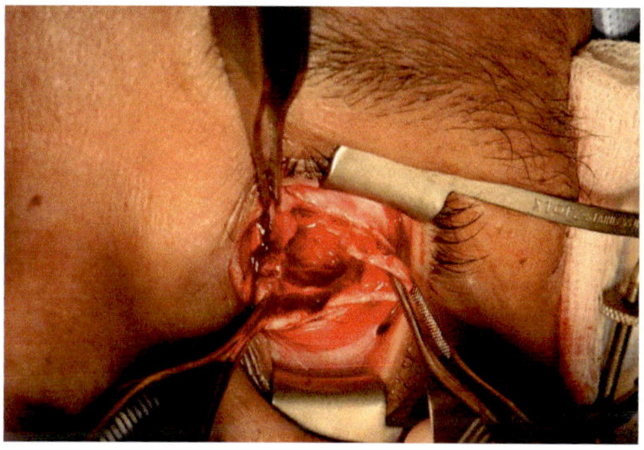

Fig. 39.8 The posterior sclera is opened and the retrobulbar, intraconal space is visualized

This stab incision is extended in the 6 or 12 o'clock meridian, leaving 2mm of sclera on each end (Fig. 39.7). This allows for palpation of the orbit for any foreign bodies or masses, as well as to determine appropriate size for an intraconal spherical implant (Fig. 39.8).

A spherical implant, most commonly silicone, is then placed in the intraconal space (Fig. 39.9). The posterior sclera is closed with 5–0 polyglactin suture in an interrupted fashion (Fig. 39.10). The anterior sclera is closed with 5–0 polyglactin suture in a buried interrupted fashion (Fig. 39.11). This allows for double scleral wall closure and protection over the spherical implant, reducing risk of migration or extrusion [5]. The conjunctiva is closed with 6–0 polyglactin or plain gut suture

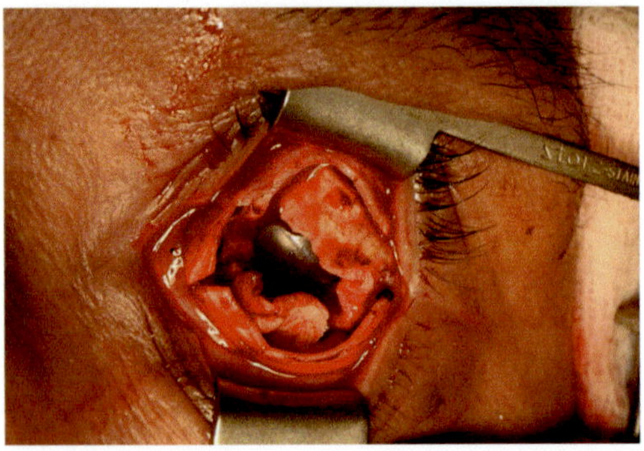

Fig. 39.9 A spherical silicone implant is implanted to the intraconal space

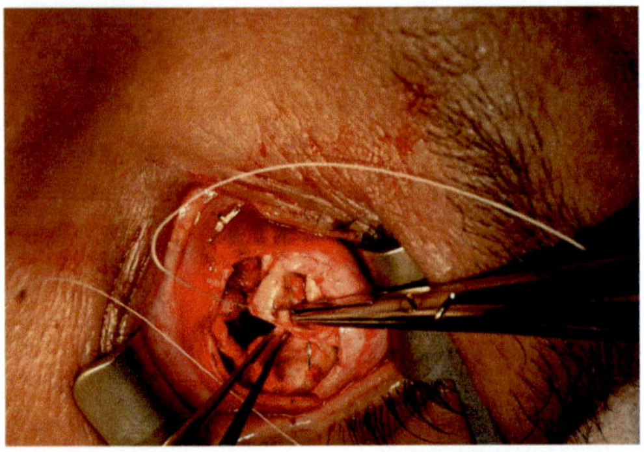

Fig. 39.10 The posterior sclera is closed with interrupted 5-0 polyglactin suture

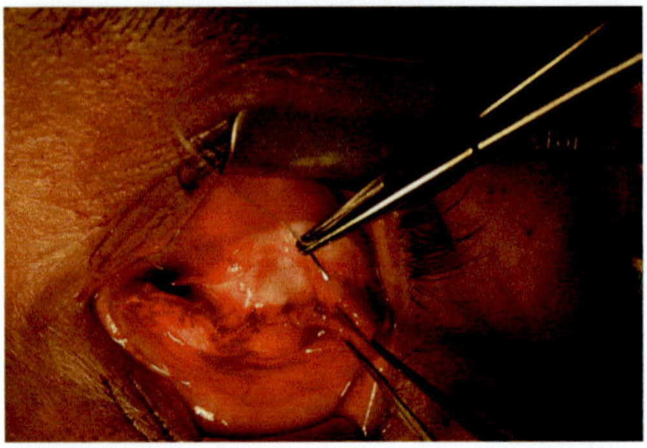

Fig. 39.11 The anterior sclera is closed with interrupted 5-0 polyglactin suture

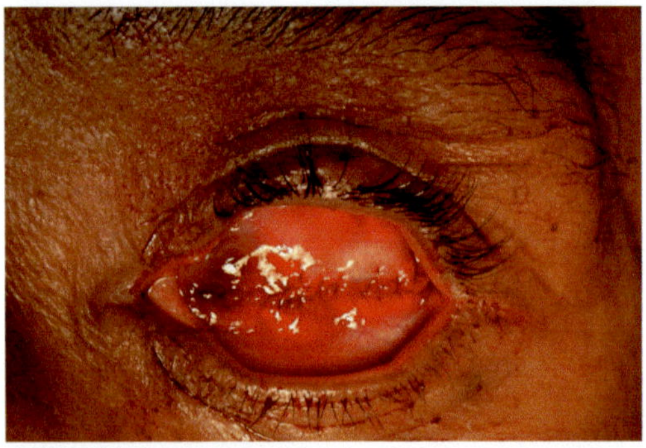

Fig. 39.12 The conjunctiva is closed with 6-0 polyglactin or chromic suture

(Fig. 39.12). A silicone or acrylic conformer is then placed on the conjunctiva surface to preserve the lid fornices (Fig. 39.13). A temporary tarsorraphy can then be performed to maintain the conformer position and limit postoperative swelling. A retrobulbar block of 0.75% bupivacaine with 1:100,000 epinephrine can give a 4 to 6 h block to help with postoperative discomfort (Fig. 39.14). A retrobulbar injection of liposomal bupivicaine can also be considered, if available, and may provide a longer lasting postoperative block. A pressure patch is then placed to apply firm pressure to prevent postoperative hematoma (Fig. 39.15).

Evisceration with Intrascleral Implant (Video 39-1)

Similar steps are performed, but a smaller spherical implant is placed in the intraocular space. Alternately, posterior scleral relaxing incisions can be placed to expand the intraocular space, allowing for a larger intraocular implant. Anterior sclera is then closed with similar 5-0 polyglactin suture. This is preferred in patients with significant medical comorbidities as well as those unable to stop anticoagulation, with active intraocular infection, or unable to tolerate significant anesthesia (6–8).

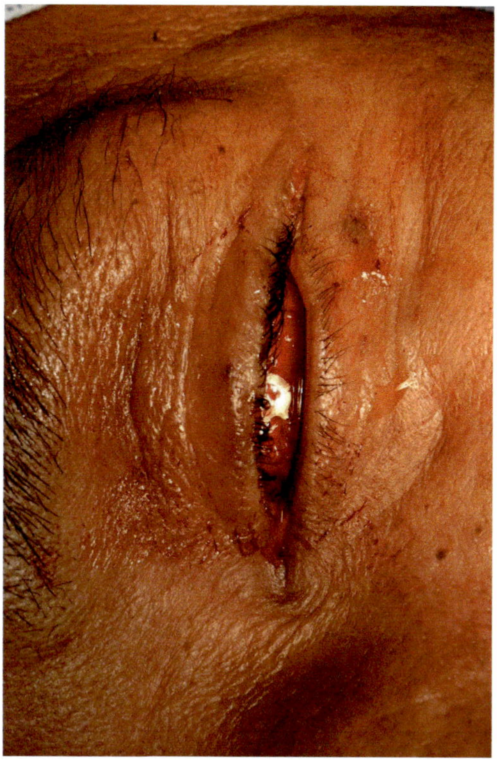

Fig. 39.13 Plastic conformer placed

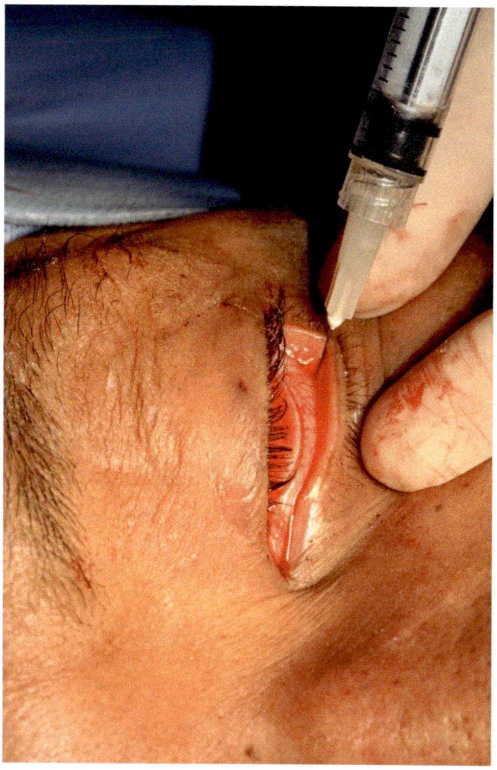

Fig. 39.14 Retrobulbar block (0.75% bupivicaine with 1:100,000 epinephrine) administered

Postoperative Management

The procedure is typically performed in the outpatient surgery setting. Antibiotics should be considered in cases of endophthalmitis and otherwise on a case-by-case basis. Postoperative pain can be significant, but mostly controlled with oral narcotics, in conjunction with antiemetics. Pressure patching can be removed as soon as the next day, but longer patching may reduce recovery time. Patients are typically seen one week after surgery to evaluate the degree of edema. Ocularist consultation for an ocular prosthetic occurs between 6 and 10 weeks after surgery. Annual socket checks should be performed to assess the socket mucosal lining for any fornix foreshortening as well as to rule out any implant exposure or extrusion. Anophthalmic sockets can have chronic mucopurulent discharge, and antibiotic steroid ointment can be used as needed to quell these symptoms.

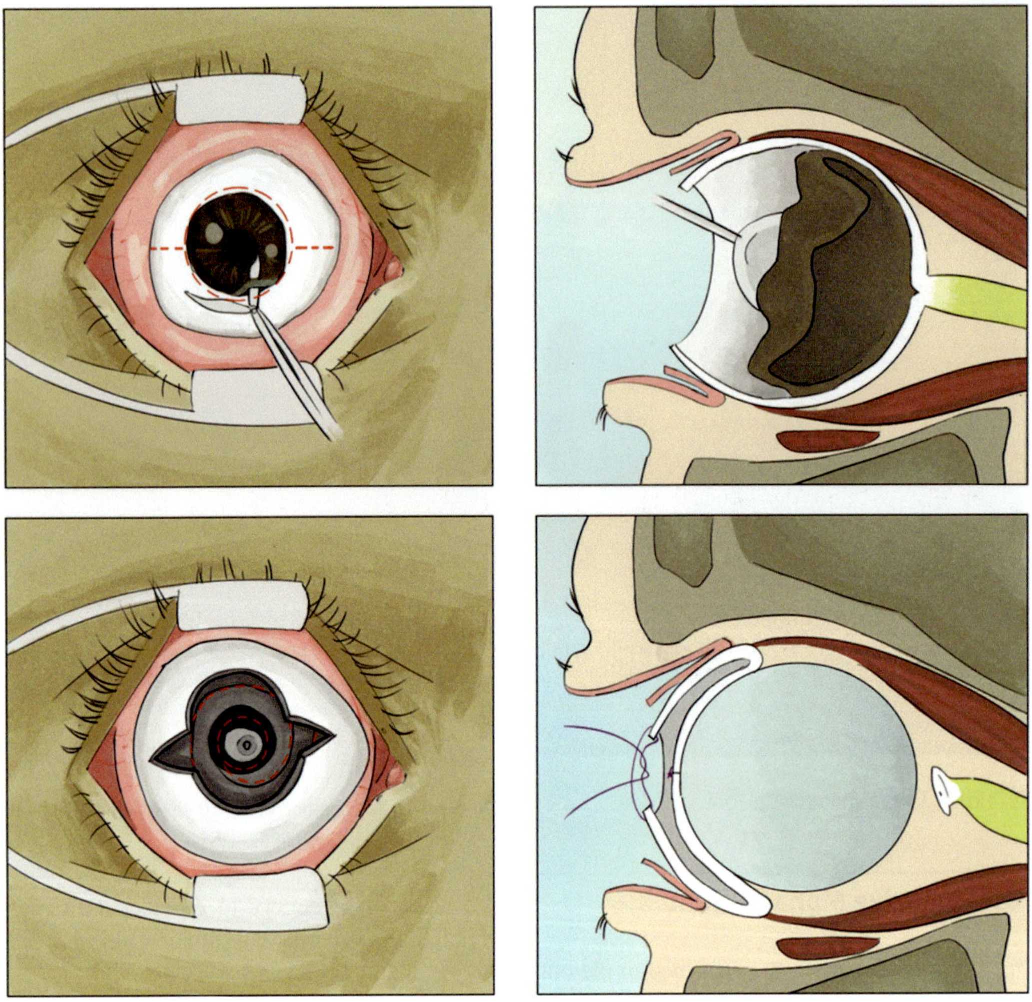

Fig. 39.15 Illustration depicting steps of evisceration with placement of alloplastic sphere implant deep to posterior sclera

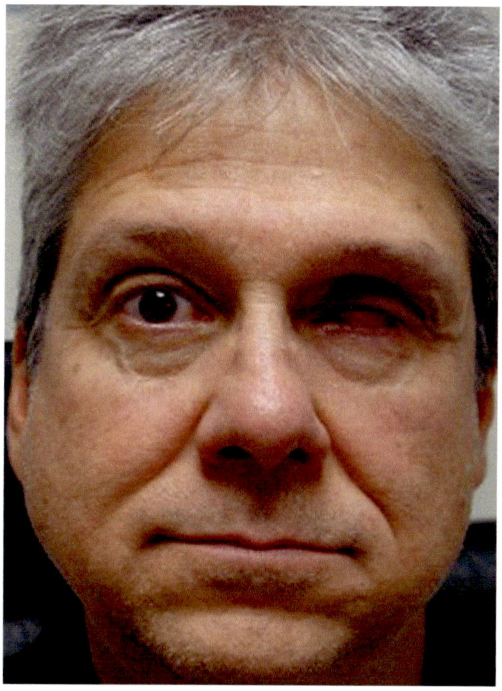

Fig. 39.16 Patient status post left evisceration with a healthy socket and prosthesis out

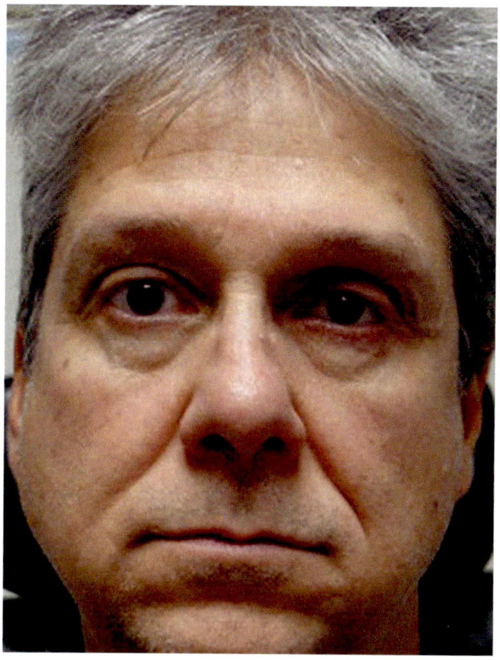

Fig. 39.17 Patient in Fig. 39.16 wearing a well-fitting left eye prosthesis. Note very subtle deep superior sulcus owing to slight volume deficiency in the orbit. Photo credit: Jeremiah Tao

Conclusions

Evisceration is an efficient method of eye removal. It is contraindicated if intraocular malignancy is suspected but otherwise is an ideal treatment for endophthalmitis and other conditions in which there is no vision potential. Prosthetic motility may be optimal, and results may be good but there may exist some limitations in size of sphere implant that can be inserted with evisceration (Figs. 39.16 and 39.17).

References

1. Nakra T, Simon GJ, Douglas RS, Schwarcz RM, McCann JD, Goldberg RA. Comparing outcomes of enucleation and evisceration. Ophthalmology. 2006;113(12):2270–5. https://doi.org/10.1016/j.ophtha.2006.06.021. PMID: 16996606.
2. Dave TV, Das AV, Mohapatra S, Bansal O, Ganguly A. Outcomes and complications of evisceration with primary implant: an electronic medical record driven analytics of 1800 cases. Orbit. 2022;41(6):717–25. https://doi.org/10.1080/01676830.2021.1998915. PMID: 34783616.

3. Long JA, Tann TM 3rd, Girkin CA. Evisceration: a new technique of trans-scleral implant placement. Ophthal Plast Reconstr Surg. 2000;16(5):322–5. https://doi.org/10.1097/00002341-200009000-00003. PMID: 11021379.
4. Dave TV, Ezeanosike E, Basu S, Ali MJ, Kaliki S, Naik MN. Effect of optic nerve disinsertion during evisceration on nonporous implant migration: a comparative case series and a review of literature. Ophthal Plast Reconstr Surg. 2018;34(4):336–41. https://doi.org/10.1097/IOP.0000000000000987. PMID: 28863119.
5. Lai KKH, Kuk AKT, Au AKH, Wong KKH, Wang T, Tsang A, Tai JHT, Ong THL, Ko STC, Chan E, Ko CKL. Single or double? A comparison of evisceration techniques. Int Ophthalmol. 2022. https://doi.org/10.1007/s10792-022-02578-x. PMID: 36482132.
6. Tripathy D, Rath S. Evisceration with primary orbital implant in fulminant endophthalmitis/panophthalmitis. Orbit. 2015;34(5):279–83. https://doi.org/10.3109/01676830.2015.1078366. PMID: 26308681.
7. Ozgur OR, Akcay L, Dogan OK. Primary implant placement with evisceration in patients with endophthalmitis. Am J Ophthalmol. 2007;143(5):902–4. https://doi.org/10.1016/j.ajo.2006.11.029. PMID: 17452189.
8. Chiu SJ, Tan JHY, Currie ZI. To implant or not to implant: emergency orbital eviscerations with primary orbital implants. Eye. 2021;35(11):3077–86. https://doi.org/10.1038/s41433-020-01382-0. PMID: 33432166; PMCID: PMC8526810.

Enucleation and Dermis Fat Grafting

40

Jordan Miller O'Dell and Jason A. Sokol

Abstract

Enucleation is indicated for an ocular malignancy, a blind painful eye, a disfiguring blind eye, or as sympathetic ophthalmia prophylaxis. The procedure is performed under general anesthesia and includes detaching the extraocular muscles and severing the optic nerve. An implant or dermis fat graft is usually inserted to restore orbital volume. When the socket is healed, the patient may be fitted for an ocular prosthesis.

Keywords

Enucleation · Eye removal · Eye prosthesis · Ocular prosthesis · Anophthalmia · Anophthalmic socket · Dermis fat graft · Eye socket surgery

Supplementary Information The online version contains supplementary material available at https://doi.org/10.1007/978-3-031-63178-8_40.

J. M. O'Dell · J. A. Sokol (✉)
University of Kansas, Kansas City, MO, USA
e-mail: jsokolmd@gmail.com

J. M. O'Dell
e-mail: jordanemiller09@gmail.com

Introduction

Enucleation is surgery to remove the entirety of the eye. This procedure is indicated for an ocular malignancy, a blind painful eye, a disfiguring blind eye, or as sympathetic ophthalmia prophylaxis. Enucleation is favored to evisceration in cases of intraocular tumor or malignancy, or if there is concern for sympathetic ophthalmia, as evisceration may leave uveal tissue [1]. It has been purported that performing enucleation within 10–14 days of a traumatic injury may reduce the incidence of sympathetic ophthalmia [1, 2]. However, the evidence supporting this protocol may lacking and each eye removal decision should be individualized weighing multiple factors including co-morbidities and the patient's own desires. Enucleation is also preferred to evisceration in cases where the sclera may be abnormal, such as scleromalacia, staphyloma, or phthisis.

Presurgical counseling is important prior to enucleation surgery. There is a significant psychological impact to having one's eye removed permanently [1]. In cases of trauma, attempted repair of the globe is usually warranted, not only to in an attempt to preserve the eye, but also to reinforce the ocular prognosis. It is important to remember that patients may experience depression or other psychological disturbances following enucleation. Formal psychiatric assessment and care is appropriate for many patients [1]. It

J. Tao (ed.), *Efficient Oculofacial Surgery*, https://doi.org/10.1007/978-3-031-63178-8_40

is also advisable to refer patients to local vision rehabilitation programs, which may be able to provide tools and aids for monocular vision. Cautioning the patient to protect their healthy eye with full-time use of protective glasses is imperative [1].

Anatomic Considerations

When preparing to remove the globe, it is important to consider the position of the extraocular muscles, anatomy of the optic nerve, and dimensions of the average globe. The optic nerve is approximately 25 mm long within the orbit. The spiral of Tillaux outlines extraocular muscle insertion sites in relation to the cornea. The medial rectus is approximately 5.5 mm posterior to the limbus, the inferior rectus 6.5 mm posterior, the lateral rectus 6.9 mm posterior, and the superior rectus 7.7 mm posterior. The inferior oblique attaches to the globe overlying the macula, about 8 mm inferior to the insertion of the lateral rectus. The inferior oblique and inferior rectus are contained in a fascial layer that is continuous with the capsulopalpebral fascia, and sends fascial attachments to the inferior fornix, the inferior tarsus, and the lower lid skin. Manipulation of extraocular muscles or clamping the optic nerve may lead to an oculocardiac reflex. Intraoperative communication between the surgeon and anesthesiologist is important to ensure there are no cardiac or systemic complications. The average volume of an adult globe is 7.0 mL. A 20 mm spherical implant, once wrapped in donor sclera and paired with a prosthetic eye, will closely approximate the volume of an average adult globe [1].

Technique (Video 40-1)

General anesthesia is commonly necessary for this procedure that is usually very painful. Subconjunctival local anesthetic as well as a retrobulbar block reduce the oculocardiac reflex, and help with post-operative pain control.

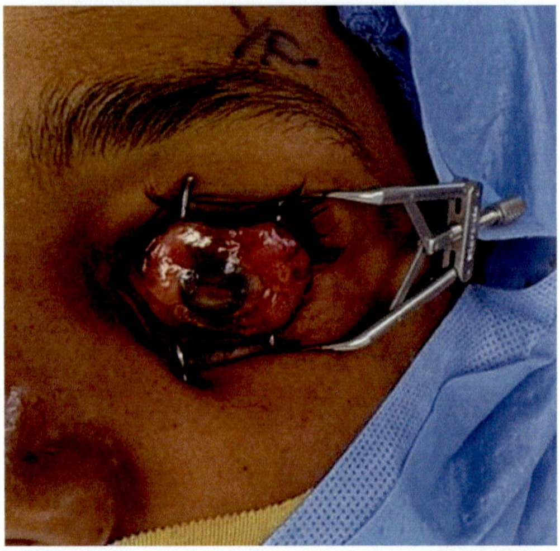

Fig. 40.1 Exposed globe

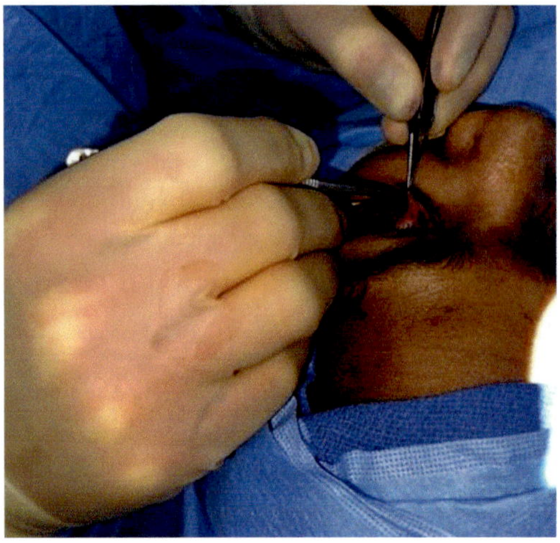

Fig. 40.2 360° peritomy

A frontal nerve block and inferior fornix block may also be helpful [1, 2].

An eyelid speculum is placed (Fig. 40.1) and 360-degree peritomy is made using scissors (Fig. 40.2). Tenons fascia is undermined to the equator to identify the rectus muscles. Each rectus muscle, beginning with the medial rectus and advancing to inferior, lateral, and then superior is isolated using a muscle hook (Fig. 40.3) and secured with a double armed 5-0 polyglactin suture. The muscle is then detached from the

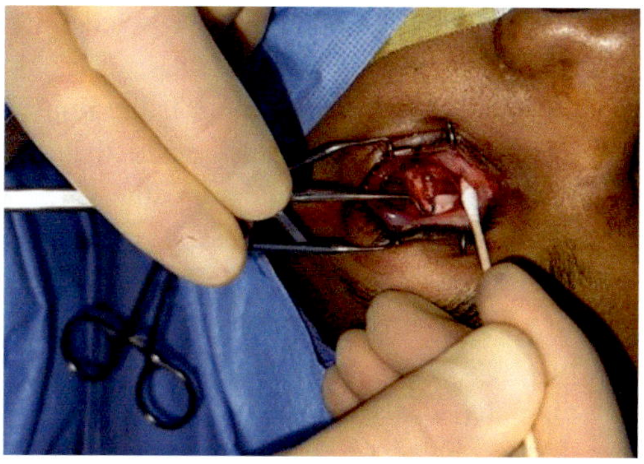

Fig. 40.3 Medial rectus isolated on Jameson hook

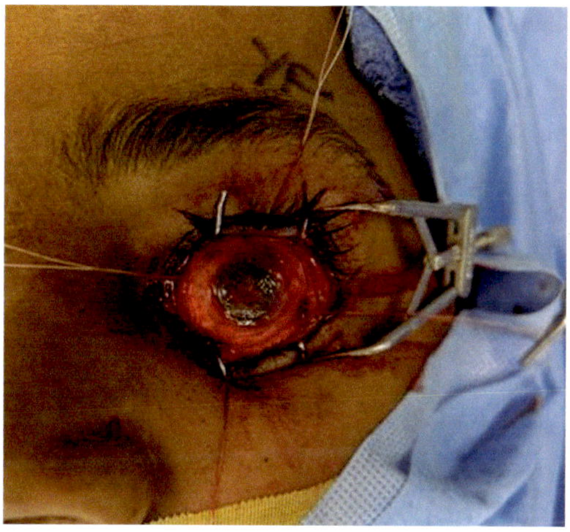

Fig. 40.4 Rectus muscles isolated on suture

globe with sharp dissection, being careful not to disrupt the intermuscular septum and muscle sheaths (Fig. 40.4). The superior oblique and inferior oblique are isolated with a Jameson muscle hook and released from the eye. The inferior oblique may be tagged with suture for later placement. The distal superior oblique is usually not secured and allowed to retract in the orbit.

With the extraocular muscles detached, the globe is then gently pulled anteriorly and rotated laterally to expose the optic nerve medially. A snare with an 18-gauge wire is used to encircle the globe and then the optic nerve. Tightening of the snare achieves detachment of the optic nerve to the globe with minimal blood loss. Alternatively, a curved hemostat can then be applied to clamp the optic nerve several millimeters posterior to the globe. This is left in place for three minutes to cut off flow through the central retinal artery. Curved Metzenbaum scissors or enucleation scissors are used to incise the nerve between the globe and the hemostat. In cases or tumor or malignancy, the globe and resected optic nerve should be thoroughly examined, and, in cases of retinoblastoma, intraoperative frozen sections may be employed to ensure the optic nerve is free of tumor extension. After complete tumor excision, the cut end of the optic nerve can be lightly cauterized, and the clamp removed. Digital pressure may be useful to aid in hemostasis (Fig. 40.5) [1, 2].

A spherical silicone implant wrapped in autogenous temporal fascia, fascia lata, or donor sclera is placed in the open socket (Fig. 40.6). The extraocular muscles are attached to the implant in their near normal anatomic positions using the previously attached double armed suture (Fig. 40.7). Good alternatives to a silicone sphere include acrylic or PMMA that share the nonporous, nonadherent, non reactive attributes. Porous implants are used by some surgeons, but the authors feel these introduce excessive cost and may increase morbidity due to greater incidence of infection, exposure, or pain. Porous implants afford an ability to place a peg that, through coupling with a subsequent

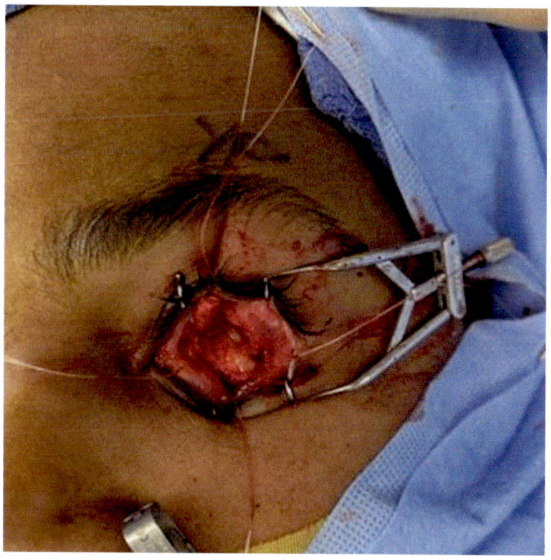

Fig. 40.5 Enucleated socket

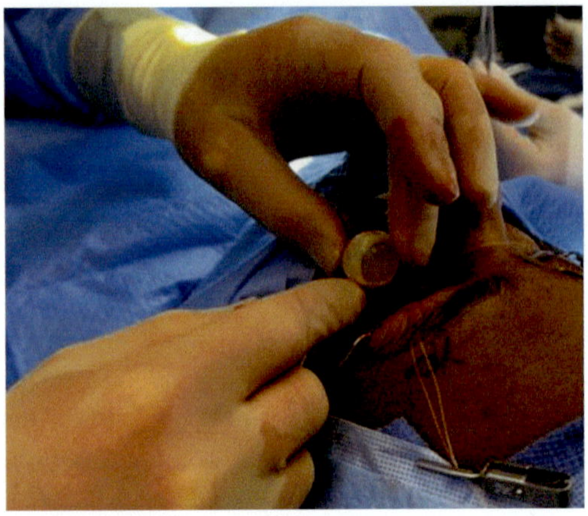

Fig. 40.6 Silicone implant wrapped in donor sclera

eye prosthesis, may achieve improved motility. However, pegs are associated with extremely high rates of infection and subsequent socket deterioration, and the risk to benefit ratio may be too high.

An optional step is to secure the inferior oblique head to either the lateral aspect of the implant or alternatively anterior. An anterior placement, achieves an additional barrier to prevent extrusion or erosions underneath the socket site of the subsequent prosthesis.

The size of the sphere in normal sized adults is usually 20 mm in diameter. In select cases, the implant may be larger or smaller. If the implant is too small, enophthalmos may ensue that may be associated with a poor ocular prosthesis fit.

Alternatively, to an alloplastic implant, a dermis fat graft may be used. (Video 40-2) The benefits of a dermis fat graft are an autologous and integrated volume replacement. In cases of conjunctival scarring or short fornices, the bare dermis can serve as a spacer to expand the socket (the bare dermis is slowly overgrown with conjunctiva). Drawbacks include a second surgical site and unpredictable results with tissue absorption (occasionally fat growth), which may require reoperation.

A dermal fat graft is harvested from the lower abdomen, flank, or the lateral gluteal region. A circle or an ellipse approximately 15 mm in diameter is marked, incised, and dissected about 2 cm deep and resected. The donor area is transformed into an ellipse for closure in 3 layers. The subcutaneous fat is closed with 3-0 polyglactin, the subcutaneous layer is closed with 4-0 polyglactin, and the skin is closed with 5-0 absorbable suture. The epidermal layer is removed from the resected tissue before being

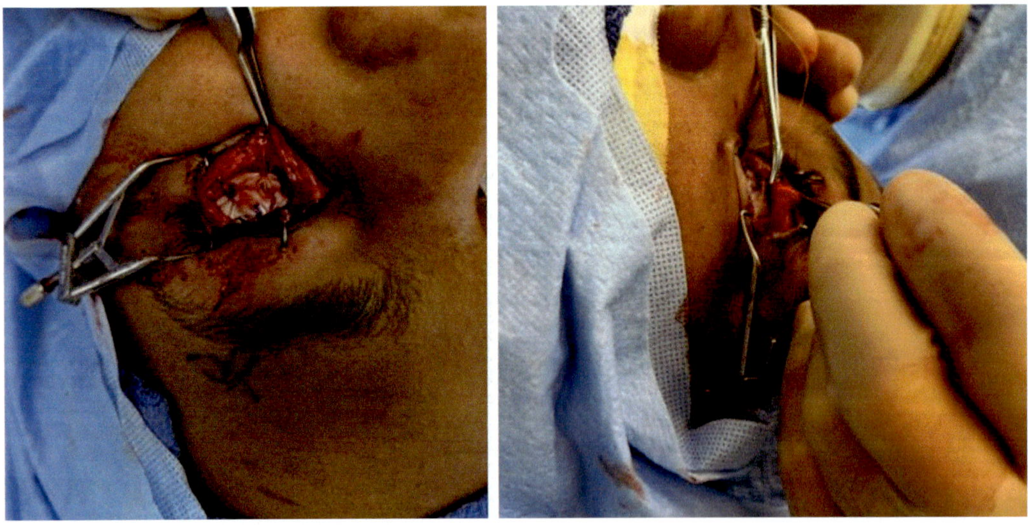

Fig. 40.7 Attach rectus muscles to implant

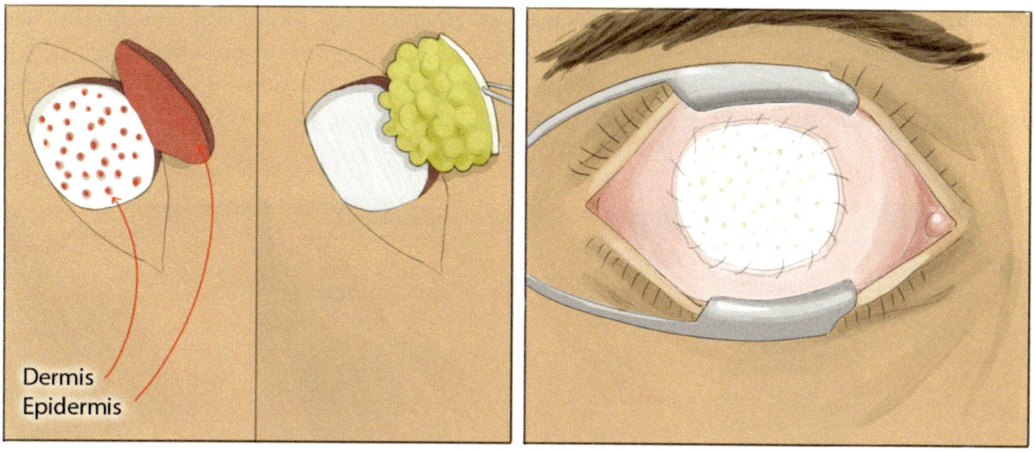

Fig. 40.8 Dermis fat graft, illustration courtesy of Michael Han MD

placed into the orbital defect. The epidermis may be removed with a shave technique using a blade. Alternatively, and when a thicker dermal component is desired, such as when additional conjunctival surface area is needed, the epidermis may be removed with a diamond burr. The dermal region is sutured to the conjunctiva using 5-0 or 6-0 polyglactin or plain gut suture [2] (Fig. 40.8).

Dermis fat grafts are sewn into the orbit with absorbable sutures (e.g., 4-0 or 5-0 polyglactin). The rectus muscles can be sewn to the nearest normal anatomic site in relation to the fat graft. In cases with adequate conjunctiva, the graft can be entirely or mostly buried. When additional socket and forniceal space is needed, the dermis is left exposed with the conjunctiva sewn 1–2 mm on to the edge of the dermis.

In cases of prior radiation, when the conjunctiva and tenons are contracted and fragile, it has been demonstrated that spreading the rectus muscles out and suturing them together with 5-0 running polyglactin can create another layer over the implant to prevent the occurrence of extrusion [3]. The anterior tenons capsule and orbital tissues are closed using interrupted non-absorbable suture securing inferotemporal to superonasal tissue and superotemporal to inferonasal tissue (Fig. 40.9). The overlying conjunctiva is then closed using 6-0 fast or plain gut suture (Fig. 40.10). An acrylic conformer placed to maintain the fornices and antibiotic ointment

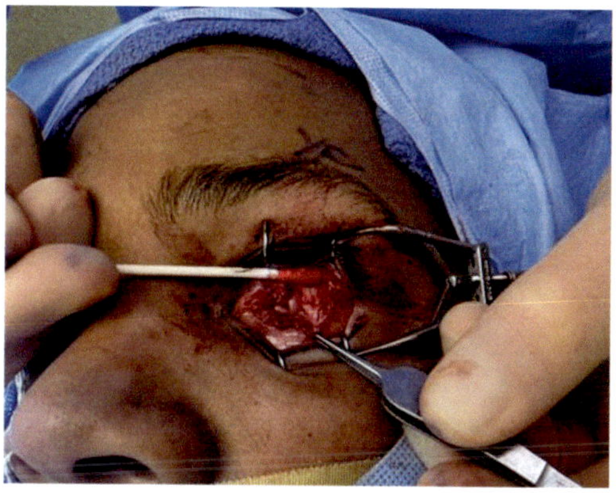

Fig. 40.9 Closure of tenons and orbital tissues

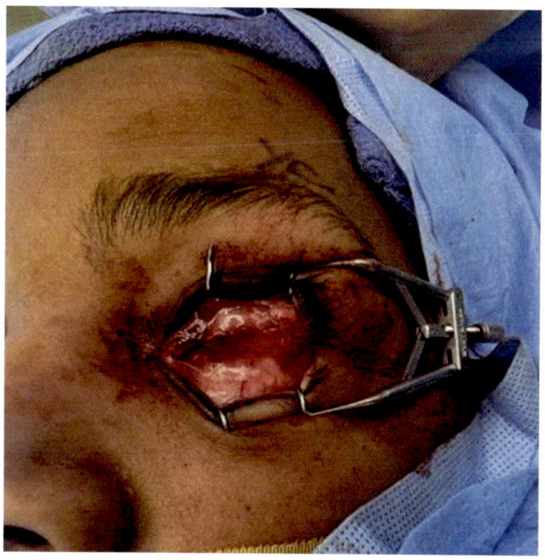

Fig. 40.10 Closure of conjunctiva prior to placement of acrylic conformer

is applied into the fornices. A light pressure bandage is placed.

The patient should be placed on an oral antibiotic for five days and encouraged to use frequent ice packs. Pain medication and antiemetics may also be prescribed. At 1–3 days post-operative, the dressing can be removed, and the patient instructed on daily care and

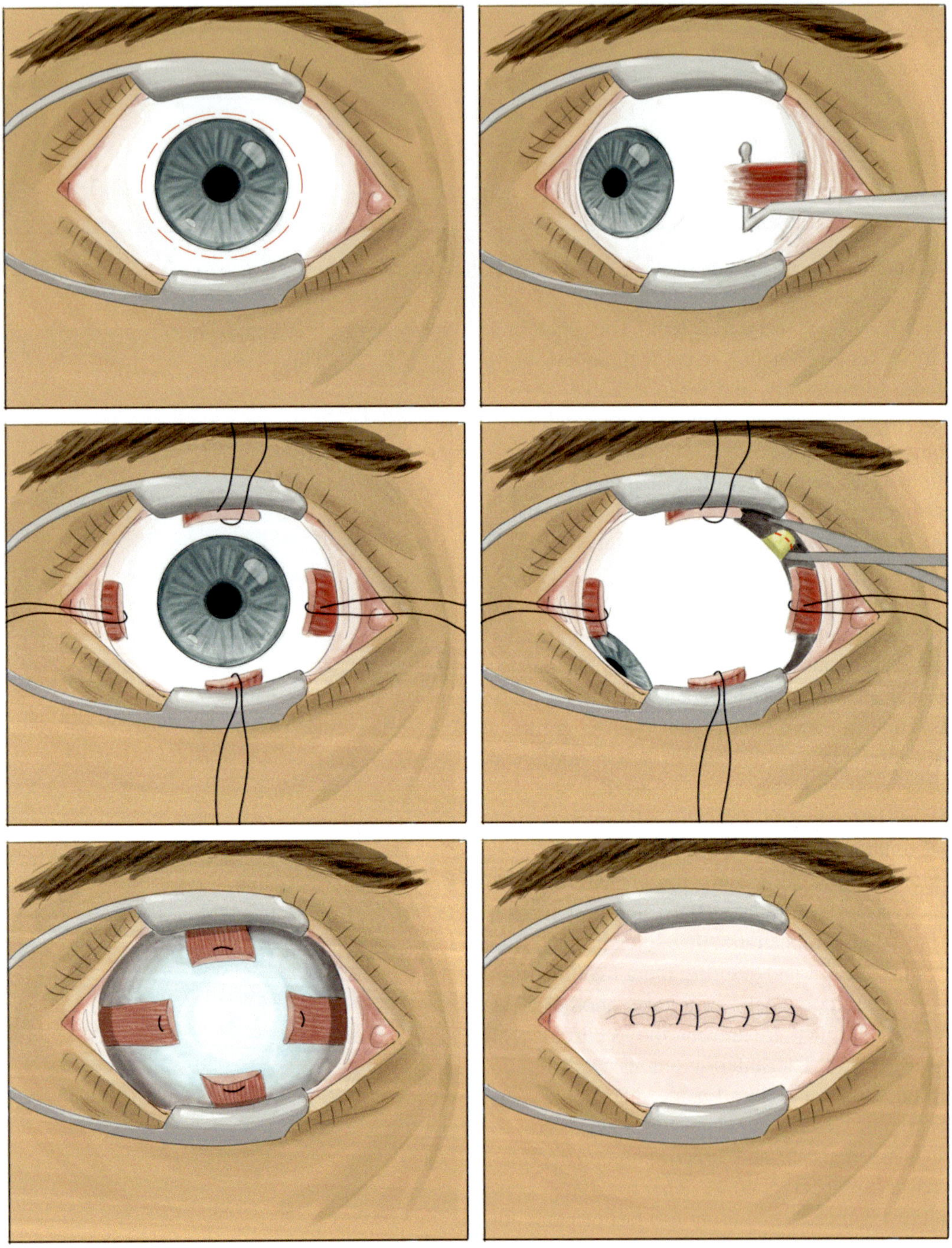

Fig. 40.11 Schematic drawing of enucleation technique, courtesy of Michael Han MD

placement of antibiotic ointment four times daily. Prosthetic fitting can be arranged in 6–8 weeks [1, 2].

Conclusion

Enucleation is a necessary procedure for many patients. Psychological factors should not be overlooked when removing an eye. Good technique with attempts to preserve extraocular muscle anatomy and physiology combined with and adequate volume replacement with an implant or dermis fat graft can achieve good results (Fig. 40.11). With adequate orbital volume and preservation of eyelid and surrounding soft tissue anatomy, patients can wear a prosthesis that restores a symmetric facial appearance (Figs. 40.12 and 40.13).

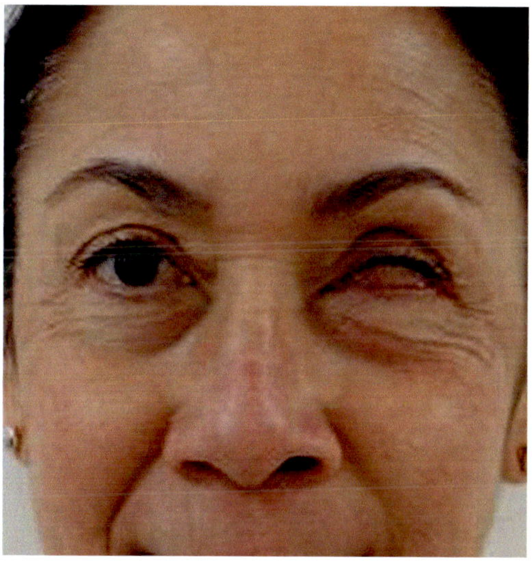

Fig. 40.12 Left healthy anophthalmic socket with with prosthesis out

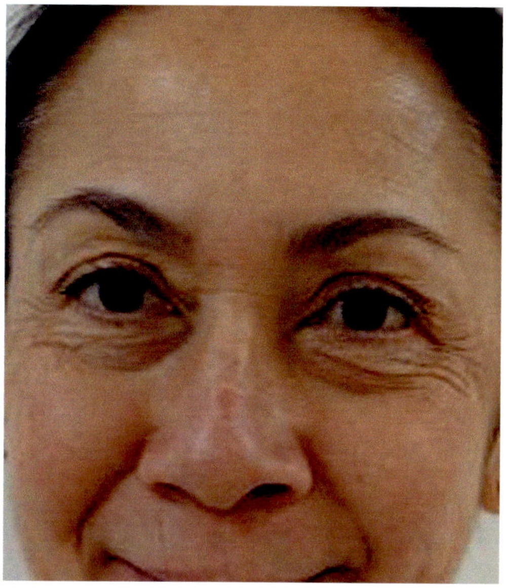

Fig. 40.13 Patient in Fig. 40.12 wearing a well-fitting left eye prosthesis

References

1. McCord CD, Tanenbaum M, Nunery W, Chen WP. Enucleation, evisceration, and exenteration. In: Oculoplastic surgery. Essay. Raven Press; 1995. pp. 581–591.
2. Reinheimer WT. Techniques of enucleation and evisceration. Operative techniques in otolaryngology-head and neck surgery. https://www.sciencedirect.com/science/article/pii/S1043181018300848. Accessed 7 Jan 2022.
3. Chu HY, Liao YL, Tsai YJ, Chu YC, Wu SY, Ma L. Use of extraocular muscle flaps in the correction of orbital implant exposure [published correction appears in PLoS One. 2013;8(11). https://doi.org/10.1371/annotation/d77a80cc-f8bc-4140-b0b3-c9f05c861776]. *PLoS One*. 2013;8(9):e72223. https://doi.org/10.1371/journal.pone.0072223

Orbital Exenteration

41

Jan P. Ulloa Padilla, Kenneth Morgenstern, and Cat Burkat

Abstract

Orbital exenteration (OE) is the surgical removal of the eye and all surrounding orbital and periocular structures. In select cases, an extended exenteration that removes surrounding bone, may be necessary. OE is usually indicated for aggressive malignancy that is otherwise untreatable with other modalities. In this chapter, the authors describe indications and surgical technique for OE.

Keywords

Exenteration · Eye removal · Orbital malignancy · Orbital mucormycosis

Introduction

One of the most disfiguring and psychologically impacting surgery in ophthalmology remains orbital exenteration (OE). The first OE documented is accredited to Georg Bartisch, who performed the procedure and described it in 1583. It consists of removing the orbital contents with or without the eyelids. Primary intraocular, cutaneous, or sinus malignancies that invade the orbital tissues and primary orbital malignancies that require margin free excision are the most common indications for orbital exenteration (OE). Obtaining margin-free excisions of these lesions tend to be difficult due to the nature of the orbital fat and the involvement of other extraocular structures.

Cutaneous basal cell carcinoma and squamous cell carcinoma are the most common tumors that invade the orbit and require exenteration. Squamous cell carcinoma is the most common entity originating from the sinus that may necessitate OE. Sebaceous carcinoma is particularly prevalent in the Asian population. Intraocular malignancies such as choroidal melanoma rarely involves the orbit, with OE a very rare management option as studies have not demonstrated improved survival with OE. Adenoid cystic carcinoma of the lacrimal gland is a primary orbital malignancy that has traditionally been commonly managed with OE; however other oncologic managements have emerged. Optic nerve tumors, soft tissues sarcomas, sinus tumors and orbital bony wall tumors might also necessitate OE, depending on presentation, extension, and behavior of the tumor.

Supplementary Information The online version contains supplementary material available at https://doi.org/10.1007/978-3-031-63178-8_41.

J. P. U. Padilla · C. Burkat (✉)
University of Wisconsin, Madison, WI, USA
e-mail: cburkat@wisc.edu

K. Morgenstern
Morgenstern Center for Orbital and facial Plastic Surgery, Philadelphia, PA, USA

J. Tao (ed.), *Efficient Oculofacial Surgery*, https://doi.org/10.1007/978-3-031-63178-8_41

Orbital exenteration may rarely be a treatment modality for severe inflammatory conditions, trauma, and developmental abnormalities. It is worth noting that some malignancies are not treated with OE, such as lymphocytic tumors or rhabdomyosarcomas. Lastly, severe infections such as mucormycosis and, less commonly, aspergillosis require generous debridement, and in some cases exenteration [1–4].

The evaluation of a patient with an invasive orbital process is extensive and commonly requires a multispecialty approach. Orbital exenteration sometimes spans related disciplines of otolaryngology, neurosurgery, dermatology, maxillofacial surgey, or craniofacial surgery. Ophthalmological care for and attention to the uninvolved eye is also a critical.

Neuro-imaging with CT or MRI is usually warranted to determine the extent of the malignancy, including evidence of sinus or intracranial invasion. Definitive tissue diagnosis is a requirement, as this will give valuable information in terms of prognosis, survival, and additional systemic work up coordinated with an oncologist. Once it has been determined that OE is indicated, an approach must be determined. In this chapter the authors describe the most common and accessible OE techniques, complications, and postoperative orbital socket management.

Techniques

The surgical approach and technique depend on the origin, localization, and extent of the primary disease process. Numerous nomenclatures have been proposed. This chapter employs a modified classification system per Meyer and Zaoli and the terms: total exenteration, subtotal exenteration and extended exenteration.

Orbital exenteration and any removal of diseased tissues are often performed with the secondary goal of minimizing loss of healthy tissue, and thus several surgical approaches to these orbital tumors are warranted. It is also important to note that OE can be of curative or palliative benefit for extensive tumors, and reconstruction of the exenteration defects can often be quite challenging.

Total exenteration is defined as the removal of all intraorbital content including the globe, extraocular muscles, lacrimal gland, and drainage system along with the optic nerve. Subtotal exenteration can be defined as a removal of certain orbital components. This is most useful for tumors or pathologic entities that the clinician is certain to only be involving a specific anatomical space such as the anterior orbit. Subtotal exenteration is customized to each patient, and the benefit to this approach is the preservation of other anatomical structures such as a remnant of the optic nerve, and posterior orbital tissues in the orbital apex, if the offending tumor is only involving the anterior orbit. For mass lesions not involving the orbit apex, exenteration may be performed to remove tissue anterior to the anatomical delineation of the posterior globe. This is often used for eyelid skin and conjunctival tumors. The technique allows for faster orbital healing and a better fitting prosthetic.

An extended orbital exenteration involves the removal of the intraorbital content and additional removal of orbital bones or facial tissues [5]. This sometimes is approached in a multidisciplinary manner and may involve otolaryngology, plastic surgery, and neurosurgery specialists.

Total Exenteration (Video 41-1)

Orbital exenteration is performed under general anesthesia. The face prepped and draped in sterile fashion.

1. An oval shaped marking around the surgical eye is made, placed superiorly and inferiorly to the upper and lower eyelid lashes, respectively and preserving as much skin as possible. These markings extend and join at the medial and lateral canthus (Fig. 41.1A). In some orbital disease processes eyelid skin not spared and the initial incisions start on the orbital rim circumferentially.

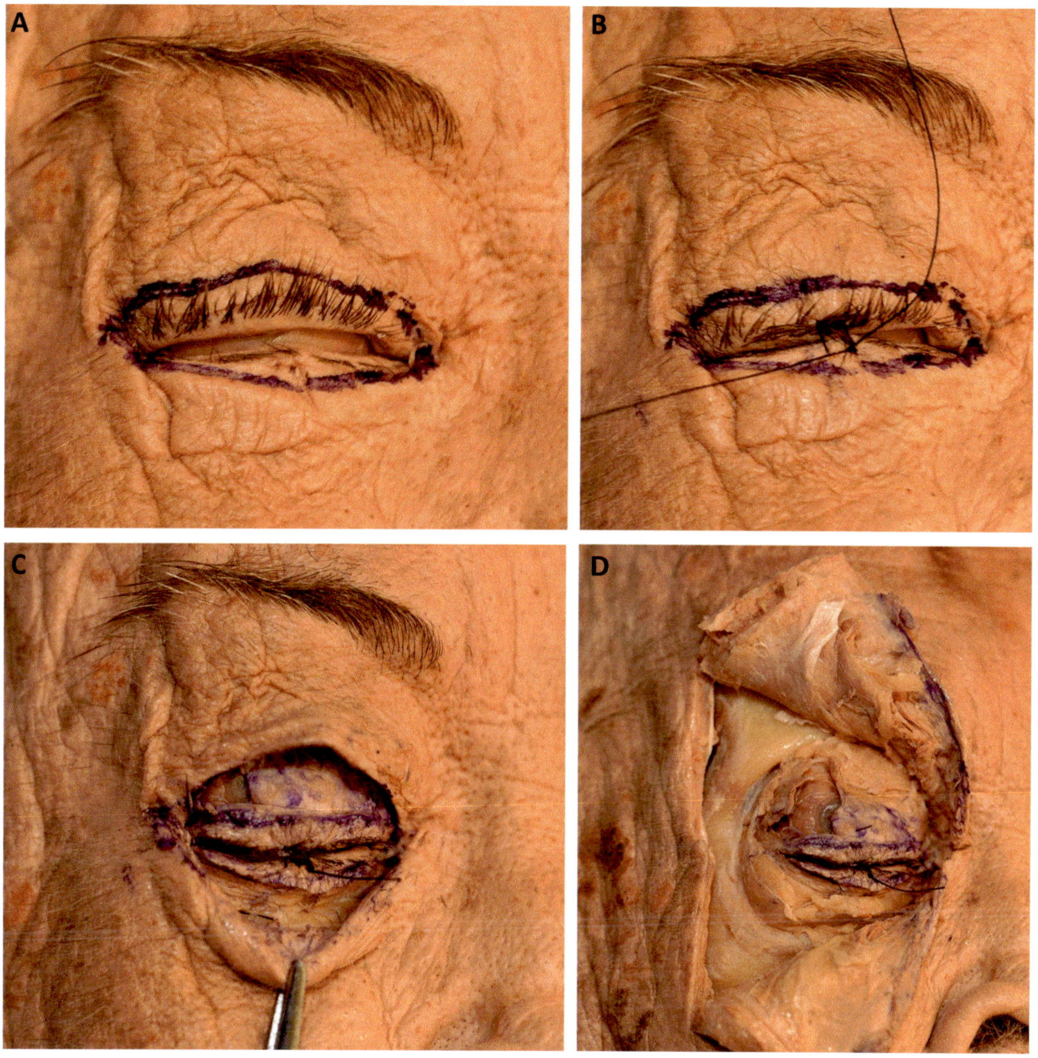

Fig. 41.1 Total exenteration—non eyelid sparing. **A** The incision markings are made approximately 2 mm superiorly to the lashes in the upper eyelid and inferiorly to the lashes in the lower eyelid. These markings are joined at the lateral and medial canthal areas, forming an oval shape around the eyelid margins. **B** Marginal traction sutures are placed in a horizontal mattress fashion. One is presented in this specimen; however, 2–3 traction sutures are recommended for adequate tension. **C** The incisions are made with a #15 Bard-Parker blade or electrosurgical cautery along the previously made markings. **D** After the initial incision is made, dissection is continued under the orbicularis oculi towards the periosteum at the level of the orbital rim. **E** The periosteum is incised along the orbital rim, and dissection is continued in a subperiosteal plane towards the orbital apex (temporal vertical incision made here to demonstrate the lateral orbital rim). **F** The medial canthal tendon (over the probe) is a structure of particular importance, as it is intrinsically joined with the periosteum at the level of the medial orbital wall. Aggressive dissection in this medial orbital wall area may cause significant bleeding or an orbital fracture. **G** The supraorbital neurovascular bundle is exposed as it passes over the medial orbital rim, or through a separate supraorbital foramen. This structure may be cut, and dissection continued towards the orbital apex. **H** The posterior ethmoidal artery courses through the posterior ethmoidal foramina displayed in this photo. Care must be taken with this artery as well as the anterior ethmoidal artery which courses approx. 10 mm anterior to the posterior ethmoidal artery. **I** The lacrimal fossa with the dissection probe within the connection of the orbit to the inferior meatus, where the lacrimal duct drains. **J** and **K** The orbital apex after removal of the exenteration specimen. The optic nerve and ophthalmic artery are visible. The dissection probe is showing the optic nerve and inferiorly the ophthalmic artery. **L–N** The orbital content specimen. Anterior (1L), lateral (1M), and posterior (1N) views

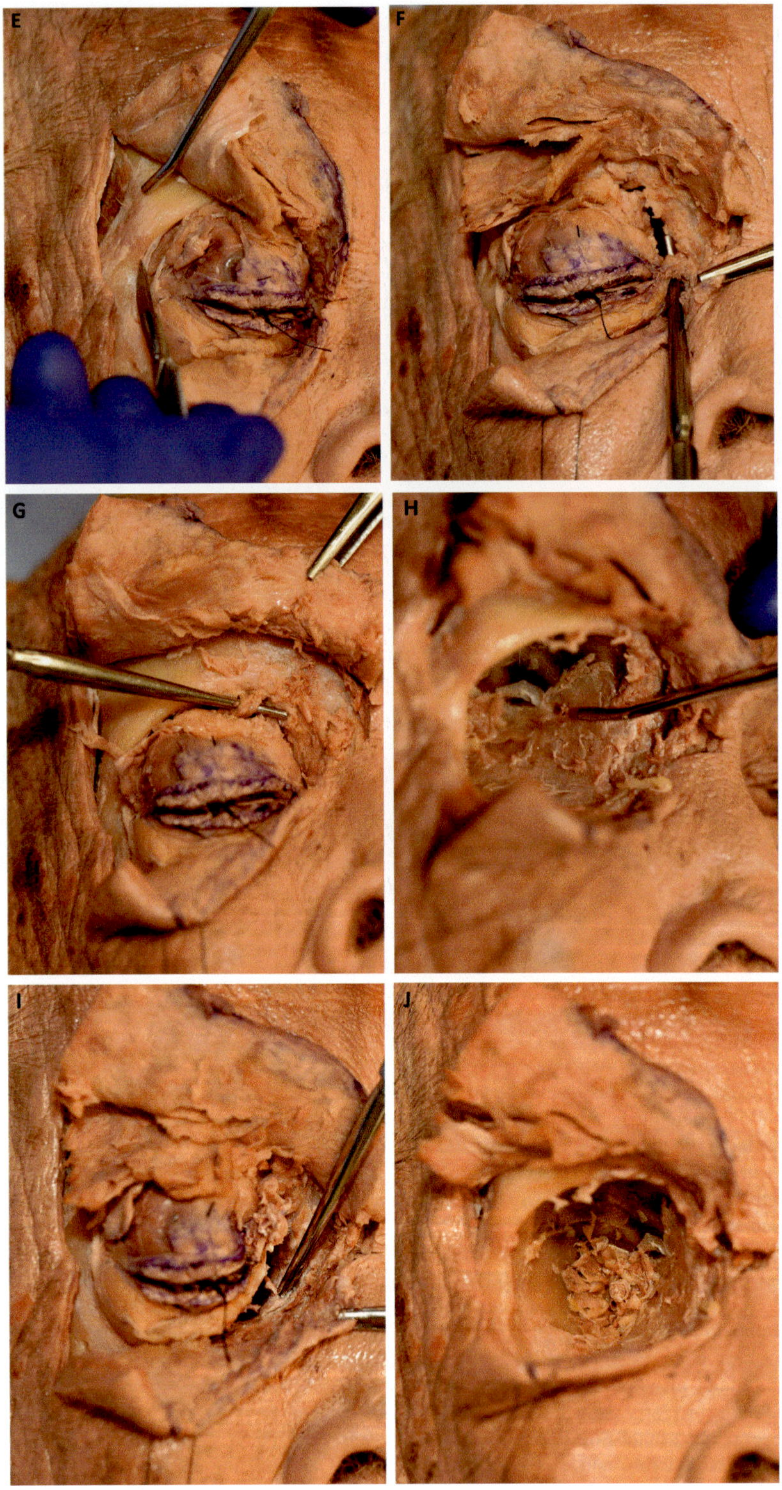

Fig. 41.1 (continued)

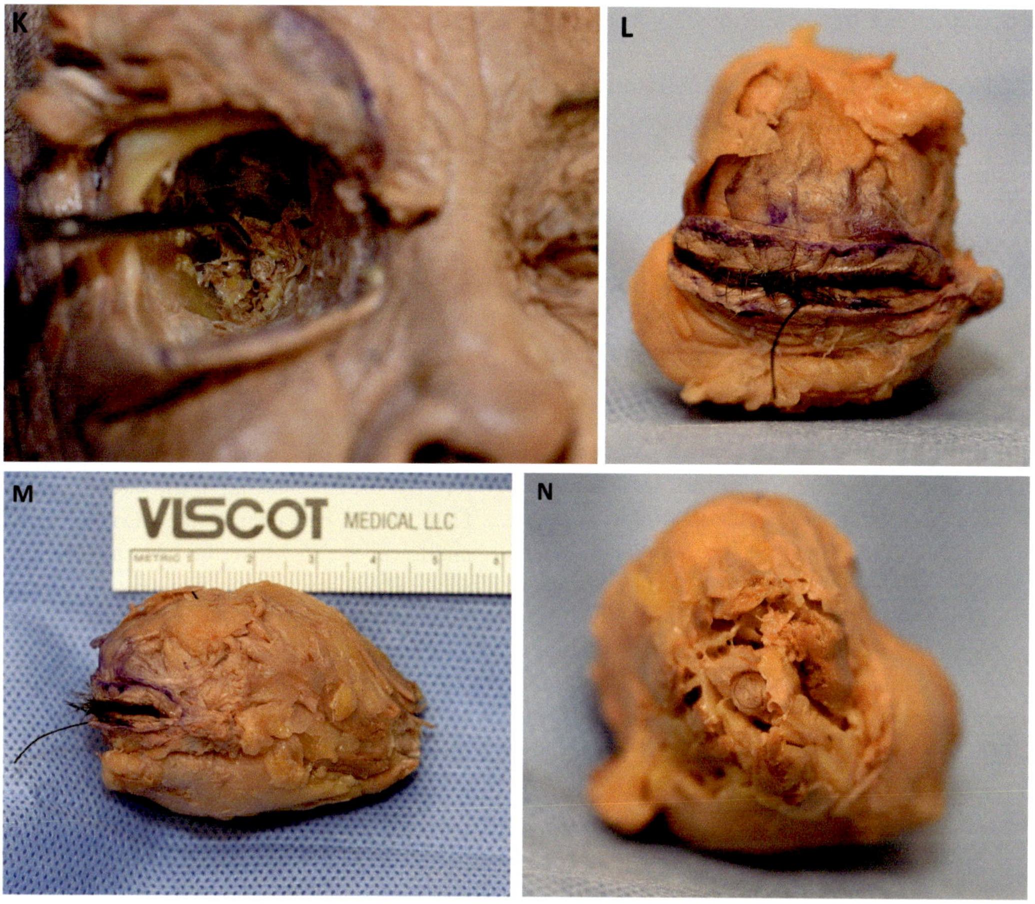

Fig. 41.1 (continued)

2. Two to three silk 4-0 traction sutures may be placed through the eyelid margins (Fig. 41.1B).
3. An incision is made with the #15 Bard-Parker blade along the skin markings (Fig. 41.1C).
4. Dissection is performed in the suborbicularis oculi muscle plane, anterior to the orbital septum, towards the superior and inferior orbital rim until periosteum is seen (Fig. 41.1D).
5. Once the orbital rim periosteum is exposed, an incision (using a blade or cutting cautery) through periosteum is made circumferentially at the level of the arcus marginalis (Fig. 41.1E).
6. Periosteal elevators are used to separate the periosteum from the orbital walls, from the orbital rim towards the apex. The periosteum is most tightly adherent to the orbital sutures such as the frontozygomatic suture, medial canthal tendon (Fig. 41.1F), and orbital fissures- special care around these areas is recommended to avoid fractures to the orbital walls. The periosteal elevator may inadvertently fracture the orbital walls, especially the thin medial orbital wall (lamina papyracea). When dissecting the orbital roof, excessive force may cause a fracture with cerebrospinal fluid leak.
7. Along the superonasal orbital rim, the neurovascular bundle that arises from the

supraorbital foramen or notch can be cauterized and cut (Fig. 41.1G).

8. Hemostasis is achieved with electrocautery. Several anatomical landmarks are released or transected to free the orbital soft tissues from the bone including the inferior oblique muscle origin, trochlea, anterior and posterior ethmoidal arteries (Fig. 41.1H) at the level of the medial wall and inferior orbital fissure.
9. In the inferomedial orbit, the lacrimal sac is dissected from the lacrimal fossa and separated from the nasolacrimal duct. The duct is trasected and cauterized (Fig. 41.1I).
10. In the inferotemporal orbit, the inferior orbital fissure is identified, with cautious dissection and cautery of the vessels.
11. Once the orbital apex has been reached, a right-angled clamp or hemostat can be applied to the apical tissues which include the optic nerve and superior orbital fissures contents. Enucleation scissors can then be used to transect the posterior orbital tissues.
12. Significant bleeding from the ophthalmic artery and other large posterior orbital vesselsare managed with pressure, ligation, or cautery. If cautery is used at the apex, bipolar is advised (Fig. 41.1J and K).
13. Once hemostasis is achieved, the exenterated tissues are submitted to pathology for further analysis, with marked margins for proper identification by the pathologist. Frozen section may be useful in some instances of cutaneous origin carcinomas to ensure that the perimeter of resected tissues are free of tumor (Fig. 41.1L–N).
14. The remnant upper and the lower eyelid skin are folded into the orbit. The orbital walls may be left to heal by second intention or a skin graft (split or full thickness) may be used to line the cavity. Fenestration of the graft aids in allowing it to fit within the concave confines of the interior orbit (Fig. 41.2).

Subtotal Exenteration

Orbital exenteration is performed under general anesthesia. The correct surgical site is properly identified, and the face prepped and draped in sterile fashion.

1. Traction sutures may be placed at the eyelid margins.
2. An incision is made through skin and orbicularis muscle using a #15 Bard-Parker blade or electrosurgical cautery towards the orbital rim periosteum. Dissection proceeds in the subperiosteal place on the orbital walls posteriorly, usually starting at the lateral margin. Care should be taken in the medial canthus and lower eyelid where the large angular vessels (which pass approximately 8–12 mm inferomedially to the medial canthal angle) may cause significant bleeding.
3. The oval or circular incision is carried down to the orbital rim periosteum which is then incised and carefully separated from the orbital walls using a periosteal (Freer) elevator. Special attention must be given to the tight adhesions of the periosteum to the orbital sutures, and to important landmarks such as lacrimal sac, trochlea, and inferior orbital fissure to avoid orbital fractures.
4. Dissection is continued posteriorly towards the orbital apex.
5. The periosteum/periorbita is incised behind the globe, to enter the retrobulbar conal space behind the diseased tissues.
6. A right-angled clamp or hemostat can be applied to the posterior margin of the exenteration. Enucleation scissors are then used to cut above the clamp.
7. The traction sutures are used to lift and remove the anterior orbital content.
8. Hemostasis can be achieved with bipolar cautery and pressure to the posterior orbital apex tissue edges.
9. At the end of the case, remnant apical tissues remain in the posterior orbit.

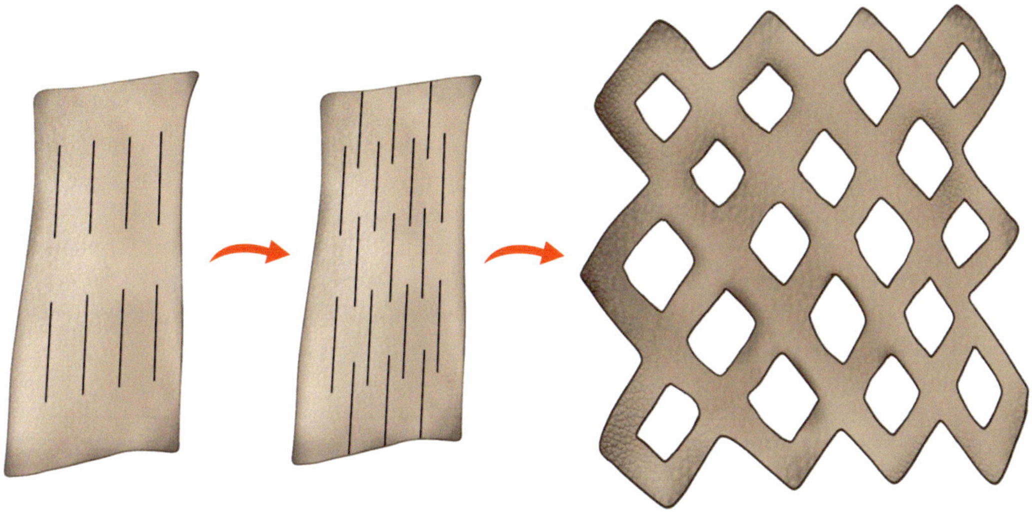

Fig. 41.2 Schematic illustration of manual meshing of the skin graft. Incisions are placed in a staggered linear fashion to allow for spreading of the graft

Extended Orbital Exenteration

An extended orbital exenteration is usually required when the malignancy involves the orbital bones. A radical exenteration involves removal of adjacent structures such as paranasal sinuses. A multispecialty approach is often utilized. Once the orbital exenteration has been performed, it is extended to remove the extension of the tumor, be that in the maxillary sinus, ethmoid sinus, cheek, lacrimal fossa, or cranial fossa. A more complex reconstruction strategy is usually warranted with free flaps, temporalis muscle flaps, dermis fat grafts, artificial dermis grafts or regional flaps [6–9].

Orbit Cavity Reconstruction

Granulation

The orbit cavity may be left to heal by spontaneous granulation. Delayed healing is common with this method; however, it is inexpensive, permits the development of a bowl-shaped cavity and has no second surgical site morbidity. At the end of surgery, the socket is packed, and antibiotic ointment applied. The dressings are changed every few days until granulation is observed.

Skin grafting

An orbital exenteration is performed in the same manner as described previously. Appropriate donor sites from which to harvest a graft include the thighs, trunk, or supraclavicular area; in general, large areas of skin without hair is preferred.

- Measure the appropriate graft size at the donor site, or with slight oversizing for anticipation of graft contracture.
- If harvesting with a dermatome, apply mineral oil or petrolatum.
- Pull the donor site in opposite directions parallel to the path of the dermatome, making the donor site taught.
- Bring the dermatome into contact with the skin at a 45-degree angle. Flatten the dermatome to be parallel with the skin as the graft is being harvested.
- Once the desired length has been achieved, angle the dermatome upwards to exit at a 45-degree angle to the skin surface.

- Carefully remove the graft from the donor site, paying special attention to the orientation, as the dermis side must be sutured towards the wound bed in the recipient site.
- Place the graft on a gauze soaked in normal saline until it is ready to be meshed. Apply an epinephrine-soaked gauze to the donor site for hemostasis.
- The process of meshing a graft allows the graft to spread out more, to cover a larger surface area with the same graft size. Utilizing a mesher, pass the graft with the desired ratio (typical ratios used include 3/8 to 1, 1 to 1, 2 to 1, 3 to 1 and even 6 to 1).
- If a mesher is not available, the graft can be manually meshed by placing the skin graft on a flat surface and using a 11 or 15 scalpel blade to create lines of small incisions in the graft. The adjacent lines of holes should be staggered so that the graft will fit the concave configuration of the orbit (Fig. 41.2). If a ridged or multi-grooved derma carrier is available, the graft can be placed on top, and the blade used to draw lines perpendicular to the grooves—this results in equidistant perforations at the tops of the ridges, and areas of intact skin in the valleys, thus resulting in a meshed pattern more efficiently.
- Once the graft has been meshed, secure the graft to the remaining eyelid skin with a 6-0 plain gut suture so that it covers the orbital cavity. Once the graft is in position, line the graft with petrolatum gauze and pack the orbit tightly with nonadherent gauze (e.g., telfa or adaptic) under xeroform dressing (or ribbon impregnated with antibiotic ointment) so that the graft remains seated smoothly and firmly on the bony surfaces. Secure the orbit with eyepatches and tape to achieve gentle pressure.
- The advantages include obtaining a bowl-shaped socket with more rapid healing and epithelialization. The donor site may be covered with a mesh gauze. The patient will be ready for a prosthesis approximately 2 months after surgery.

If eyelid skin was largely spared and the orbital cavity does not require a large skin graft, a full thickness skin graft harvested with a scalpel may suffice. This obviates a need for a dermatome and a mesher. Full thickness skin may be manually thinned with scissors and pie crusted with several blade incisions.

Biologic Dermal Matrix Graft

The use of a dermis xenografts may obviate second surgical site morbidity with the use of autologous skin grafts [10]. Composed of 2 layers, the dermal layer is usually made of bovine collagen and the epidermal layer is made of silicone. The graft can be secured to the orbital skin and packet in the usual fashion, significantly reducing surgical time. The silicone layer is subsequently removed, and the socket may be left to epithelialize.

Flap Reconstruction

Several flaps are useful for the reconstruction of an orbital socket post-exenteration including: paramedian frontalis flap, frontalis flap, glabellar flap, superficial temporalis flap and temporalis muscle flap. The temporalis muscle flap is particularly useful. It is commonly employed when covering the anterior cranial fossa or the sinuses, and results in a full orbital socket.

Free Flaps

In some instances free flaps are useful in dealing with complex orbital and facial defects. These are especially useful if vital structures adjacent to the orbit are exposed, namely the intracranial space. Possible flaps include the radial forearm flap, anterolateral thigh flap, latissimus dorsi, and microvascular scapular flap. The description of these flaps is beyond the scope of this chapter; however, the main complications associated with free flaps include surgical morbidity, flap necrosis, and the need for additional debulking surgery. The mass effect obliterates the necessary cavitary seat for an exenteration prosthesis.

Temporalis Muscle Flap

The temporalis muscle flap is an excellent technique for orbital reconstruction, as it provides adequate volume, and vascularity allowing for faster healing of the orbital socket. The temporalis muscle is in the temporal fossa, and it originates from the parietal and frontal bones of the fossa as well as the deep temporalis fascia and it inserts in the ramus of the mandible. It has an intricate anatomical relation with the superficial and deep temporalis fascia with significant surgical considerations.

1. An incision is made anteriorly to the tragus and extends superiorly and posteriorly along the temporalis muscle in an arc configuration (Fig. 41.3A).
2. Dissection is performed towards the temporalis fascia and continued superficially to this plane to raise the skin flap and expose the temporalis muscle which occupies the temporalis fossa (Fig. 41.3B).
3. Exposure of the zygomatic arch and lateral orbital wall are also needed (Fig. 41.3C).
4. An orbital wall osteotomy with a bone drill is performed on the orbital process of the zygoma on the lateral orbital wall, leaving the rim intact, as the muscle flap will reach the orbit through this osteotomy (Fig. 41.3C, red arrow shows the osteotomy).
5. Once the temporalis muscle is exposed, the fascia is incised at the superior edge of the muscle, and a subperiosteal dissection is performed to separate the muscle from the bone (Fig. 41.3D).
6. The anterior and posteriors edges of the muscle are also detached as needed to allow adequate movement of the muscle towards the osteotomy and orbit (Fig. 41.3E).
7. At the end of the dissection, the temporalis muscle must have a hinge at the level of the coronoid to allow adequate vascularization of the muscle.
8. The temporalis muscle is passed through the tunnel; (Fig. 41.3F) in this manner, a prominent orbital rim is avoided which can be seen when passing the muscle flap over the orbital rim instead.
9. Once the muscle is within the orbit, (Fig. 41.3G) it must be sutured to the edges of the orbital rim tissues, such as the eyelid skin (if preserved). In a total exenteration, a skin graft can be placed over the muscle flap.

Complications

Graft necrosis or failure

Hemorrhage or blood clots under the graft and a low-grade infection are the most common causes of graft failure. It can be managed conservatively, however if a chronic infection is suspected it should be managed with antibiotics to allow proper healing of the orbit.

Numbness

Facial numbness is usually caused after damage to the trigeminal nerves sectioned at the superior orbital fissure. In some cases, numbness improves months after the surgery; however, it can rarely be permanent. In subtotal exenterations, especially for processes in the inferior

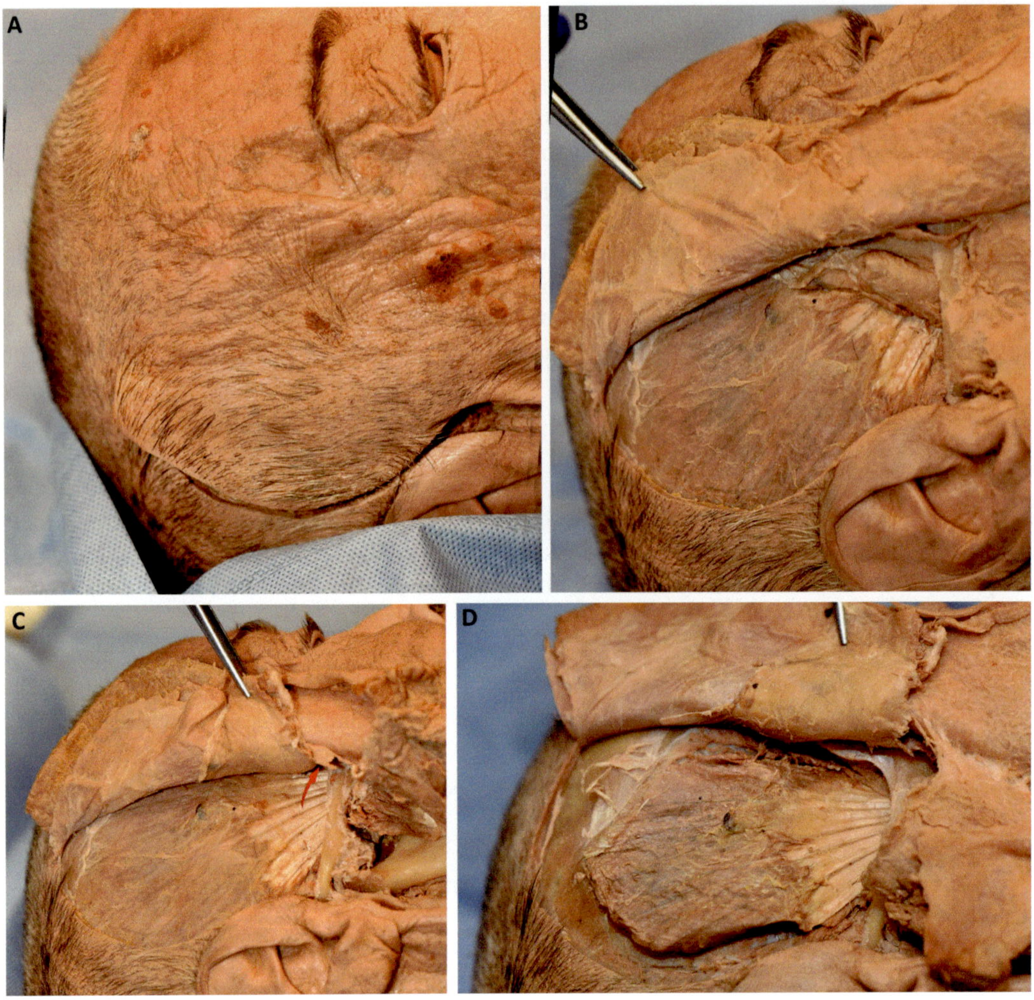

Fig. 41.3 Temporalis muscle flap. **A** An incision is made anterior to the tragus and extending superiorly along the temporalis fossa. **B** Dissection is then performed towards the temporalis fascia, and the superficial plane of the muscle is observed. Complete exposure of the muscle is required. **C** Dissection is continued inferiorly to expose the zygomatic arch. In the inner aspect of the zygomatic arch and its connection to the lateral orbital wall is the site for the osteotomy (marked with X), which can be achieved with a bone drill. **D** The dissection is continued along the superior edge of the temporalis muscle in a subperiosteal place to separate the entire temporalis flap from the fossa. **E** The attachments of the flap to the fascia are also incised to allow adequate mobilization of the flap as seen here. **F** The temporalis flap is then inserted through the osteotomy. **G** The muscle is draped inside the orbit over the bone, which provides vascularized tissue and volume to the orbit. The muscle may be sutured to the orbital rim periosteum to secure it in place. Additionally, a skin graft or dermis fat graft can also be placed over the temporalis flap for additional volume restoration

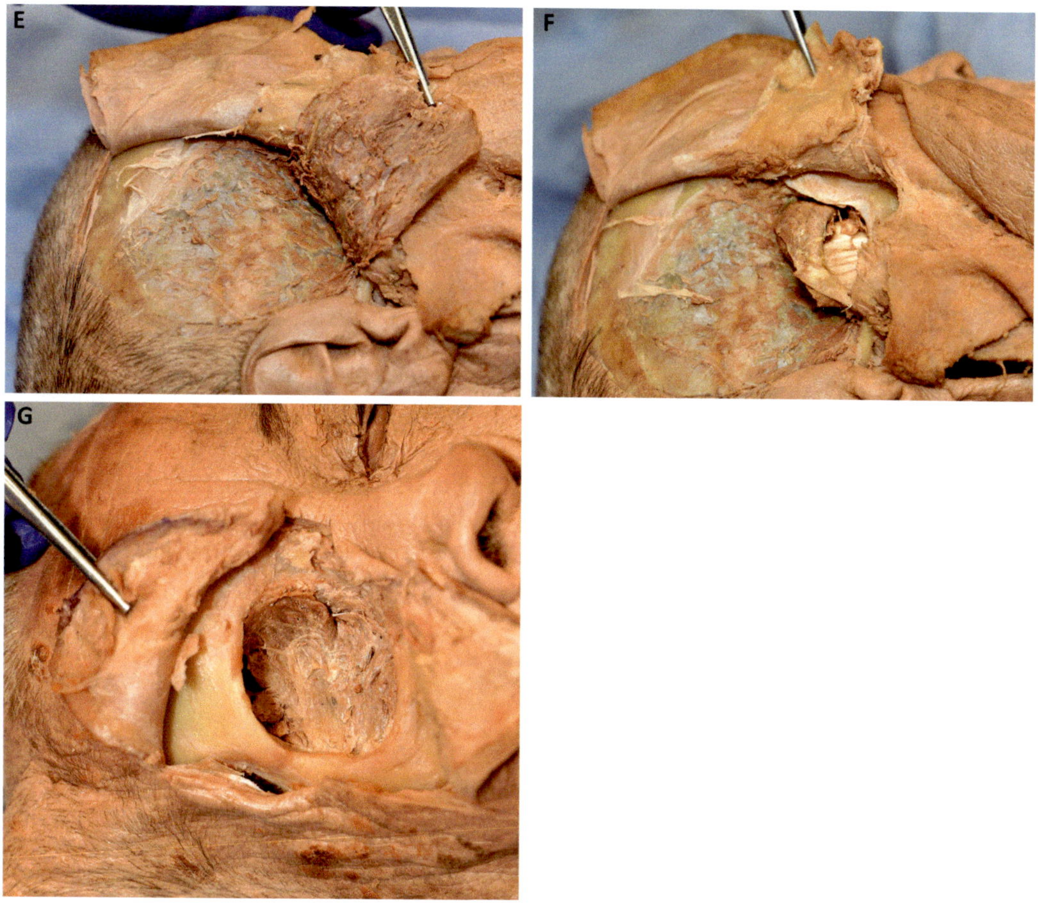

Fig. 41.3 (continued)

orbit, the supraorbital nerves may be spared to maintain forehead and head sensation.

Sino-orbital fistulas

This is a common post-exenteration complication [11]. Frequently caused during the dissection of the periosteum of the orbital walls, a small connection may be created between the orbit and the sinuses, usually the ethmoid sinus. This may lead to infections and graft failure, but rarely requires closure as they spontaneously close. If continued discharge is noted, and difficulty wearing or sizing a prosthesis develops, then a flap or a temporalis muscle transplantation may be performed over the fistula.

CSF leak and Meningitis

Meningitis following exenteration is associated with immediate or delayed cerebrospinal fluid (CSF) leak. This most commonly occurs when dissecting the orbital content off the roof of the orbit. It can be managed in conjunction with neurosurgery with a lumbar drain, medications to reduce intracranial pressure, or direct surgical

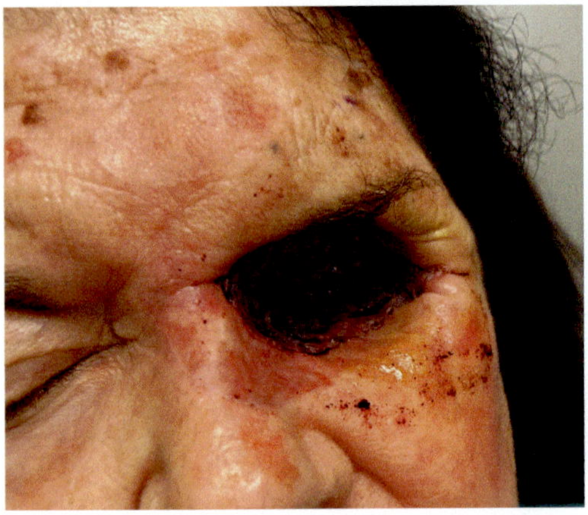

Fig. 41.4 1 week postoperative appearance of an exenteration with packing removed and meshed full thickness skin graft visible. The orbit should be packed with xeroform gauze over a nonadherent dressing to allow the skin graft to integrate to the orbit cavity

closure. An intraoperative CSF leak may be managed with direct suture, fibrin glue, fat or flap interposition, bone graft or bone wax.

Conclusions

Orbital exenteration is a necessary procedure for aggressive tumors or infectious processes of the orbit. The extent of the exenteration can be customized. In general, the orbital cavity is lined with skin and an orbital prosthesis can later be fit for cosmesis that can provide reasonable facial symmetry (Fig. 41.4, 41.5A and B) [12]. Flap coverage of the orbital defect is an option but large flaps, including free flaps, often obliterate a proper seat for the orbital prosthesis.

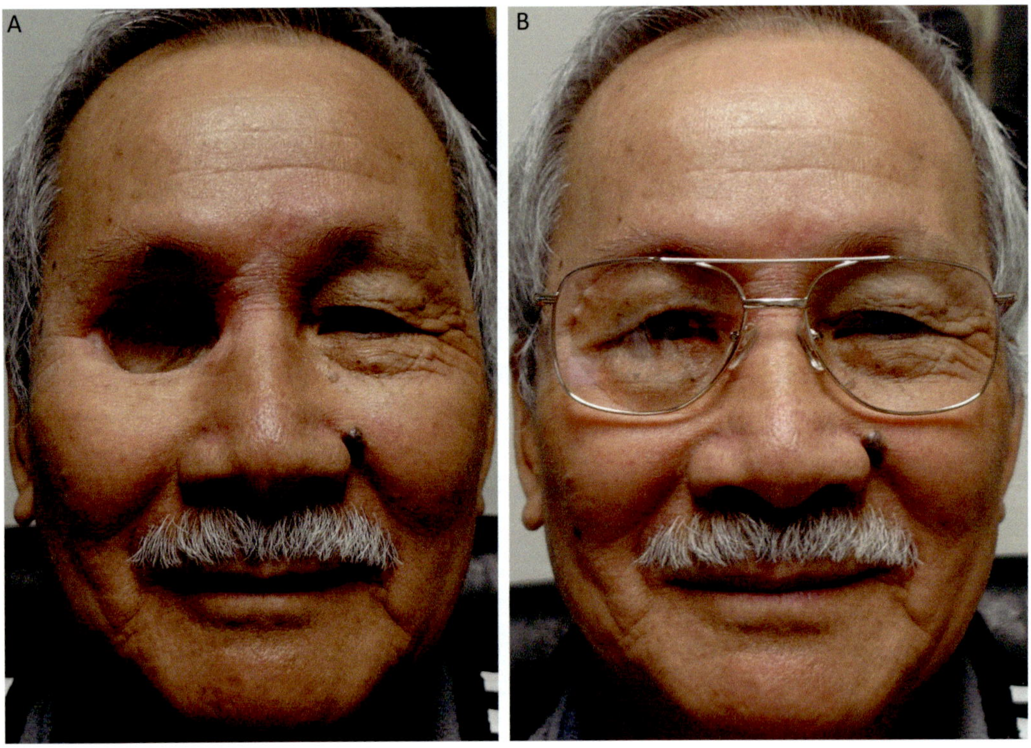

Fig. 41.5 (**A**) A patient with a healed right exenterated socket and orbital prosthesis removed. **B** Patient in **A** wearing a well-fitting right orbital prosthesis (Spectacles can further improve cosmesis by partial coverage of the prosthesis)

References

1. Martel A, Baillif S, Nahon-Esteve S, et al. Orbital exenteration: an updated review with perspectives. Surv Ophthalmol. 2021;66(5):856–76.
2. Nerad JA. Techniques in ophthalmic plastic surgery: a personal tutorial. Philadelphia, PA: Saunders; 2010.
3. Aryasit O, Preechawai P, Hirunpat C, Horatanaruang O, Singha P. Factors related to survival outcomes following orbital exenteration: a retrospective, comparative, case series. BMC Ophthalmol. 2018;18(1):186. https://doi.org/10.1186/s12886-018-0850-y.
4. Bartley GB, Garrity JA, Waller RR, Henderson JW, Ilstrup DM. Orbital exenteration at the Mayo Clinic. 1967–1986. Ophthalmology 1989;96(4):468–73.
5. Fomete B, Omeje KU, Agbara R, Adebayo E, Ikhekuamen E, Amole O. Extended orbital exenteration: proposal for modification of Meyer and Zaoli's classification. Nig J Dent Res. 2022;7(2):97–102. https://doi.org/10.4314/njdr.v7i2.4.
6. Shore JW, Burks R, Leone CR, McCord CD. Dermis-fat graft for orbital reconstruction after subtotal exenteration. Am J Ophthalmol. 1986;102(2):228–36.
7. Martel A, Hamedani M, Lagier J, Bertolotto C, Gastaud L, Poissonnet G. L'exentération orbitaire a-t-elle encore sa place en 2019 Journal Français d'Ophtalmologie. 2020;43(2):152–74.
8. Jategaonkar A, Vernon D, Byrne P. Regional reconstruction of orbital exenteration defects. Semin Plast Surg. 2019;33(02):120–4.
9. Badhey A, Haidar Y, Genden E. Soft tissue microvascular reconstruction of orbital exenteration defects. Semin Plast Surg. 2019;33(2):125–31. https://doi.org/10.1055/s-0039-1685480.
10. Ameloot F, Mezzine H, Khairallah G, et al. Reconstruction of exenteration socket with Integra® dermal substitute and skin graft. J Fr Ophtalmol. 2019;42(7):746–52. https://doi.org/10.1016/j.jfo.2019.03.023.
11. Al-Hity A, Gregory ME, Kemp EG. The intraoperative use of polydioxanone foil to reduce the risk of sino-orbital fistula formation in orbital exenteration. Orbit Amst Neth. 2018;37(2):140–4. https://doi.org/10.1080/01676830.2017.1383463.
12. Ariani N, Visser A, van Oort RP, et al. Current state of craniofacial prosthetic rehabilitation. Int J Prosthodont. 2013;26(1):57–67. https://doi.org/10.11607/ijp.3220.

Anophthalmic Socket Surgery

42

Maria Belen Camacho, Jenny N. Wang, and Jeremiah P. Tao

Abstract

The goals of anophthalmic socket rehabilitation are to provide sufficient underlying orbital volume and conjunctival surface area that permit a patient to wear a comfortable and realistic eye prosthesis. In this chapter, the authors describe common clinical scenarios and detail surgical interventions for the anophthalmic socket. These include mucous membrane grafting, fornix formation, dermis fat grafting, and volume implants, among others.

Keywords

Anophthalmic socket · Enophthalmos · Fornix reconstruction · Volume loss · Spacer graft · Eyelid retraction

Introduction

Anophthalmic socket reconstruction aims to restore orbital volume and achieve adequate conjunctiva surface area to allow the socket to retain an acceptable ocular prosthesis.

After enucleation or evisceration, loss of orbital volume, along with rotation or displacement of remnant orbital contents or a prior implant can impair the fit of an ocular prosthesis.

Shifts in orbital soft tissues can translate to eyelid positional changes owing to interfascial connections. For example, a shift in the superior orbit soft tissues may lead to the retraction of the superior rectus/levator muscle complex.

Other anatomical changes can include a shallow inferior fornix, volume loss, and a contracted socket, which can cause the eye socket to appear anophthalmic with a deep superior sulcus. A volume implant may ultimately extrude, requiring replacement of volume (Figs. 42.1 and 42.2) with inadequate underlying orbital volume, external changes include upper eyelid ptosis and lower eyelid retraction [1] (Fig. 42.3).

There is no universal treatment for socket contracture or volume deficiency. However, successful rehabilitation of an anophthalmic socket that retains a cosmetically acceptable eye prosthesis requires identify underlying pathology causing orbital volume shortage or socket contracture or both.

Supplementary Information The online version contains supplementary material available at https://doi.org/10.1007/978-3-031-63178-8_42.

M. B. Camacho · J. P. Tao (✉)
Divison of Oculofacial Plastic and Orbital Surgery, University of California, Irvine, CA, USA
e-mail: jeremiat@hs.uci.edu

J. N. Wang
School of Medicine, University of California, Irvine, CA, USA

J. Tao (ed.), *Efficient Oculofacial Surgery*, https://doi.org/10.1007/978-3-031-63178-8_42

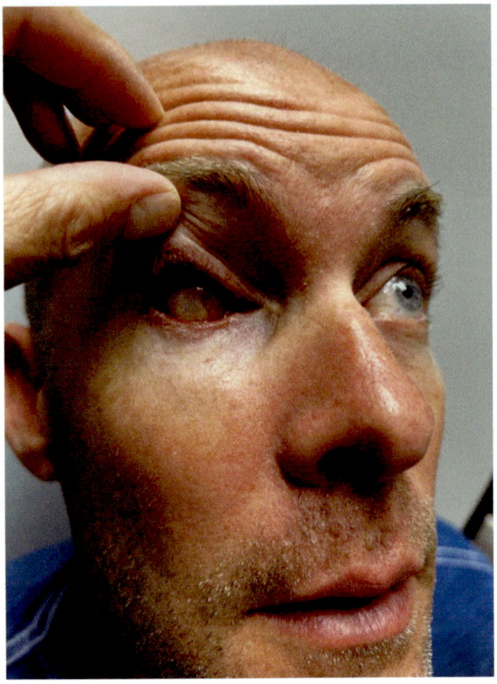

Fig. 42.1 Conjunctival thinning and anterior migration of an orbital sphere implant

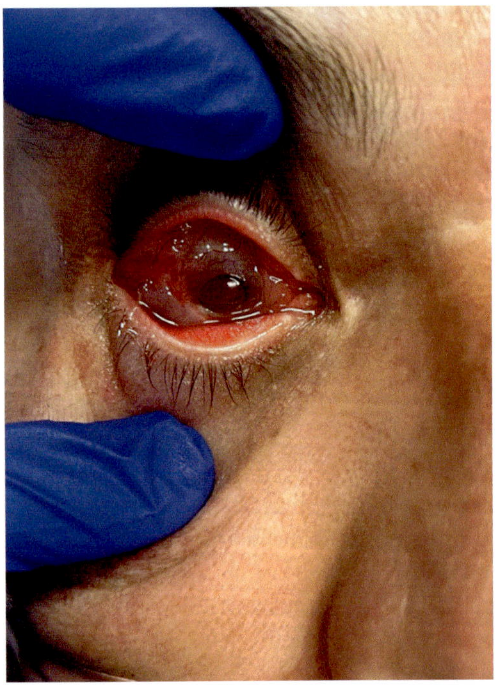

Fig. 42.2 An impending extrusion of a sphere implant (conjunctiva injected with local anesthetic)

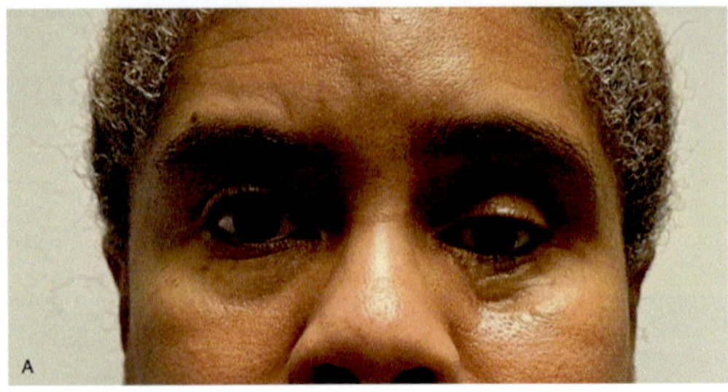

Fig. 42.3 Left deep superior sulcus, ptosis, and a slightly low seated prosthesis due to enophthalmos in an anophthalmic socket

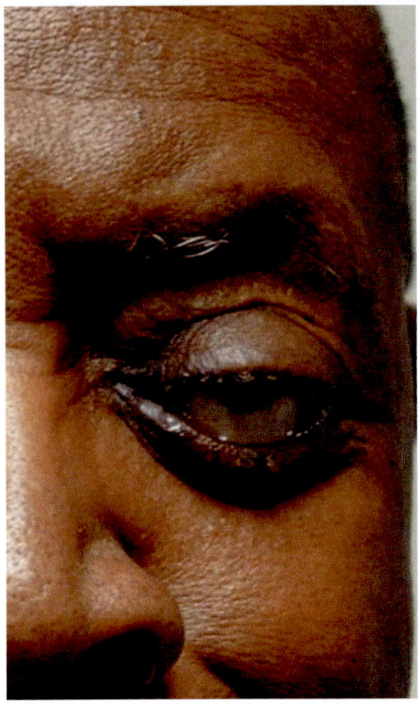

Fig. 42.4 Low seated prosthesis due to excessive device bulk and weight

For cases of mild contracture or eyelid malposition, non-surgical options exist: an ocularist may be able to adjust the prostheses. For blepharoptosis, a thicker superior prosthesis or a ptosis crutch (rigid extension) can suffice [1]. However, the added ocular prosthesis bulk may lead to other problems, such as a low seated prosthesis owing to excess weight (Fig. 42.4).

The conjunctiva should be assessed for sufficient surface. For cases of moderate or severe socket contraction, surgical reconstruction may be indicated (Figs. 42.5 and 42.6). In

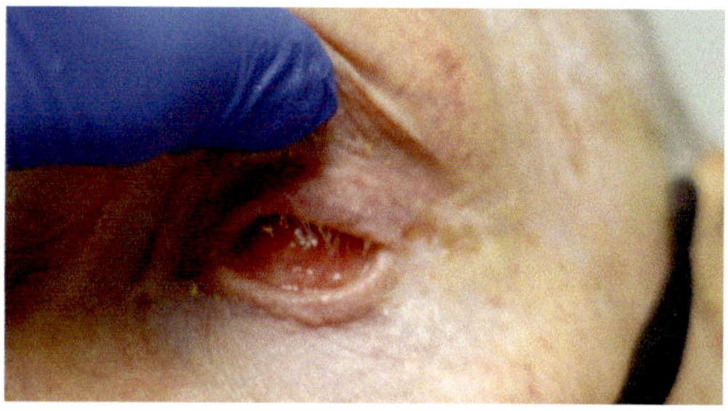

Fig. 42.5 An irradiated socket with conjunctival contracture and obliterated inferior fornix causing an inability to retain a prosthesis

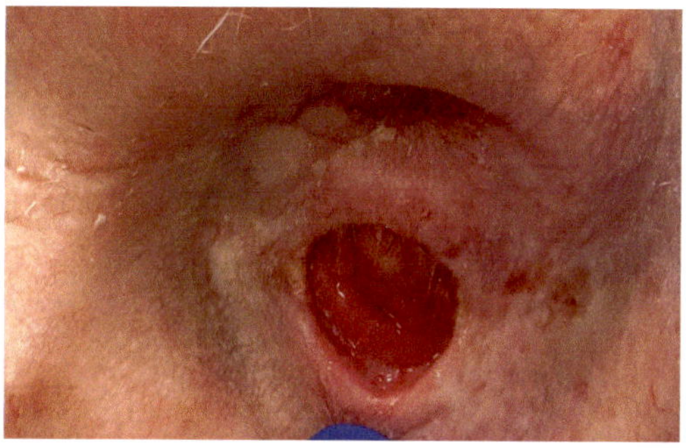

Fig. 42.6 Socket in Fig. 42.5 after fornix re-deepening using a mucous membrane graft harvested from the mouth

this chapter, the authors describe various surgical techniques for the rehabilitation of the anophthalmic socket including those for conjunctival and fornix contracture as well as those for orbital volume loss.

Surgical Management of Socket Conjunctival Contracture

With the shortening of the posterior lamella of the upper and/or lower eyelids or the central socket, an ocular prosthesis has an inadequate seat underneath the eyelids. Even if an eye prosthesis can be fit to tight confines, the foreshortened fornices can cause an inability to blink or close the eyelids.

For lower eyelid retraction accompanied by lower fornix contraction, the insertion of a spacer graft to lengthen the posterior lamella may be useful. This is detailed in other chapters, but the identical principles apply to the anophthalmic socket. Various materials, including homologous, synthetic, and autogenous options, have been used as spacers to achieve posterior lamellar lengthening and deepening of the inferior fornix. Historically, homologous materials such as donor sclera have been utilized, but their use carries a potential risk of infectious disease transmission. Synthetic eyelid implants like porous polyethylene can also be used, but they are associated with a high risk of complications, including exposure, extrusion, and infection. Autogenous materials, such as buccal mucosa, hard palate, and auricular cartilage, may be preferable to lengthen the posterior lamella [2].

Buccal or Labial Mucosa Graft (Video 42-1)

While it less optimally treats lower eyelid retraction since they lack rigidity, a buccal mucosa effectively increases conjunctiva surface area (Fig. 42.7). An appropriately sized mucous membrane graft is harvested from the inside of the lower lip. Graft size depends on the defect size of the contracted socket and generally should be about 40–50% larger than the anticipated defect owing to expected contracture. While harvesting the graft, it is important to avoid causing trauma to the lip margin, gums, and opening of the parotid duct (Stenson's duct) adjacent to the second molar tooth. The defect is closed with 4 0 or 5-0 chromic suture.

Attention is directed to the socket where a horizontal incision is fashioned through scarred socket conjunctiva. The conjunctiva is further dissected, and adhesions are released to slide superiorly and inferiorly into the fornixes.

The mucosal graft is thinned with scissors and then it is placed into the previously developed conjunctival wound. The graft is sutured to the conjunctival edges with a running or interrupted 6-0 polyglactin or chromic suture. Inferiorly, additional large caliber mattress

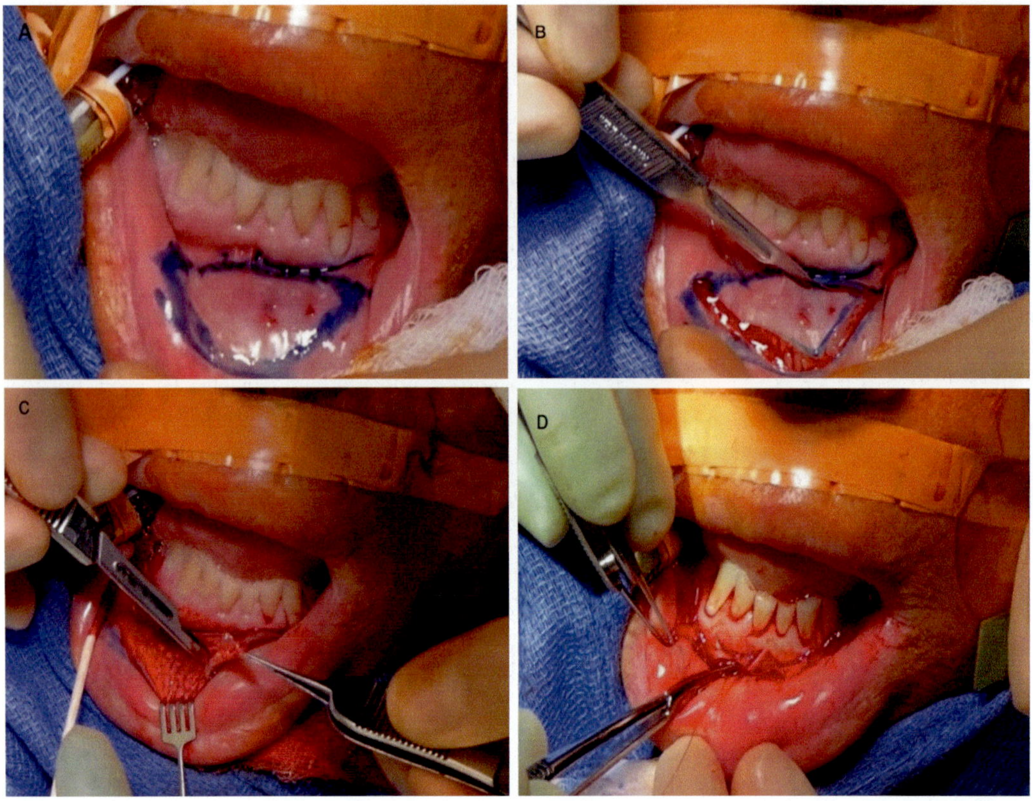

Fig. 42.7 Intraoperative photos of harvesting the mucous membrane graft from the mouth. **A**, **B**) Large mucous membrane graft incision on inner lower lip marked and initial incision with a #15 blade; **C**; Oral mucous membrane graft harvested with a scalpel; **D**) Harvest site closed with interrupted, buried 5-0 chromic gut sutures

sutures (4-0, 5-0 polyglactin) may be useful to further deepen the fornix. Double armed sutures are passed through the graft into the fornix, engaging the inferior rim periosteum prior to exiting skin and tied externally (Fig. 42.8).

Hard Palate and Auricular Cartilage Grafts

While buccal or labial mucosal grafts increase conjunctival surface area, hard palate or cartilage grafts aim to elevate the eyelid mechanically in addition to adding mucosal surface area. Although these are associated with a second surgical site and donor site morbidity, these grafts are well tolerated, elevate the eyelid, and end can help elongate a shortened inferior conjunctival fornix [3, 6].

A hard palate graft is described in another chapter but briefly, the graft is harvested with a #15 blade or a crescent blade. The dimension of the graft is approximately 3–5 mm by 8–12 mm. With the incision site lateral to midline, the graft is dissected in the submucosal plane. The crescent blade offers aids in achieve the appropriate angle for submucosal dissection in the oral surgical cavity confines (Fig. 42.9). The harvested hard palate graft is trimmed of submucosal tissue and sewn into the posterior eyelid defect with interrupted 6-0 chromic suture.

Auricular cartilage grafts (also described in detail another chapter) may be harvested from the retroauricular region through a 2–3 cm

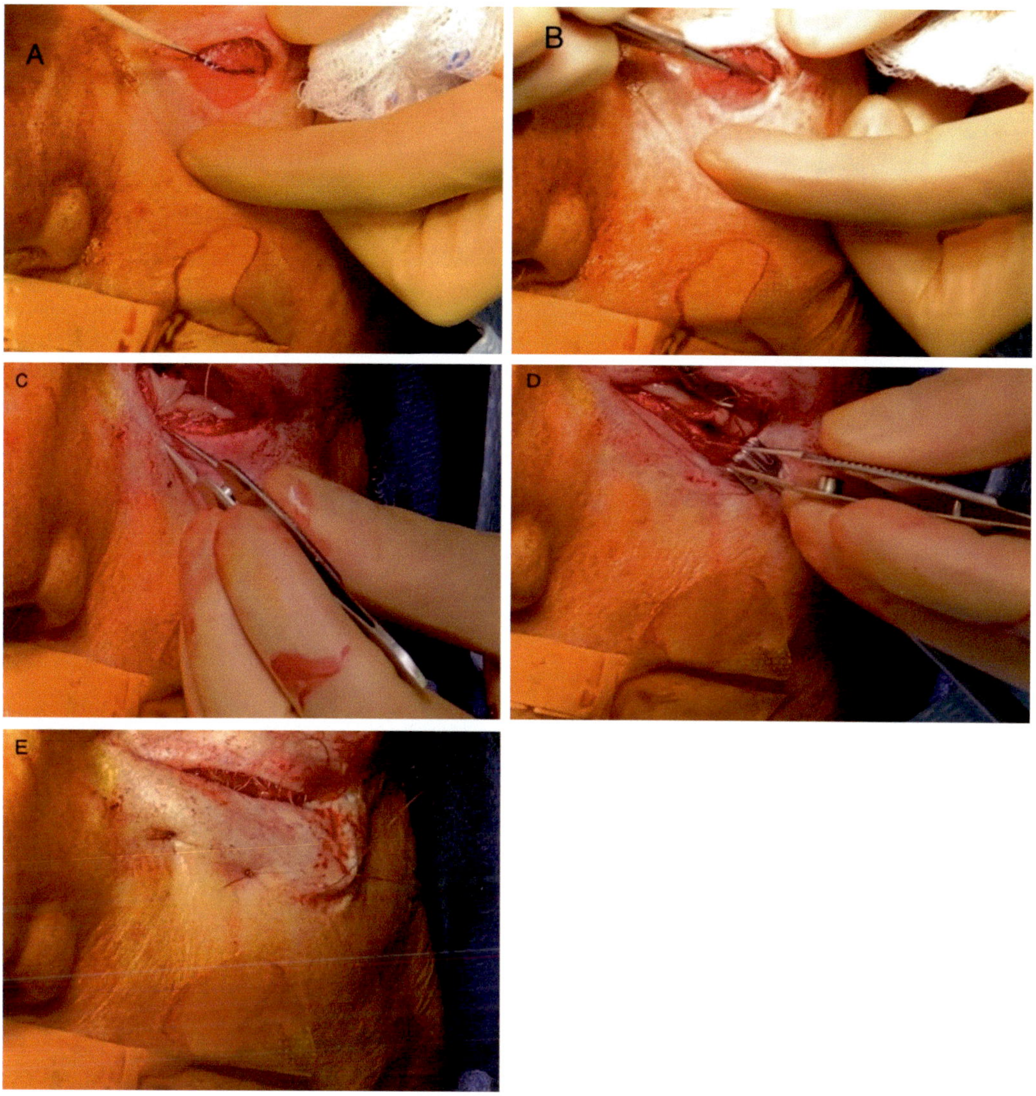

Fig. 42.8 Intraoperative photos of mucous membrane graft placed in a contracted socket. **A**, **B**) #15 blade used to incise the conjunctiva in the left lower fornix; **C**) After release of adhesions, the oral mucous membrane graft secured to the conjunctival defect using 6-0 polyglactin sutures; **D**, **E**) Double armed 4-0 chromic sutures passed to through the central graft engaging inferior rim periosteum prior to external skin knots to encourage fornix redeepening

incision (Fig. 42.10). With the skin incised and dissected, the underlying cartilage is sharply dissected and harvested. The harvest site defect is closed with buried 5-0 vicryl sutures and 5-0 chromic sutures to the skin.

Hard palate or cartilage lower eyelid graft procedures are generally accompanied by a lateral canthotomy and canthoplasty. A small #15 blade skin incision is created. The incision is carried along the inferior tarsal border to incise the conjunctiva and lower eyelid retractors from the inferior tarsal border. The graft is sewn into the lower eyelid conjunctiva after lysing cicatricial bands. The graft is secured into the defect with interrupted 6-0 chromic suture. The eyelid is usually placed on upwards stretch with a Frost suture tarsorrhaphy.

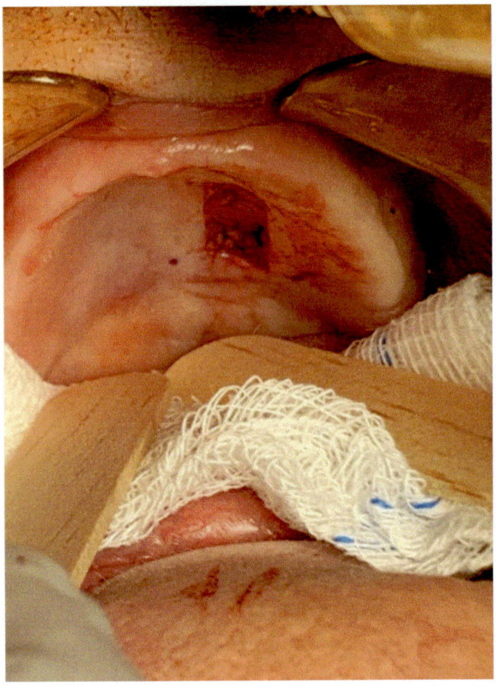

Fig. 42.9 Intraoperative photo of hard palate graft harvest

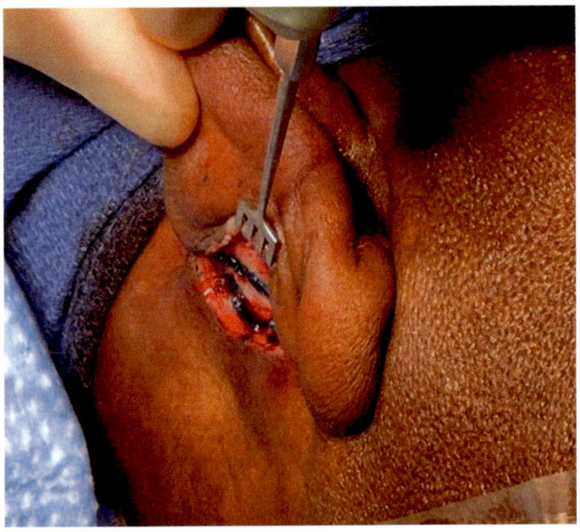

Fig. 42.10 Intraoperative photo of auricular cartilage graft harvest

Dermis Fat Graft (Video 42-2)

In patients presenting with both socket contraction and socket volume deficiency, a dermis fat

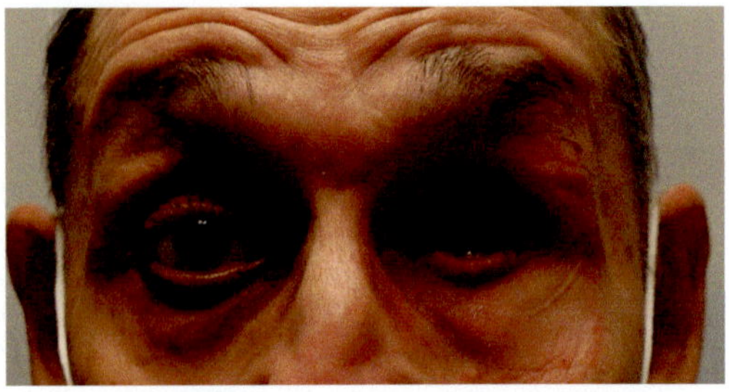

Fig. 42.11 Enophthalmos with short fornices and conjunctival scarring causing a poorly fitting prosthesis

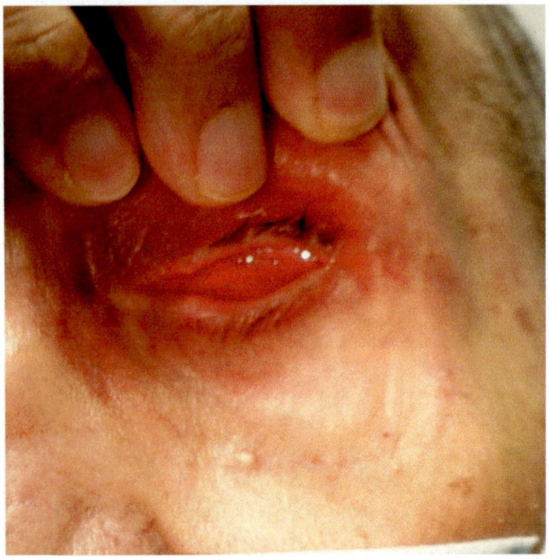

Fig. 42.12 Foreshortened fornices in sunken, enophthalmic orbit

grafts may be ideal (Figs. 42.11 and 42.12) [5]. These grafts are readily available and provide volume in the form of fat and support in the dermal component. The dermis also provides a suturing substrate to keep the graft in the desired position. Dermis fat grafts are often useful secondarily if a prior sphere implant extrudes or gets exposed. Caution should be exercised when using dermis fat grafts in cases with a history of previous socket irradiation or severe socket scarring that may have insufficient vascular supply.

The dermis fat graft is harvested from the buttock or abdomen, ideally in a non-hair bearing area (Fig. 42.13). A diamond burr or a #15 blade is used to de-epithelialize the graft.

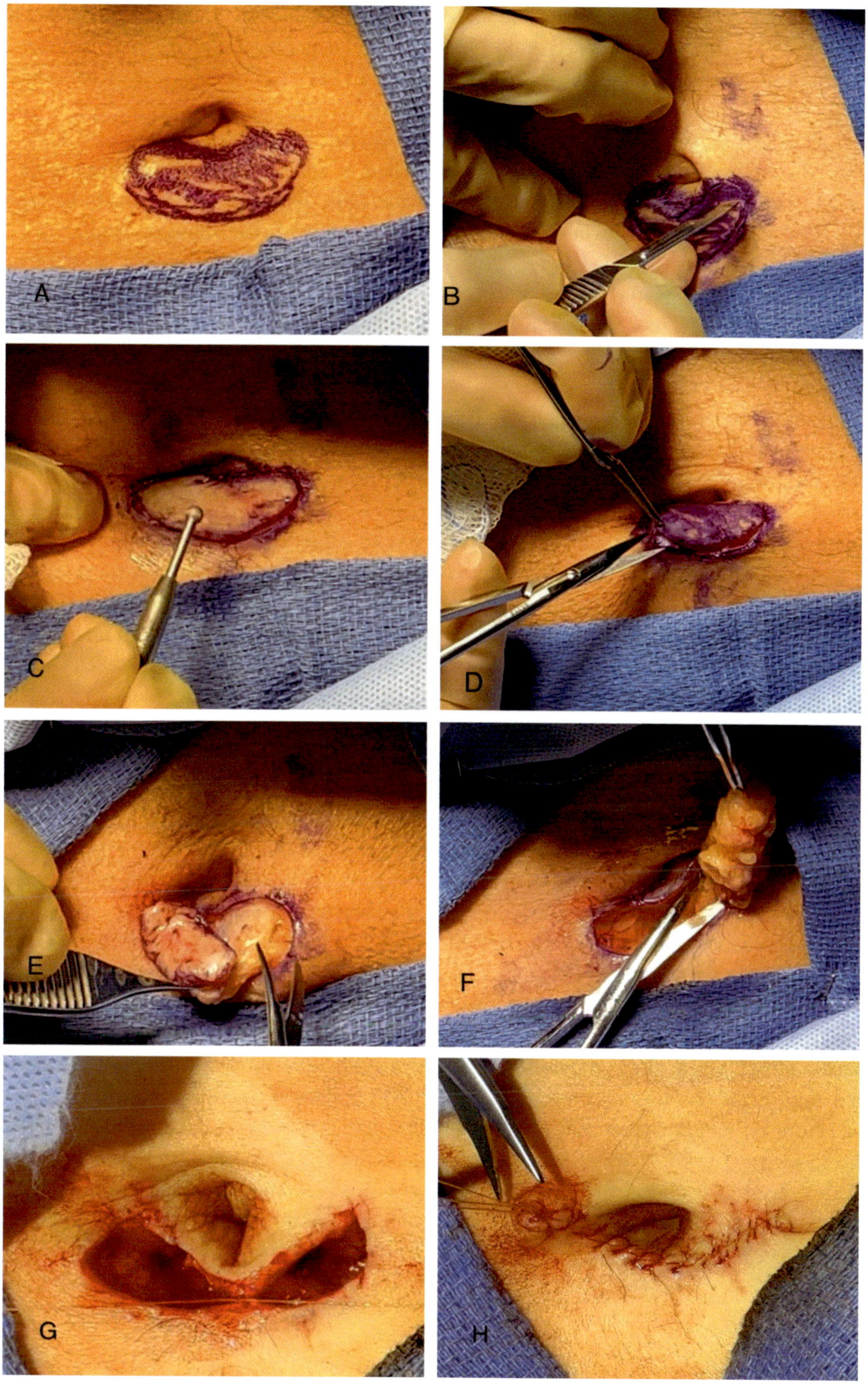

Fig. 42.13 Intraoperative photos of dermis fat graft harvest. **A**) Periumbilical harvest site marked (inking epidermis aids in maintaining graft orientation); **B**) Incision with a #15 blade; **C**) Diamond burr used to de-epithelialize the graft (#15 blade may be used but the burr helped maintain a thicker dermal component; **D**) Perimeter of dermis severed from underlying fat; **E**, **F**) fat resected from surrounding host site; **G**, **H**) Harvest wound closed in layers

Scissors are used to harvest the dermis and subcutaneous fat. The wound is closed with 3-0 polyglactin deep sutures, followed by 4-0 monofilament synthetic absorbable suture to the subcuticular plane. Tissue glue (e.g., Dermabond™) is useful to reinforce the wound. The anterior surface of the graft should have a diameter between 20–24 mm and a thickness of about 20 mm.

Attention is directed to the socket where a #15 blade is used to create a conjunctival incision. Dissection is carried into the orbit to lyse of adhesions. If a prior implant is present, it is removed along with its surrounding capsule. The scarred conjunctiva is opened, and wide conjunctival undermining is performed to release submucosal bands. The dermis component is secured to the cut ends of the conjunctiva and tendons using 5-0 polyglactin interrupted sutures. Additional 4-0 polyglactin mattress sutures are placed in the cardinal directions to secure the central aspect of the graft to the underlying orbital tissues (Fig. 42.14). A double-armed 4-0 silk suture tarsorrhaphy is secured centrally over a conformer dressed with antibiotic ophthalmic ointment. A gentle pressure patch is placed.

Minor complications, including pyogenic granulomas, cysts, and fistulas can be addressed with surgical excision. Necrosis of the graft or lost volume due to absorption may be addressed with another dermis fat graft.5· 6

Skin Grafts

In special situations, a skin graft (described in detail in another chapter) may be indicated. Trauma, burn, or radiation can induce anterior lamella shortage. In the setting of sufficient conjunctiva, scarred eyelids can be lengthened anteriorly to reform fornices. Skin grafts can be harvested from another eyelid, the auricular, or supraclavicular region, among others (Fig. 42.15).

Alloplastic volume implants (Video 42-3)

When a sphere extrudes, displaces, or otherwise fails, attempts can be made to reposition or replace with the same or similar device. As an alternative to a dermis fat graft or another sphere, an alloplastic wedge volume implant can be placed outside the muscle cone, namely along the orbit floor or medial wall (Fig. 42.16). The authors generally prefer silicone that can be preshaped or hand carved with a #15 blade. These may have utility in the setting of orbit volume expansion due to severe trauma (Fig. 42.17).

Eyelid surgery

Blepharoptosis repair and lower eyelid ectropion repair as described in detail in other chapters also have roles in the setting of anophthalmos to improve prosthesis fit or appearance (Fig. 42.18). The same general principles apply, but eyelid surgery in the anophthalmic socket may be less predictable due to variability in underlying anatomic relationships after an eye has been removed. The physiology of extraocular muscles and communicating eyelid connective tissue bands is common altered with prior surgery and implants or grafts.

Conclusion

Anophthalmic socket surgery is indicated to allow a patient to wear a cosmetically acceptable ocular prosthesis. Each case presents unique pathology and treatment is customized. The general surgical aims are restoring orbit volume and conjunctival surface area, including fornices).

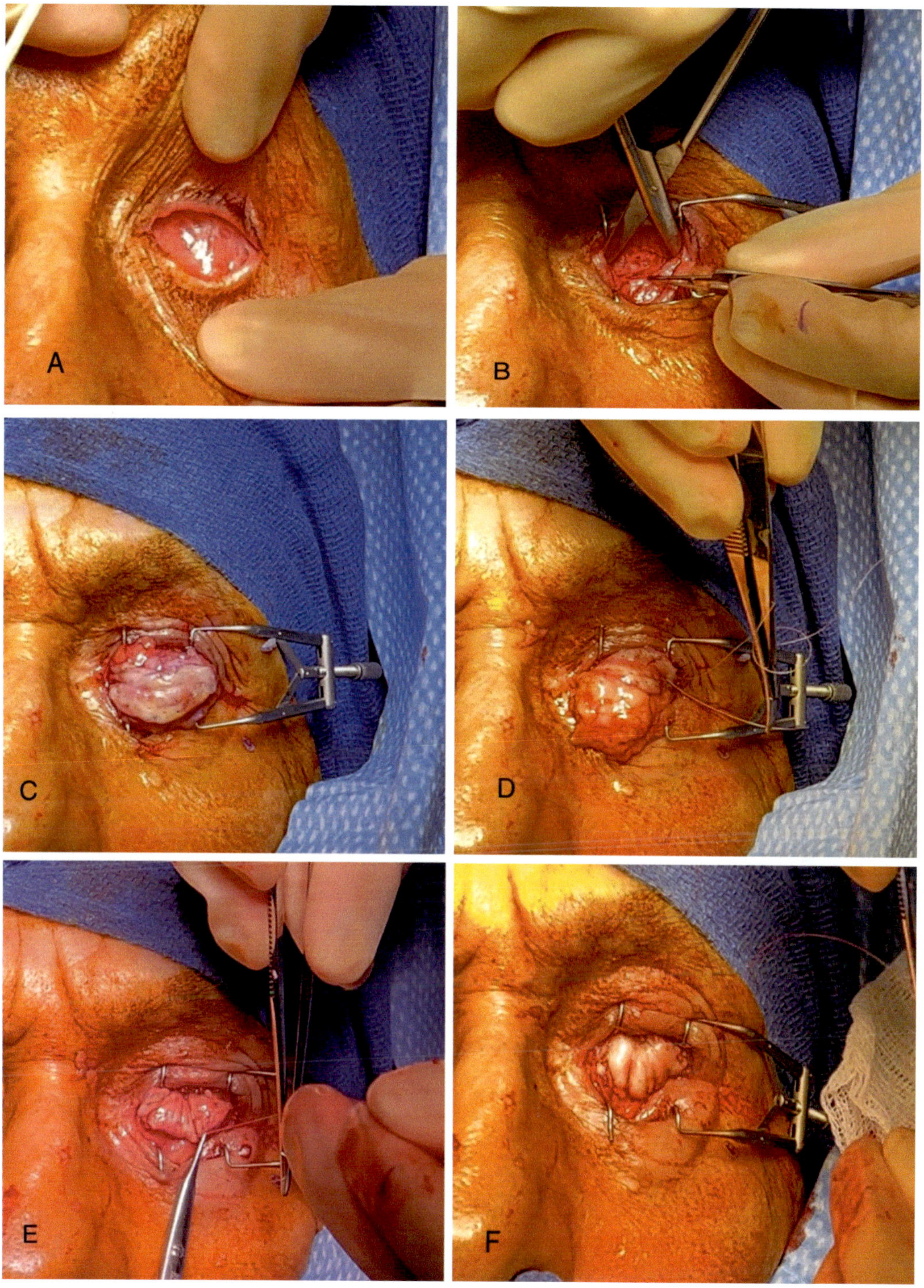

Fig. 42.14 Intraoperative photos of dermis fat graft placement into orbit. **A**, **B**) Central socket opened with sharp dissection and conjuntival undermining was performed to release cicatricial bands; **C**, **D**) The dermis fat graft positioned and secured to the perimeter of the conjunctiva defect using 5-0 polyglactin interrupted sutures; **E**, **F**) 4-0 polyglactin mattress sutures were placed in the cardial directions to secure the central aspect of the graft to the underlying orbital tissues; **G**) A double-armed 4-0 silk suture tarsorrhaphy secured centrally over a conformer dressed with antibiotic ointment

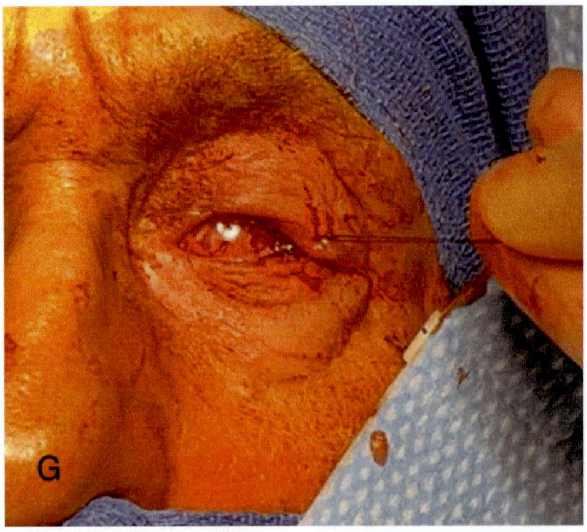

Fig. 42.14 (continued)

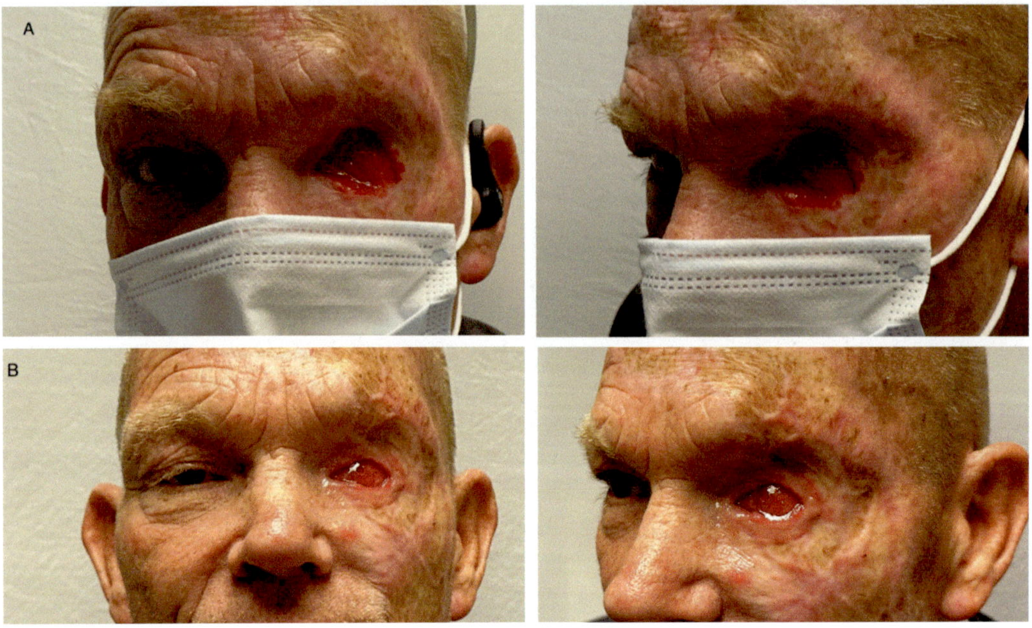

Fig. 42.15 (**A**) Patient who lost the left eye and has significant periocular skin loss and shortage due to a burn (**B**) After supraclavicular skin grafts to replace the anterior lamella of the left upper and lower eyelids to reform eyelids with posterior fornices

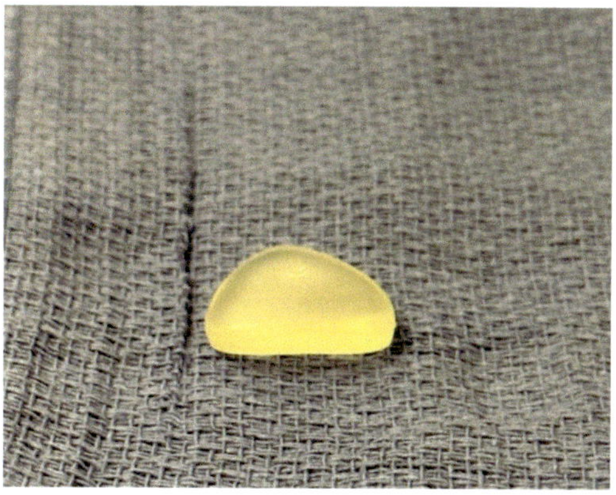

Fig. 42.16 Photo of a silicone orbital wedge implant

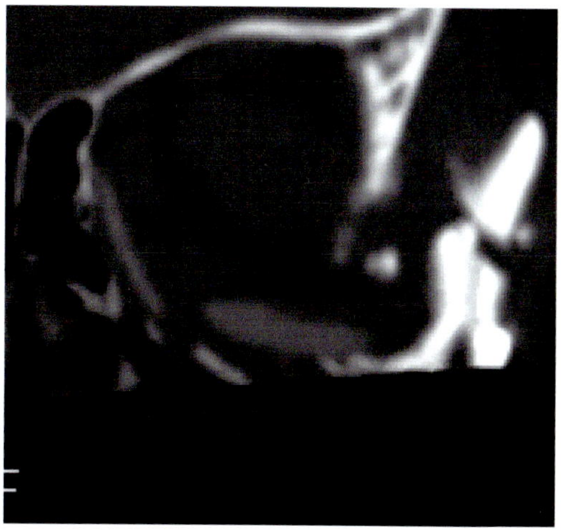

Fig. 42.17 Coronal computed tomography image demonstrating a silicone wedge implants along both the orbital floor and medial wall to treat orbital volume expansion due to severe orbital wall trauma

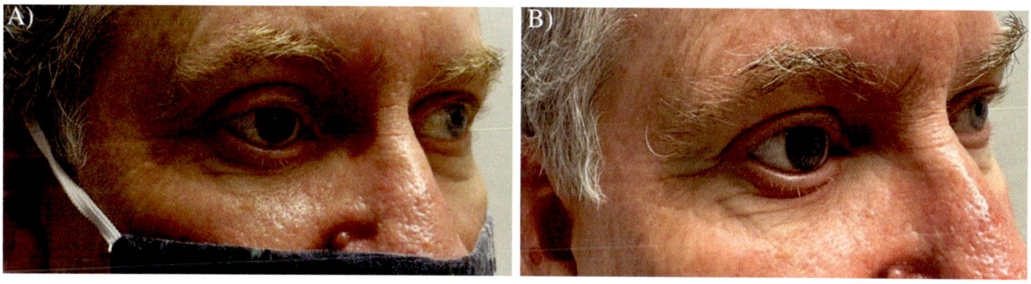

Fig. 42.18 **A**) Right anophthalmos with mild ptosis contributing an unsatisfactory appearance (prosthesis otherwise fit well). **B**) After Muller muscle conjunctival resection posterior ptosis repair, and improvement of blepharoptosis.

References

1. Javier Servat J, Black EH, Nesi FA. Smith and Nesi's ophthalmic plastic and reconstructive surgery; 2021.
2. Molgat YM, Hurwitz JJ, Webb MC. Buccal mucous membrane-fat graft in the management of the contracted socket. Ophthal Plast Reconstr Surg. 1993;9:267–72.
3. Holck DE, Foster JA, Dutton JJ, Dillon HD. Hard palate mucosal grafts in the treatment of the contracted socket. Ophthal Plast Reconstr Surg. 1999;15:202–9.
4. Choi CJ, Tran AQ, Tse DT. Hard palate-dermis fat composite graft for reconstruction of contracted anophthalmic socket. Orbit. 2019;38(3):199–204.
5. Jovanovic N, Carniciu AL, Russell WW, Jarocki A, Kahana A. Reconstruction of the orbit and anophthalmic socket using the dermis fat graft: a major review. Ophthal Plast Reconstr Surg. 2020;36(6):529–39.
6. Hashikawa K, Terashi H, Tahara S. Therapeutic strategy for the triad of acquired anophthalmic orbit. Plast Reconstr Surg. 2007;119:2182–8. https://doi.org/10.1097/01.prs.0000260706.07368.f1.
7. Li D, Jie Y, Liu H, Liu J, Zhu Z, Mao C. Reconstruction of anophthalmic orbits and contracted eye sockets with microvascular radial forearm free flaps. Ophthal Plast Reconstr Surg. 2008;24(2):94–7.
8. Mombaerts I, Groet E. Upper eyelid ptosis surgery using a preparatory ocular prosthesis. Ophthalmic Plast Reconstr Surg. 2009;25(2):90–3.

External Dacryocystorhinostomy

43

Sammie E. Fung, Liane O. Dallalzadeh, and Catherine Y. Liu

Abstract

Nasolacrimal duct obstruction is a common cause of epiphora. In addition to symptomatic excess tears, it may be associated with infection (dacryocystitis). Surgical bypass of a nasolacrimal duct obstruction via dacryocystorhinostomy (DCR) may be indicated to treat epiphora or infection or both. The external approach has an extensive history and remains a key oculofacial surgical procedure. In this chapter, the authors describe indications and surgical techniques for external DCR.

Keywords

Epiphora · Tearing · Dacryocystitis · Nasolacrimal duct obstruction · Lacrimal sac · Dacryocystorhinostomy (DCR) · External DCR

Supplementary Information The online version contains supplementary material available at https://doi.org/10.1007/978-3-031-63178-8_43.

S. E. Fung · L. O. Dallalzadeh · C. Y. Liu (✉)
UC San Diego, San Diego, CA, USA
e-mail: catherine.liu@gmail.com

Introduction

Obstruction of the nasolacrimal duct (NLDO) can lead to epiphora and/or acute or chronic dacryocystitis. Acquired NLDO occurs most frequently during middle age, with women about twice as likely as men to be affected [1, 2].Dacryocystorhinostomy (DCR) surgery is recommended for complete nasolacrimal duct obstruction to relieve epiphora and infection in acquired cases, and after multiple failed attempts at probing in congenital cases.

The procedure is thought to have been described early as the times of ancient Mesopotamia in the Code of Hammurabi, but the first well documented description of the DCR technique was in 1893, when Caldwell described a procedure to correct chronic stenosis of the nasolacrimal duct from an endonasal approach [3]. Subsequently, an external approach was described by Toti in 1904 using an external nasal skin incision. Advantages of the external approach include direct visualization and access, low cost, high success rates, and ability to identify a lacrimal sac tumor if suspected [3–5]. Disadvantages include scarring at the incision line, which can be minimized with various skin approaches. The authors acknowledge that many surgeons favor an endoscopic DCR approach. However, it is not described owing to the added complexity, cost, and instrumentation needs that do not conform to the

J. Tao (ed.), *Efficient Oculofacial Surgery*, https://doi.org/10.1007/978-3-031-63178-8_43

objectives of this book, not to mention its much lower success rate. In this chapter, the authors describe an external approach that has the highest DCR success rate and that is not associated with a conspicuous scar in the majority of cases.

Preoperative Evaluation

A thorough medical and surgical history should be conducted in preparation for surgery. A history of chronic sinusitis or poorly-controlled inflammatory conditions such as granulomatosis with polyangiitis (GPA) or sarcoidosis can lead to reduced DCR success rates; success rates can improve with systemic immunosuppressive therapy [6–9]. Any patient with a history of blood-stained epiphora or mass above the medial canthal tendon should undergo maxillofacial imaging to evaluate for a potential neoplasm. Prior sinus surgeries or radiotherapy can change the surgical anatomy, or delay healing. Exposure to phospholine iodide, 5-fluorouracil, or docetaxel can lead to stenosis of the canaliculus, puncta, or nasolacrimal duct [4, 10].

Pre-operative evaluation should include nasolacrimal irrigation testing to localize the obstruction. Dye retention test (Fig. 43.1) or Jones test I/II can also help with the diagnosis. A complete eye exam is important to address other potential causes of tearing, such as eyelid malposition, ocular surface disease, and weakened orbicularis (such as CN VII palsy) that can reduce the lacrimal pump function.

Importantly, patients with obstructive sleep apnea and require a continuous positive airway pressure (CPAP) device should be identified. While tear drain surgery is not absolutely contraindicated, post DCR, positive airway pressure may force air retrograde through the nasolacrimal drainage pathway and irritate or dry the eye. A full face mask CPAP is one solution should this occur, but patients should be counseled on this side effect of a successful DCR (Fig. 43.2).

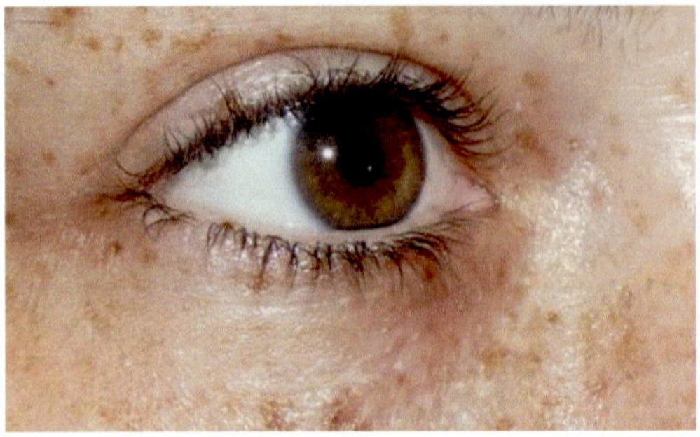

Fig. 43.2 External scar at site of incision, 3 months post-surgery

Success Rates

Success rates for external DCR are generally greater than 90–95% [5, 11–13]. Failure is typically secondary to closure of the surgical ostomy from fibrosis, scarring, or granulation tissue; this may be mitigated by initially removing a larger portion of the bone, which allows for creating a larger soft tissue opening, or the creation of mucosal flaps [14]. Additional factors which may decrease the success of DCR include chronic sinusitis and other inflammatory conditions [14]. Acute dacryocystitis should be treated with antibiotics and/or incision and drainage to reduce inflammation, if possible,

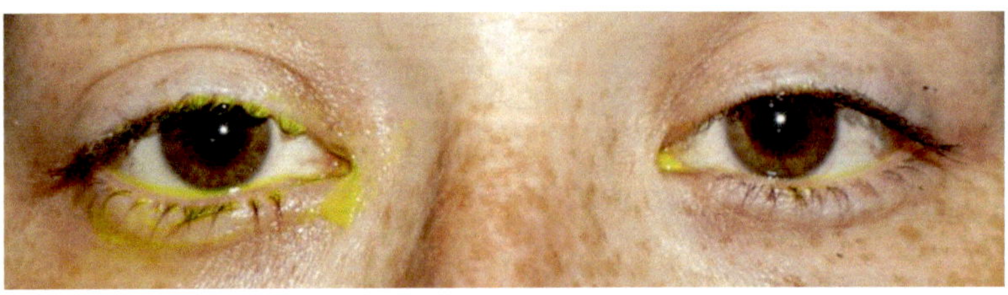

Fig. 43.1 Dye retention test shows an obstruction in the right nasolacrimal system

before proceeding with DCR, to improve outcomes. Repeated attempts at DCR or endonasal approaches carry lower rates of success [14, 15].

Surgical Technique (Videos 43-1 and 43-2)

With the help of a nasal speculum and headlight, local anesthetic solution containing 1:200,000 parts epinephrine is injected into the nasal mucosal tissue near the uncinate process of the middle turbinate using a 22-gauge spinal needle (Fig. 43.3). The nose is packed with Afrin-soaked neurosurgical cottonoids to help achieve hemostasis. The skin is prepped in a sterile and aseptic fashion.

A 12–15 mm (8–10 mm in children) curvilinear mark along the nasojugal fold as shown in Fig. 43.4. Further local anesthesia may be injected into the region overlying the lacrimal sac with a 27-gauge needle as well as to the lateral nasal sidewall mucosa with the needle introduced from the nares. An ethmoidal nerve block is optional.

The skin and orbicularis is incised with a #15 scalpel blade over the previously marked incision line. A Z or W configuration, with the major incisions within the oblique skin tension lines of the lateral nose can help forestall web

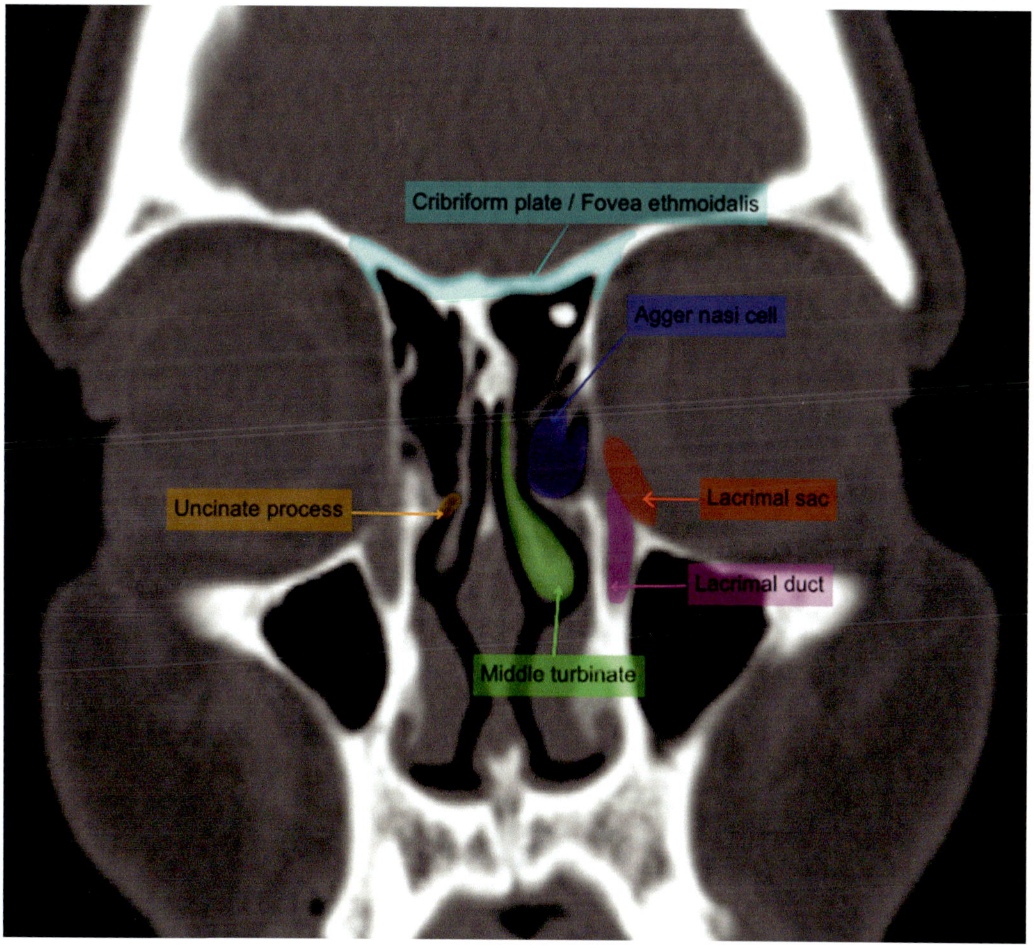

Fig. 43.3 Landmarks and overview. A coronal view of the sinuses using a computed tomography (CT) scan is depicted to present the relevant anatomical landmarks for a DCR. Note that the lacrimal sac is at and below the medial canthal tendon, which lies about 15 to 20 mm (mm) from the inferior-most part of the cribriform plate [16].

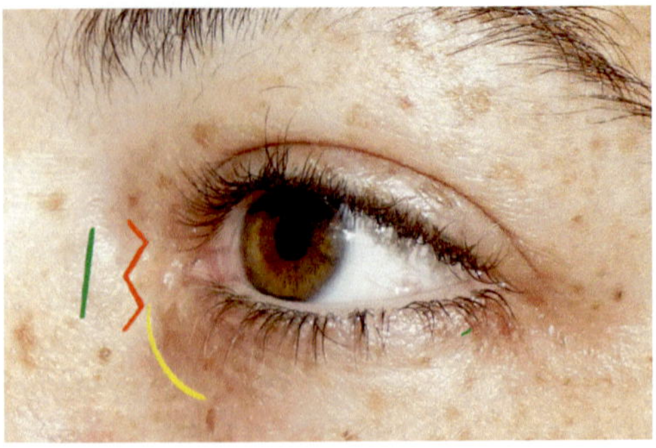

Fig. 43.4 Incision planning. A common external DCR incision is an approximately 10–15 mm vertical incision placed 10 mm medial to the insertion of the medial canthal tendon and lateral to the angular vessels. Variations exist in incision placement to improve scar concealment. These include the tear trough incision (yellow) placed in a curvilinear fashion along the nasojugal skin fold, linear nasal incision (green), and the modified W incision (orange) to fit relaxed skin tension lines

formation by breaking up the wound and also keeping more of the wound in the direction of the relaxed tension lines. (Vertical incisions have been traditionally described, but since they cross the horizontal or oblique-horizontal tension lines at the medial canthus due to the orbicularis oculi and levator labii alaeque nasi muscles, are more prone to web formation and a conspicuous scar).

A curved Stevens scissors is used to bluntly dissect through the orbicularis and expose the orbital rim and anterior face of the maxilla. The angular vessels typically lie medial to the wound. Electrocautery should be minimal here to avoid injury to facial nerve branches that supply the medial eyelids in addition to the vascular structures. The anterior medial canthal tendon can be released for better exposure of the lacrimal sac (Figs. 43.5, 43.6, 43.7, 43.8, 43.9, 43.10 and 43.11).

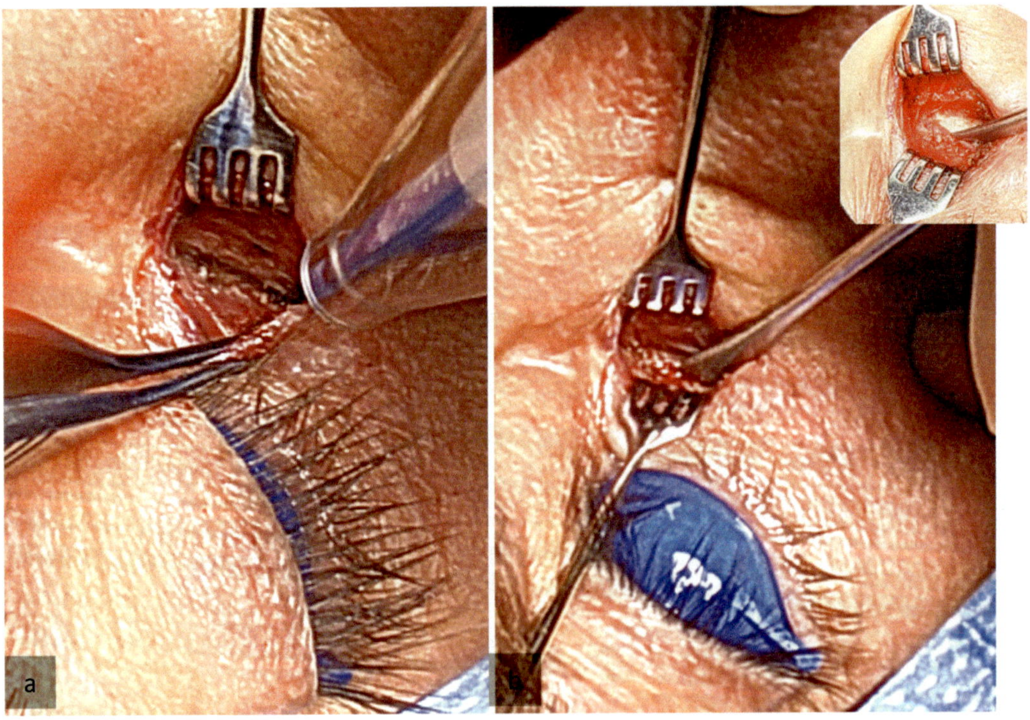

Fig. 43.5 Periosteum incised at the orbital rim and lateral nasal area. Using a #15 scalpel blade or cutting cautery a 10 mm vertical incision through the periosteum medial to the anterior lacrimal crest (5**a**). An elevator is used to lift the periosteum at the orbital rim (5**b** and inset)

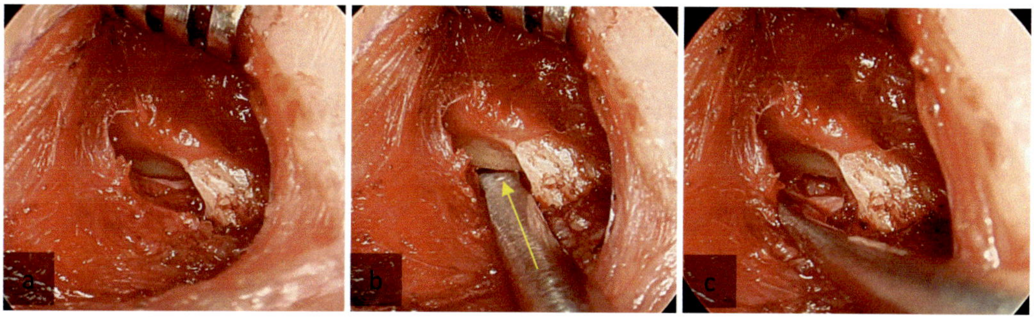

Fig. 43.6 Lacrimal fossa exposed. Dissect in the subperiosteal plane into the orbit and expose the lacrimal sac fossa widely from the canthal tendon to the nasolacrimal duct entrance (6**a**). An osteotomy is initiated with a drill or using gentle pressure with a Freer elevator at the lacrimal bone (yellow arrow, 6b; osteotomy depicted in 6**c**)

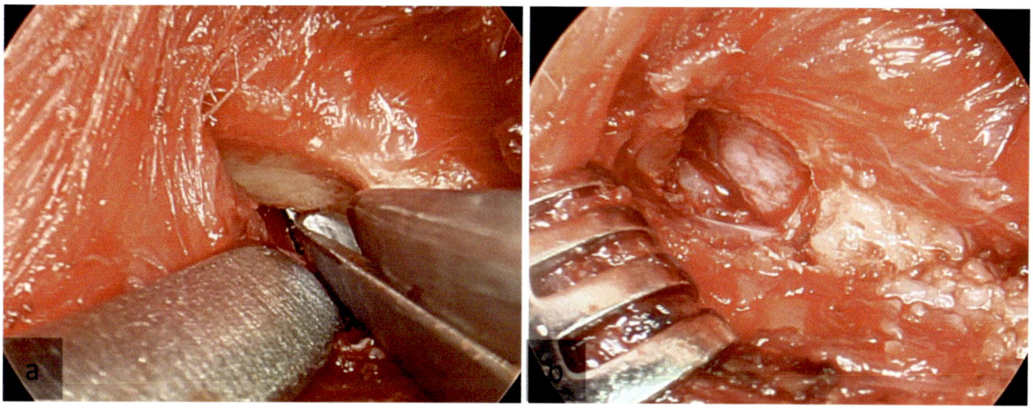

Fig. 43.7 Osteotomy enlarged. The osteotomy is enlarged to 10–25 mm wide with serially larger Kerrison rongeurs (1 mm, 2 mm, 3 mm; 7**a**). (A drill may be useful to initiate the osteotomy and to remove thicker bone that is more difficult to remove with rongeurs). Care must be taken not to torque the instrument while removing bone in order to minimize risk of fracture extension. The nasal mucosa is now visualized (7**b**). A cotton tip applicator may be inserted in the nasal cavity to tent the exposed nasal mucosa to confirm clear passage. In some patients, an anterior agger nasi cell of the ethmoid sinus can block the creation of a fistula between the lacrimal sac and the nasal cavity. The pre-placed nasal packing is removed

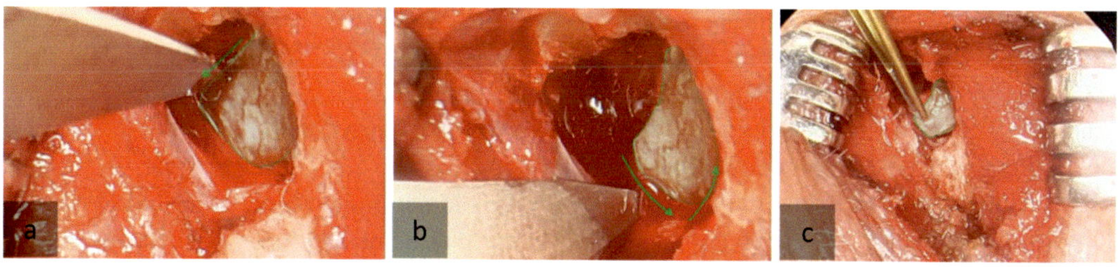

Fig. 43.8 Create an anterior nasal mucosa flap. An anterior flap in the nasal mucosa is fashioned with sharp dissection (highlighted in green). Cuts are oriented superiorly (arrow in 8**a**), deep, and inferiorly (arrows in 8**b**). The nasal mucosa flap is shown in Fig. 43.8**c**. An optional posterior oriented flap can also be fashioned

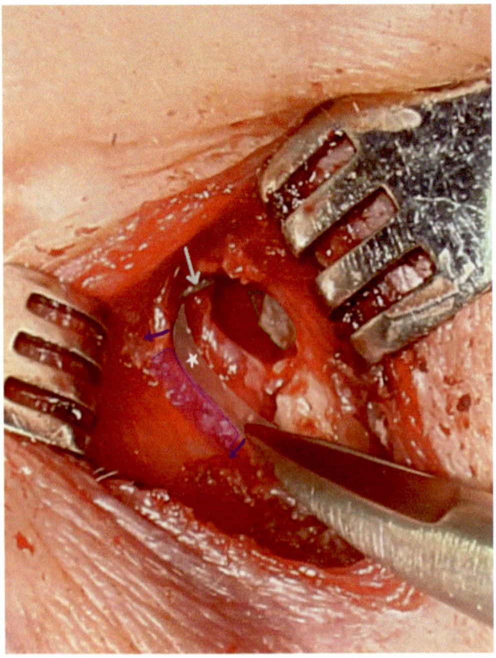

Fig. 43.9 Anterior lacrimal sac flap creation. With the help of a Bowman probe or Crawford lead wire inserted in the canaliculus to tent the lacrimal sac, a crescent blade or sickle knife is used to make an incision along the vertical length of the lacrimal sac that is extended with scissors. The lacrimal sac should be opened to above the level of the common canaliculus and continued inferiorly to the entrance of the nasolacrimal duct. White star denotes the view into the inside of the lacrimal sac. Grey arrow denotes the Bowman probe entering from the canaliculus used to tent and identify the sac. Green highlight denotes the anterior flap of the nasal mucosa. Purple highlight denotes location of the anterior flap of the lacrimal sac, with purple arrows denoting the back cuts to be made

Superior and inferior back cuts are made with scissors to fashion an anterior flap of the lacrimal sac (purple). A posterior flap can also be fashioned. The nasal mucosa flaps are sutured using 5-0 polyglactin suture on a small semicircular needle (e.g. P2) to reflect the nasal flap to allow for passage of the stent.

The silicone stent should not be under significant tension at the puncta to prevent canalicular cheesewiring. The stent is tied in the nose with 2 square knots and the tails are trimmed (Fig. 43.12).

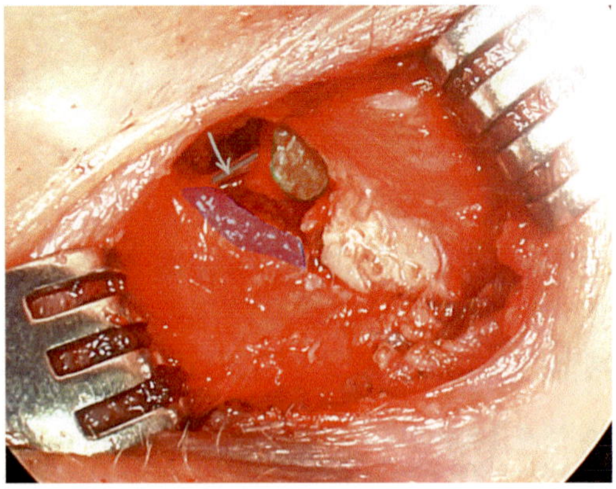

Fig. 43.10 Insertion of a bicanalicular silastic stent. A bicanalicular silicone stent (grey arrow) is advanced through each canaliculus, the newly created osteotomy, and into the nose. Retrieval of the stent can be aided by using a hemostat inserted through the nose

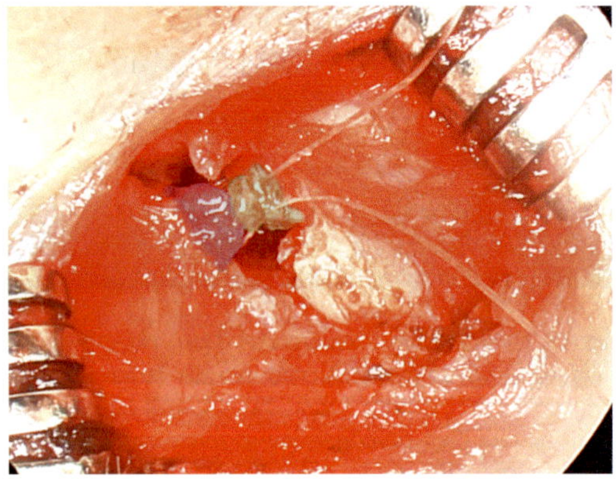

Fig. 43.11 Approximation of the nasal mucosal and lacrimal sac flaps. The anterior flaps of the nasal and lacrimal sac mucosa are secured using 5-0 polyglactin suture. (Posterior flaps, if available are secured to each other in advance of suturing of the anterior flaps)

Postoperative Care

A steroid-antibiotic ointment should be applied to the suture line two times daily for seven days. In addition, a steroid-antibiotic combination solution should be applied to the eye four times daily for seven days. Fluticasone nasal spray can be used daily for 1 month. Patients should be instructed to avoid blowing their nose for

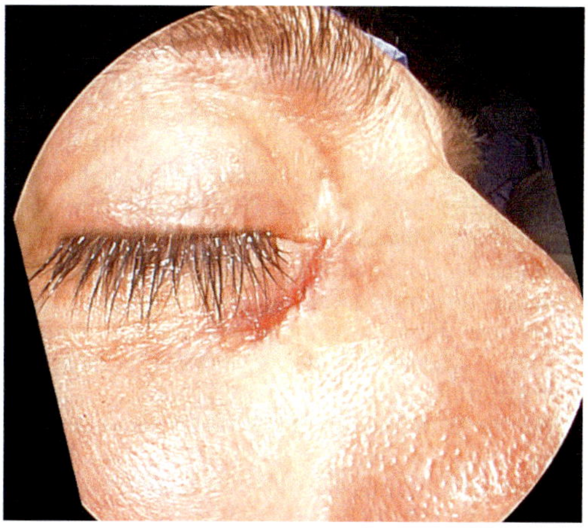

Fig. 43.12 Skin closure. The orbicularis is secured with deep buried 5-0 or 6-0 vicryl and the skin is closed with 6-0 gut sutures

five days and counseled that epiphora may continue while the silicone stent remains in place. The silicone tube can typically be removed after three months.

Potential Complications

Potential complications include epistaxis, wound infection, recurrent obstruction, and sump syndrome.

- **Epistaxis:** Intraoperative epistaxis can be managed with pressure, cottonoids soaked in local anesthesia with epinephrine and tranexamic acid, or oxymetazoline, or use of a hemostatic agent. The head of the bed can be elevated. Communication with the anesthesiologist is also important for proper blood pressure control. Post-operative bleeding, while unusual, can be managed with nasal compression and head elevation.
- **Wound infection:** Wound infection is rare, and more likely when operating during acute dacryocystitis. Systemic antibiotics and wound cultures are indicated.
- **Persistent epiphora:**
  - **Silastic stent placement**: The presence of the silicone stent in a stenotic canalicular system can yield persistent epiphora post-operatively. Patient should be informed of this possibility pre-operatively and assessed once the silicone stent is removed for resolution.
  - **Sump syndrome:** This is an uncommon complication where the inferior portion of the nasolacrimal sac is not opened, instead collecting tears, and leading to residual epiphora. It can be diagnosed endoscopically or with a dacryocystogram and generally requires a revision of the DCR to remove the sump and extend the osteotomy.
  - **Failed DCR:** Failure is typically secondary to closure of the surgical osteotomy from fibrosis, scarring, or granulation tissue; this may be mitigated by initially removing a larger portion of bone. Once identified, a revision DCR can be performed, albeit with lower success rate. In some revision cases, or cases with upper lacrimal drainage stricture the editor places double silicone stents.
- **Silastic stent extrusion:** If a silastic stent extrudes, it should be removed with care to avoid corneal injury and ocular surface irritation. It does not require replacement since early extrusion has not been associated with a higher rate of DCR failure.
- **Lagophthalmos:** A rare complication due to damage to the peripheral fibers of the zygomatic and buccal branches of the facial nerve within the medial canthal area during incision formation resulting in orbicularis oculi weakness. In a prior study, lagophthalmos was temporary and typically resolved in 3.5 months [17].

Conclusion

External dacryocystorhinostomy is the gold standard treatment for nasolacrimal duct obstruction [18–20]. With thoughtfulness about wound design and good surgical technique, facial scarring is minimal.

References

1. Phan L, McCulley T. Age related gender differences in the occurrence of acquired nasolacrimal duct obstruction in Saudi Arabia. Invest Ophthalmol Vis Sci. 2013;54(15):5347.
2. Shen GL, Ng JD, Ma XP. Etiology, diagnosis, management and outcomes of epiphora referrals to an oculoplastic practice. Int J Ophthalmol. 2016;9(12):1751–5. https://doi.org/10.18240/ijo.2016.12.08.
3. Ullrich K, Malhotra R, Patel BC. Dacryocystorhinostomy. In: StatPearls. StatPearls Publishing; 2020. http://www.ncbi.nlm.nih.gov/books/NBK557851/. Accessed 28 July 2020.
4. Mansur C, Pfeiffer ML, Esmaeli B. Evaluation and management of chemotherapy-induced epiphora, punctal and canalicular stenosis, and nasolacrimal duct obstruction. Ophthalmic Plast Reconstr Surg. 2017;33(1):9–12. https://doi.org/10.1097/IOP.0000000000000745.
5. Sobel RK, Aakalu VK, Wladis EJ, Bilyk JR, Yen MT, Mawn LA. A Comparison of endonasal dacryocystorhinostomy and external dacryocystorhinostomy: a report by the American academy of ophthalmology. Ophthalmology. 2019;126(11):1580–5. https://doi.org/10.1016/j.ophtha.2019.06.009.
6. Hardwig PW, Bartley GB, Garrity JA. Surgical management of nasolacrimal duct obstruction in patients with Wegener's granulomatosis. Ophthalmology. 1992;99(1):133–9. https://doi.org/10.1016/s0161-6420(92)32026-3.
7. Stewart CM, Rose GE. External dacryocystorhinostomy in patients with granulomatous polyangiitis. Eye. 2020;34(8):1382–5. https://doi.org/10.1038/s41433-019-0662-1.
8. Stewart CM, Rose GE. External dacryocystorhinostomy in patients with systemic sarcoidosis. Ophthalmology. 2019;126(8):1200–2. https://doi.org/10.1016/j.ophtha.2019.02.017.
9. Lee BJ, Nelson CC, Lewis CD, Perry JD. External dacryocystorhinostomy outcomes in sarcoidosis patients. Ophthal Plast Reconstr Surg. 2012;28(1):47–9. https://doi.org/10.1097/IOP.0b013e3182364ad2.
10. Kintzel PE, Michaud LB, Lange MK. Docetaxel-associated epiphora. Pharmacother J Human Pharmacol Drug Therapy. 2006;26(6):853–867. https://doi.org/10.1592/phco.26.6.853.
11. Yener HI, Ozcimen M. Long-term results in transcanalicular laser and external dacryocystorhinostomy. Beyoglu Eye J. 2020;5(1):22–5. https://doi.org/10.14744/bej.2019.70299.
12. Jawaheer L, MacEwen CJ, Anijeet D. Endonasal versus external dacryocystorhinostomy for nasolacrimal duct obstruction. Cochrane Database Syst Rev. 2017;2:CD007097. https://doi.org/10.1002/14651858.CD007097.pub3.
13. Savino G, Battendieri R, Traina S, et al. External vs. endonasal dacryocystorhinostomy: has the current view changed? Acta Otorhinolaryngol Ital. 2014;34(1):29–35.
14. Altin Ekin M, Karadeniz Ugurlu S, Aytogan H, Sahin Atik S. Failure in revision dacryocystorhinostomy: a study of surgical technique and etiology. J Craniof Surg. 2020;31(1):193–96. https://doi.org/10.1097/SCS.0000000000005829.
15. Korkut AY, Teker AM, Ozsutcu M, Askiner O, Gedikli O. A comparison of endonasal with external dacryocystorhinostomy in revision cases. Eur Arch Otorhinolaryngol. 2011;268(3):377–81. https://doi.org/10.1007/s00405-010-1339-3.
16. Ugurbas SH, Sargon MF, Zilelioglu G. Anatomical risk margins in dacryocystorhinostomy. Ann Ophthalmol. 2000;32(1):50–3. https://doi.org/10.1007/s12009-000-0012-7.
17. Vagefi MR, Winn BJ, Lin CC, et al. Facial nerve injury during external dacryocystorhinostomy. Ophthalmology. 2009;116(3):585–90. https://doi.org/10.1016/j.ophtha.2008.09.050.
18. Korn BS, Kikkawa DO. Video Atlas of oculofacial plastic and reconstructive surgery. 2nd ed. Elsevier; 2017.
19. Dutton JJ. Atlas of oculoplastic and orbital surgery. 1st ed. Lippincott Williams & Wilkins; 2013.
20. Riordan-Eva P, Augsburger JJ. Vaughn & Asbury's general ophthalmology. 19th ed. McGraw-Hill Education, Inc.; 2018.

Conjunctivodacryocystorhinostomy (CDCR) with Jones Tube

44

Lisa Y. Lin and Michael K. Yoon

Abstract

In cases of epiphora due to upper lacrimal system obstruction, a canalicular bypass surgery or conjunctivodacryocystorhinostomy (CDCR) with placement of a glass or Pyrex® (Jones) tube may be indicated. Glass or Pyrex® is requisite owing to capillary attraction. These may be implanted with or without an external incision and with or without an endoscope. Complications include migration or occlusion of the tube. Cleaning or tube exchange is usually necessary over time. Successful Jones tubes achieve significant epiphora relief for many patients. In this chapter, the authors detail CDCR surgical technique.

Keywords

Jones tube · Lester Jones tube · Conjunctivodacryocystorhinostomy (CDCR) · Epiphora · Upper lacrimal obstruction

Supplementary Information The online version contains supplementary material available at https://doi.org/10.1007/978-3-031-63178-8_44.

L. Y. Lin · M. K. Yoon (✉)
Harvard University, Boston, MA, USA
e-mail: michael_yoon@meei.harvard.edu

Introduction

Epiphora is the overflow of tears at the eyelid margin and can cause a serious impact on a patient's quality of life. In the absence of an obvious etiology for reflex tearing or a lacrimal pump problem, the presence of constant epiphora suggests an obstruction of the lacrimal drainage system.

An obstruction of the lacrimal drainage system can occur at any point, from the puncta to the valve of Hasner. Depending on the location of the obstruction, surgical management can include punctoplasty, canalicular stenting, dacryocystorhinostomy (DCR), and in cases of severe upper lacrimal system obstruction, a canalicular bypass surgery with placement of a Jones tube can be performed.

A Jones tube is a Pyrex® glass tube that acts as a sump drain, carrying tears from the conjunctival cul de sac into the nose, while bypassing the obstructed canaliculus. The tear drainage via the Jones tube is chiefly capillary attraction but aided by a slight pressure gradient created in the nose during inhalation. A Jones tube can be placed in conjunction with a standard external or endonasal DCR, known as a conjunctivodacryocystorhinostomy (CDCR), or it can be placed with direct puncture from the caruncle into the nasal cavity, with or without endoscopic guidance. In this chapter, the authors describe

J. Tao (ed.), *Efficient Oculofacial Surgery*, https://doi.org/10.1007/978-3-031-63178-8_44

surgical methods of Jones tube placement as well as preoperative assessment, patient selection, and postoperative management.

History of the Jones Tube

Dr. Lester E. Jones introduced the Jones tube in 1965 [1]. Prior to this invention, management of upper lacrimal obstructions included reiterative probing and canalicular stenting, which had poor success rates. In collaboration with a glassblower, Gunther Weiss, Jones designed a Pyrex® tube with an internal diameter of 0.8 mm and a 30-degree beveled tip, determined to have optimal capillary action for tear drainage [1, 2].

The Jones tube has become the most common method for treating upper lacrimal obstruction. The original design, intended to have minimal friction for easy in-office removal for cleaning, remains popular, but tube migration remains the most common complication.

Several design modifications of the Jones tube aim to reduce migration. These include the Putterman Gladstone tube, which has an intranasal dilation of the tube, frosted tubes, extended angle tubes, polyporous ethylene coated tubes, and the StopLoss Jones tube which has a silicone intranasal flange [2–4]. Figure 44.1 demonstrates a variety of Jones tube sizes and modifications.

Preoperative Assessment and Patient Selection

Jones tube placement is indicated for patients with an upper lacrimal drainage system obstruction affecting long segments of the lacrimal canaliculus or lacrimal punctum or both. Patients may develop these obstructions from several different etiologies. Acquired fibrosis and scarring can occur after recurrent infection (particularly after herpetic infection), autoimmune processes, Stevens-Johnson syndrome, or neoplasms. Iatrogenic obstruction can occur after chemotherapy, such as docetaxel, or radiation therapy, and trauma to the canalicular system can lead to obstruction if improperly repaired. In children, congenital canalicular agenesis can be an etiology for epiphora [5].

Pre-operative patient assessment may involve several steps. First, evaluation of epiphora can be performed using the dye disappearance test. Next, the patency of the upper and lower caniculär can be assessed with a lacrimal probe with or without irrigation using a lacrimal cannula. Lastly, a nasal examination should be performed to assess for intranasal abnormalities or tumors that could be causing distal obstructions [6]. The requirement of continuous positive airway pressure (CPAP) is a relative contraindication for Jones tube placement or dacryocystorhinostomy in general since ocular irritation by airflow is a concern. A full facemask CPAP system or temporary wax occlusion of the tube may obviate problems with a Jones tube in these patients.

Surgical Approach

There have been several modifications of the surgical approach to Jones tube implantation, including the use of lasers or endoscopes [7–9]. In this chapter, the authors focus on minimally invasive and minimally equipment intensive CDCR [9].

External DCR Approach (Video 44-1)

An external DCR approach provides direct and open visualization of the osteotomy and the distal Jones tube in relation to the surrounding tissues. No special instrumentation is required. A medial canthal incision is fashioned (with the primary incisions in the oblique medial canthus relaxed skin lines is helpful to avoid webbing and to better camouflage the wound; see chapter on external DCR). Dissection is carried down to the level of the periosteum, which is incised and elevated. An osteotomy site was created with a burr and rongeurs. The nasal mucosa is opened, with or without the creation

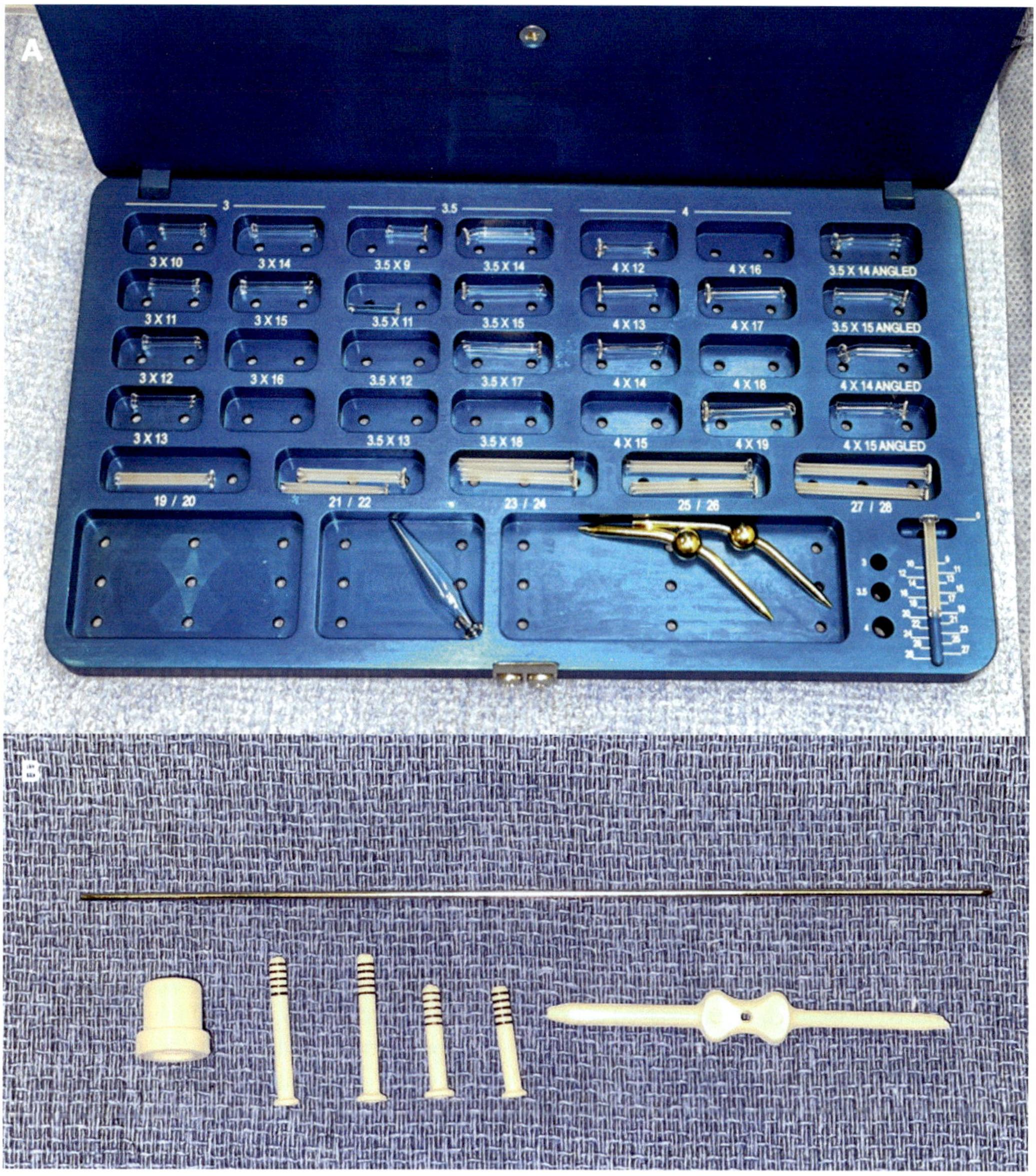

Fig. 44.1 **A** shows a collection of Jones tubes of varying sizes and external coatings. **B** shows the StopLoss Jones tube sizing and insertion kit, which includes a guide wire (upper), button cap (left lower), dilator with narrow and broad ends (right lower), and 4 sizing tubes (middle lower)

of flaps. The distance from the caruncle to just past the nasal mucosa is estimated. Sharp dissection is fashioned at the caruncle and with the aid of a guide wire, an appropriately sized Jones tube is advanced. The tube is visualized through the medial canthus wound where the distal end is seated past the lateral nasal mucosa in the nose, ensuring the distal end is not against the septum and is otherwise free from obstruction. Positioning is re-inspected from nares with the aid of a headlight or an adjustable overhead light and nasal speculum (this internal inspection can be performed with an endoscope, if available). 5-0 polyglactin suture may be used to secure nasal mucosa flaps away from the distal tube end or the tube can be seated through the incision through the mucosa. The tube collar and proximal end is secured with 5-0 polyglactin to the surrounding caruncle. The skin wound is closed with 6-0 plain sutures.

An alternative option is the StopLoss Jones tube. This device has a traditional external (i.e. proximal) flange but has an added internal silicone flange bonded 2 mm from the distal tip. The tube comes in varied lengths, ranging from 9.0 to 22.0 mm, with the most common lengths being 17.0 and 18.0 mm. The external flange is available in 3.5 and 4.0 mm diameters.

The sizing and insertion kit (Fig. 44.1B) comes with a guide wire with a sharp and blunt end and a dilator with narrow and broad ends. There are also 4 sizing tubes (15.0 and 20.0 mm lengths, and 3.5 and 4.0 mm external flanges) that have 5 rings with 1 mm increments from the distal tip.

Closed Approach

A closed approach obviates an external facial wound, but visualization is variable. Unlike the external approach that can always be performed without an endoscope, the closed approach sometimes requires the additional endonasal visualization afforded by this equipment. The nose is packed with a decongestant, such as cocaine-soaked or oxymetazoline-soaked cottonoid pledgets (typically 0.5 × 3 inch). Local anesthetic may be administered to the soft tissues surrounding the osteotomy. Then the patient is prepped and draped in routine fashion.

Direct visualization into the nose is performed with the aid of a nasal speculum and headlight or an endoscope, if available. Video endoscopy allows for illuminated and magnified visualization of the nasal anatomy as well as ultimate positioning of the distal end of the tube. A 0-degree ridged endoscope is used to visualize the middle meatus (Fig. 44.2A). At this stage, out fracture of the middle turbinate or a partial turbinectomy can be performed to create more space within the middle meatus.

First, the cap is placed over the blunt end of the Jones tube guide wire inserter. The inserter is placed at the posterior caruncle, aiming the wire to pass through the lacrimal sac (Fig. 44.3A and B). The wire is advanced through the soft tissue down to the lacrimal bone, then through the bone, and into the nasal cavity. The button cap is removed. The distal (sharp) end can be visualized within the middle meatus in the nose (Fig. 44.2B). The Jones tube dilator is then passed over the guide wire inserter (Fig. 44.3C). First the narrow end of the dilator should be used, and then reversed to use the broad end to further widen the tract (if desired). Keeping the wire guide in place, the dilator is removed, and the Jones tube sizer (Figs. 44.2C and 44.3D) is threaded over the guidewire and into place. The sizer has 1 mm increment hash marks to allow for estimating the proper measurement of the tube as well as appropriate positioning. Based on the sizing tube length, the number of rings visible in the nose is subtracted from the length of the sizer to approximate the length needed for the tube (i.e., the length of the tissue tract is the length of the sizing tube minus the number of visible rings). Then, add back 4 mm so that the tube allows for 2 mm of distance from the nasal wall to the internal wall, and 2 mm from the flange to the tip of the tube.

The appropriately sized Jones tube is then inserted over the guide wire. Care should be taken while sliding the Jones tube into position to avoid excess force onto the tube which may break. Once the tube is inserted, the guide wire is removed. With endonasal visualization the internal flange should be confirmed to be intact, and both the proximal and distal end should be assessed for good positioning (Figs. 44.2D, 44.3E, and F). The distal end should be seated approximately 2 mm from the lateral nasal wall and not touching the septum. In some cases, the tube may be fixated to the medial canthus with a dissolvable suture.

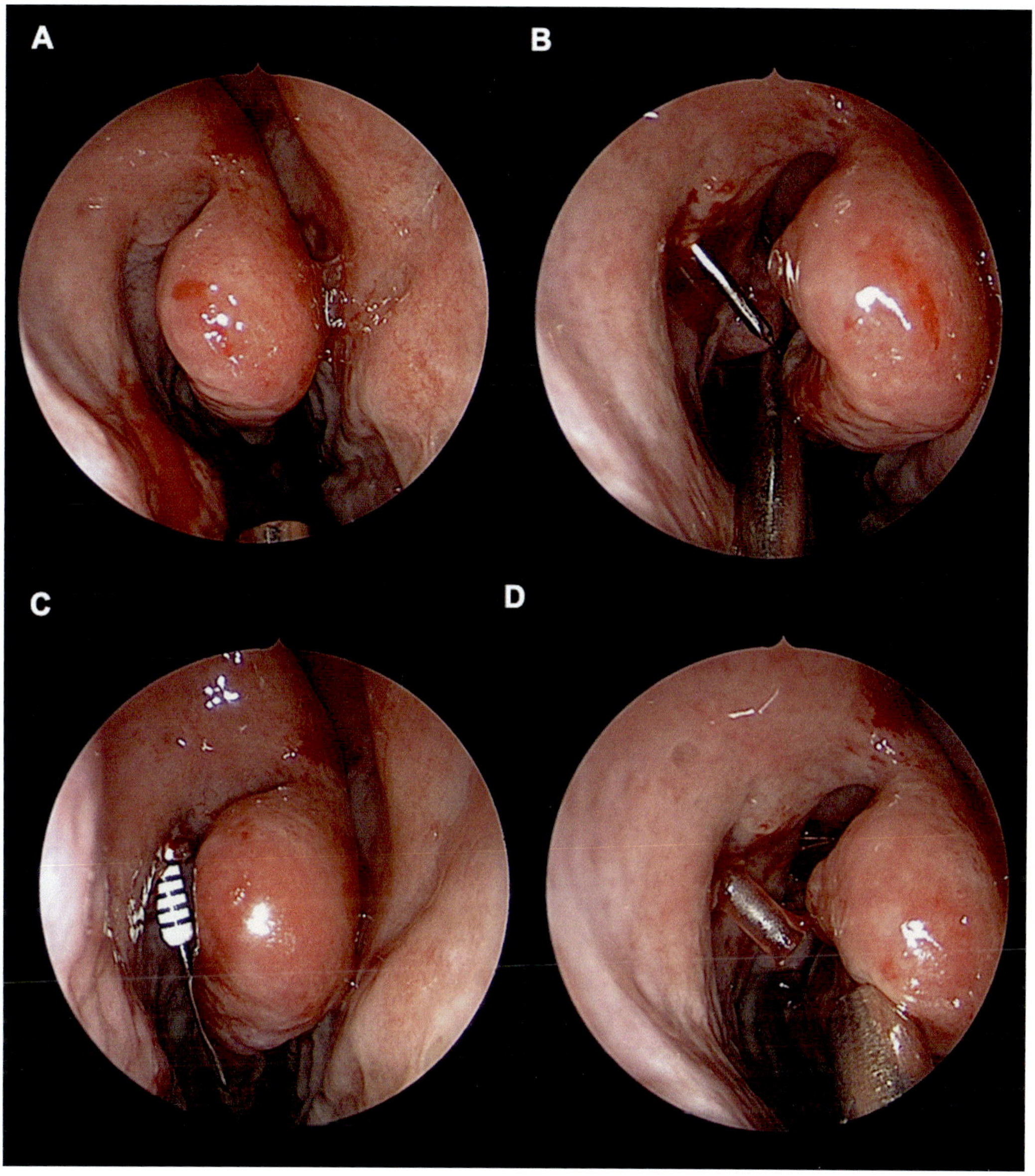

Fig. 44.2 Endoscopic photographs of minimially invasive Jones tube placement. **A** demonstrates the middle turbinate, **B** shows the guide wire inserted, **C** shows the sizing tube inserted over the guide wire, and **D** shows the Jones tube

Post Operative Management

Post Operative Care

Post operative assessment is namely to assess for proper tube positioning. In the immediate post-operative period, a topical antibiotic ointment can be placed on the caruncle. Ultimately, the flanged proximal end of the Jones tube should be flat within the caruncle and should avoid contact with the ocular surface (Fig. 44.4).

Patients with a Jones tube require counseling on lifelong maintenance and care of the tube.

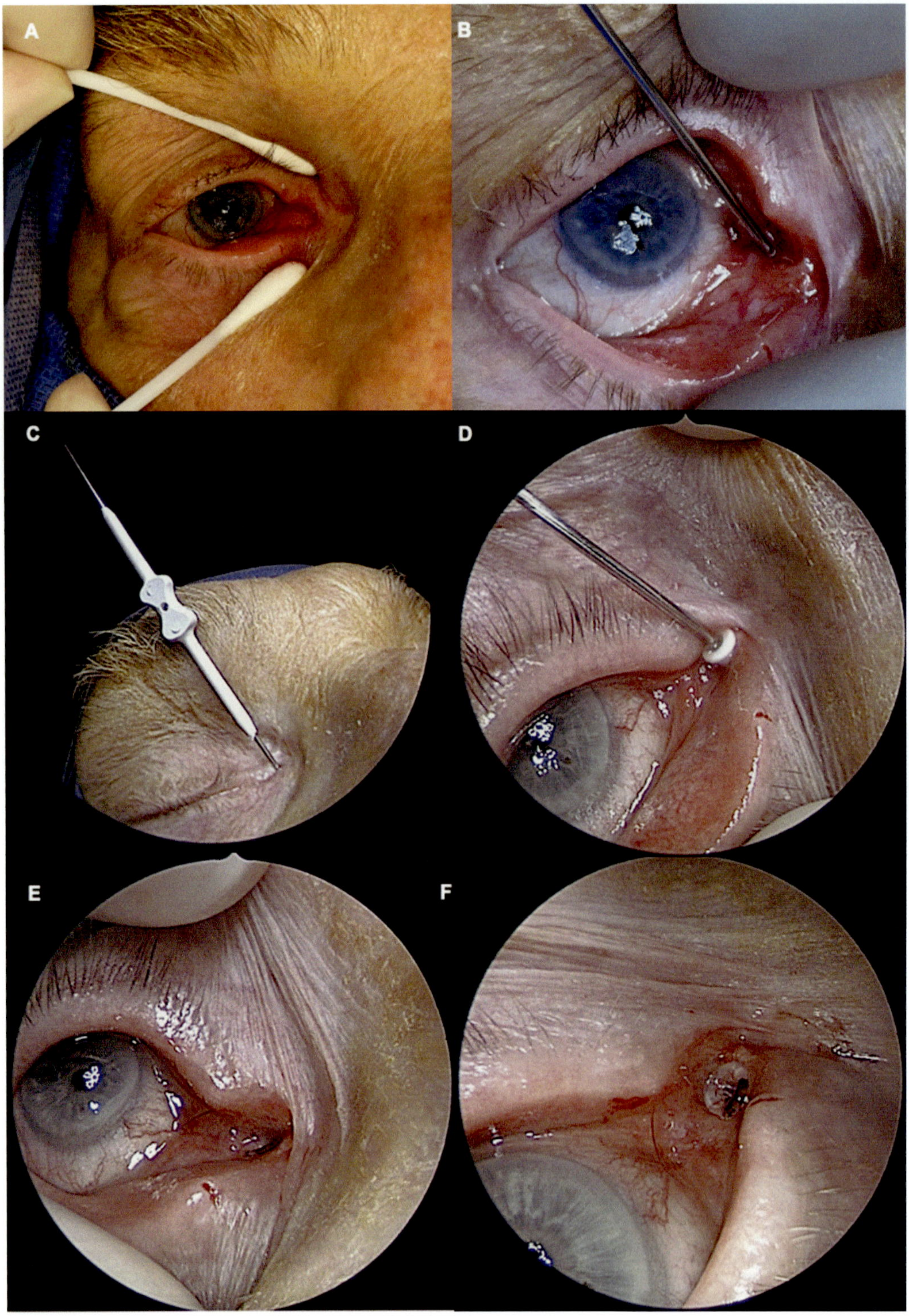

Fig. 44.3 Intraoperative photographs. **A** and **B** demonstrate the positioning of the guide wire. **C** shows the dilator over the guide wire, **D** shows the sizing tube over the guide wire, and **E** and **F** show a well seated Jones tube

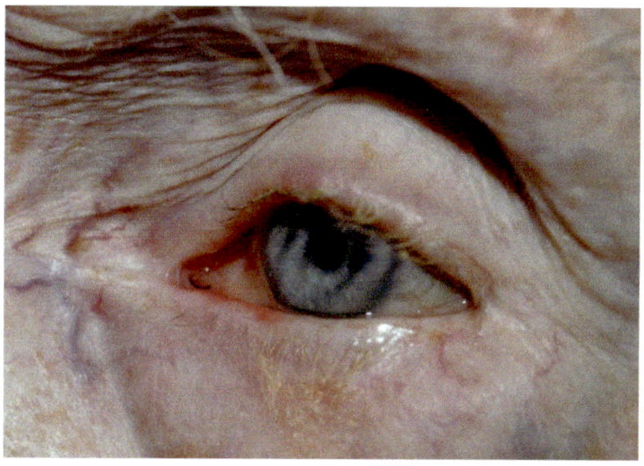

Fig. 44.4 Post-operative external photograph demonstrating a well seated Jones' tube

To prevent expulsion or migration of the tube, patients should lightly cover the tube when sneezing. It is also suggested to use intranasal saline sprays and artificial tears frequently to prevent mucoid buildup within the tube.

Complications

One of the most common complications of Jones tubes is migration or malposition of the tube. This can occur immediately after surgery or years later. Some studies suggest that the majority of tube failures occur within the first three months, and conversely, the tube can be tolerated and remain effective at symptom management for several decades [10, 11]. The tube can migrate either medially into the nose or laterally out of the caruncle. Tube migration can occur due to poor fit of the tube, external manipulation or trauma, or scarring. If the tube is still present but in an improper position, it may need to be repositioned back into place or replaced with a tube of a different length and diameter for a better fit.

Jones tubes may also become obstructed, or more rarely, the lacrimal sac may become infected [11]. The tube itself can become clogged with mucus, which can be flushed with irrigation to relieve the obstruction. An interdental brush may be useful. Some tubes become increasingly associated with infection, due to accumulation of biofilm. In these instances, tube exchange may be necessary if conservative measures such as antibiotic drops, cleaning and syringing the tube are unsuccessful. However, there may be other sources of obstruction at either the distal or proximal ends of the tube. Proximally, the flange may become buried under the conjunctiva, and distally, the end may become obstructed with scar tissues or pyogenic granulomas, or it may be abutting nasal tissue. If the tube is obstructed by nasal mucosa due to improper fit, the tube may need to be exchanged.

Conclusion

The management of epiphora requires careful evaluation to determine the underlying etiology. In cases of upper lacrimal drainage system obstruction, CDCR, or Jones tube, can be performed to bypass the obstructed pathway and create an alternative drainage system. Patients and surgeons should understand that there is an almost universal need for subsequent management including tube cleaning, repositioning, or replacement.

References

1. Jones LT. Conjunctivodacryocystorhinostomy. Am J Ophthalmol. 1965;59:773–83. https://doi.org/10.1016/0002-9394(65)93004-7.
2. Steele EA. Conjunctivodacryocystorhinostomy with Jones tube: a history and update. Curr Opin Ophthalmol. 2016;27(5):439–42. https://doi.org/10.1097/ICU.0000000000000287.
3. Gladstone GJ, Putterman AM. A modified glass tube for conjunctivodacryocystorhinostomy. Arch Ophthalmol. 1985;103(8):1229–30. https://doi.org/10.1001/archopht.1985.01050080141036.
4. Bagdonaite L, Pearson AR. Early experience with the StopLoss Jones Tube. Orbit. 2015;34(3):132–6. https://doi.org/10.3109/01676830.2015.1014507.
5. Weber A, Yen MT. Conjunctivodacryocystorhinostomy. In: Freitag SK, Lee NG, Lefebvre DR, Yoon MK, editors. Ophthalmic plastic surgery: tricks of the trade. 1st ed. Thieme; 2019.
6. Nerad JA. Diagnosis and management of the patient with tearing. In: Techniques in ophthalmic plastic surgery: a personal tutorial. 2nd ed. Elselvier; 2020.
7. Athanasiov PA, Madge S, Kakizaki H, Selva D. A review of bypass tubes for proximal

lacrimal drainage obstruction. Surv Ophthalmol. 2011;56(3):252–66. https://doi.org/10.1016/j.survophthal.2011.02.009.

8. Eisenbach N, Karni O, Sela E, et al. Conjunctivodacryocystorhinostomy (CDCR) success rates and complications in endoscopic vs non-endoscopic approaches: a systematic review. Int Forum Allergy Rhinol. 2021;11(2):174–94. https://doi.org/10.1002/alr.22668.
9. Nowak R, Rekas M, Ali MJ. Long-term quality of life in patients following minimally invasive conjunctivodacryocystorhinostomy with StopLoss Jones tube. Ophthal Plast Reconstr Surg. 2022;38(2):170–5. https://doi.org/10.1097/IOP.0000000000002017.
10. Scawn RL, Verity DH, Rose GE. Can Lester Jones tubes be tolerated for decades? Eye. 2018;32(1):142–5. https://doi.org/10.1038/eye.2017.168.
11. Sekhar GC, Dortzbach RK, Gonnering RS, Lemke BN. Problems associated with conjunctivodacryocystorhinostomy. Am J Ophthalmol. 1991;112(5):502–6. https://doi.org/10.1016/s0002-9394(14)76849-7.

Optic Nerve Sheath Fenestration

45

Vivek R. Patel

Abstract

An optic nerve sheath fenestration (ONSF) surgery aims to create a pathway for egress of CSF from the immediate retrobulbar optic sheath to de-pressurize this region, potentially resulting in normalization of the translaminar pressure gradient. In this chapter the author describes a medial transconjunctival approach to ONSF.

Keywords

Optic nerve sheath fenestration · Idiopathic intracranial hypertension · Pseudotumor cerebri

Introduction

Papilledema is a well-known and important manifestation of intracranial hypertension, irrespective of the underlying cause. Left untreated, papilledema can lead to significant visual field loss and even blindness. In general, management is first treating the underlying cause (i.e. tumor, infection, hydrocephalus). In idiopathic intracranial hypertension (IIH), an imbalance exists between cerebrospinal fluid (CSF) production and absorption. Medical management involves reducing CSF synthesis whereas surgical options (shunting, venous sinus stenting, and optic nerve sheath fenestration (ONSF) aim to improve CSF outflow.

Given the contiguity of CSF compartments within the central nervous system, subarachnoid fluid freely communicates with the peri-optic regions. There is an elaborate network of arachnoid trabeculations within the retrobulbar CSF spaces [1], allowing for further sequestration of fluid, ultimately resulting in anterior bowing of the lamina cribrosa due to the retrobulbar CSF pressure exceeding the intraocular pressure (translaminar gradient).

The goal of ONSF surgery is to create a pathway for egress of CSF from the immediate retrobulbar optic sheath to de-pressurize this region, potentially resulting in normalization of the translaminar pressure gradient. Given the lack of prospective evidence demonstrating superiority of one surgical approach over another, the choice of procedure is typically made on a case by case basis. Commonly, when visual compromise due to papilledema occurs out of proportion to symptoms of elevated

Supplementary Information The online version contains supplementary material available at https://doi.org/10.1007/978-3-031-63178-8_45.

V. R. Patel (✉)
UC Irvine, Irivne, CA, USA
e-mail: vivekrp@hs.uci.edu

J. Tao (ed.), *Efficient Oculofacial Surgery*, https://doi.org/10.1007/978-3-031-63178-8_45

intracranial pressure (pulsatile tinnitus, headache), ONSF is the procedure of choice [2, 3].

Once OSNF is chosen as the most appropriate surgical option, the next step is to decide whether unilateral or bilateral surgery is warranted. Although the decision is nuanced and varies based on factors specific to each case, the following general principles apply. Unilateral surgery can impact the contralateral side given interconnections between the CSF spaces throughout the central nervous system. Hence, many surgeons first operate on the more severely affected eye (4). However, in cases where both eyes demonstrate significant swelling and/or visual compromise, bilateral surgery may be necessary to maximize the effect on the translaminar gradient behind both eyes.

Technique (Video 45-1 and 45-2)

ONSF can be performed via a superomedial eyelid crease incision or medially through a transconjunctival incision. In this chapter the author describes the medial approach to ONSF. This can be performed with (video 45-1) or without (video 45-2) medial rectus muscle disinsertion. The procedure can be performed with or without an operating microscope.

Following induction of general anesthesia, the eye is prepped and draped in the usual fashion for eye muscle surgery. A 120 degree limbal conjunctival peritomy is fashioned to permit access to the medial rectus muscle. This incision is deliberately wider than generally used for strabismus surgery so that subconjunctival tissue surrounding the medial rectus muscle does not limit access to the deep retro-equatorial space. The medial rectus muscle is then imbricated at its insertion site using 6-0 polyglactin suture. It is then detached from the eye at the insertion and reflected medially with some tension on the sutures to reduce the chances of inadvertent injury to the under surface of the muscle. Another 6-0 polyglactin suture is used to weave a continuous, running anchoring bucket handle stitch through the medial rectus insertion. This is performed by creating a series of partial thickness scleral passes, and tying the two ends together, providing strength to the anchoring suture (Fig. 45.1). The surgeon or assistant can then use this suture to abduct the eye with great leverage and control, affording improved and safer access to the retrobulbar nerve sheath where the penetrating incision is ultimately made.

The operating microscope is moved into place, with the primary surgeon seated temporally and first assistant superiorly. Magnification is increased and focus is optimized to allow clear resolution of the small, often engorged blood vessels within the optic nerve sheath at its insertion with the globe. Since abduction of the eye can put significant strain on the eye and potentially compromise blood flow to the eye, a timer is set so that the eye is in the abducted position for a maximum of 90 s at a time, followed by a 60 s break before resuming abduction for another 90 s. A quarter inch malleable retractor is bent to a right angle configuration, and gently placed by the primary region, parallel and lateral to the reflected medial rectus muscle, into the surgical space to expose the retrobulbar optic nerve sheath. Retrobulbar fat invariably occludes direct visualization of the optic nerve sheath, but careful use of the retractor assists in revealing the semi-translucent dural tissue

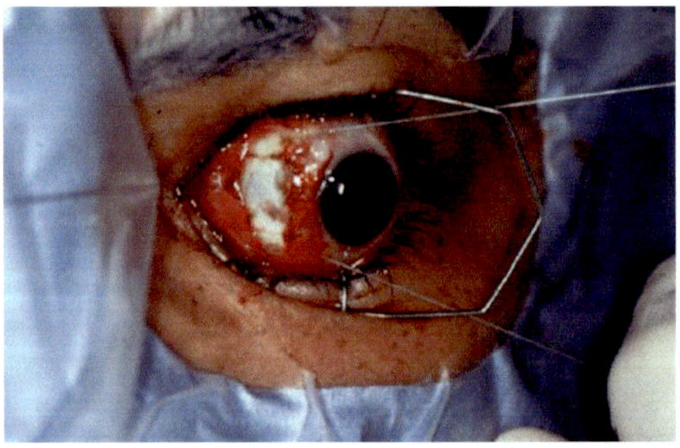

Fig. 45.1 A 6-0 polyglactin suture on a spatulated needle was woven through the medial rectus insertion along its entire width, using partial thickness scleral passes. The ends are tied together to create an anchoring bucket handle stitch to permit secure and controlled manipulation of the eye

which will ultimately be the site of the fenestration (Fig. 45.2). Large intervening blood vessels can be pushed aside using long wooden cotton tips, offering a space wide enough to create the fenestration. Once a desired site for the initial incision into the nerve sheath is chosen and visualized, a 20-gauge super-sharp blade is used to penetrate the sheath. The incision must be deep enough to enter the CSF space, evidenced by visual egress of CSF which may be under significant pressure (Fig. 45.3). At this point a nerve or Sinskey hook is used to enter the incised area and strip away subdural arachnoid granulations and trabeculations to widen the area of filtration. Long neurosurgical or fine tipped Westcott scissors are used to carefully remove some of the incised dural sheath, effectively creating the desired "window." Alternatively, a Kelly glaucoma punch may be utilized to fashion a sheath window. Minimum bleeding should be expected, but if it does occur, tamponade of culprit vessels using long cotton tips or neurosurgical patties is typically enough, making cautery unnecessary.

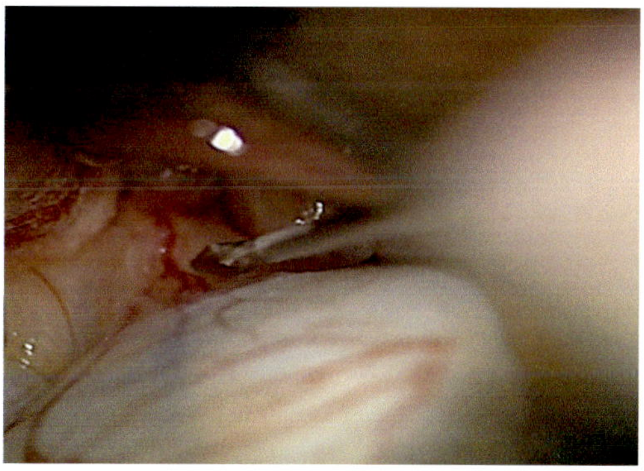

Fig. 45.2 View through the operating microscope demonstrating the site of initial penetration of the optic nerve sheath, using a 20 gauge super-sharp blade. Note the longitudinal greyish band (long ciliary nerve) coursing along the sclera, offering a useful landmark to follow along the convexity of the globe, leading to the point where the nerve sheath intersects with the globe

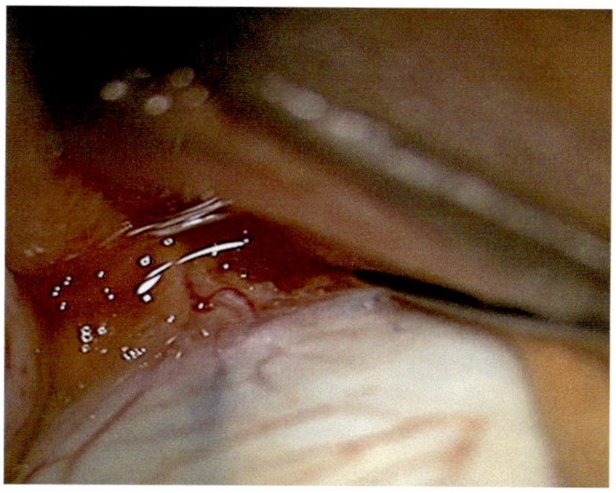

Fig. 45.3 Following effective penetration of the dural covering and further stripping of the arachnoid trabeculations, the retrobulbar optic nerve region is seen bathed in straw-colored CSF

The anchoring suture is then removed, medial rectus muscle repositioned and fastened to the original insertion site, and the conjunctiva is closed. A patch is placed over one eye and removed roughly 30 min after emergence from general anesthesia. Topical steroid and antibiotic drops are given for one week, and the patient is instructed to continue acetazolamide if relevant. The patient should be carefully monitored over the next several weeks to follow his or her clinical course and treatment response.

Conclusion

In summary, ONSF is a powerful technique, offering direct decompression of the retrobulbar optic nerve sheath, and reduction of papilledema (Figs. 45.4 and 45.5). The optic nerve can be accessed from a medial bulbar transconjunctival approach with or without disinsertion of the medial rectus muscle.

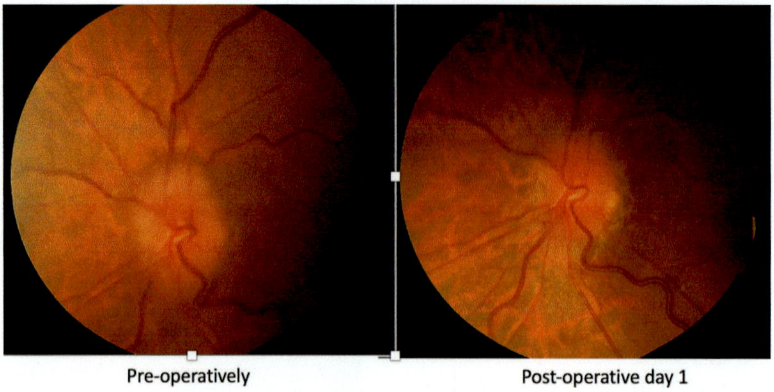

Fig. 45.4 Papilledema before (left) and after (right) ONSF

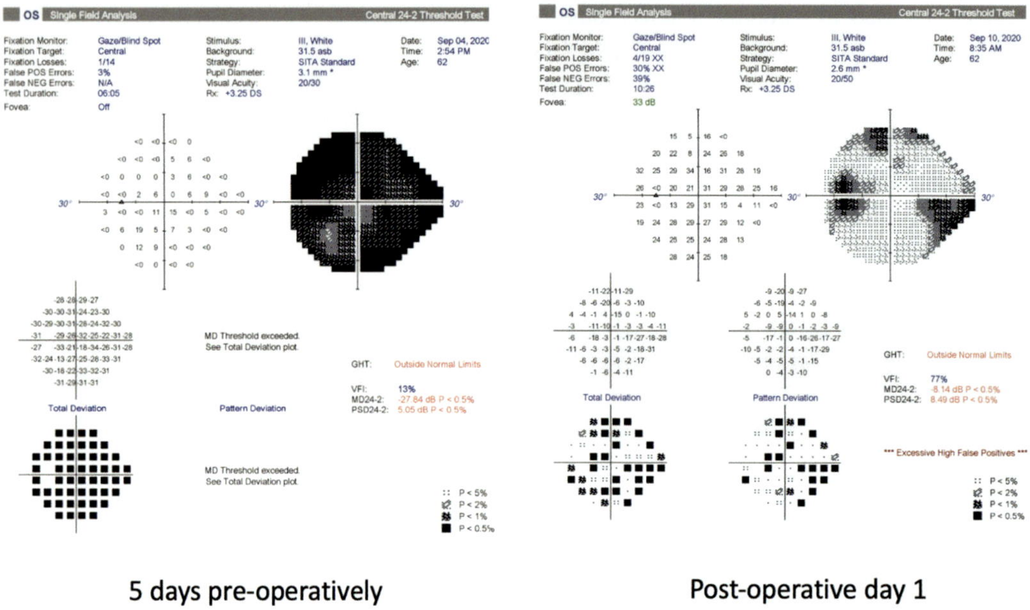

Fig. 45.5 Humphrey visual field before (left) and after (right) ONSF

References

1. Liu KC, Fleischman D, Lee AG, Killer HE, Chen JJ, Bhatti MT. Current concepts of cerebrospinal fluid dynamics and the translaminar cribrosa pressure gradient: a paradigm of optic disk disease. Surv Ophthalmol. 2020;65(1):48–66.
2. Feldon SE. Visual outcomes comparing surgical techniques for management of severe idiopathic intracranial hypertension. Neurosurg Focus. 2007;23(5):E6. https://doi.org/10.3171/FOC-07/11/E6. PMID: 18004968.
3. Fonseca PL, Rigamonti D, Miller NR, Subramanian PS. Visual outcomes of surgical intervention for pseudotumour cerebri: optic nerve sheath fenestration versus cerebrospinal fluid diversion. Br J Ophthalmol. 2014;98(10):1360–3. https://doi.org/10.1136/bjophthalmol-2014-304953. PMID: 24820047.
4. Alsuhaibani AH, Carter KD, Nerad JA, Lee AG. Effect of optic nerve sheath fenestration on papilledema of the operated and the contralateral nonoperated eyes in idiopathic intracranial hypertension. Ophthalmology. 2011;118(2):412–4. https://doi.org/10.1016/j.ophtha.2010.06.025. PMID: 20801522.

Index

J. Tao (ed.), *Efficient Oculofacial Surgery*, https://doi.org/10.1007/978-3-031-63178-8

MIX
Papier aus verantwortungsvollen Quellen
Paper from responsible sources
FSC® C105338

If you have any concerns about our products,
you can contact us on
ProductSafety@springernature.com

In case Publisher is established outside the EU,
the EU authorized representative is:
Springer Nature Customer Service Center GmbH
Europaplatz 3, 69115 Heidelberg, Germany

Printed by Libri Plureos GmbH
in Hamburg, Germany